# COMPUTED TOMOGRAPHY

## Physical Principles, Clinical Applications, and Quality Control

**FOURTH EDITION**

**Dr. EUCLID SEERAM**, PhD, MSc, BSc, FCAMRT
Medical Imaging and Radiation Sciences
University of Sydney; Monash University;
Charles Sturt University
Australia

ELSEVIER

ELSEVIER

3251 Riverport Lane
St. Louis, Missouri 63043

COMPUTED TOMOGRAPHY: PHYSICAL PRINCIPLES, CLINICAL APPLICATIONS, AND QUALITY CONTROL, FOURTH EDITION

ISBN: 978-0-323-31288-2



**Notices**

Knowledge and best practice in this field are constantly changing. As new research and experience broaden our understanding, changes in research methods, professional practices, or medical treatment may become necessary.

Practitioners and researchers must always rely on their own experience and knowledge in evaluating and using any information, methods, compounds, or experiments described herein. In using such information or methods they should be mindful of their own safety and the safety of others, including parties for whom they have a professional responsibility.

With respect to any drug or pharmaceutical products identified, readers are advised to check the most current information provided (i) on procedures featured or (ii) by the manufacturer of each product to be administered, to verify the recommended dose or formula, the method and duration of administration, and contraindications. It is the responsibility of practitioners, relying on their own experience and knowledge of their patients, to make diagnoses, to determine dosages and the best treatment for each individual patient, and to take all appropriate safety precautions.

To the fullest extent of the law, neither the Publisher nor the authors, contributors, or editors, assume any liability for any injury and/or damage to persons or property as a matter of products liability, negligence or otherwise, or from any use or operation of any methods, products, instructions, or ideas contained in the material herein.

**Library of Congress Cataloging-in-Publication Data**

Seeram, Euclid, author.
Computed tomography : physical principles, clinical applications, and quality control / Dr. Euclid Seeram. -- Fourth edition.
p. ; cm.
Includes bibliographical references and index.
ISBN 978-0-323-31288-2 (pbk. : alk. paper)
I. Title.
[DNLM: 1. Tomography, X-Ray Computed. WN 206]
RC78.7.T6
616.07'572--dc23

2015020943

*Content Strategist:* Sonya Seigafuse
*Content Development Specialist:* Laura Goodrich
*Publishing Services Manager:* Hemamalini Rajendrababu
*Project Manager:* Kamatchi Madhavan
*Design Direction:* Amy Buxton
*Marketing Manager:* Kristen Conrad

Printed in the United States of America

Last digit is the print number: 9 8 7 6 5 4 3 2 1

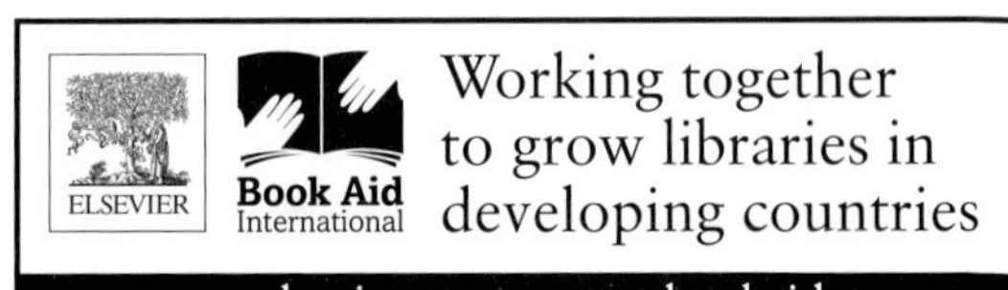

# DEDICATION

This book is dedicated with love and affection to my beautiful, smart, and overall cute and witty granddaughter

**CLAIRE.**

You bring so much joy and happiness to our lives.

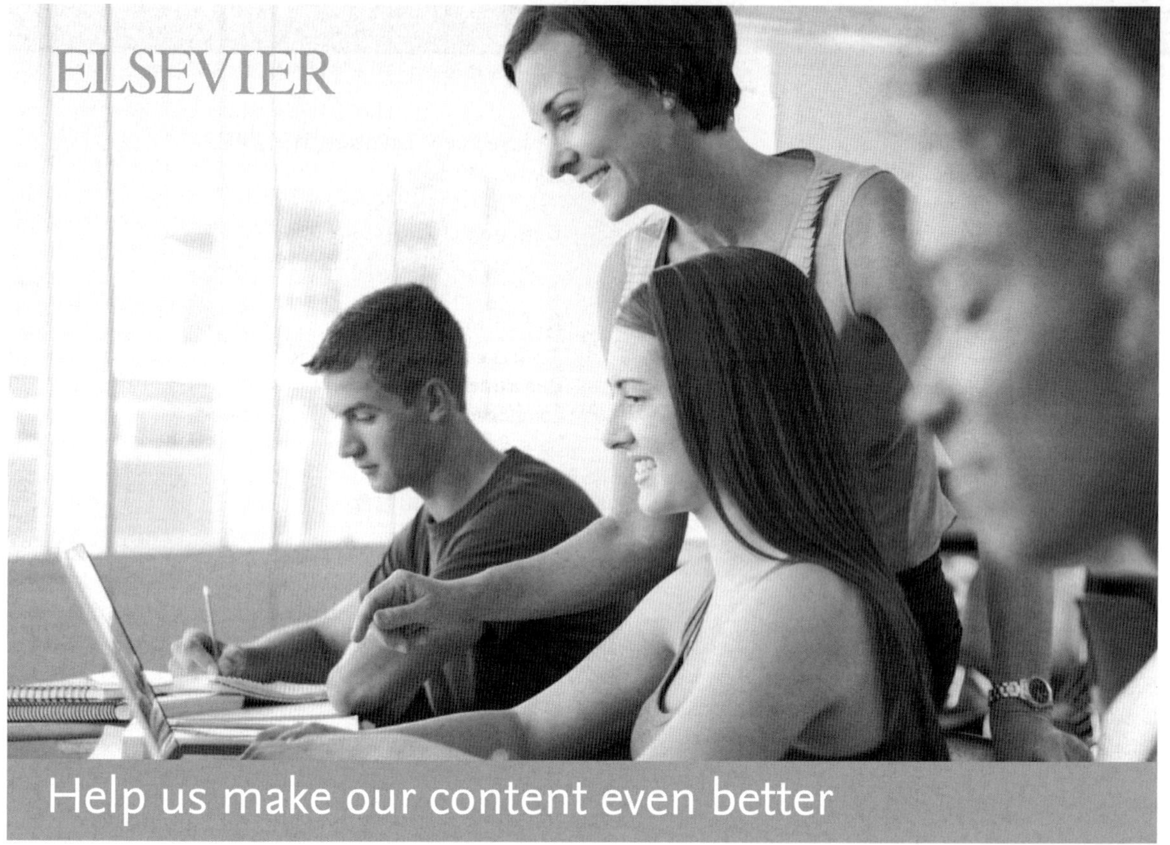
ELSEVIER
Help us make our content even better

# CONTRIBUTORS

**Dr Frederic H. Fahey, D.Sc**
Director of Nuclear Medicine/PET Physics
Division of Nuclear Medicine
Children's Hospital
Boston, MA

**Dr Jiang Hsieh, PhD**
Chief Scientist, Applied Science Lab
General Electric Healthcare Technologies
Waukesha, WI

**Dr Matthew D. Palmer, PhD**
Radiology
Harvard Medical School
Nuclear Medicine Physicist
Beth Israel Deaconess Medical Center
Boston, MA

*The author and publisher would also like to acknowledge the following individuals for contributions to the previous editions of this book:*

**Dr Borys Flak, MD**
Associate Clinical Professor
Department of Radiology, University of British Columbia
Vancouver, British Columbia, Canada

**Dr Jocelyne S. LaPointe, MD, FRCPC**
Neuroradiologist
Department of Radiology
Vancouver General Hospital
Vancouver, British Columbia, Canada

**Dr Scott Lipson, MD**
Associate Director of Imaging
Department of Radiology
Long Beach Memorial Medical Center
Long Beach, CA

**Dr Son Nguyen, MD**
Staff Radiologist
Miller's Children's Hospital
Long Beach Memorial Medical Center
Long Beach, CA

# REVIEWERS

**Jeff L. Berry, MS, RT (R) (CT)**
Associate Professor, Radiography Program Director
Department of Medical Imaging & Radiation Sciences
College of Allied Health
University of Oklahoma Health Sciences Center
Oklahoma City, OK

**Rebecca Blankley, MFA, RT (R) (M) (CT), MRI**
Lecturer III
University of New Mexico
Albuquerque, NM

**Patricia M. Davis, BS Medical Imaging Technology, RT (R) (MR)**
Assistant Clinical Professor, Clinical Liaison
Indiana University Kokomo
Kokomo, IN

**Nicole B. Dhanraj, PhD, RT (R) (CT) (MR)**
Continuing Education
Puyallup, WA

**Kerry Greene-Donnelly, MBA, RT (R) (M) (CT) (QM)**
Assistant Professor
Upstate Medical University
Syracuse, NY

**Caroline J. Khazei, RTR**
Instructor, CT Technologist
Vancouver General Hospital/ British Columbia Institute of Technology
Vancouver, BC

**Diana E. Mishler, MBA-HM, RT (R) (S), RDMS**
Director and Clinical Assistant Professor
Medical Imaging Technology Program
Indiana University Kokomo
Kokomo, IN

**Leanna Neubrander, MS, RT (R) (CT) (ARRT)**
Assistant Professor, Department of Radiologic Sciences
Adventist University of Health Sciences
Orlando, FL

**Kamau Nkenge, M.S.R.S, RRA, RT (CT) (R) (ARRT)**
Registered Radiologist Assistant
MedStart Good Samaritan Hospital;
Professor
Community College of Baltimore County Essex Campus
Baltimore County, MD

**Amanda L. Pedrick, BS, RT (R) (CT) (MR) (ARRT)**
CT and MRI Programs Manager and Instructor
Eastern Florida State College
Cocoa, FL

**Taryn Price, BS RS, RT (R) (CT)**
CT Instructor (faculty)
New Mexico State University–Dona Ana Community College
Las Cruces, NM

**Kristi K. Rayman, BS, RT (R) (M) (CT) (MR)**
Advanced Medical Imaging Program Coordinator
Mitchell Technical Institute
Mitchell, SD;
Circuit Lecturer
Stronger Links Medical Imaging Education
Spearfish, SD

**Robin Annette Rayman, CNMT, PET, RT (N), EMT-B**
Certified Nuclear Medicine and PET Technologist
Sanford USD Medical Center
Sioux Falls, SD

**Adam J. Stevens, MA, RT (R) (CT) (MR)**
Computed Tomography Program Director
University of Nebraska Medical Center, School of Allied Health Profession
Omaha, NE

**Ronald Walker, MBA, CNMT, PET**
Assistant Professor
The University of Findlay
Findlay, OH

**Timothy Whittaker, MS, RT (R) (CT) (QM)**
Professor of Radiography
Hazard Community and Technical College
Hazard, KY

# FOREWORD

Computed tomography (CT) still remains one of the most important diagnostic tools in medicine and health. What is still amazing is that development of CT has not abated over recent years and the clinical applications continue to grow rapidly with increasing benefit for patients and clinicians. While CT is one of many diagnostic imaging tools, it will maintain its position in the forefront of radiologic departments.

Such an effective tool requires competent and reflective operators. Initially it would appear that the usability of radiologic equipment becomes easier with subsequent technological generations, but this appearance substantially undermines the responsibilities generated by the advancement in CT techniques. The plethora of data generated, the expectation of useful image reconstructions by clinical staff, the move to automated segmentation and quantification procedures, sophisticated quality assurance procedures, and the huge potential for excessive patient exposure requires that technological staff are highly efficient and knowledgeable about the opportunities that this device offers. Regarding the latter point, radiation dose, it has never been so necessary for clinicians and health professionals to have a solid and working knowledge of dose-reducing measures.

The name Euclid Seeram has become synonymous with learning and teaching in CT and other areas of medical imaging. This fourth edition of his very well-known text, *Computed Tomography—Physical Principles, Clinical Applications, and Quality Control*, expands on previous editions. This textbook still covers the topics of the previous editions and now brings the reader up to date with the latest technologies, including iterative reconstruction algorithms, detector and x-ray tube design and technologies, spectral imaging, and updates on SPECT/CT and PET/CT. Importantly, there is an increased focus on CT dose-optimization strategies and approaches. It also informs the reader of methods for ensuring that these new technologies are implemented for the patient's greatest benefit. The focus of the previous editions has been on educating students; now this text will serve as a fundamental reference to current radiographers and clinicians so that they can update their CT knowledge.

Dr Seeram is a distinguished and rigorous academic who has a proven track record in providing understandable and comprehensive radiologic manuscripts. A hallmark of his approach is the ability to convey complex topics in an easy-to-read and manageable way, and this work is no exception. He presents his topics in an organized, progressive, and comprehensive manner so that at the end of each clearly defined chapter, learning objectives are met and the reader comes away with a solid and supported knowledge of specific topics. Euclid has decades of experience in the teaching of CT and medical imaging and during this time has gained worldwide respect as an educator. Both clinicians and physicists in the field of medical imaging are in agreement with the high level of influence Euclid has on medical imaging education and on the profession as a whole. He is simply a global leader in his field, and policy makers, health service providers, the industry, and patients everywhere should be grateful for the impact Dr Seeram has had on radiologic science and technology education.

Euclid has the gift of being able to explain difficult concepts in a way that students can grasp. This ability has made the previous versions of this text highly desirable reading in the learning of CT. Earlier editions can be found on the syllabuses of all leading education institutions in the world that teach medical imaging; hence, the influence Euclid has had over a generation of CT users is immeasurable.

The previous text became essential reading within undergraduate and graduate curricula, and the fourth edition will be essential reading for students and should be an essential text for all CT departments globally. We again congratulate the author for adding another first-class tome to his already impressive collection. We would highly recommend this textbook to students studying medical imaging, those in allied fields where CT is becoming more important such as nuclear medicine and radiation therapy, and to those already in the field who need an update or just want a great reference text.

A great textbook by a great educator.

***Patrick Brennan, PhD***
*Professor Diagnostic Imaging*
*Medical Imaging and Radiation Sciences*
*Faculty of Health Sciences*
*The University of Sydney, Australia*
***Stewart Carlyle Bushong, ScD, FAAPM, FACR***
*Professor of Radiologic Science*
*Baylor College of Medicine*
*Houston, Texas*
***Rob Davidson, PhD, MAppSc(MI), BBus, FIR***
*Professor in Medical Imaging*
*Head, Discipline of Medical Radiations*
*University of Canberra*
*Canberra, Australia*

# PREFACE TO THE FOURTH EDITION

The motivation for the fourth edition of *Computed Tomography—Physical Principles, Clinical Applications, and Quality Control* stems from the continued technical evolution of computed tomography (CT) to meet the needs of the clinical environment.

The continued evolution of CT is marked by the refinement of current physical principles, the introduction of new principles, and the development of engineering tools to make these scanners perform at such high levels. Such performance meets the needs of various clinical imaging requirements. One such notable technical evolution is the introduction of iterative reconstruction algorithms for use in routine practice. These algorithms play a role in the improvement of image quality and reduced radiation dose to the patient. All CT manufacturers offer iterative reconstruction algorithms for implementation on their scanners. The fourth edition, of course, adds more scope to the content of the third edition by elaborating on new elements of the evolution and deleting elements that some may consider "obsolete." This is mandatory to bring the textbook "up to date."

## NEW TO THIS EDITION

The chapters in this book have been updated to address the continued technical evolution and major technology trends in CT. Furthermore, a set of updated articles have been cited to support the inclusion of the following:

- The design and implementation of *iterative reconstruction (IR) algorithms*. A new chapter has been added to the contents of this book and addresses the concepts that are important to the CT technologist such as the assumptions made to derive the filtered back-projection (FBP) algorithm, noise reduction techniques, IR without modeling, modeling approaches in IR, examples of IR algorithms, and the performance evaluation studies on IR algorithms. Today all major CT manufacturers have implemented IR algorithms on their scanners.
- *Design innovations in CT detector technology* such as the NanoPanel Prism Detector (Philips Healthcare), the Gemstone Clarity Detector (GE Healthcare), the Stellar Detector (Siemens Healthcare), and PureVISION and the Quantum Vi detectors (Toshiba Medical Systems) are described. In addition, detector technologies are discussed such as *new scintillation crystals* (such as, for example, GE's Gemstone garnet of the type $(Lu,Gd,Y,Tb)_3(Ga,Al)_5O_{12}$ detector) and *miniaturized detector electronics* through the use of *integrated microelectronic circuitry* such as the *application-specific integrated circuit* (ASIC) for analog-to-digital conversion. Furthermore, detectors are described in the categories of the conventional energy integration (EI) detector, the dual-layer detector, and the direct conversion detector (photon counting detector). *Detector-based spectral CT*, the purpose of which is to exploit the transmitted x-ray photons through the patient using energy weighting and material decomposition approaches, is also briefly described.
- *Alternative x-ray tube designs* for multislice CT (MSCT), such as the recent directly cooled x-ray tubes (direct anode cooling)
- *The use of graphics processing unit (CPU) computing in CT* for image reconstruction, image processing, dose calculations, and treatment plan optimization in imaging and radiation therapy
- *Medical image fusion overview* (definitions, medical image fusion areas of studies, steps in medical image fusion, major medical image fusion algorithms, and clinical applications)
- *Single-photon emission computed tomography (SPECT/CT)* has been added to the PET/CT chapter.
- RSNA and ACR statements on the *future of CT screening*
- *Increased focus on CT dose optimization strategies and approaches*
- CT Dose Index Registry, Image Wisely, and Image Gently
- Use of *bismuth shields* in CT including the AAPM Position Statement on the Use of Bismuth Shielding
- Equipment and *phantoms for QC testing, the ACR CT accreditation QC tests, and QC concepts from the International Atomic Energy Agency (IAEA)*

In addition to updated content, a set of learning outcomes and key terms to watch for and remember have been added to the beginning of each chapter. Ten multiple choice questions are provided at the end of each chapter for students to check their understanding of the materials studied.

The fourth edition keeps up with the latest advances in CT imaging where each chapter from the previous edition has been expanded and updated to include state-of-the-art technology and the most up-to-date information on physical principles, instrumentation, clinical applications, and quality control. The addition of numerous new images demonstrates the achievements of these technological advances. New line drawings provide a better representation of important concepts in the text, and a new page layout makes it easier to locate information. Last but not least, a reasonable effort has been made to keep the cited literature current. These references are important since they serve a twofold purpose:

1. To validate the statements made in the textbook regarding CT principles and applications
2. To guide the student to the primary and secondary sources of information that serve as the fundamental basis for pursuing their own research and presentations

Multislice CT has revolutionized CT scanning and has resulted in a wide range of new clinical applications that are examined in this book. This growth of CT technology and its clinical applications have resulted in a new, expanded edition of *Computed Tomography—Physical Principles, Clinical Applications, and Quality Control* that reflects the current state of CT technology.

### Ancillaries

New ancillaries have also been added to this edition (available online on Evolve), including:

- A test bank of approximately 600 questions available in ExamView format
- A practice test to help students reinforce what they have learned and prepare for the ARRT CT Registry Examination
- An image collection of the figures from the book

## PURPOSE

The fourth edition has grown by including descriptions of new technology and elaboration of some previous content to accommodate all the recent advances in CT, and in this regard, the text remains dedicated to its original manifold purposes:

1. To provide comprehensive coverage of the physical principles of CT and its clinical applications for both adults and children
2. To lay the theoretical foundations necessary for the clinical practice of CT scanning
3. To enhance communication between the CT technologist and other related personnel, such as radiologists, medical physicists, and CT vendors
4. To promote an understanding of 2D and 3D anatomic images as they relate to CT

## CONTENT AND ORGANIZATION

The content and organization of the book has not been changed significantly; however, certain chapters have been deleted completely and some content has been reshaped and added to "new" chapters. For example, in the third edition, Chapter 2, an Introduction to Computers, has been deleted; however, some relevant content from this chapter has been used and included in the new Chapter 7. Chapters 11 and 12 have been combined to create the new Chapter 11. A completely new chapter (Chapter 6) on IR algorithms has been added to the fourth edition. Chapter 15 has been included in the new Chapter 13.

The content and organization of the fourth edition are as follows:

Chapter 1 lays the foundations of computed tomography by reviewing its history, including the introduction of the CT scanner as a diagnostic medical imaging tool. Chapter 2 examines the topic of image processing and representation and explores the relevancy of CT to the technology of digital image processing.

Chapter 3 begins with a discussion of the limitations of radiography and conventional tomography followed by a more in-depth examination of the physical principles of CT, radiation attenuation, the meaning of CT numbers, and other technological considerations and concludes with a list of the advantages and limitations of CT. Chapter 4 addresses the concepts of data acquisition and the first step in image production and also includes a description of CT detectors. Chapter 5 focuses on what the CT technologist needs to know to understand the process of image reconstruction and introduces the notion of cone-beam reconstruction. Chapter 6 is the new chapter on IR algorithms and deals with not only the basic principle of an IR algorithm but also provides examples of several IR algorithms from the major CT manufacturers. Furthermore, performance evaluation studies on IR algorithms from 2012 to 2015 are included in this chapter.

Chapter 7 is devoted to basic CT instrumentation and includes a description of the data acquisition, computer, and image display, storage, and communication systems. In addition this chapter has essential elements from Chapter 2 in the third edition, including an overview of computer systems, computer applications in radiology, and finally the components of picture archiving and communication systems (PACS) and three-dimensional (3D) imaging. The discussion of image manipulation and visualization tools continues in Chapter 8, which includes an introduction to multiplanar reconstruction and 3D imaging. Chapter 9 describes the essentials on image quality and includes a discussion of image artifacts in CT. Chapter 10, on the other hand, deals with radiation dose in CT and provides an increased focus on CT dose optimization strategies and approaches, including examples of several dose optimization research studies.

Chapters 11 through 13 are devoted to the physical concepts of volume CT scanning. Chapter 11 details the evolution and fundamentals of multislice spiral/helical CT (also called *volume CT*). This chapter is considered a pivotal chapter in the book, since most of the recent developments in multislice CT are described here. Chapter 12 furthers the discussion by presenting other technical applications of multislice spiral/helical CT and includes a description of CT angiography (CTA), CT fluoroscopy, applications of radiation therapy, medical image fusion, flat-detector CT (FD-CT), CT screening, breast CT imaging, quantitative CT, and portable multislice CT scanning. Chapter 13 examines in-depth three-dimensional concepts in CT imaging, since the advances in spiral/helical CT have resulted in an increased use of 3D display of sectional anatomy. Additionally, virtual reality imaging concepts are included in this chapter. Chapter 14 presents a description of single-photon emission computed tomography/CT (SPECT/CT) as well as positron emission tomography CT (PET/CT).

The next three chapters include coverage of the clinical applications of CT: Chapter 15, "CT of the Head, Neck, and Spine"; Chapter 16, "CT of the Body"; and Chapter 17, "Pediatric CT." Included are a set of updated references that are key to these chapters.

The final chapter in the book, Chapter 18, presents updated information on CT quality control, including a description of CT phantoms and the ACR CT Accreditation QC Tests. Three appendices summarize some of the historical and technical developments in CT, the use of the terms *spiral* and *helical,* a detailed description of the physics of cardiac CT imaging.

## USE AND SCOPE

This comprehensive text is written to meet the wide and varied requirements of its users, students and instructors alike, and meets the many different educational and program needs. *Computed Tomography—Physical Principles, Clinical Applications, and Quality Control* can be used as the primary text for introductory CT courses at the diploma, associate, and baccalaureate degree levels; it serves as a resource for continuing education programs; it functions as a reference text for the CT technologist and other imaging personnel; and it provides the necessary overview of the physical and clinical aspects of CT, which is a prerequisite for graduate-level (Master's Degree) courses in CT.

The content is intended to meet the educational requirements of various radiologic technology professional associations including the American Society of Radiologic Technologists, the American Registry for Radiologic Technologists, the Canadian Association of Medical Radiation Technologists, and the College of Radiographers in the United Kingdom and those in Africa, Asia, Australia, and continental Europe.

CT has become an integral part of the education of radiologic technologists who play a significant role in the care and management of patients undergoing sophisticated CT imaging procedures.

Read on, learn, and enjoy. *Your patients will benefit from your wisdom.*

**Euclid Seeram, PhD, MSc, BSc, FCAMRT**
**British Columbia, Canada**

# ACKNOWLEDGMENTS


The single most important and satisfying task in writing a book of this nature is to acknowledge the help and encouragement of those individuals who perceive the value of its contribution to the imaging sciences literature. It is indeed a pleasure to express sincere thanks to several individuals whose time and efforts have contributed tremendously to this fourth edition. First and foremost, I must thank all my contributors—four radiologists, three medical physicists—who gave their time and expertise to write selected chapters in this book. They are listed on a separate page. In particular, I am indebted to Jiang Hsieh, PhD, Chief Scientist with General Electric Healthcare, and Frederic H. Fahey, DSc and Matthew R. Palmer, PhD, both from Harvard Medical School.

The content of this book is built around the works and expertise of several noted medical physicists, radiologists, computer scientists, and biomedical engineers who have done the original research. In reality, they are the tacit authors of this text, and I am truly grateful to all of them. In this regard, I owe a good deal of thanks to Dr Godfrey Hounsfield and Dr Allan Cormack, both of whom shared the Nobel Prize for Medicine and Physiology for their work in the invention and development of the CT scanner. I have been in personal communication with Dr Hounsfield and he has graciously provided me with details of his biography and his original experiments, and signed his Nobel Lecture, which he sent to me. He will always be remembered in the world of medical imaging education and clinical practice as the one who provided a significant diagnostic tool for use in medicine, and especially for those who work in CT. His signature is included in the textbook as an illustration shown in Figure 1-8. I am also grateful to several other physicists from whom I have learned much about CT physics through their writings. These include Professor Willi Kalender, PhD, Institute of Medical Physics in Germany; Mahadevappa Mahesh, PhD, Chief Physicist, Johns Hopkins Hospital in Baltimore; Michael McNitt-Gray, PhD, University of California; Cynthia McCollough, PhD, Mayo Clinic; Thomas Flohr, PhD, Siemens Medical Solutions, Germany; and last but not least, Shinichiro Mori, PhD, National Institutes of Radiologic Sciences, Japan. Another notable medical physicist to whom I owe thanks is John Aldrich, PhD, Vancouver General Hospital, University of British Columbia, whose seminars on radiation dose in CT and other topics have taught me quite a bit. Thanks John.

In addition, I must acknowledge the efforts of all the individuals from CT vendors who have assisted me generously with technical details and photographs of their CT scanners and accessories for use in the book. In particular, I am grateful to the following CT manufacturers and their representatives: Wes Henschel, Samantha Barr, and Amit Yadav of GE Healthcare; Michael Regan of Philips Healthcare, Canada; Charles Uh and Monica Ramsuran of Siemens Healthcare, Canada; and David McDougall, MRT(R) of Toshiba of Canada, Medical Systems Division. Equally important are the individuals who provided me with several CT images for use in the third edition of the text that are still being used in the fourth edition. Thanks so much for this assistance. These individuals are acknowledged in the respective figure legends and include Hon Jin Chang and Mark Pulaski of Neurologica Corporation, Danvers, MA; Magan Stalter of The Phantom Laboratory, Incorporated, Salem, NY; Pamela Durden of Gammex Inc., Middleton, WI; and Ville Dollhofer of Venturetec Mechatronics GmbH, Germany.

In this book I have used several illustrations and quotes from original papers published in the professional literature, and I am indeed thankful to all the publishers and the authors who have done the original work and have provided me with permission to reproduce them in this textbook. I have purposefully used several quotes so as not to detract from the authors' original meaning. I personally believe that these quotes and illustrations have added significantly to the clarity of the explanations. In this regard, I am appreciative of the Radiological Society of North America for use of materials from *Radiographics* and *Radiology*; Springer Science and Business Media for materials from *European Radiology*; and Elsevier for figures from *Physica Medica*. Furthermore, I must acknowledge the assistance of Yeon Hyeon Choe, MD, Editor-in-Chief, of the *Korean Journal of Radiology*; as well as the American Association of Physicists in Medicine, for materials from *Medical Physics*; Wiley-Blackwell Publishers Inc., for materials from *Australian Radiology*; ImPACT Scan from the United Kingdom, especially Sue Edyvean; and the American Thoracic Society. There are several radiologists who graciously gave their permission as well, and I would like to list some of their names here: Dr Dalrymple, Dr Silva, Dr Kalra, and Dr Van der Molen. Furthermore, I am grateful to the following authors for the use of their illustrations: Alex Pappachen James,

PhD, and Belur Dasarathy, PhD, Faculty in Electrical and Electronic Engineering, Nazarbayev University, Astana for information on medical image fusion; Guillem Pratx, PhD, Assistant Professor, Radiation Oncology, Physics, Stanford University; Dr Caterina Ghetti of Azienda Ospedaliero-Universitaria, Parma, Italy; Hyun Woo Goo, MD; Willi A. Kalender, PhD, of the Institute of Medical Physics Germany for his current photograph; Dr Marcel Beister, Dr Daniel Kolditz, and Dr Willi A. Kalender of the Institute of Medical Physics Germany for use of information from their seminal paper on iterative reconstruction algorithms; and last but certainly not least, Michael Lell, MD, Professor of Radiology, Department of Radiology, University Erlangen, Germany. I trust that I have not forgotten any other individuals who have shaped the technical content of this book to its present form. Thank you all for your gracious generosity in supporting the development of this book.

Additionally, I must acknowledge the work of the 16 reviewers of this book (listed separately) who offered constructive comments to help improve the quality of the chapters. Their efforts are very much appreciated.

The people at Elsevier, Health Professions Division, deserve special thanks for their hard work, encouragement, and support of this project. They are Sonya Seigafuse, Executive Content Strategist; Laura Goodrich, Content Development Specialist; and Kamatchi Madhavan, Project Manager, Health Science, Book Production, Chennai Elsevier India. They have all offered sound and good advice in bringing this book to fruition. I must also thank the individuals in the production department at Elsevier for doing a wonderful job on the manuscript to bring it to its final form. In particular, I am grateful to members of the production team who have worked exceptionally hard during the production of this book, especially in the page-proof stage.

My family deserves special mention for their love, support, and encouragement while I worked into the many hours of the day on this manuscript. I appreciate the efforts of my lovely wife, Trish, a warm, caring, and very special person in my life, and the cutest chaplain I know; our handsome and brilliant son David, a special young man of strength and heart; and our beautiful daughter-in-law, Priscilla, a very smart and hard-working young woman. Thanks for everything, especially for thinking that I am the greatest husband and Dad. Dave and Priscilla are now caring and devoted parents to my beautiful, smart, and overall cute and witty granddaughter Claire. This book is dedicated to her with all my love.

Furthermore, there are three more individuals who have always put me on a pedestal: Patrick Brennan, PhD, and Rob Davidson, PhD, from the University of Sydney and formerly of Charles Sturt University in Australia, respectively; and Stewart Bushong, DSc, of Baylor College of Medicine, Houston, TX. They have honored me by writing the Foreword. Both Patrick and Rob have also been instrumental in getting me honorary senior lecturer and adjunct professor appointments at the University of Sydney and Charles Sturt University, respectively. Additionally, Professor Marilyn Baird, PhD, Head, Department of Medical Radiation Sciences at Monash University in Australia, played a major role in getting me the appointment of adjunct associate professor at Monash University.

To my good friend and colleague Anthony Chan, PhD, MSc, PEng, CEng, a Canadian award-winning biomedical engineer, I am grateful for the stimulating and useful discussions of various CT topics. Last, but not least, I wish to express sincere appreciation to Peter Kench, PhD, for making me a part of the University of Sydney's CT specialization component of the Master's Degree in Medical Imaging. I am also grateful to the thousands of students who have diligently completed my CT Physics course. Thanks for all the challenging and stimulating questions. Keep on learning and enjoy the pages that follow.

**Euclid Seeram, PhD, MSc, BSc, FCAMRT**
*British Columbia, Canada*

# CONTENTS

## Appendices

1

# Computed Tomography: An Overview

## OUTLINE



## LEARNING OBJECTIVES

On completion of this chapter, you should be able to:

1. state the meaning of the terms
   - "transverse axial tomography"
   - "image reconstruction from projections."
2. state terms synonymous with CT.
3. outline three steps that constitute the CT process.
4. identify major components of a CT scanner and briefly explain how a CT scanner works.
5. trace the significant developments in the history of CT including the contributions of Hounsfield and Cormack.
6. identify the essential elements of a digital imaging system.
7. identify several applications of volume CT scanning.
8. identify major technology trends in CT technology.
9. identify several features of CT product data.
10. state the meaning of digital image processing.

## KEY TERMS TO WATCH FOR AND REMEMBER

The following key terms/concepts are important to your understanding of this module.

**americium**
**computed tomography (CT)**
**CT screening**
**data acquisition**
**digital imaging system**
**dose descriptors**
**dose optimization**
**emission CT**
**gantry**
**generation**
**graphics Processing Unit (GPU)**
**high-speed CT**
**image reconstruction**
**positron emission tomography (PET) scanner**
**quality control**
**rendering**
**scanning**
**single-photon emission tomography (SPECT)**
**spectral CT imaging**
**transmission CT**
**transverse axial tomography**
**volume CT**

Medical imaging has experienced significant changes in both the technological and clinical arenas. Innovations are commonplace in the radiology department, and today the introduction of new ideas, methods, and refinements in existing techniques is clearly apparent. The goal of these developments is to optimize the technical parameters of the examination to provide the acceptable image quality at reduced radiation doses needed for diagnostic interpretation and, more importantly, to provide improved patient care management. One such development, **computed tomography (CT),** is a revolutionary tool of medicine, particularly in medical imaging. This chapter explores the meaning of CT through a brief description of its fundamental principles and historical perspectives. Furthermore, it summarizes the growth of CT from its introduction in the 1970s to today's technology, with an emphasis on the physical and technical aspects of CT imaging.

## MEANING

The word *tomography* is not new. It can be traced back to the early 1920s, when a number of investigators were developing methods to image a specific layer or section of the body. At that time, terms such as "body section radiography" and "stratigraphy" (from *stratum*, meaning "layer") were used to describe the technique. In 1935 Grossman refined the technique and labeled it tomography (from the Greek *tomos*, meaning "section"). A conventional tomogram is an image of a section of the patient that is oriented parallel to the film.

In 1937, Watson developed another tomographic technique in which the sections were transverse (cross sections); this technique was referred to as **transverse axial tomography.** However, these images lacked enough detail and clarity to be useful in diagnostic radiology, preventing the technique from becoming fully realized as a clinical tool.

### Image Reconstruction from Projections

CT overcomes limitations in detail and clarity by using the mathematical construct of **image reconstruction** from **projections** to produce sharp, clear images of cross-sectional anatomy. Image reconstruction from projections had its theoretic roots in 1917 when the Austrian mathematician Radon proved it possible to reconstruct or build up an image of a 2D or 3D object from a large number of its projections from different directions. This procedure has been used in a number of fields, ranging from astronomy to electron microscopy; for example, in astronomy images of the sun have been reconstructed, and in microscopy images of the molecular structure of bacteria can be reconstructed.

Similarly, images of the human body can be reconstructed by using a large number of projections from different locations (Fig. 1-1). In simplified terms, radiation passes through each cross section in a specific way and is projected onto a detector that sends signals to a computer for processing. The computer produces clear, sharp images of the internal structure of the object.

A more complete definition of this technique has been given by Herman (1980), who stated: "Image reconstruction from projections is the process of producing an image of a two-dimensional distribution (usually some physical property) from estimates of its line integrals along a finite number of lines of known locations." The CT scanner uses this process to produce a variety of images ranging from cross-sectional 2D and 3D images to virtual reality images of the anatomy or organ system under study.

Image reconstruction from projections finally found practical application in medicine in the 1960s through the work of investigators such as Oldendorf,

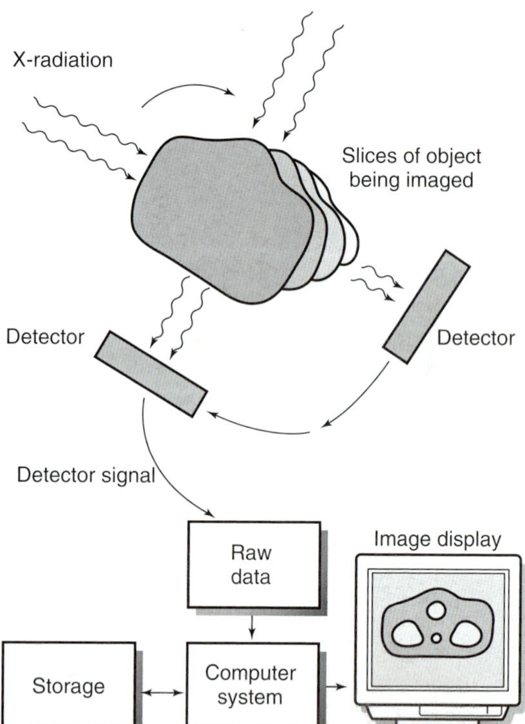


**FIGURE 1-1** Image reconstruction from projections. From many different locations, radiation passes through each slice or cross section of the object being imaged. This radiation is projected onto a detector that sends signals to a computer for processing into an image that reveals the internal structure of the object.

Kuhl, and Edwards, who studied problems in nuclear medicine. In 1963, Cormack also applied reconstruction techniques to nuclear medicine, and in 1967, Hounsfield finally applied reconstruction techniques to produce the world's first clinically useful CT scanner for imaging the brain (Fig. 1-2).

These studies resulted in two types of CT systems: **emission CT,** in which the radiation source is inside the patient (e.g., nuclear medicine), and **transmission CT,** in which the radiation source is outside the patient (e.g., x-ray imaging). Both involve image reconstruction. Image reconstruction has also been used in diagnostic medical sonography and **magnetic resonance imaging (MRI).** This book discusses only the fundamental principles and technology of x-ray transmission CT.

### Evolution of Terms

Hounsfield's work produced a technique that revolutionized medicine and diagnostic radiology. He called the technique *computerized transverse axial scanning* (tomography) in his description of the system, which was first published in the *British Journal of Radiology* in 1973. Since then a number of other terms have appeared in the literature. Terms such as "computerized transverse axial tomography," "computer-assisted tomography or computerized axial tomography," "computerized transaxial transmission reconstructive tomography," "computerized tomography," and "reconstructive tomography" were not uncommon. The term computed tomography was established by the Radiological Society of North America (RSNA) in its major journal *Radiology.* In addition, the *American Journal of Roentgenology* accepted this term, which has now gained widespread acceptance within the radiologic community. Throughout the remainder of this book the term computed tomography and its acronym, CT, are used.

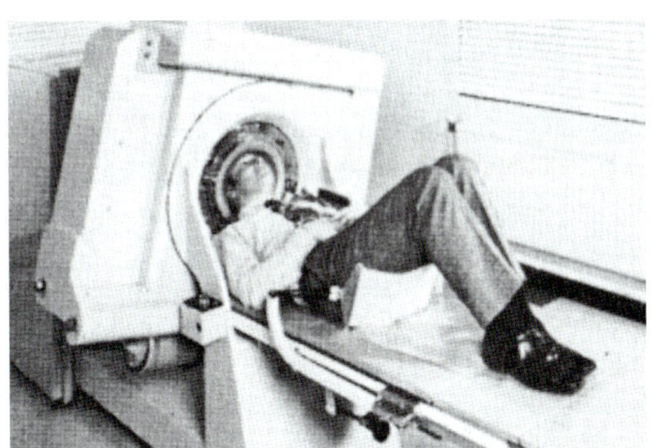

**FIGURE 1-2** First-generation model of a CT head scanner. (Courtesy Thorn EMI, London, United Kingdom.)

## PROCESS

The formation of CT images by a CT scanner involves three steps: **data acquisition; image reconstruction; and image display, image post processing, image storage, and communication** (Fig. 1-3). Image communication and storage of CT images are functions of the Picture Archiving and Communication System (PACS).

### Data Acquisition

The term **data acquisition** refers to the collection of x-ray transmission measurements from the patient. Once x rays have passed through the patient, they fall onto special electronic detectors that measure the transmission values, or **attenuation** values. Enough transmission measurements or data must be recorded to meet the requirements of the reconstruction process. The first brain CT scanner used a data acquisition scheme where the **x-ray tube** and detectors moved in a straight line, or translated, across the patient's head, collecting a number of transmission measurements as they moved from left to right

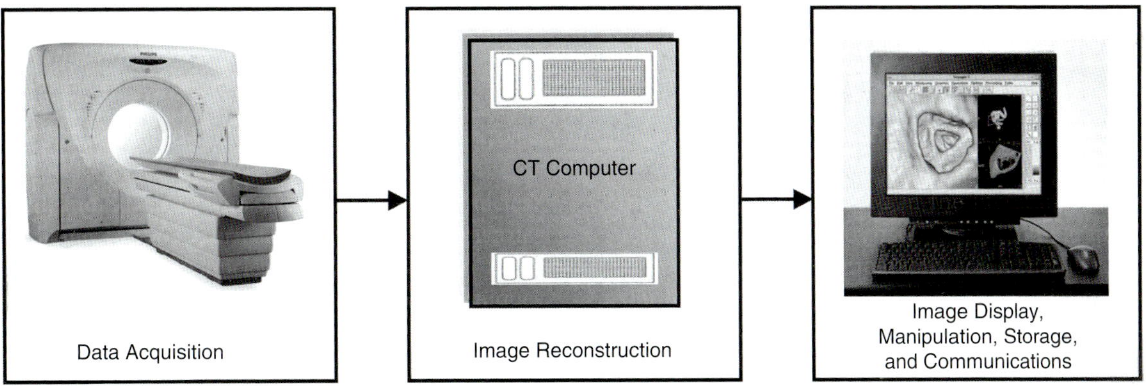


**FIGURE 1-3** Steps in the production of a CT image. (See text for further explanation.)

(Fig. 1-4). Then the x-ray tube and detector rotated 1 degree and started again to move across the patient's head, this time from right to left. This process of translate-rotate-stop-rotate, referred to as ***scanning***, is repeated over 180 degrees.

The fundamental problem with this method of data collection was the length of time required to obtain enough data for image reconstruction. Later, more efficient schemes for scanning the patient were introduced (see Chapter 4). These schemes involve rotating the x-ray tube and detectors continuously as the patient moves through the scanner simultaneously. This process results in scanning a volume of tissue rather than a single slice of tissue, which was characteristic of the early CT scanners. Acquiring a volume of tissue during the scanning is now referred to as **volume scanning**. The **continuous rotation** of the x-ray tube and detectors and the simultaneous movement of the patient result in a *spiral/helical* path traced by the x-ray beam. The goal of volume scanning is not only to improve the volume coverage speed but to provide new tools for clinical applications.

Data acquisition also involves the conversion of the electrical signals obtained from the electronic detectors to digital data, which the computer can use to process the image.

## Image Reconstruction

After enough transmission measurements have been collected by the detectors, they are sent to the computer for processing. The computer uses special mathematical techniques to reconstruct the CT image in a finite number of steps called **image reconstruction algorithms** (see Chapters 5 and 6). For example, the image reconstruction algorithm used by Hounsfield to develop the first CT scanner was called the *algebraic reconstruction technique*, belonging to a class of algorithms referred to as iterative reconstruction algorithms.

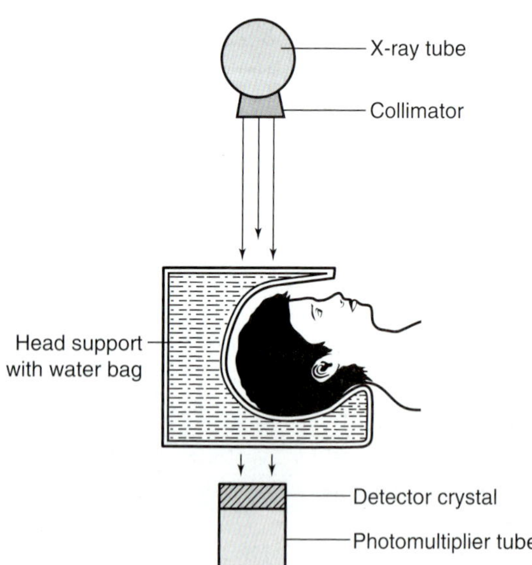


**FIGURE 1-4** Data collection scheme in the first CT brain scanner.

Analytical reconstruction algorithms have also been developed for spiral/helical **volume CT** scanners. These include fan beam-filtered **back-projection** algorithms and **interpolation** algorithms, as well as **cone-beam** *image reconstruction algorithms*. Today, all new CT scanners use *iterative reconstruction algorithms*. These algorithms will be described in Chapter 6.

A computer is central to the CT process. In general, this involves a minicomputer and associated microprocessors for performing a number of specific functions. In some CT scanners, **array processors** perform high-speed calculations, and specific microprocessors perform **image-processing** operations. Therefore, in this regard, computers are described briefly in Chapter 7.

## Image Display, Processing, Storage, Recording, and Communications

After the computer has performed the image reconstruction process, the reconstructed image can be displayed and recorded for subsequent viewing and stored for later analysis. The image is usually displayed on a cathode ray tube, although other display technologies are now available; for example, touch screen technology is used for scan setup and control in some scanners. However, the cathode ray tube remains the best device for the display of grayscale imagery, although LCDs are now used. Display monitors are mounted onto control consoles that allow the technologist (operator's console) and radiologist (physician's console) to manipulate, store, and record images.

Image manipulation or **digital image processing** (see Chapter 2), as it is often referred to by some authors, has become popular in CT, and many computer **software** packages are now available. Images can be modified through image post processing to make them more useful to the observer for diagnostic interpretation; for example, transverse axial images can be reformatted into coronal, sagittal, and paraxial sections. In addition, images can also be subjected to other image-processing operations such as image smoothing, edge enhancement, grayscale manipulation, and 3D image processing.

Images can be recorded and subsequently stored in some form of archive. In the past, images were recorded on x-ray film because of its wider grayscale compared with that of instant film. Such recording is accomplished by multiformat video cameras, although laser cameras are now common in radiology departments. It is important to note, however, that film-based recording has become obsolete.

CT images can be stored on magnetic tapes and magnetic disks. More recently, optical storage technology has added a new dimension to the storage of information from CT scanners. In optical storage the stored data are read by optical means such as a laser beam. In this case, storage is referred to as *laser storage*. Optical storage media include at least three formats: disk, tape, and card (see Chapter 7).

In CT, **communications** refers to the electronic transmission of text data and images from the CT scanner to other devices such as laser printers; diagnostic workstations; display monitors in the radiology department, intensive care unit, and operating and trauma rooms in the hospital; and computers outside the hospital. Electronic communications in CT require a standard protocol that facilitates **connectivity** (networking) among multimodalities (CT, MRI, digital radiography, and fluoroscopy) and multivendor equipment. The standard used for this purpose is the Digital Imaging and Communication in Medicine standard established by the American College of Radiology (ACR) and the National Electrical Manufacturers Association. CT departments now operate in a PACS environment that allows the flow of CT data and images among devices and people not only in the radiology department but throughout the hospital as well. Additionally, the PACS is connected to a Radiology Information System, which in turn is connected to the Hospital Information System. (Networking and PACS are described in Chapter 7.)

## HOW CT SCANNERS WORK

To enhance understanding of the early experiments and current technology, the technologist must be familiar with the way a CT scanner works (Fig. 1-5). The technologist first turns on the scanner's power and performs a quick test to ensure that the scanner is in good working order. The patient is in place in the scanner opening, with appropriate positioning for the particular examination. The technologist sets up the technical factors at the control console. Scanning can now begin.

When x rays pass through the patient, they are attenuated and subsequently measured by the detectors. The x-ray tube and detectors are inside the **gantry** of the scanner and rotate around the patient during scanning. The detectors convert the x-ray photons (attenuation data) into electrical signals, or **analog signals,** which in turn must be converted into digital (numerical) data for **input** into the computer. The computer then performs the image reconstruction process. The reconstructed image is in numerical form and must be converted into electrical signals for the technologist to **view** on a television monitor. The images and related data are then sent to the

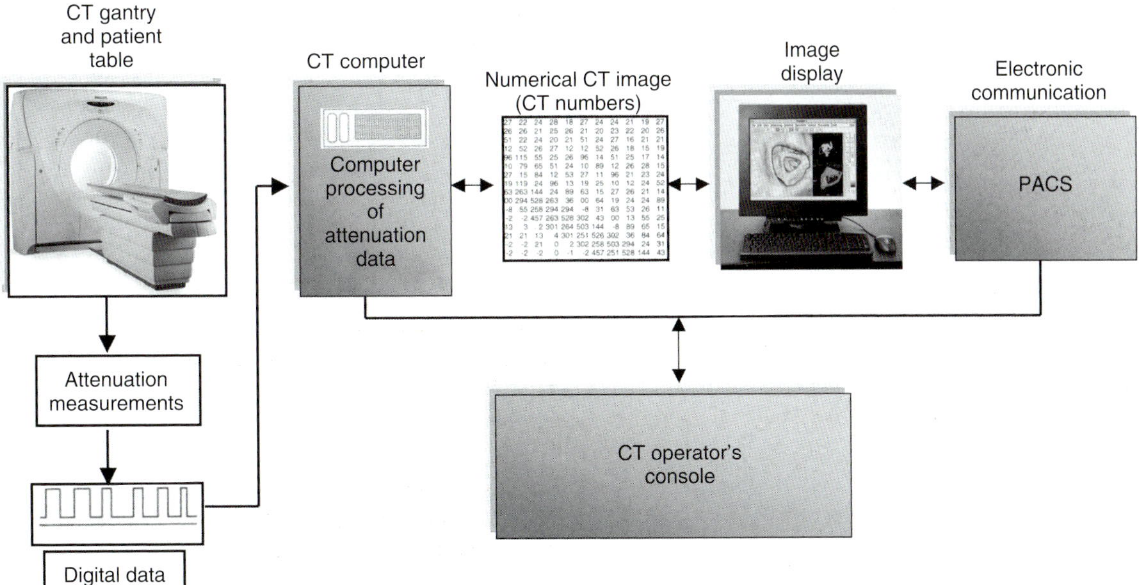


**FIGURE 1-5** A CT scanner showing the main components. The data communications component is not shown.

PACS, where a radiologist will be able to retrieve and interpret them. Finally, the image can be stored on optical disks.

## HISTORICAL PERSPECTIVES

### Early Experiments

The invention of the CT scanner has revolutionized the practice of radiology. CT is so remarkable that in many cases it generates a dramatic increase in diagnostic information compared with that obtained by conventional x-ray techniques. This extraordinary invention was made possible through the work of several individuals, most notably Godfrey Newbold Hounsfield and Allan MacLeod Cormack (Bates et al., 2012; Beckmann, 2006).

#### Godfrey Newbold Hounsfield

Godfrey Newbold Hounsfield (Fig. 1-6) was born in 1919 in Nottinghamshire, England. He studied electronics and electrical and mechanical engineering. In 1951, Hounsfield joined the staff at EMI Limited (now Thorn EMI; manufacturer of records and electronics, and recorded The Beatles under the EMI Label) in Middlesex, where he began work on radar systems and later on computer technology. His research on computers led to the development of the EMIDEC 1100, the first solid-state business computer in Great Britain. For an interesting short commentary on the relationship between EMI and The Beatles, the reader should refer to a book titled *X-Ray Vision—The Evolution of Medical Imaging and Its Human Significance* by Gunderman (2013).

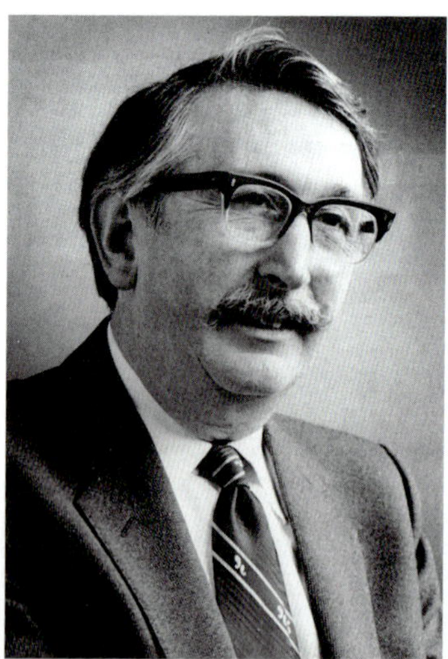

**FIGURE 1-6** The inventor of clinical computed tomography, Dr. Godfrey Hounsfield. (Courtesy Thorn EMI, London, United Kingdom.)

In 1967, Hounsfield was investigating pattern recognition and reconstruction techniques by using the computer. (In image processing, pattern recognition involves techniques for the observer to identify, describe, and classify various features represented in an image or a signal.) From this work, he deduced that, if an x-ray beam was passed through an object from all directions and measurements were made of all the x-ray transmission, information about the internal structures of that body could be obtained. This information would be presented to the radiologist in the form of pictures that would show 3D representations.

With encouragement from the British Department of Health and Social Security, an experimental apparatus was constructed to investigate the clinical feasibility of the technique (Fig. 1-7). The radiation used was from an **americium** gamma source coupled with a crystal detector. Because of the low radiation **output,** the apparatus took about 9 days to scan the object. The computer needed 2.5 hours to process the 28,000 measurements collected by the detector. Because this procedure was too long, various modifications were made and the gamma radiation source was replaced by a powerful x-ray tube. The results of these experiments were more accurate, but it took 1 day to produce a picture (Hounsfield, 1980).

To evaluate the usefulness of this machine, Dr. James Ambrose, a consultant radiologist at Atkinson-Morley's Hospital, joined the study. Together, Hounsfield and Ambrose obtained readings from a specimen of human brain. The findings were encouraging in that tumor tissue was clearly differentiated from gray and white matter and controlled experiments with fresh brains from bullocks showed details

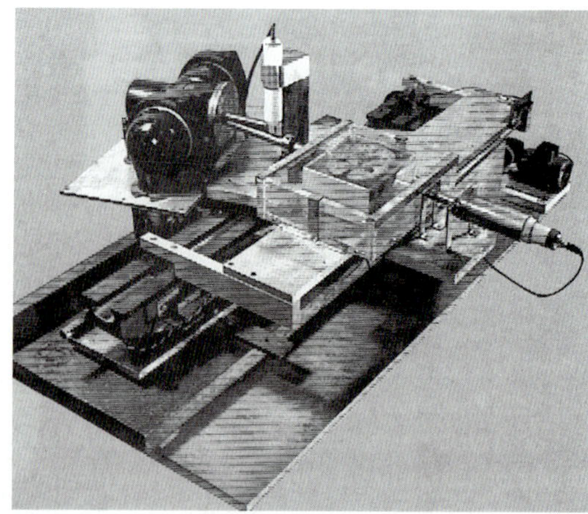

**FIGURE 1-7** The original lathe bed scanner used in early CT experiments by Hounsfield. (Courtesy Thorn EMI, London, United Kingdom.)

such as the ventricles and pineal gland. Experiments were also done with kidney sections from pigs.

In 1971 the first clinical prototype CT brain scanner (EMI Mark 1) was installed at Atkinson-Morley's Hospital and clinical studies were conducted under the direction of Dr. Ambrose. The processing time for the picture was reduced to about 20 minutes. Later, with the introduction of minicomputers, the processing time was reduced further to 4.5 minutes.

In 1972 the first patient was scanned by this machine. The patient was a woman with a suspected brain lesion, and the picture showed clearly in detail a dark circular cyst in the brain. From this moment on, and as more patients were scanned, the machine's ability to distinguish the difference between normal and diseased tissue was evident (Hounsfield, 1980).

Dr. Hounsfield's research resulted in the development of a clinically useful CT scanner for imaging the brain. For this work, Hounsfield received the McRobert Award (akin to a Nobel Prize in engineering) in 1972. During the same year, he became a Fellow of the Royal Society and subsequently was awarded the Lasker Prize in the United States and, in 1977, Dr. Hounsfield was appointed Commander of the British Empire. In 1979, Hounsfield shared the Nobel Prize in medicine and physiology with Allan MacLeod Cormack, a physics professor at Tufts University in Medford, Massachusetts, for their contributions to the development of CT. Figure 1-8 shows a note sent to the author from Dr. Hounsfield in response to several questions. After receiving this prestigious prize, he was knighted by her majesty Queen Elizabeth and became an Honorary Fellow of the Royal Academy of Engineering. Dr. Hounsfield died on August 12, 2004, at age 84 (Isherwood, 2004). By developing the first practical CT scanner, Dr. Hounsfield opened up a new domain for technologists, radiologists, medical physicists, engineers, and other related scientists.

For a more detailed account of Hounsfield's pioneering work, the interested reader should refer to the book *Godfrey Hounsfield: Intuitive Genius of CT* by Stephen Bates, Liz Beckmann, Adrian Thomas, and Richard Waltham (2012), who were friends of Hounsfield and worked with him at EMI. This book includes a description of Hounsfield's life, work, awards, and publications.

## Allan MacLeod Cormack

Allan MacLeod Cormack (Fig. 1-9) was born in Johannesburg, South Africa, in 1924. He attended

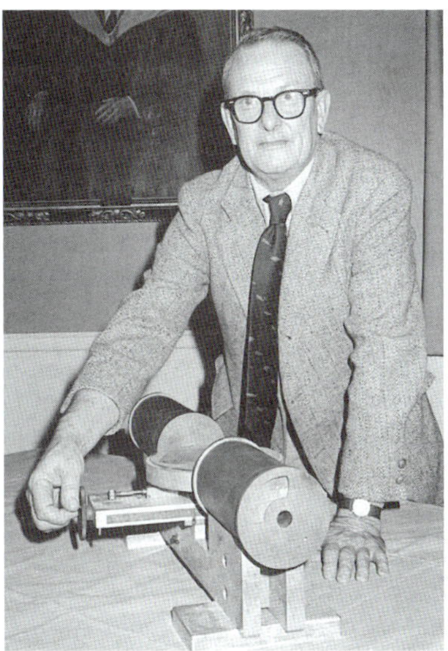

**FIGURE 1-9** Allan MacLeod Cormack shared the Nobel Prize with Godfrey Hounsfield for his mathematical contributions to the problem in CT. (Courtesy Tufts University, Medford, Mass.)

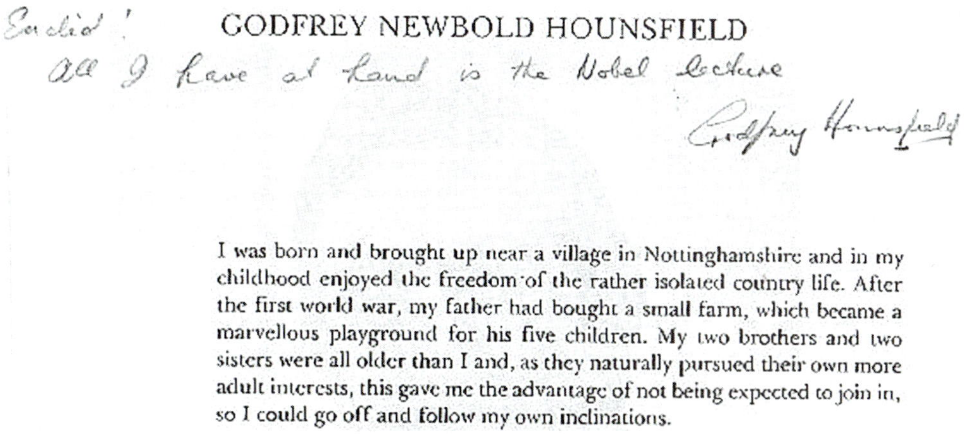

Euclid!

GODFREY NEWBOLD HOUNSFIELD

All I have at hand is the Nobel lecture

Godfrey Hounsfield

I was born and brought up near a village in Nottinghamshire and in my childhood enjoyed the freedom of the rather isolated country life. After the first world war, my father had bought a small farm, which became a marvellous playground for his five children. My two brothers and two sisters were all older than I and, as they naturally pursued their own more adult interests, this gave me the advantage of not being expected to join in, so I could go off and follow my own inclinations.

**FIGURE 1-8** A personal note from Dr. Godfrey Hounsfield to the author, Euclid Seeram.

the University of Cape Town where he obtained a Bachelor of Science in Physics in 1944 and earned a Master of Science in Crystallography in 1945. He subsequently studied nuclear physics at Cambridge University before returning to the University of Cape Town as a physics lecturer. He later moved to the United States and was on sabbatical at Harvard University before joining the physics department at Tufts University in 1958.

Professor Cormack developed solutions to the mathematical problems in CT. Later, in 1963 and 1964, he published two papers in the *Journal of Applied Physics* on the subject, but they received little interest in the scientific community at that time. It was not until Hounsfield began work on the development of the first practical CT scanner that Cormack's work was viewed as the solution to the mathematical problem in CT (Cormack, 1980). Cormack died at age 74, in Massachusetts on May 7, 1998. Additionally, back in South Africa, Dr. Cormack was granted the Order of Mapungubwe, South Africa's highest honor, in December 2002, for his contribution to the invention of the CT scanner.

## Growth

### First 10 Years

Between 1973 and 1983 the number of CT units installed worldwide increased dramatically. Perhaps the first significant technical development came in 1974 when Dr. Robert Ledley (Fig. 1-10), a professor of radiology, physiology, and biophysics at Georgetown University, developed the first whole-body CT scanner. (Hounsfield's EMI scanner scanned only the head.)

Dr. Ledley graduated with a doctorate in dental surgery from New York University in 1948, and in 1949 he earned a master's degree in theoretical physics from Columbia University. He holds more than 60 patents on medical instrumentation and has written several books on the use of computers in biology and medicine. In 1990 he was inducted into the National Inventors' Hall of Fame for the invention of the automatic computed transverse axial CT scanner.* In 1997, Dr. Ledley won the National Medal of Technology, an honor awarded by the President of the United States for outstanding contributions to science and technology (Ledley, 1999). He also served as president of the National Biomedical Research Foundation at Georgetown University Medical Center, and passed away in 2012.

These pioneering works were followed by the introduction of three **generations** (a term used to refer to the method of scanning) of CT scanners. In 1974 a fourth-generation CT system was developed (Fig. 1-11).

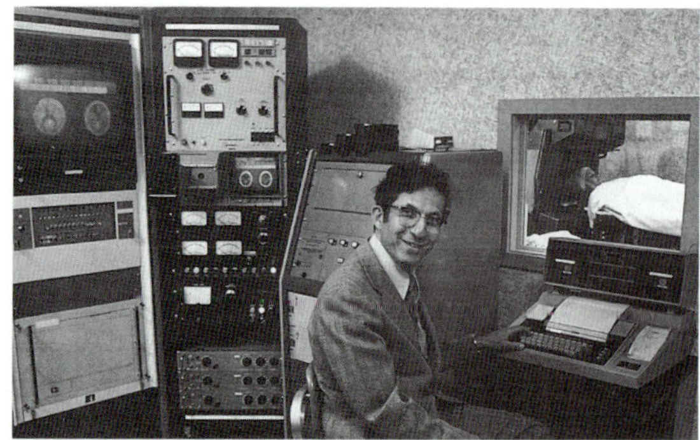

**FIGURE 1-10** Dr. Robert Ledley developed the first whole-body CT scanner, the automatic computed transverse axial CT scanner. (Courtesy Robert Ledley, Washington, D.C.)

A computer capable of performing multiple functions is central to the CT system. The CT computer has undergone several changes over time (see Chapter 7). Image quality is another significant development as a result of technological changes. Although earlier images appeared "blocky," images acquired later were remarkably improved (Fig. 1-12). Improvements in image quality included improved **spatial resolution,** decreased scan time, increased density resolution, and changes to the x-ray tube to facilitate the increased loadability required of whole-body scanners. For example, the **matrix** size in 1972 was 80 × 80; in 1993, it was 1024 × 1024. In addition, the spatial resolution and scan time in 1972 were reported to be three line pairs per centimeter (lp/cm) and 5 minutes, respectively, compared with 15 lp/cm and 1 second, respectively, in 1993 (Kalender, 1993). Increased loadability resulted in scanners capable of dynamic CT examinations that took a series of scans in rapid succession. Later-model CT scanners could operate in several modes such as the prescan localization mode, which produced a survey scan of the region of interest. Rapid reformatting of the axial scans into coronal, sagittal, and oblique sections also became possible.

### High-Speed CT Scanners

In 1975, the first **high-speed CT** scanner, the dynamic spatial reconstructor (DSR) was installed in the biodynamics unit at the Mayo Clinic. The goal of the DSR was to perform dynamic volume scanning to accommodate imaging of the dynamics of organ systems and the functional aspects of the cardiovascular and pulmonary systems with high **temporal resolution** as well as imaging anatomic details (Ritman et al., 1991; Robb & Morin, 1991). Research on this unit has since been discontinued.

In the mid-1980s, another high-speed CT scanner was introduced that used electron beam technology,

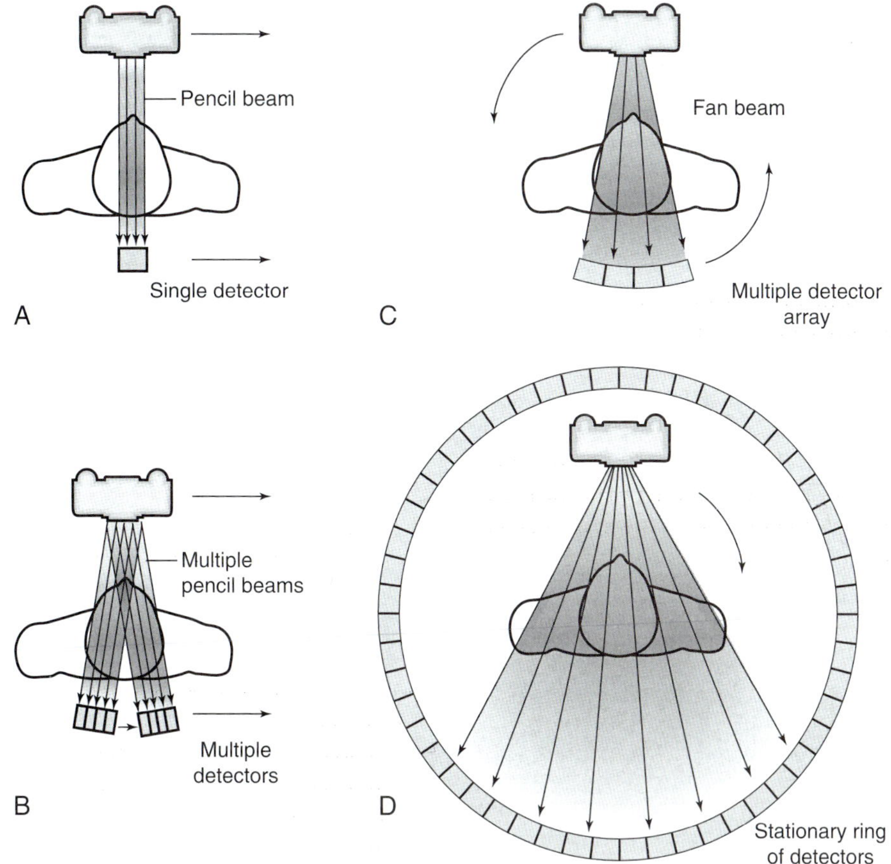


**FIGURE 1-11** Four basic scanning methods or systems: **A,** first generation; **B,** second generation; **C,** third generation; **D,** fourth generation.

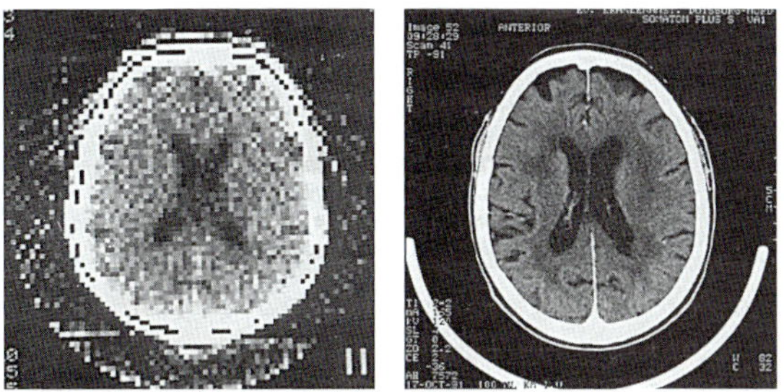

**FIGURE 1-12** The appearance of early CT images (*left*) compared with those produced by a more recent CT scanner (*right*). The difference in image quality is apparent. (From Schwierz, G., & Kirchgeorg, M. (1995). *Electromedica, 63*, 2–7.)

a result of work by Dr. Douglas Boyd and colleagues during the late 1970s at the University of California at San Francisco. The scanner was invented to image the cardiovascular system without **artifacts** caused by motion. At that time the scanner was called the *cardiovascular CT scanner*. Later, this scanner was acquired and marketed by Siemens Medical Systems under the name Evolution and was subsequently referred to as the electron beam CT (EBCT) scanner. The most conspicuous difference between the EBCT scanner and conventional CT is the absence of moving parts. At that time, the EBCT scanner was capable of acquiring multislice images in as little as 50 and 100 ms.

The U.S. Food and Drug Administration (FDA) cleared the EBCT scanner in 1983. As of 2007, the EBCT scanner is marketed by General Electric (GE) Healthcare under the name e-Speed and it now features proprietary technologies that play a significant role in imaging the heart. In October 2002, the e-Speed CT scanner received FDA clearance and it is now capable of 33-ms, 50-ms, and 100-ms true temporal resolution to produce images at up to 30 frames per second (GE Healthcare, personal communication, 2007).

Because nearly 20 manufacturers made CT scanners between 1973 and 1983, a number of developments unique to particular manufacturers were also introduced. The evolution of CT continued after 1983, with nearly 10 manufacturers competing for the CT market. (Box 1-1 highlights the developments

### BOX 1-1 Milestones in Computed Tomography Development from Philips Medical Systems

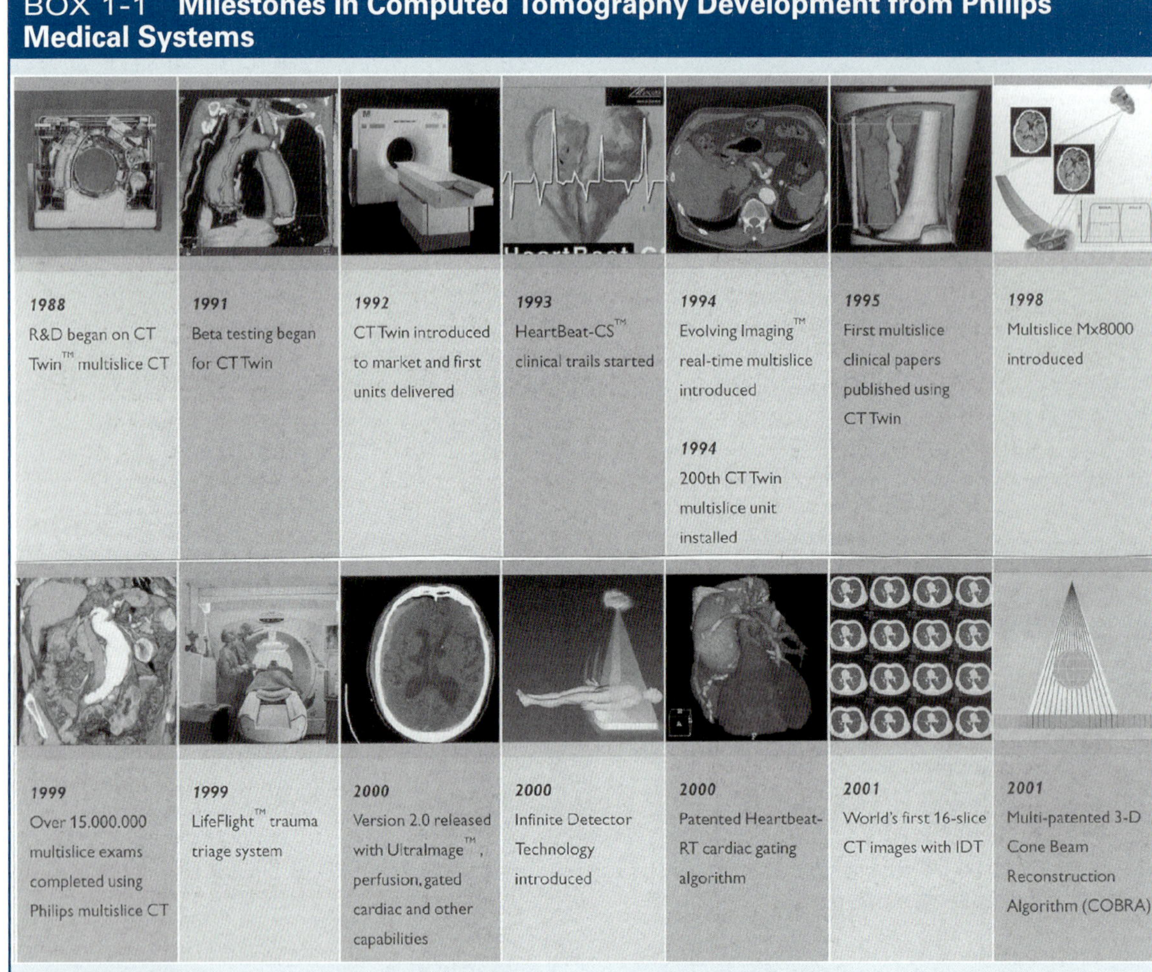


Courtesy Philips Medical Systems.

from a major manufacturer actively involved in the research and development of the CT scanner between 1988 and 2001.)

## Spiral/Helical CT Scanners: Volume Scanning

In conventional CT the patient is scanned one slice at a time. The x-ray tube and detectors rotate for 360 degrees or less to scan one slice while the table and patient remain stationary. This slice-by-slice scanning is time-consuming; therefore, efforts were made to increase the scanning of larger volumes in less time. This notion led to the development of a technique in which a volume of tissue is scanned by moving the patient continuously through the gantry of the scanner while the x-ray tube and detectors rotate continuously for several rotations. As a result, the x-ray beam traces a path around the patient (Fig. 1-13). Although some manufacturers call this **beam geometry** *spiral CT* (the beam tracing a spiral path around the patient), others refer to it as *helical CT* (the beam tracing a helical path around the patient). This book uses both terms synonymously.

The idea of this approach to scanning can be traced to three sources (Kalender, 1995). In 1989, the first report of a practical spiral CT scanner was presented at the RSNA meeting in Chicago by Dr. Willi Kalender (Fig. 1-14). Dr. Kalender has made significant contributions to the technical development and practical implementation of this approach to CT scanning. His main research interests are in the areas of diagnostic imaging, particularly the development and introduction of volumetric spiral CT. His work is documented in more than 900 scientific papers, more than 300 original publications among these, and more than 30 patents (Kalender, personal communications, 1999, 2006, 2014).

Dr. Kalender was born in 1949 and studied medical physics in Germany. Subsequently, he continued his studies at the University of Wisconsin in the United States. He later worked with Siemens Medical

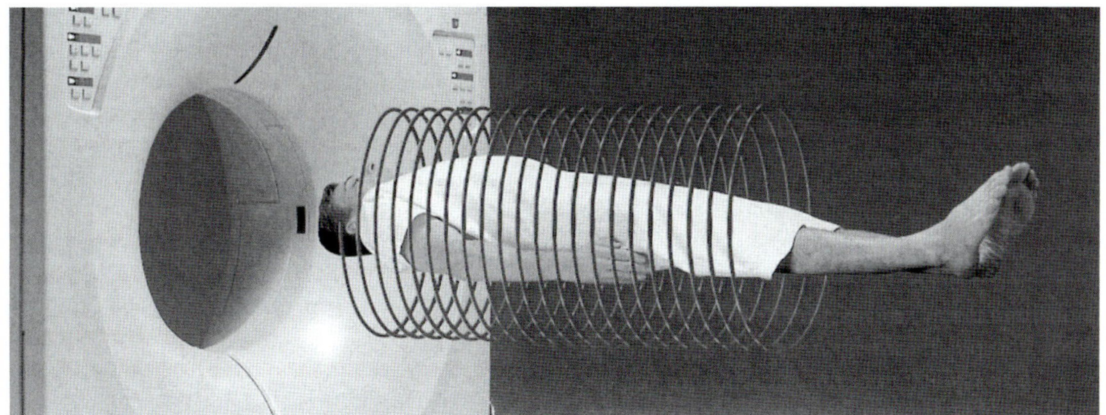

**FIGURE 1-13** With volume CT scanners, the x-ray tube and detectors rotate continuously as the patient moves continuously through the gantry. As a result, the x-ray beam traces a path (beam geometry) around the patient. This method of scanning the patient is referred to as helical or spiral CT. (Courtesy Toshiba America Medical Systems, Tustin, Calif.)

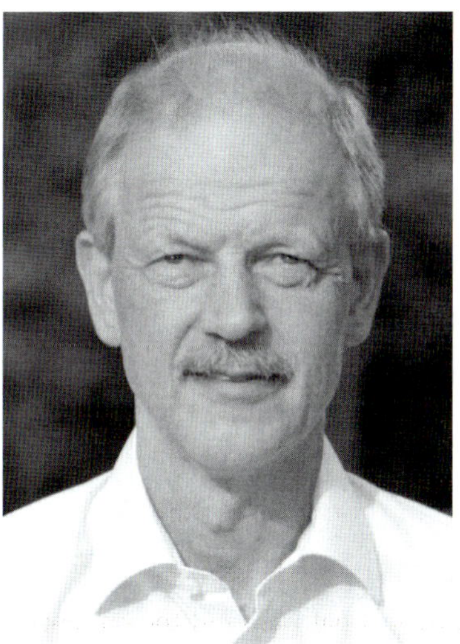

**FIGURE 1-14** Dr. Willi Kalender has made significant contributions to the introduction and development of volume spiral CT scanning. (Courtesy Willi Kalender, Nürnberg, Germany.)

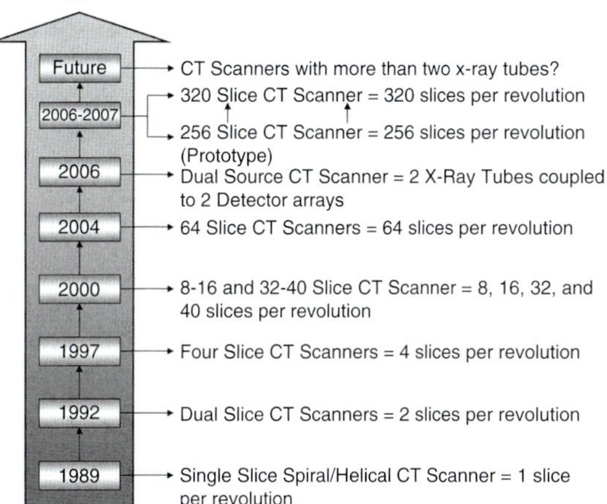


**FIGURE 1-15** The evolution of MSCT scanners, including the DSCT scanner.

Solutions in the area of CT, and in 1995 he became professor and chairman of the Institute of Medical Physics, which is associated with the University of Erlanger, Nürnberg, Germany. Dr. Kalender has several awards including the prestigious Cross of the Order of Merit of the Federal Republic of Germany (Kalender, 2014) by the President of the Federal Republic of Germany, 2004.

The spiral/helical CT scanners developed after 1989 were referred to as *single-slice spiral/helical* or **volume CT** *scanners*. In 1992 a dual-slice spiral/helical CT scanner (volume CT scanner) was introduced to scan two slices per 360-degree rotation, thus increasing the volume coverage speed compared with single-slice volume CT scanners.

In 1998 a new generation of CT scanners was introduced at the RSNA meeting in Chicago. These scanners are called **multislice CT (MSCT)** scanners because they are based on the use of multidetector technology to scan four or more slices per revolution of the x-ray tube and detectors, thus increasing the volume coverage speed of single-slice and dual-slice volume CT scanners. The number of slices per revolution has been increasing at a steady pace, as outlined in Figure 1-15. In 2004, a 256-slice prototype CT scanner was undergoing clinical tests and, more recently, a comparison of the doses from the 256-slice CT scanner and a 16-slice CT scanner has been reported (Mori et al., 2006). The cone beam geometry of the 256-slice prototype CT scanner is shown in Figure 1-16. The number of detectors is 912 (transverse) x 256 (cranio-caudal) and the cone angle is about 120, and a gantry rotation time of 1 sec.

In addition to the improvements in the performance characteristics—such as minimum scan time, data per 360° scan, image matrix, **slice thickness,** and spatial and contrast resolution—from 1972 to 2004, MSCT scanners are now based on new technologies. These include new x-ray tube and detector technologies to accommodate high-speed imaging, large-bore gantry apertures to facilitate ease of patient positioning and patient access, improved **z-axis** resolution, radiation **dose optimization** with dose modulation techniques, integrated software featuring multiple software platforms, and intuitive interfacing and software for data management such as workflow optimization and image processing. Two notable new concepts for MSCT, particularly for scanners that have 16 or greater detector rows, are the reconstruction algorithm and the definition of an important parameter called the **pitch.** These scanners now use cone-beam image reconstruction algorithms to address the cone-beam geometry as the detector width increases to accommodate 16–320 detector rows. The pitch for volume scanners has now been defined by the International Electrotechnical Commission (IEC), after much debate in the literature as to what the exact definition should be. The IEC states that the pitch for MSCT scanners is the ratio of the table feed per revolution of the x-ray tube to the total width of the collimated beam. Pitch is described in a subsequent chapter.

One of the central goals in the development of the CT scanner is to achieve **isotropic** *resolution*, where the voxel is a perfect cube (equal length, width, and height) as opposed to *nonisotropic resolution*, where the voxel is not a perfect cube, as is clearly illustrated in Figure 1-17. The impact of isotropic resolution on CT images has improved image quality in all three dimensions; hence, 3D images are sharp in appearance and do not exhibit the stair-step artifacts seen in nonisotropic resolution 3D images. Scanners can now achieve isotropic resolution of <0.4 mm.

### Dual-Source CT Scanner

In 2005, Siemens Medical Solutions announced a new type of CT scanner at the RSNA, called the SOMATOM Definition. This is a dual-source CT (DSCT) scanner that features two x-ray tubes and two detectors (Fig. 1-18) specifically intended for

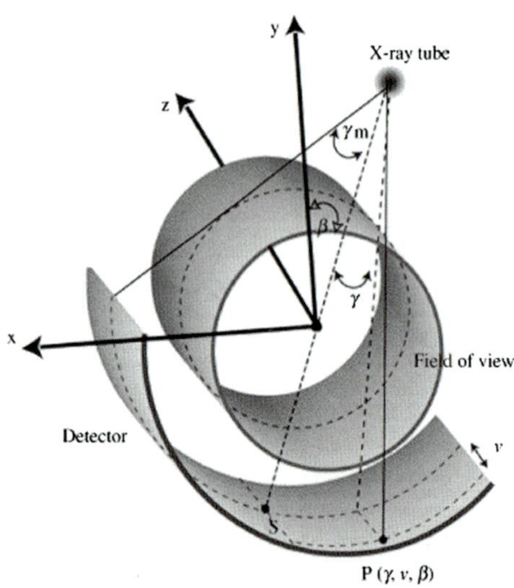


**FIGURE 1-16** Cone beam geometry of the prototype 256-detector row Multi-slice CT scanner, which makes use of a wide cylindrical 2 dimensional detector. The number of detectors is 912 (transverse) x 256 (cranio-caudal) and the cone angle is about 120, and a gantry rotation time of 1 sec. (From Mori S et al: Noise properties for three weighted Feldkamp algorithms using a 256-detecotor row CT-scanner: Case study for hepatic volumetric cine imaging. *European Journal of Radiology*, 59 (2); 289–294, 2006. Reproduced by permission.)

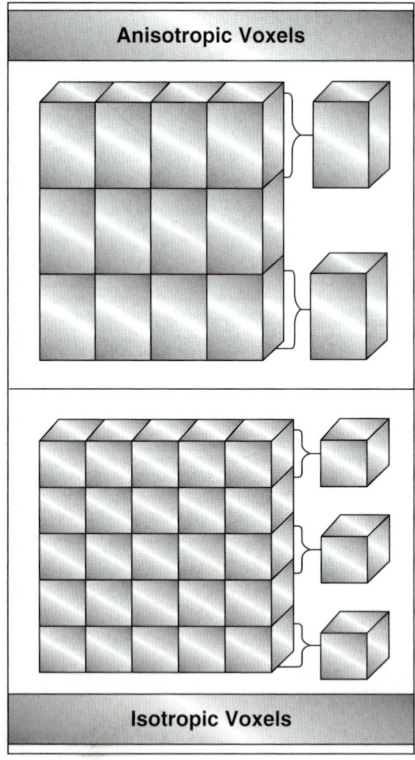


**FIGURE 1-17** Isotropic resolution in CT implies that voxels are perfect cubes with all dimensions being equal, as opposed to anisotropic resolution where all dimensions are not equal.

imaging cardiac patients in a very short time. As illustrated in Figure 1-19, the performance of the DSCT scanner compared with the single-source CT (SSCT) scanner in imaging the beating heart at a low and stable heart rate (60 beats/min) is improved because of the higher temporal resolution of the DSCT scanner (Fig. 1-19, *A*). Furthermore, as the heart rate increases to 100 beats/min, the DSCT scanner offers much better image quality (sharpness) in both systolic and diastolic phases compared with the SSCT scanner (Fig. 1-19, *B*).

DSCT is also referred to as dual-energy CT since the two x-ray tubes operate at different energies. In this regard, the term *spectral CT* is also used synonymously to refer to dual-energy CT.

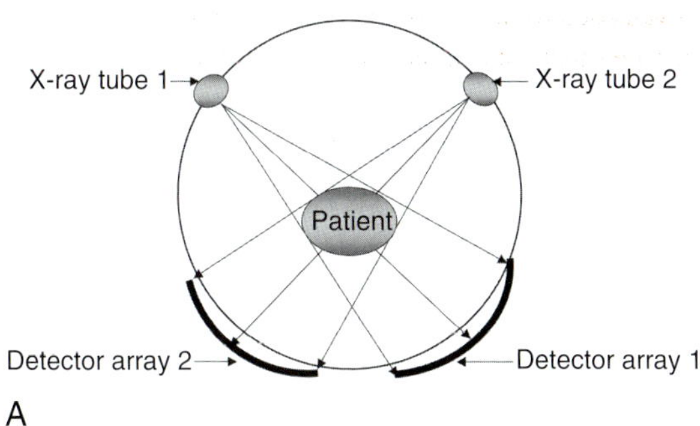


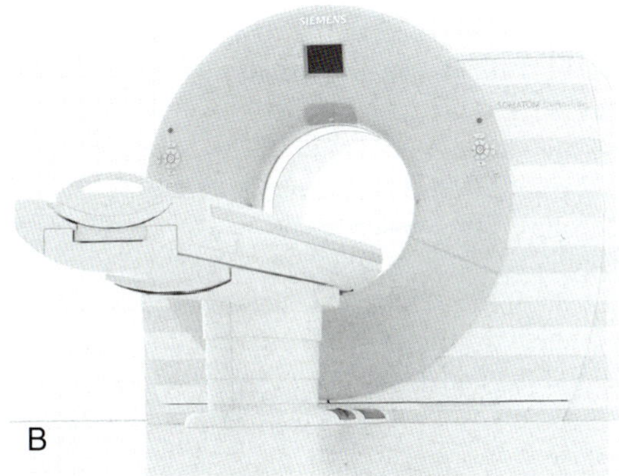


**FIGURE 1-18** The basic concept of the DSCT scanner **(A)** and a full view of the scanner **(B)** introduced by Siemens Medical Solutions. (Courtesy Siemens Medical Solutions.)

## Other Technical Applications of Volume CT

Volume CT scanning has resulted in a wide range of applications such as **CT fluoroscopy, CT angiography,** 3D imaging, virtual reality imaging, and more recently improved cardiac CT imaging. CT has found applications in radiation therapy and nuclear medicine technologies as well. In radiation therapy, for example, the CT scanner is now used in CT simulation processes (Fig. 1-20). As noted, the *CT simulator* includes the CT scanner, which is specially equipped with a flat table top and lasers that facilitate accurate positioning of the patient and is coupled to the radiation treatment planning virtual simulator. As noted by Mutic et al. (2003), "the scanner is accompanied by specialized software which allows treatment planning on volumetric patient CT scans in a manner consistent with conventional radiation therapy simulators." This scanner can either be installed in the radiology department or in the radiation therapy department. In nuclear medicine, the CT scanner is combined with a **positron emission tomography (PET) scanner** (Ell, 2006) and **single-photon emission tomography (SPECT)** to form single units referred to as a PET/CT scanner and a SPECT/CT scanner (Jones et al., 2013). SPECT/CT and PET/CT are described in detail in Chapter 14.

## Portable CT

A unique event in the evolution of CT technology was the development of a mobile CT scanner to image patients who are too ill or physically

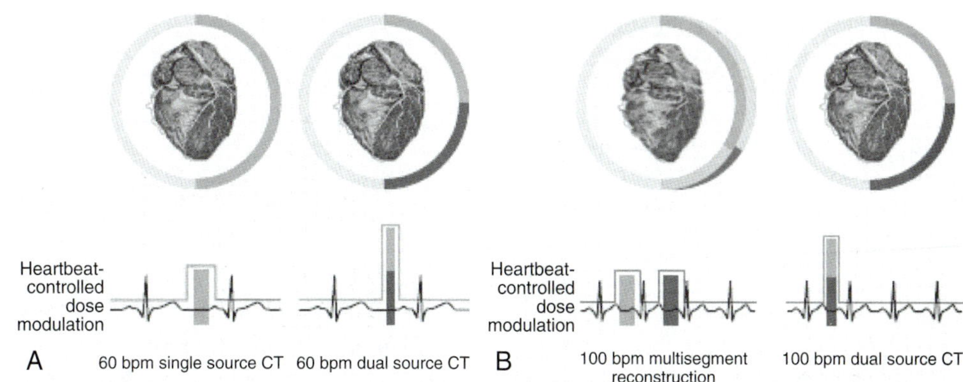


**FIGURE 1-19** A visual comparison of the image quality of an SSCT scanner **(A)** and the DSCT scanner **(B)** in cardiac imaging. (Courtesy Siemens Medical Solutions.)

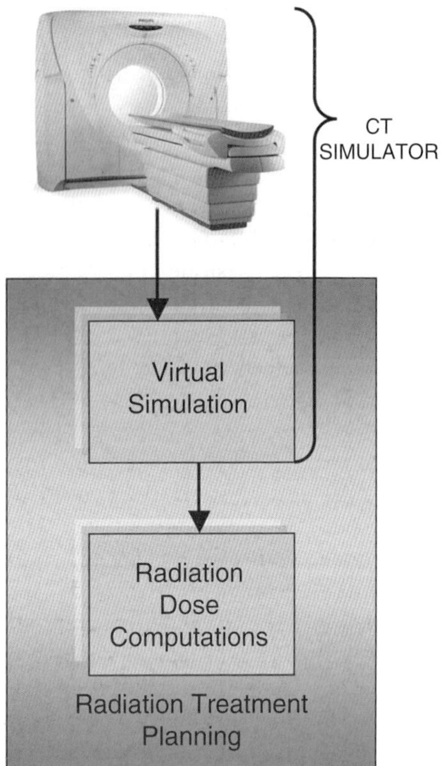


**FIGURE 1-20** The CT simulation process in radiation therapy with a CT scanner.

traumatized to be transported to a fixed CT. Philips Medical Systems introduced this type of scanner specifically for use in the operating room, intensive care unit, and emergency trauma unit. The portable CT scanner is compact and mounted on wheels to facilitate transportation of the unit to remote locations in the hospital by technologists. Other portable CT scanners are commercially available from NeuroLogica, a subsidiary of Samsung Electronics (http://www.neurologica.com/products/ceretom).

## Clinical Efficacy Studies

The term *efficacy* is synonymous with effectiveness, **efficiency,** and performance. A number of investigators designed efficacy studies to test the clinical usefulness of this new diagnostic technique. Studies reported the results of scanning the brain, spinal cord, neck, thorax, abdomen, retroperitoneum, pelvis, and extremities.

CT became well established in the diagnosis of diseases of the central nervous system, and in some cases, it eliminated the need for examinations such as pneumoencephalography and reduced the frequency of cerebral angiography. Disorders such as gliomas, metastases, intracranial lesions, aneurysms, infarctions, hemorrhage, and atrophy have been successfully detected by CT. Later, whole-body clinical applications (see later chapters) became effective. In addition, CT proved useful in radiation treatment planning to provide accurate isodose curves and in other areas, such as determination of the mineral salt content in bones, or quantitative CT. Studies using MSCT scanners clearly demonstrated their usefulness in a wide range of clinical applications, including playing a central role in cardiac imaging in applications such as coronary angiography, assessment of ventricular function and pulmonary veins, and calcium scoring (DeRoos, 2006).

## Radiation Dose Studies

A fundamental goal of any new imaging technique is to provide maximum information content with the minimum radiation dose to the patient. Perry and Bridges (1973) measured both the cranial radiation dose and the gonadal radiation dose for a series of scans. Their results provided a foundation for future studies. Initially, the radiation dose to the patient was thought to be negligible because the beam in CT was tightly collimated, but the patient **exposure** for a series of CT scans usually exceeds that of film radiography of the same area.

Radiation dose is an integral topic in CT technology, because the CT beam geometry and method of acquiring images differ from those of conventional radiography. Several imaging parameters in CT affect dose, including slice thickness, **noise,** resolution detector efficiency, reconstruction algorithm, **collimation,** and **filtration.** Various dose studies have explored the ways in which these factors influence the dose.

These studies have also led to the development of special ways to measure and describe the dose (Kalender, 2005; McNitt-Gray, 2002; Seeram, 1999, 2014). Ionization chambers or thermoluminescent **dosimeters** are used to measure the dose. **Dose descriptors** include the single-scan dose profile, multiscan dose profile, CT dose index, multiscan average dose, and isodose curves.

Additionally, manufacturers have developed various schemes to reduce the dose in CT. One scheme uses three elements to keep the patient dose to a minimum during **data acquisition:** (1) combined applications to reduce exposure, a prepatient filtering technique that reduces the dose by about 15% compared with conventional CT; (2) new ultrafast ceramic detectors that reduce the dose by another 25%; and (3) online dose modulation, whereby the milliamperage (mA) is optimized to the patient characteristics (diameter and absorption) to reduce the dose. This particular development in CT dose reduction is referred to as *automatic tube current modulation technique* (Iball et al., 2006; Rizzo et al., 2006). Different manufacturers have different methods to do *automatic exposure control* in CT.

## Quality Control

As with any medical **imaging system,** CT scanners are subject to **quality control** procedures and tests. These **quality control (QC)** tests must meet both quantitative and qualitative criteria, which indicate that the scanner is in perfect working condition. Testing system performance is vital to maintain optimal image quality and minimize the production of image artifacts. Because the CT system consists of several mechanical and electronic components, many quality control tests are currently available. These range from simple tests, which the technologist can perform by using various phantoms provided by the manufacturers, to more complex tests that may require the expertise of the radiologic physicist or biomedical engineer. More recently, the ACR has introduced a CT phantom referred to as the ACR phantom, as illustrated in Figure 1-21, to be used for any CT QC program. The phantom basically consists of four sections that can be imaged simultaneously to generate several test results. Quality control for CT scanners will be described in detail in a later chapter.

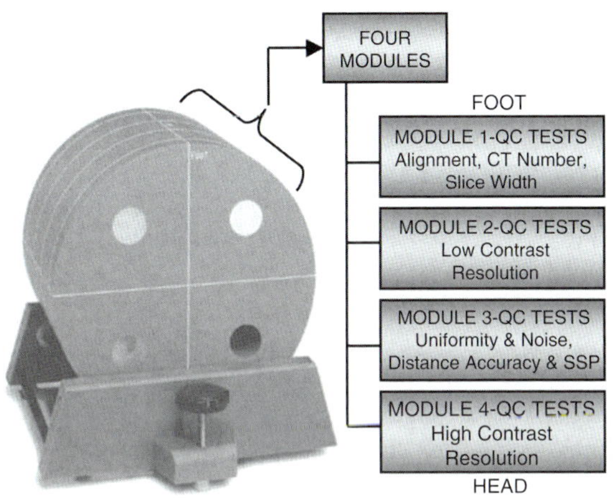


**FIGURE 1-21** The ACR phantom used for CT quality control. The phantom consists of four sections (modules) for performing several quality control tests.

## Other Uses

CT is useful in areas other than medicine. For example, CT can be used to study *internal log defects.* Funt and Bryan (1987) investigated the use of CT technology in a sawmill. They developed and tested algorithms that automatically interpreted CT images of logs and stated, "The computer program uses the high density and elliptical shape of knots to distinguish them from good wood, and the low density and rough texture of rotten areas to separate rotten wood from sound wood." Habermehl and Ridder (1997) detailed the use of a portable CT scanner to take images of trees to determine wood rots; locate knots, hollows, and other defects; and determine water distribution inside the tree trunk (Fig. 1-22). These portable tree CT scanners use a cesium 137 gamma radiation source with a fan beam falling on an array of about 30 sodium iodide detectors.

CT has also been used in *paleoanthropology.* Zonneveld et al. (1989) found that CT can visualize internal anatomy of completely preserved Egyptian

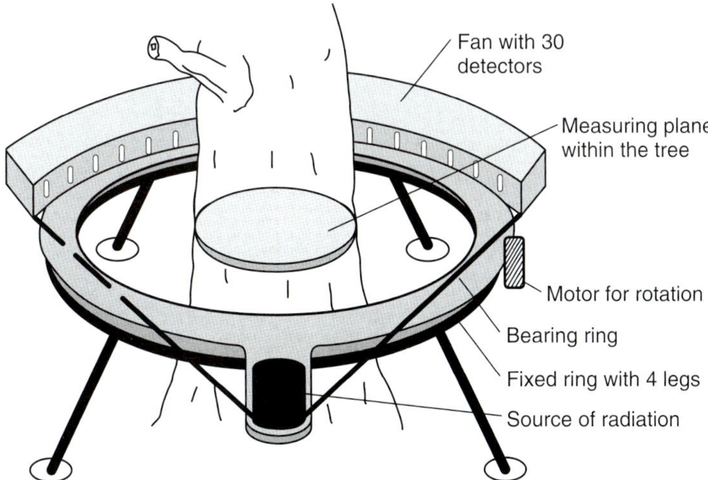


**FIGURE 1-22** A portable CT scanner for imaging trees. (From Habermehl, A., & Ridder, H. W. (1997). γ-Ray tomography in forest and tree sciences. In U. Bonse (Ed.), *Developments in x-ray tomography: proceedings of the SPIE*, pp. 234–243.)

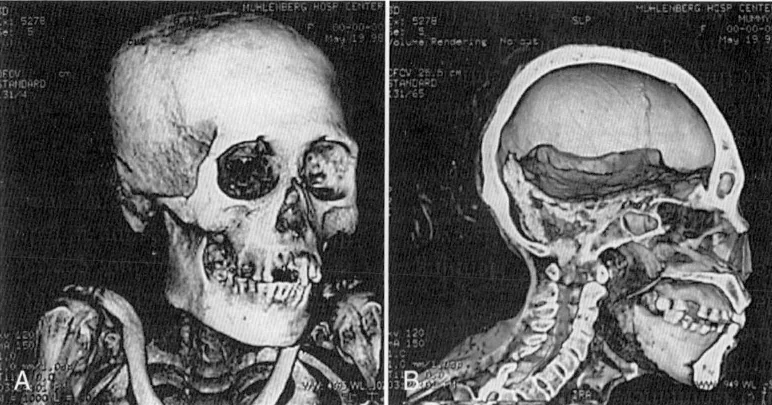


**FIGURE 1-23** CT can be used to image mummies without destroying the bandages or plaster in which they are wrapped. **A,** 3D CT image of a 1000-year-old Peruvian mummy using volume rendering with a bone and detail filter. **B,** A lateral view of the same mummy shows residual brain in the posterior fossa. (Courtesy John Posh, personal communication, Bethlehem, Pa.)

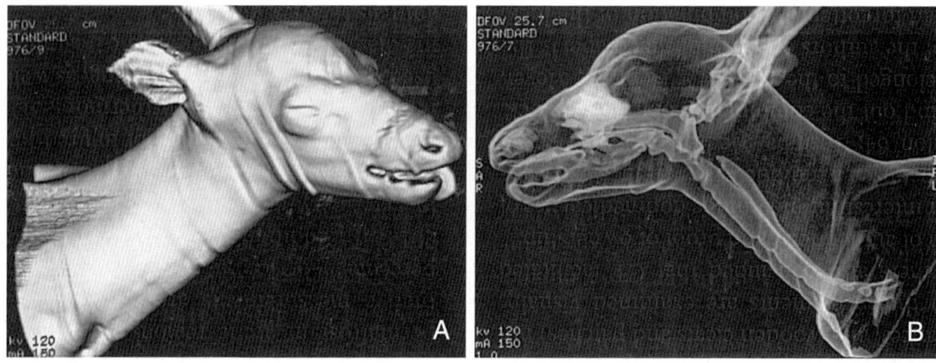


**FIGURE 1-24** **A,** 3D surface rendering of a 2-month-old whitetail fawn mauled by a mountain lion. **B,** The same fawn examined by CT with a 3D transparency program to demonstrate the airways and other air-filled cavities. (Courtesy John Posh, personal communication, Bethlehem, Pa.)

mummies (Fig. 1-23; Yasuda et al., 1992). Additionally, Hoffman et al. (2002) reported the use of CT in what they refer to as *paleoradiology*. Recently, a CT system for dedicated imaging of mummies has become available and will be used in a major research project planned by the Egyptian Supreme Council of Antiquities in conjunction with Siemens Medical Solutions (who donated an MSCT scanner) and the National Geographic Society.

Several cases report the use of CT in paleo-ornithology, oil exploration, fat stock breeding, and other animal investigations (Fig. 1-24). In fat stock breeding, pigs are scanned to determine the meat quality defined as the best combination of water, protein, and fat, thus eliminating the need to kill the pigs for this determination (Fig. 1-25).

Sirr and Waddle (1999) used CT to evaluate bowed stringed instruments such as violins. The scans demonstrated varying degrees of internal damage

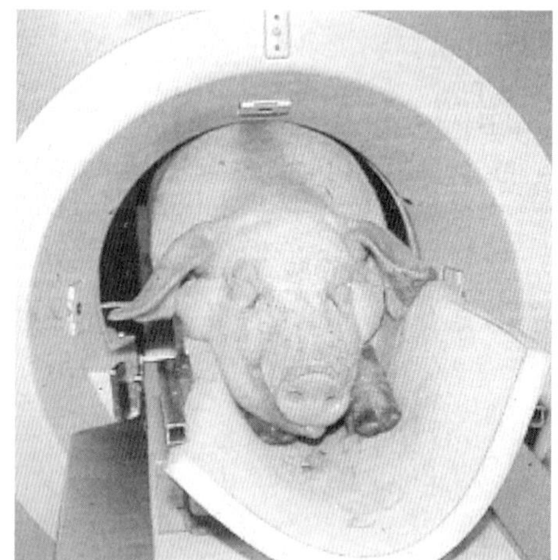

**FIGURE 1-25** CT scanning of pigs in fat stock breeding to determine meat quality. (Courtesy Siemens Medical Systems, Iselin, NJ.)

(e.g., wormholes, air gaps, and plastic deformities of wood) or those resulting from repair (e.g., glue lines, filler substances, and wooden cleats and patches) not seen when the instruments are examined visually. The researchers also concluded that CT facilitated verification of authenticity and proof of ownership.

Another interesting and unique nonmedical use of CT is one that used a multidetector 64-slice CT scanner (Aquillon 64; Toshiba Medical Systems, Nasu, Japan) to find out the combination of a bicycle lock. The lock belonged to the son of Dr Henning Meyer, MD (one of the authors of the published paper). The little boy had forgotten the combination of the lock. Fortunately the lock was not on the bicycle.

The lock was scanned using 0.5-mm detector collimation and 350 mA, 120 kV, pitch of 0.33, and 0.4-second rotation time. Additionally, the CT images were reconstructed using a smooth abdominal kernel, and the reconstruction was performed with 0.5-mm section thickness in 0.4-mm increments. The authors indicated that "Orthogonal multiplanar reformations were viewed with the scanner's workstation to identify the correct code combination"

Resulting images were published by Henning Meyer, MD, Marc Dewey, MD, Ahi Sema Issever, MD, and Patrick Rogalla, MD., from the Department of Radiology, Charite´ Universitatsmedizin Berlin, Germany, in Radiology (Meyer et al, 2007)

The authors reported that they used "an unorthodox method to tackle this problem. As conventional radiographs deliver only a superimposed image of the complete lock, we here describe for the first time how multidetector CT helped in identifying the combination of a German-made high-quality bicycle lock" (Meyer et al, 2007).

In preparation for CT imaging, "the positions of the dials were prepared to show digit 0 on the right side of the lock. The positions of all other digits are shown on an overlay. By following the position of each notch, one can clearly identify the combination of the lock.

A set of four CT images showed the notches of the lock (dark blotches on the each of four images) and clearly revealed that the combination was 1789. This result must have made the little boy very happy.

More recently, CT scanners are now used at major airports for *automated explosives detection*. As baggage is scanned, the CT data (numbers) of the contents obtained as a result of the scanning are compared with **CT numbers** of known explosives or contraband. If the two sets of CT numbers correspond, an alarm is sounded.

The CT scanner is also used in the heavy oil and oil sands industry in Alberta, Canada, to obtain quantitative data on carbonates and oil sands when investigating sites for oil extraction from tar sands. Furthermore, the CT scanner is being used to study permafrost in arctic regions of the world. Quantitative measurements are used to determine the percentage of ice in permafrost cores (Cameron, 2014). In addition, the CT scanner has been used in veterinary medicine at Charles Sturt University in Australia since 2012. In particular, the scanner is useful in providing images of injured horses, birds, reptiles, and mammals. Furthermore, 3D imaging is used to assist in surgical planning, as well as providing diagnoses and managing the treatment of injured animals (Davies, 2014).

## APPLICATIONS OF VOLUME SCANNING

Volume scanning from either single-slice spiral/helical or multislice spiral/helical CT generates vast amounts of data compared with slice-by-slice conventional CT scanning. Several new applications provide radiologists and other physicians with additional tools for taking images of patients with CT and enhancing their own diagnostic effectiveness. These new applications include continuous imaging or CT fluoroscopy, 3D imaging and visualization, CT angiography, and virtual reality imaging.

### CT Fluoroscopy

CT fluoroscopy, or continuous imaging, depends on spiral/helical data acquisition methods, high-speed processing, and a fast image-processing algorithm for image reconstruction. In conventional CT, the time lag between data acquisition and image reconstruction makes real-time display of images impossible. CT fluoroscopy allows for the reconstruction and display of images in real time with variable frame rates. In 1996 the U.S. FDA approved real-time CT fluoroscopy as a clinical tool for use in radiology (Katada et al., 1996).

CT fluoroscopy is based on three advances in CT technology: (1) fast, continuous scanning made possible by spiral/helical scanning principles; (2) fast image reconstruction made possible by special **hardware** performing quick calculations and a new image reconstruction algorithm; and (3) continuous image display by use of cine mode at frame rates of two to eight images per second (Daly & Templeton, 1999).

Other support tools were developed to facilitate **interventional procedures** in CT fluoroscopy. One such tool, the Fluoro Assisted Computed Tomography System, uses a unique flat-panel amorphous silicon digital detector coupled with an x-ray tube by a C-arm, which is a part of the CT gantry.

## Three-Dimensional Imaging and Volume Visualization

3D imaging is a popular technique in CT because of the availability of large amounts of digital data. It is now possible on CT scanners and the results have been promising (Fishman et al., 1991). 3D CT is already used in radiation treatment planning, craniofacial imaging, surgical planning, and orthopedics.

3D images can be obtained by a hardware-based or a software-based approach. The hardware-based approach uses specialized equipment such as electronic computer display units to execute algorithms for 3D imaging, and the software-based approach uses computer programs or software-coded algorithms. These algorithms, or **rendering** techniques, transform the transaxial CT data into simulated 3D images. In general, two classes of techniques are available for the transformation: surface and volume based. Each technique consists of three steps: volume formation, classification, and image projection. Although volume formation involves stacking images to form a volume with some preprocessing, classification refers to determining the tissue types in the slices. According to Fishman (1991), image projection consists of "projecting the classified volume data in such a manner that a two-dimensional (2D) representation or simulation of the 3D volume is formed." Additionally, Fishman (2004) reviewed the essentials of 3D rendering describing the evolution and progress through the years.

Computer graphics has played a role in the evolution and refinement of 3D imaging (Rhodes, 1991). Computer graphics involves the creation, manipulation, and display of pictures or images with the computer. It allows the user to express ideas and information in a visual format and includes various ways to represent data to create and display images by use of graphics programming languages and image-processing techniques.

3D CT has created a new area of interest for technologists (Seeram, 2004) who have the opportunity to participate in its development. Today, 3D articles are appearing more often in the literature to support the increasing 3D applications that can make full use of the large datasets generated by the new MSCT scanners (Bolan, 2013; Dalrymple et al., 2005).

***Volume visualization*** is a term used in the discussion of the display of images in CT. It involves the use of computer programs, or **visualization tools,** that provide the observer-diagnostician with additional information from the image to facilitate diagnosis. These tools can be simple (e.g., image contrast and brightness [**windowing**] tools) or advanced (e.g., 3D imaging, interactive, and **cine visualization tools**). Examples of current state-of-the art CT images are shown in Figure 1-26. A comprehensive review article on volume visualization is written by Zhang et al. (2011).

## CT Angiography

**CT angiography** is defined as CT imaging of blood vessels opacified by **contrast media** (Kalender, 1995). During contrast injection, the entire area of interest is scanned with spiral/helical CT and images are recorded when vessels are fully opacified to show arterial or venous phases of enhancement.

CT angiography uses 3D imaging principles to display images of the vasculature through intravenous injection of contrast media compared with those of intra-arterial angiograms. Four essential elements are patient **preparation;** selection of acquisition parameters (total spiral/helical scan time, slice thickness, table speed) to optimize the imaging process; contrast media injection; and postprocessing techniques and visualization tools such as algorithms to display 3D images in interactive cine modes, multiplanar reconstruction, maximum intensity projection, shaded surface display, and **volume rendering** (Zhang et al., 2011).

## CT Endoscopy: Virtual Reality Imaging

Virtual reality is a branch of computer science that immerses users in a computer-generated environment and allows them to interact with 3D scenes. The application of virtual reality concepts to the creation of inner views of tubular structures is called *virtual endoscopy* (DeWever at al., 2005; Vining, 1999). Volume CT scanners produce large datasets (2D axial images) compared with their conventional slice-by-slice counterparts. Subsequently, volume CT scanners have improved 3D imaging, CT fluoroscopy, CT angiography, and CT virtual endoscopy (Fig. 1-27).

## Cardiac CT Imaging

To image the beating heart with the goal of reducing motion artifacts and a loss of both spatial and contrast resolution, fast CT scanners such as the EBCT scanner were introduced to overcome these problems and produce good diagnostic images of the heart. Alternatively, the patient's electrocardiogram (ECG) is used to provide prospective imaging, after it is recorded at the same time with the scanning with stop and go scanners. Subsequently, retrospective imaging has been developed where the ECG is correlated with image reconstruction in spiral/helical CT scanning.

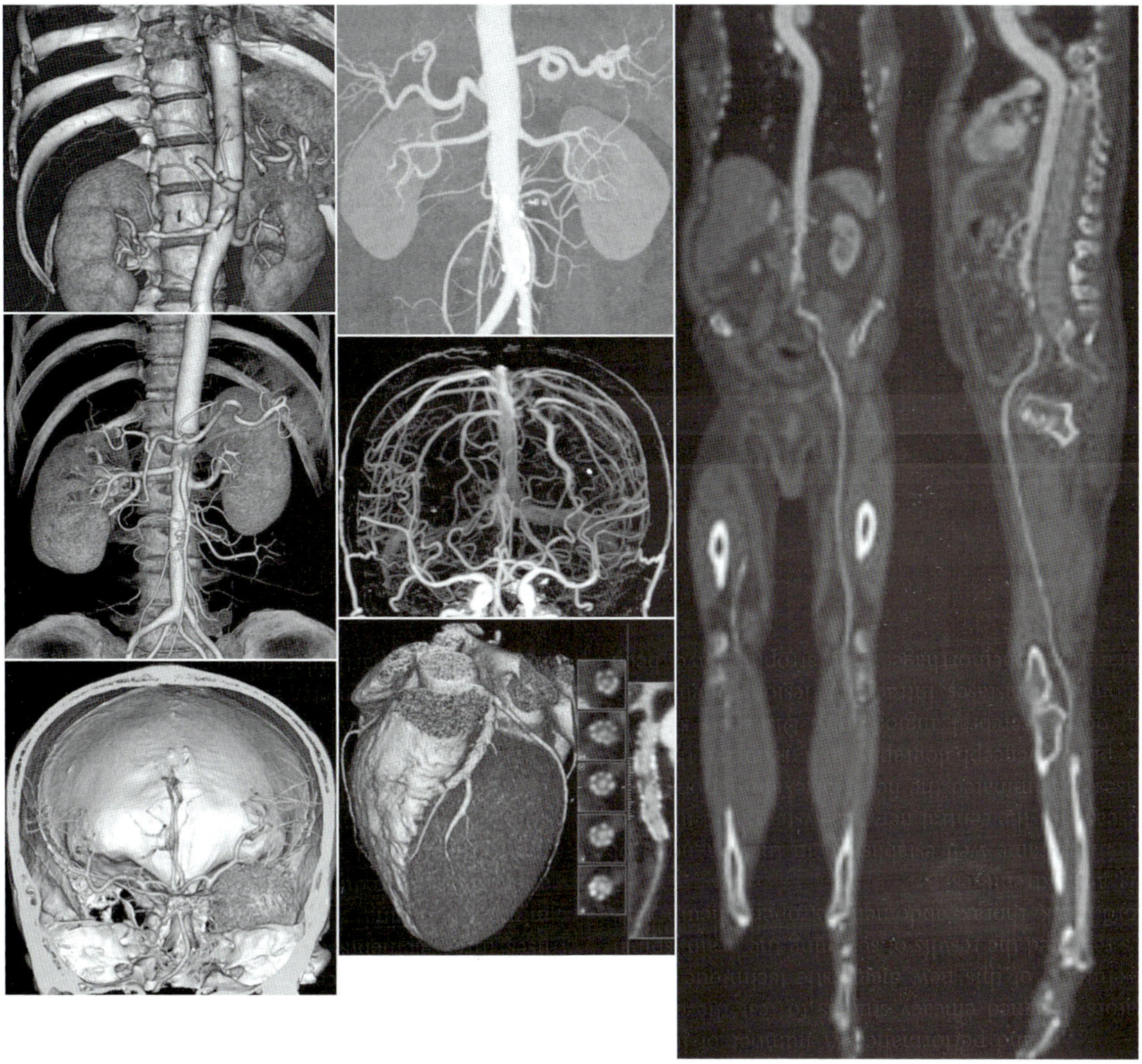

**FIGURE 1-26** Examples of current state-of-the-art CT images. Note the 3D nature of these images. (Courtesy Toshiba Medical Systems.)

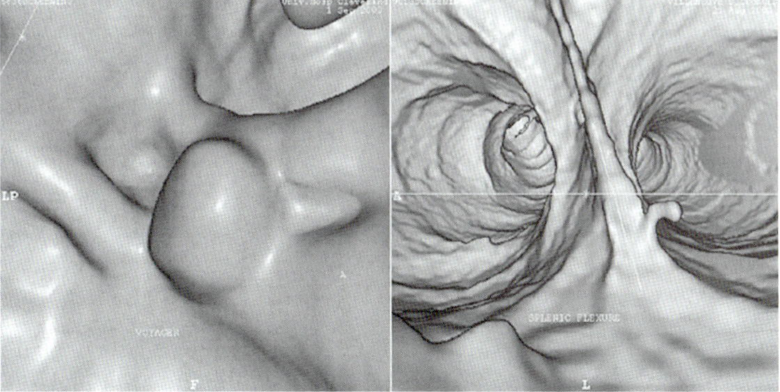


**FIGURE 1-27** Virtual CT endoscopy images. (Courtesy Philips Medical Systems.)

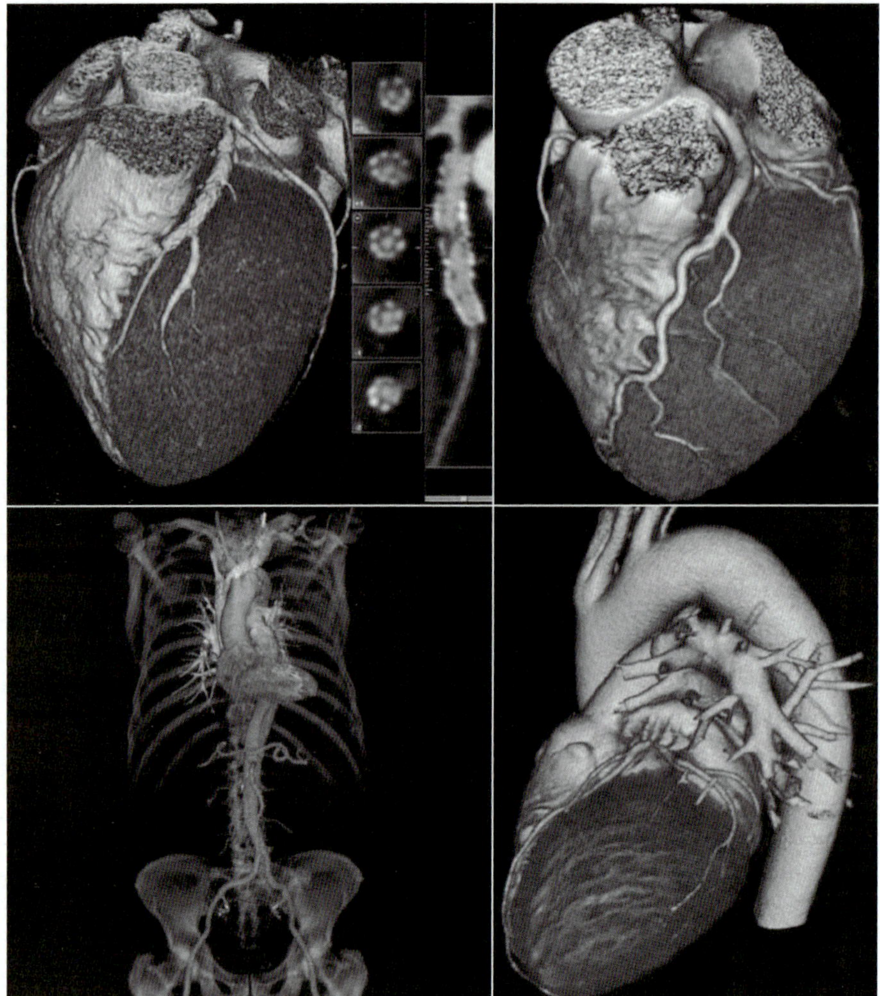

**FIGURE 1-28** Examples of 3D images of the heart and great vessels. (Courtesy Toshiba Medical Systems.)

The recent technical developments in MSCT scanners and the introduction of the DSCT scanner open up a whole new avenue for successful imaging of the heart with excellent image quality based on meeting several technical requirements. These include **low-contrast resolution** to visualize small differences in tissue contrast, high-contrast resolution (spatial resolution) to visualize small structures in the anatomy scanned, and temporal resolution to image fast-moving objects to reduce motion artifacts. These have all been made possible by fast data acquisition and dedicated reconstruction algorithms, such as the segmented (multiple) algorithms that "allow for merging synchronized transmission data from successive heart cycles. The more heart cycles that can be included in the reconstruction, the better the temporal resolution" (DeRoos et al., 2006). In addition, a low pitch factor (to be discussed later) is needed "to record at least two heart cycles and to achieve a temporal resolution in the order of magnitude of 100 ms for typical heart rates between 60-80 beats per minute (BPM)" (DeRoos et al., 2006).

Finally, scan times in cardiac CT may vary from <30 s "but preferably below 20 s." Current 64-slice MSCT scanners are capable of shorter than 20-second scan times. For example, imaging for calcium scoring and coronary angiography use scan times of 2.5 and 10 seconds, respectively (DeRoos et al., 2006). Cardiac CT applications include quantitative assessment of coronary artery calcifications, ventricular function assessment, and coronary angiography assessment of pulmonary veins. Figure 1-28 illustrates a set of cardiac images from a current MSCT scanner. The essential technical considerations of cardiac CT imaging is described in Appendix B.

## CT Screening

The excellent image quality and speed of current MSCT scanners has opened up yet another application of CT for imaging "healthy people as a means to screen for early disease" (Horton et al., 2004). This concept is referred to as **CT screening.** CT screening is being investigated as a potential tool for imaging asymptomatic individuals for the benefit related to cardiac screening, lung cancer screening, virtual colonoscopy, and whole-body imaging (Furtado et al., 2005) for the primary purpose of the early detection of disease. However, CT screening has experienced significant controversy and debate to date; therefore, it will not be discussed further in this text.

## MAJOR TECHNOLOGY TRENDS

The advances in CT technology continue at a rapid rate and CT manufacturers are active in providing innovative research leading to improved techniques that play important and significant roles in the care and management of the patient. Only a few major technology trends will be highlighted in this section to impress upon the reader that CT technology is a dynamic subject matter. For example, a few trends that dominate the CT scanning arena are related to iterative reconstruction algorithms, CT detector technologies, dose reduction and optimization efforts, **spectral CT imaging, graphics processing unit (GPU)** computing, and faster imaging techniques.

### Iterative Reconstruction Algorithms

**Iterative reconstruction (IR)** algorithms (detailed in Chapter 6) have resurfaced since its limited use in the early development of the CT. These initial iterative algorithms were replaced by **analytic reconstruction algorithms,** of which the **filtered back-projection (FBP)** algorithm became the workhorse of CT image reconstruction. Since 2014, all major CT manufacturers offer IR algorithms (Beister et al., 2012) in an effort to overcome the problems imposed with the FBP algorithm (see Chapter 5), such as image noise and streak artifacts on images. The goals of IR algorithms are to reduce image noise and reduce the higher radiation dose inherent in the FBP algorithm.

IR algorithms generally use the FBP CT data referred to as *measured projections* to create *simulated projections.* These simulated projection datasets are subsequently compared with the initial measured projection datasets to determine the difference in image noise. Once this difference is obtained it is applied to the simulated data to correct for inconsistencies. The system reconstructs a new image and the process repeats until the difference between the measured data and the simulated data is minor enough to be acceptable. The iterative process creates images that are true representations of the object being scanned with reduced noise and artifacts (Beister et al., 2012).

IR algorithms used by major CT manufacturers include adaptive statistical IR and model-based IR, both from GE Healthcare. Others include iterative model reconstruction (Philips Healthcare); image reconstruction in image space and sinogram-affirmed IR, both from Siemens Healthcare; and adaptive iterative dose reduction from Toshiba Medical Systems (Seeram, 2014). IR is described in more detail in Chapter 6.

### Detector Technologies

The detector is a significant component of the CT system because it detects and absorbs attenuated radiation from the patient and converts it into electrical signals that are subsequently digitized and sent to the CT computer to create the CT image. Detectors have evolved since the pioneering work of Hounsfield.

Detectors fall into two categories: solid-state detectors **(scintillation detectors)** and **gas-ionization detectors** (xenon gas). While the xenon gas detectors have become obsolete, scintillation detectors have evolved from the early sodium iodide (NaI) detectors used in the first-generation CT scanners. Essentially, these detectors consist of scintillators coupled to photodiodes. Scintillators used by recent high-end CT scanners include gadolinium oxysulfide, ceramic, gemstone, and ultrafast ceramic. The more recent advances in CT detectors are described in Chapter 4.

### Radiation Dose Optimization

Another important technology trend is optimization of the radiation dose in CT. The International Commission on Radiological Protection advocates the use of the as low as reasonably achievable (ALARA) philosophy when considering dose reduction to patients. In implementing the ALARA principle and balancing the need to maintain diagnostic quality images, the literature most often uses the terms dose reduction and dose optimization. Dose reduction means "reduce or diminish in size, amount, extent or number" (Merriam-Webster Dictionary, 2014), and optimization means "an act, process, or methodology of making something (as a design, system, or decision) as fully perfect, functional, or effective as possible" (Merriam-Webster Dictionary, 2014). Optimization therefore deals with both radiation dose reduction and image quality (Ramirez-Giraldo et al., 2014).

The research on dose optimization continues at a rapid rate and generally involves the use of various methodologies to demonstrate dose reduction without the loss of image quality; for example, these studies suggest at least four important requirements for dose-image quality optimization research (Mattsson, 2005; Seeram, 2014):

1. Ensure patient safety
2. Determine the level of image quality required for a particular diagnostic task
3. Obtain images at various exposure levels ranging from high to low
4. Use reliable and valid methodologies for the dosimetry, image acquisition, and evaluation of image quality using human observers, keeping in mind the nature of the detection task

Dose optimization in CT is described further in Chapter 10.

### Spectral CT Imaging

**Spectral CT** or dual-energy CT addresses how best to utilize the broad energy spectrum (from the x-ray tube) reaching the detector, and different approaches have been developed to examine the nature and use of such spectral information and to optimize the demonstration and visualization of structures in the object being imaged. Two such dual-energy CT systems include the Dual-Source CT system (Siemens Healthcare) and the fast-kVp switching CT system (GE Healthcare). Dual-energy and spectral CT are often used interchangeably.

Recently, another way to use the CT beam energy spectrum reaching the detector is to use a spectral detector based on a design that Philips Healthcare refers to as the Nano Panel Prism design (Philips, personal communications, 2014). Spectral CT is described in more detail in a later chapter.

### GPU Computing in CT

The GPU is now a significant platform for "computing massive parallel problems" (Pratx & Xing, 2011) in medical physics. Specifically, in CT, the GPU has been used primarily in three areas: image reconstruction, especially in iterative reconstruction algorithms; image processing; and calculation and treatment plan optimization (Pratx & Xing, 2011). The GPU is described in the Chapter 7.

## CT SCANNER PRODUCT DATA: CHARACTERISTIC FEATURES

The product data are usually obtained from the manufacturers and usually used during the purchase of a scanner. The essential features of the product include the following:

A. Application
B. Features
C. Composition
D. Performance specifications
E. Image quality
F. System components and their functions
G. Operating features
H. Compliance
I. Dimensions and mass
J. Siting requirements
K. Outline drawings

Of these characteristics, three important ones serve to provide the user with a generalized overview of the scanner in terms of components related to the practical aspects of scanning a patient. These include the performance specifications, image quality considerations, and the operating features. Identifying these characteristics in this chapter emphasizes the important topics from an educational perspective that require a good understanding to ensure a successful examination.

### Performance Specifications

Examples of these specifications generally include topics such as x-ray generation (generator, x-ray tube), x-ray detection, **data processing,** data storage, image display, image processing, system and dose management, clinical applications, and data transfer.

### Image Quality Consideration

Examples include the following image quality descriptors: noise, spatial resolution, high-contrast resolution, and high- and low-contrast detectability.

### Operating Features

The important features relate to patient handling and positioning, scanning, data processing, image display and processing, and patient throughput. The previous characteristics illustrate topics that must be included in a CT course of studies.

## DIGITAL IMAGE PROCESSING

CT is an excellent example of **digital image processing** (Fig. 1-29). The x-ray beam passes through the patient and falls onto special detectors that convert the x-ray photons into electrical signals (analog signals) converted into numerical data (digital data) for input into a digital computer.

*Digital image processing* involves the use of a digital computer to process and manipulate digital images. The computer receives an input of a digital image and performs specific operations on the data to produce an output image different from and more useful than the input image. The procedure had its origins at the National Aeronautics and Space

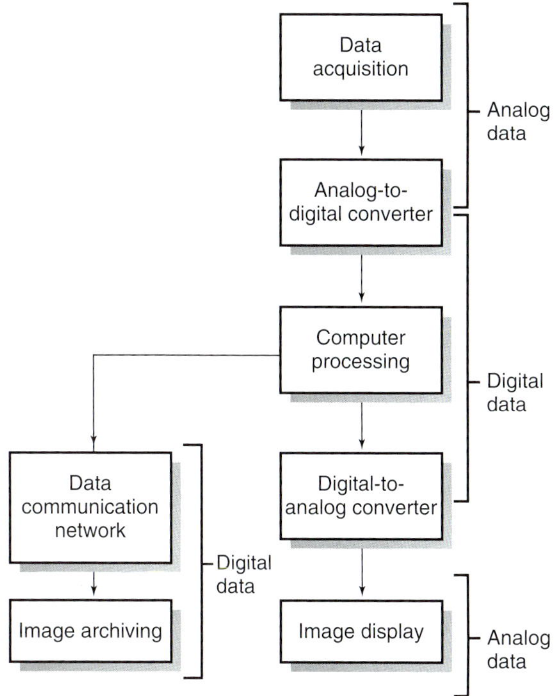


**FIGURE 1-29** Major components of the digital imaging system on which CT is based.

Administration Jet Propulsion Laboratory at the California Institute of Technology, where it was used to enhance and restore images from space. Today, the space program generates and uses the largest amount of digital data.

The digital image processing of medical images dates back to the 1970s, about the time CT was introduced to the medical community. Today, digital radiography, digital fluoroscopy, digital subtraction angiography, CT, and MRI use digital image-processing techniques. Digital image processing in radiology allows the observer to process images with use of a wide variety of algorithms to manipulate images to enhance diagnostic interpretation (Seeram, 2004; Seeram & Seeram, 2008). Such postprocessing can generate 3D images by using the stack of sectional images or the volume datasets. Various 3D images such as surface-shaded display and volume-rendered images are now commonplace (Bolan, 2013; Dalrymple et al., 2005; Zhang et al., 2011). As noted by expert CT researcher Dr. Kalender, "CT is fully 3D these days" (Kalender, 2005). The essentials of digital image processing are described further in Chapter 2.

## REVIEW QUESTIONS

Answer the following questions to check your understanding of the materials studied.

1. Which of the following does ***not*** produce a transverse axial sectional image?
   A. computed tomography
   B. conventional tomography
   C. conventional radiography
   D. computerized axial tomography
2. The acronym of choice for use in articles published in the RSNA journal, *Radiology*, is:
   A. CAT.
   B. CT.
   C. CTAT.
   D. RT.
3. Who developed the first clinically useful CT scanner?
   A. Kuhl
   B. Hounsfield
   C. Cormack
   D. Kalender
4. Which company pioneered the development of the first useful CT scanner for imaging the head?
   A. General Electric Medical Systems
   B. Siemens
   C. Elscint
   D. EMI
5. Who shared the Nobel Prize in Medicine and Physiology for his contribution to the development of CT?
   A. Kuhl
   B. Ledley
   C. Cormack
   D. Kalender
6. Who played a significant role in the development of spiral CT?
   A. Kalender
   B. Cormack
   C. Ledley
   D. Edwards
7. Which of the following is true?
   A. An analog computer is used to produce images in CT.
   B. Volume scanning involves scanning the body one slice at a time.
   C. Two essential components of a digital image processing system are the ADC and the DAC.
   D. Quality control is not so well established in CT.

## REVIEW QUESTIONS—cont'd

8. The primary goal of spiral/helical CT scanning is to:
   A. improve the volume coverage speed performance.
   B. improve the diagnostic skills of the radiologist.
   C. make use of lower mA values.
   D. scan children who are difficult to handle.
9. Which of the following applications of volume CT is based on volume formulation, classification, and image projection?
   A. CT fluoroscopy
   B. CT angiography
   C. 3D imaging
   D. CT endoscopy
10. Which of the following is based on virtual reality principles?
    A. CT fluoroscopy
    B. CT angiography
    C. 3D imaging
    D. CT endoscopy

## REFERENCES


Bates, S., Beckman, L., Thomas, A., & Waltham, R. (2012). Godfrey Hounsfield: intuitive genius of CT. *British Journal of Radiology*, *85*(1019), e1165.

Beckmann, E. C. (2006). CT scanning in the early days. *British Journal of Radiology*, *79*, 5–8.

Beister, M. (2012). Iterative reconstruction methods in x ray CT. *Physica Medica*, *28*(2), 94–108. http://dx.doi.org/10.1016/j.ejmp.2012.01.003.

Bolan, C. (2013). Routine 3D imaging becomes a reality. *Applied Radiology*, July 27–31.

Cameron, S. (2014). The usefulness of a 320-row CT scanner in the oil industry. *Visions*, *23*, 17–19.

Cormack, A. M. (1980). Early two-dimensional reconstruction and recent topics stemming from it, Nobel Award address. *Medical Physics*, *7*, 277–282.

Dalrymple, N. C., Prasad, S. R., Freckleton, M. W., et al. (2005). Introduction to the language of three-dimensional imaging with multidetector CT. *Radiographics*, *25*, 1409–1428.

Daly, B., & Templeton, P. A. (1999). Real-time CT fluoroscopy: evaluation of an interventional tool. *Radiology*, *211*, 309–315.

Davies, E. (2014). Veterinary CT with the Alexion. *Visions*, *24*, 14–17.

DeRoos, A., Kroft, L. J. M., Bax, J. J., Lamb, H. J., & Gelejins, J. (2006). Cardiac applications of multislice computed tomography. *British Journal of Radiology*, *79*, 9–16.

DeWever, W., Bogaert, J., & Verschakelen, J. A. (2005). Virtual bronchoscopy: accuracy and usefulness—an overview. *Seminars in Ultrasound CT and MRI*, *26*, 364–373.

Ell, P. J. (2006). The contribution of PET/CT to improved patient management. *British Journal of Radiology*, *79*, 23–36.

Fishman, E. K. (2004). 3D rendering: principles and techniques. In E. K. Fishman, & R. B. Jeffrey (Eds.), *Multidetector CT: principles, techniques, and clinical applications*. Philadelphia, PA: Lippincott Williams & Wilkins.

Fishman, E. K., Magid, D., Ney, D. R., et al. (1991). Three-dimensional imaging. *Radiology*, *181*, 321–337.

Funt, F., & Bryant, E. C. (1987). Detection of internal log defects by automatic interpretation of computer tomography images. *Forest Products Journal*, *37*, 56–62.

Furtado, C. D., Aguirre, D. A., Sirlin, C. B., Dang, D., Stamato, S. K., Lee, P., Sani, F., et al. (2005). Whole-body CT screening: spectrum of findings and recommendations in 1192 patients. *Radiology*, *237*, 385–394.

Gunderman, R. B. (2013). *X-ray vision-the evolution of medical imaging and its human significance*. Oxford, UK: Oxford University Press.

Habermehl, A., & Ridder, H.-W. (1997). γ-Ray tomography in forest and tree sciences. In U. Bonse (Ed.), *Developments in x-ray tomography: proceedings of the SPIE* (pp. 234–243).

Herman, G. T. (1980). *Image reconstruction from projections: the fundamentals of computerized tomography*. New York: Academic Press.

Hoffman, H., Torres, W. E., & Ernst, R. D. (2002). Paleoradiology: advanced CT in the evaluation of nine Egyptian mummies. *Radiographics*, *22*, 377–385.

Horton, K. M., et al. (2004). CT screening: principles and controversies. In E. K. Fishman, & R. B. Jeffrey (Eds.), *Multidetector CT: principles, techniques, and clinical applications*. Philadelphia, PA: Lippincott Williams & Wilkins.

Hounsfield, G. N. (1980). Computed medical imaging, Nobel Award address. *Medica Physica*, *7*, 283–290.

Iball, G. R., Brettle, D. S., & Moore, A. C. (2006). Assessment of tube current modulation in pelvic CT. *British Journal of Radiology*, *79*, 62–70.

Isherwood, I. (2004). Sir Godfrey Newbold Hounsfield–in memoriam. *European Radiology*, *14*, 2152–2153.

Jones, D. W., et al. (2013). *Practical SPECT/CT in nuclear medicine*. London: Springer.

Kalender, W. (1995). Spiral CT angiography. In L. W. Goldman, & J. B. Fowlkes (Eds.), *Medical CT and ultrasound: current technology and applications*. New London, CT: American Association of Physicists in Medicine.

Kalender, W. (2005). *Computed tomography-fundamentals, system technology, image quality, applications*. Erlangen, Germany: Publicis Corporate Publishing.

Katada, K., Kato, R., Anno, H., Ogura, Y., Koga, S., Ida, Y., Sato, M., et al. (1996). Guidance with real-time CT fluoroscopy: early clinical experience. *Radiology, 200*, 851–856.

Kelves, B. H. (1997). *Naked to the bone*. New Brunswick, NJ: Rutgers University Press.

Mattsson, S. (Ed). (2005). Optimization strategies in medical x-ray imaging. *Radiation Protection Dosimetry, 114*(1-3), 1–3. http://dx.doi.org/10.1093/rpd/nch580.

McNitt-Gray, M. F. (2002). Radiation dose in CT. *Radiographics, 22*, 1541–1553.

Merriam-Webster Dictionary. (2014). *Online English Language Dictionary*. Accessed February 2014 http:www.merriam-webster.com/dictionary.

Meyer, H., Dewey, M., Issever, A. S., & Rogalla, P. (2007). How multidetector CT can help open bike locks. *Radiology, 245*, 921.

Mori, S., Endo, M., Nishizawa, K., Murase, K., Fujiwara, H., & Tanada, S. (2006). Comparison of patient doses in 256-slice CT and 16-slice CT scanners. *British Journal of Radiology, 79*, 56–61.

Mutic, S., Palta, J. R., Butker, E. K., et al. (2004). Quality assurance for computed tomography simulators and computed tomography simulation process: report of the AAPM Radiation Therapy Committee Task Group No 66. *Medica Physica, 30*, 2762–2792.

Perry, B. J., & Bridges, C. (1973). Computerized transverse axial scanning (tomography), part 3. *British Journal of Radiology, 46*, 1048–1051.

Pratx, G., & Xing, L. (2011). GPU computing in medical physics: a review. *Medica Physica, 38*(5).

Ramirez-Giraldo, J. C. (2014). Radiation dose optimization technologies in MDCT: a review. *Medical Physics International, 2*(2), 420–430.

Rhodes, M. L. (1991). Computer graphics in medicine: the past decade. *IEEE Computer Graphics and Applications, 4*, 52–54.

Ritman, E. L., Robb, R. A., & Wood, E. H. (1991). Synchronous volumetric imaging of noninvasive vivisection of cardiovascular and respiratory dynamics: evolution of current perspectives. In E. R. Giuliani (Ed.), *Cardiology: fundamentals and practice*. St. Louis, MO: Mosby.

Rizzo, S., Kalra, M., Schmidt, B., et al. (2006). Comparison of angular and combined automatic tube current modulation techniques with constant tube current CT of the abdomen and pelvis. *American Journal of Roentgenology, 186*, 673–679.

Robb, R. A., & Morin, R. L. (1991). Principles and instrumentation for dynamic x-ray computed tomography. In M. L. Marcus, H. R. Schelbert, D. J. Skorton, & G. L. Wolf (Eds.), *Cardiac imaging: a comparison to Braunwald's heart disease*. Philadelphia, PA: WB Saunders.

Seeram, E. (1998). 3D imaging: basic concepts for radiologic technologists. *Radiologic Technology, 69*, 127–148.

Seeram, E. (1999). Radiation dose in CT. *Radiologic Technology, 70*, 534–556.

Seeram, E. (2004). Digital image processing. *Radiologic Technology, 75*, 435–452.

Seeram, E. (2014). CT dose optimization. *Radiation Technology, 85*(6), 660–675.

Seeram, E., & Seeram, D. (2008). Image postprocessing in digital radiology: a primer for technologists. *Journal of Medical Imaging and Radiation Sciences, 39*, 23–41.

Siemens Medical Solutions. (2005). Archaeology—high tech meets history. *SOMATOM, Sessions No. 16*, 33–34.

Sirr, S. A., & Waddle, J. R. (1999). Use of CT in detection of internal damage and repair and determination of authenticity in high-quality bowed stringed instruments. *Radiographics, 19*, 639–646.

Vining, D. J. (1999). Virtual colonoscopy. *Seminars in Ultrasound CT and MRI, 20*, 56–60.

Yasuda, T., Ohsihita, H., & Toriwaki, J. (1992). 3D visualization of an ancient Egyptian mummy. *IEEE Computer Graphics and Applications, 2*, 13–17.

Zhang, Q., Eagleson, R., & Peters, T. M. (2011). Volume visualization: a technical overview with a focus on medical applications. *Journal of Digit Imaging, 24*(4), 640–664.

Zonneveld, F., Spoor, F., & Wind, J. (1989). The use of the CT in the study of the internal morphology of hominid fossils. *Medicamundi, 34*, 117–127.

## BIBLIOGRAPHY

Dümmling, K. (1984). 10 years' computed tomography: a retrospective view. *Electromedica, 52*, 13–28.

Hounsfield, G. N. (1980). Computed medical imaging, Nobel Award address. *Medica Physica, 7*, 283–290.

Klingenbeck-Regn, K., & Oppelt, A. (1998). Dose in CT scanning-physical relationships and potentials for dose saving. *Electromedica, 66*, 26–30.

Schwierz, G., & Kirchgeorg, M. (1995). The continuous evolution of medical x-ray imaging, I: the technically driven stage of development. *Electromedica, 63*, 2–7.

# 2

# Digital Image Processing

## OUTLINE

**Limitations of Film-Based Imaging**
**Generic Digital Imaging System**
- Data Acquisition
- Image Processing
- Image Display, Storage, and Communication

**Historical Perspectives**
**Image Formation and Representation**
- Analog Images
- Digital Images

**What Is Digital Image Processing?**
- Definitions
- Image Domains

**Characteristics of the Digital Image**
- Matrix
- Pixels
- Voxels
- Bit Depth
- Effect of Digital Image Parameters on the Appearance of Digital Images

**Image Digitization**
- Scanning
- Sampling
- Quantization
- Analog-to-Digital Conversion
- Why Digitize Images?
- Image-Processing Techniques
- Point Operations
- Local Operations
- Global Operations
- Geometric Operations

**Image Compression Overview**
- What Is Image Compression?
- Types of Image Compression
- Visual Impact of Irreversible Compression on Digital Images

**Image Synthesis Overview**
- Magnetic Resonance Imaging
- CT Imaging
- Three-Dimensional Imaging in Radiology
- Virtual Reality Imaging in Radiology

**Image-Processing Hardware**
**CT as a Digital Image-Processing System**
**Image Processing: An Essential Tool for CT**

## LEARNING OBJECTIVES

On completion of this chapter, you should be able to:

1. trace the history of digital image processing.
2. describe the key elements of image formation and image representation.
3. define each of the following:
   - objects
   - images
   - analog image
   - digital image
   - digital image processing.
4. describe the following three steps in image digitization:
   - scanning
   - sampling
   - quantization.
5. explain how an analog-to-digital converter (ADC) works and describe the characteristics of speed and accuracy.
6. list the advantages of digitizing images.
7. list four image processing operations and explain how each works.
8. explain briefly each of the following:
   - gray-level mapping
   - look-up table
   - histogram
   - spatial frequency filtering.
9. list two ways to perform spatial frequency filtering and outline the basics of the convolution technique.
10. draw and label the components of a generic digital image-processing system.
11. describe the similarities between digital image processing and CT as a digital image-processing system.
12. list major image-processing operations used in different medical imaging modalities.
13. state the reason why image processing is an essential tool for CT technologists.

## KEY TERMS TO ... REMEMBER

The following key terms/con... ...f this Chapter.

**analog processing**
**analog signal**
**analog-to-digital conve...**
**(ADC)**
**bit**
**convolution**
**convolution kern...**
**digital processi...**
**digital signal**
**...operation**
**... table (LUT)**
**...operation**
**...ntization**
**...mpling**
**...patial frequency filtering**

## LIMIT... IMA...

Film... rad... A... tiona... **tomograph...** **ing (MRI).** All o... in the past to record ima... can make a diagnosis.

The steps in the production o... ...sed radiographic image are very familiar to r... ...ogic technologists. First, the patient is exposed to a predetermined amount of radiation needed to provide the required diagnostic image quality. A latent image is formed on the film that is subsequently processed by chemicals in a processor to render the image visible. The processed image is then ready for viewing by a radiologist, who makes a diagnosis of the patient's medical condition.

The imaging process can also result in poor image quality if the initial radiation **exposure** has not been accurately determined. For example, if the radiation exposure is too high, the film is overexposed and the processed image appears too dark, and the radiologist cannot make a diagnosis from such an image. Alternatively, if the radiation exposure is too low, the processed image appears too light and cannot be used by the radiologist. In both situations the images lack the proper image density and contrast and imaging would have to be repeated to provide the acceptable image quality needed to make a diagnosis. Additionally, the patient would be subjected to increased radiation exposure.

Despite these problems, film-based imaging has been successful for the past 100 years and it is still ...y in few departments. There are other prob... ...ociated with film-based imaging. For exam... ...n is not ideal for performing the three basic ...ions of radiation: detection, image display, and ...ge archiving.

As a radiation detector, film screen cannot show ...ifferences in tissue contrast that are <10%. This means that film-based imaging is limited in its contrast resolution. The **spatial resolution** of film-screen systems, however, is the highest of all imaging modalities, and this is the main reason that radiography has played such a significant role in imaging patients through the years.

As a display medium, the optical range and contrast for film are fixed and limited. Film can only display once—the optical range and contrast determined by the exposure technique factors used to produce the image. To change the image display (optical range and contrast), another set of exposure technique factors would have to be used, thus increasing the dose to the patient by virtue of a repeat exposure.

As an archive medium, film is usually stored in envelopes and housed in a large room. It thus requires manual handling for archiving and retrieval by an individual.

A **digital imaging system** and digital **image processing** can overcome these problems.

## GENERIC DIGITAL IMAGING SYSTEM

The major components of a generic digital imaging system for use in radiology are shown in Figure 2-1. These include **data acquisition,** image processing, image display/storage/archiving, and image communication. As noted in Chapter 1, CT consists of these major components (to be described in detail later in subsequent chapters) and can therefore be classified as a digital imaging system because it uses computers

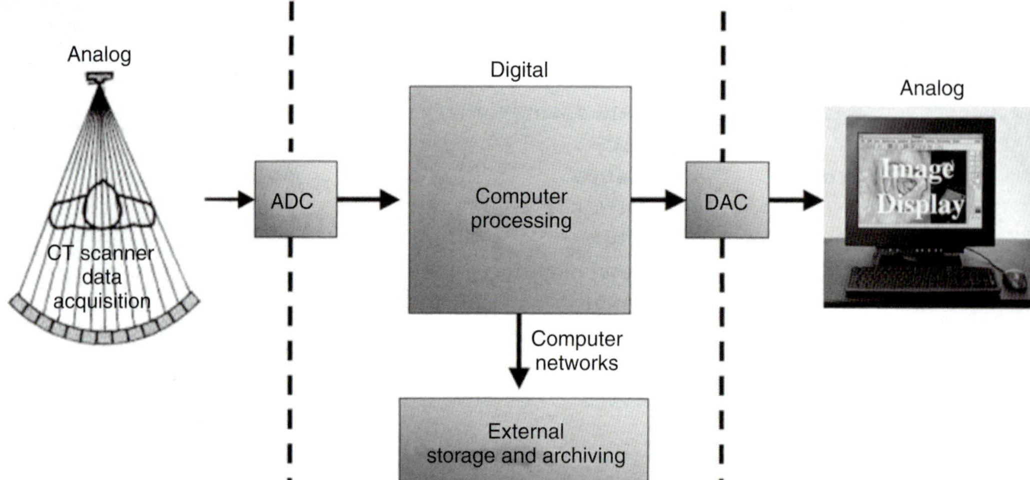


**FIGURE 2-1** The essential components of a generic digital imaging system.

to process images. Each of these components will be described briefly.

## Data Acquisition

The term *data acquisition* refers to a systematic method of collecting data from the patient. For **projection** digital radiography and CT, the data are the electron density of the tissues, which is related to the **linear attenuation coefficient** (μ) of the various tissues. In other words, it is attenuation data that are collected for these imaging modalities. Data acquisition components for these modalities include the **x-ray tube** and the digital image detectors. The output signal from the detectors is an electrical signal (an **analog signal** that varies continuously in time). Because a digital computer is used in these imaging systems, the analog signal must be converted into a **digital signal** (discrete units) for processing by a digital computer. This conversion is performed by an **analog-to-digital converter (ADC).**

## Image Processing

**Image processing** is performed by a digital computer that takes an **input** digital image and processes it to produce an **output** digital image by using the binary number system. Although we typically use the decimal number system (which operates with base 10, i.e., 10 different numbers: 0, 1, 2, 3, 4, 5, 6, 7, 8, and 9), computers use the binary number system (which operates with base 2, i.e., 0 or 1). These two digits are referred to as binary digits or **bits**. Bits are not continuous; rather they are discrete units. Computers operate with binary numbers, 0 and 1, discrete units that are processed and transformed into other discrete units. To process the word *Euclid*, it would have to be converted into digital data (binary representation). Thus the binary representation for the word *Euclid* is 01000101 01010101 01000011 01001100 01001001 01000100.

The ADC sends digital data for digital image processing by a digital computer. Such processing is accomplished by a set of operations and techniques to transform the input image into an output image that suits the needs of the observer (radiologist) to enhance diagnosis. For example, these operations can be used to reduce the **noise** in the input image, enhance the sharpness of the input image, or change the contrast of the input image. This chapter is concerned primarily with these digital image-processing operations and techniques.

## Image Display, Storage, and Communication

The output of computer processing, that is, the output digital image, must first be converted into an analog signal before it can be displayed on a monitor for viewing by the observer. Such conversion is the function of the **digital-to-analog conversion (DAC).** This image can be stored and archived on magnetic data carriers (magnetic tapes/disks) and laser optical disks for retrospective viewing and manipulation. Additionally, these images can be communicated electronically through computer networks to observers at remote sites. In this regard, **picture archiving and communication systems (PACS)** are becoming commonplace in the modern radiology department.

This chapter explores the fundamentals of digital image processing through a brief history and a description of related topics such as image representation, the digitizing process, image-processing operations, and **image-processing hardware** considerations.

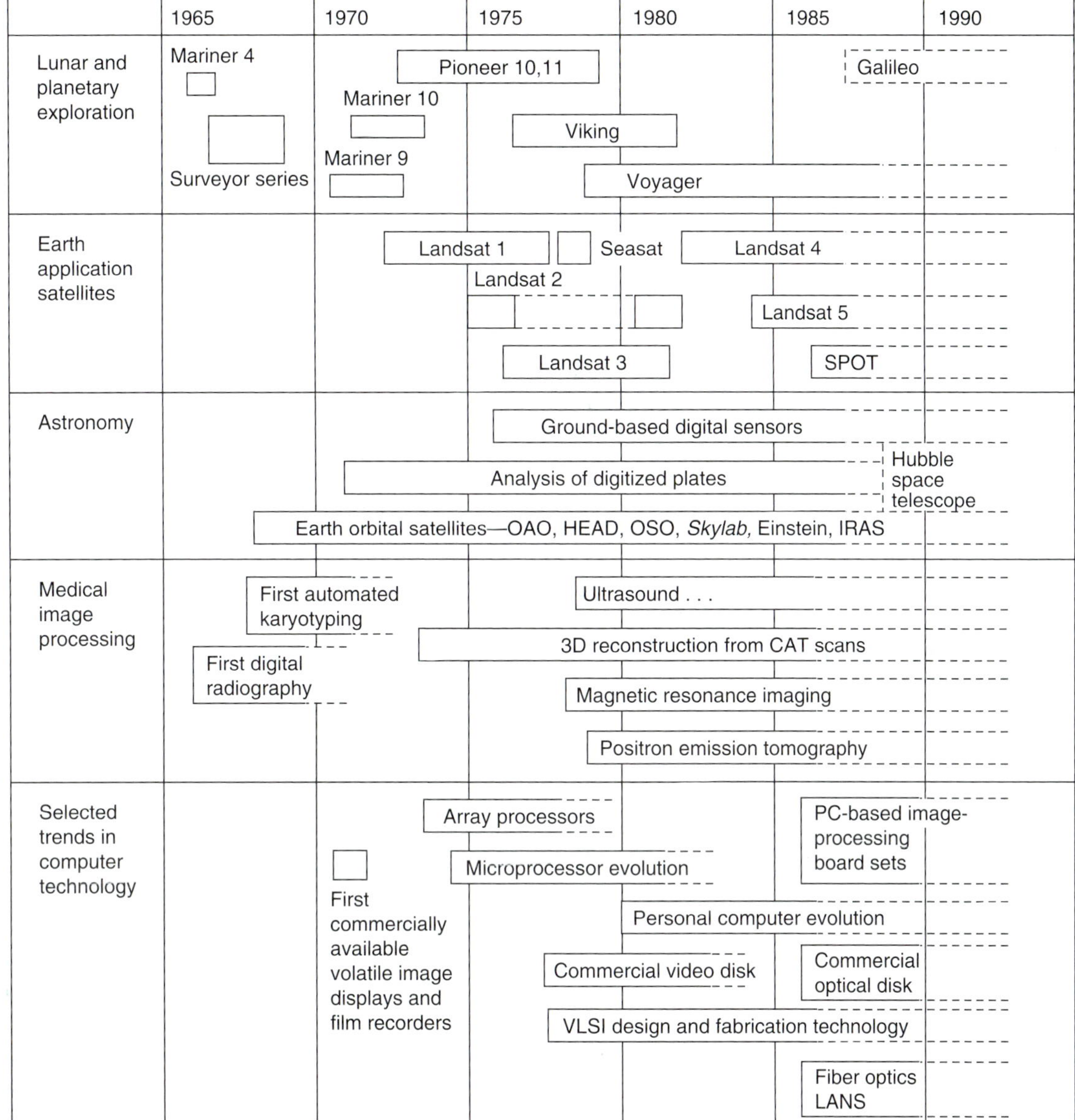


**FIGURE 2-2** Overview of the first 20 years of important developments in digital image processing. (From Green, W. B. (1989). *Digital image processing: a systems approach* (2nd ed.). New York: Van Nostrand Reinhold.)

## HISTORICAL PERSPECTIVES

The history of digital image processing dates back to the early 1960s, when the National Aeronautics and Space Administration (NASA) was developing its lunar and planetary exploration program. The Ranger spacecraft returned images of the lunar surface to Earth. These analog images taken by a television camera were converted into digital images and subsequently processed by the digital computer to obtain more information about the moon's surface.

The development of digital image-processing techniques can be attributed to work at NASA's Jet Propulsion Laboratory at the California Institute of Technology. The technology of digital processing continues to expand rapidly, and its applications extend into fields such as astronomy, geology, forestry, agriculture, cartography, military science, and medicine. (An overview of the history of digital image-processing technology is shown in Fig. 2-2.) This technology has found widespread applications in medicine and particularly in diagnostic imaging, where it has been successfully applied to ultrasound, digital radiography, nuclear medicine, CT, and MRI (Huang, 2004). Digital image processing is a multidisciplinary subject that includes physics, mathematics, engineering, and computer science.

## IMAGE FORMATION AND REPRESENTATION

An understanding of images is necessary to define digital image processing. Castleman (1996) has classified images on the basis of their form or method of **generation**. He used set theory to explain image types. According to this theory, images are a subset of all objects. Within the set of images, there are other subsets such as visible images (e.g., paintings, drawings, or photographs), optical images (e.g., holograms), nonvisible physical images (e.g., temperature, pressure, or elevation maps), and mathematical images (e.g., continuous functions and discrete functions). The sine wave is an example of a continuous function (analog signal), whereas a discrete function represents a digital image, as shown in Figure 2-3. Castleman noted that "only the digital images can be processed by computer."

### Analog Images

Analog images are continuous images. For example, a black-and-white photograph of a chest x ray is an analog image because it represents a continuous distribution of light intensity as a function of **position** on the radiograph.

In photography, images are formed when light is focused on film. In radiography, x rays pass through the patient and are projected onto x-ray film. In both cases, films are processed in chemical solutions to render them visible and the images are formed by a photochemical process. Images can also be formed by photoelectronic means, in which the images may be represented as electrical signals (analog signals) that emerge from the photoelectronic device.

### Digital Images

Digital images are numerical representations or images of objects. The formation of digital images requires a digital computer. Any information that enters the computer for processing must first be converted into digital form, or numbers (Fig. 2-4). An important component is the ADC, which converts continuous signals to discrete signals, or digital data (Luiten, 1995).

The computer receives the digital data and performs the necessary processing. The results of this processing are always digital and can be displayed as a digital image (Fig. 2-5).

## WHAT IS DIGITAL IMAGE PROCESSING?

### Definitions

In image processing it is necessary to convert an input image into an output image. If both the input image and output image are analog, this is referred to as **analog processing**. If both the input image and output image are discrete, this is referred to as **digital processing**. In cases where an analog image must be converted into digital data for input to the computer, a **digitization** system is required. CT is based on a reconstruction process whereby a digital image is changed into a visible physical image (Fig. 2-6).

Castleman (1996) defined a *process* as "a series of actions or operations leading to a desired result; thus, a series of actions or operations are performed upon an object to alter its form in a desired manner." He also defined *digital image processing* as "subjecting numerical representations of objects to a series of operations in order to obtain a desired result."

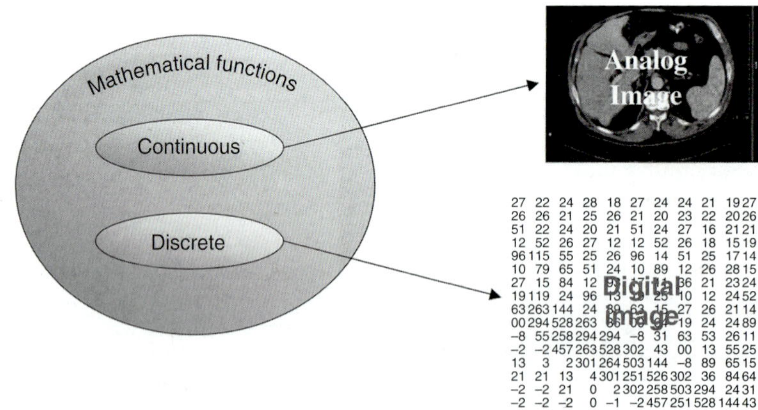


**FIGURE 2-3** Two examples of continuous and discrete images. (See text for further explanation.)

Given the variety of possible operations (Baxes, 1994), image processing has emerged as a discipline in itself (Box 2-1).

## Image Domains

Images can be represented in two domains on the basis of how they are acquired (Huang, 2004). These domains include the spatial location domain and the spatial **frequency domain**. All images displayed for viewing by humans are in the spatial location domain. Radiography and CT, for example, acquire images in the spatial location domain.

As mentioned earlier, the digital image is a numerical image arranged in such a manner that the location of each number in the image can be identified by using a right-handed *x-y* coordinate system, where the *x*-axis describes the rows or lines placed on the image and the *y*-axis describes the columns, as shown in Figure 2-7. For example, the first **pixel** in the upper left corner of the image is always identified as 0,0. The spatial location 9,4 will describe a pixel that is located nine pixels to the right of the left-hand side of the image and four lines down from the top of the image. Such an image is said to be in the spatial location domain.

Images can also be acquired in the spatial frequency domain, such as those acquired in MRI. The term *frequency* refers to the number of cycles per unit length, that is, the number of times a signal changes per unit length. Although small structures within an object (patient) produce high frequencies that represent the detail in the image, large structures produce low frequencies and represent contrast information in the image.

Digital image processing can transform one image domain into another image domain. For example, an image in the spatial location domain can be transformed into a spatial frequency domain image, as is illustrated in Figure 2-8. The **Fourier transform** (FT) is used to perform this task. The FT is mathematically rigorous and will not be covered in this article. It converts a function in the time domain (say signal intensity versus time) to a function in frequency domain (say, signal intensity versus frequency). The inverse FT denoted by $FT^{-1}$ is used to transform an image in the frequency domain back to the spatial location domain for viewing by radiologists and technologists. Physicists and engineers, on the other hand, would probably prefer to **view** images in the frequency domain.

The major reason for doing this is to facilitate image processing that can enhance or suppress

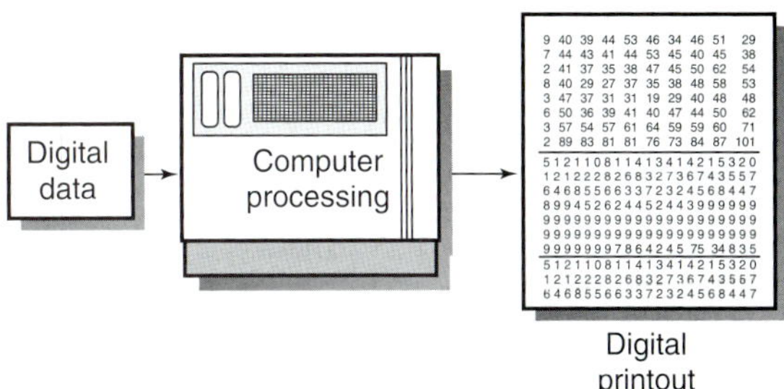


**FIGURE 2-5** Input digital data can be displayed in digital form after computer processing.

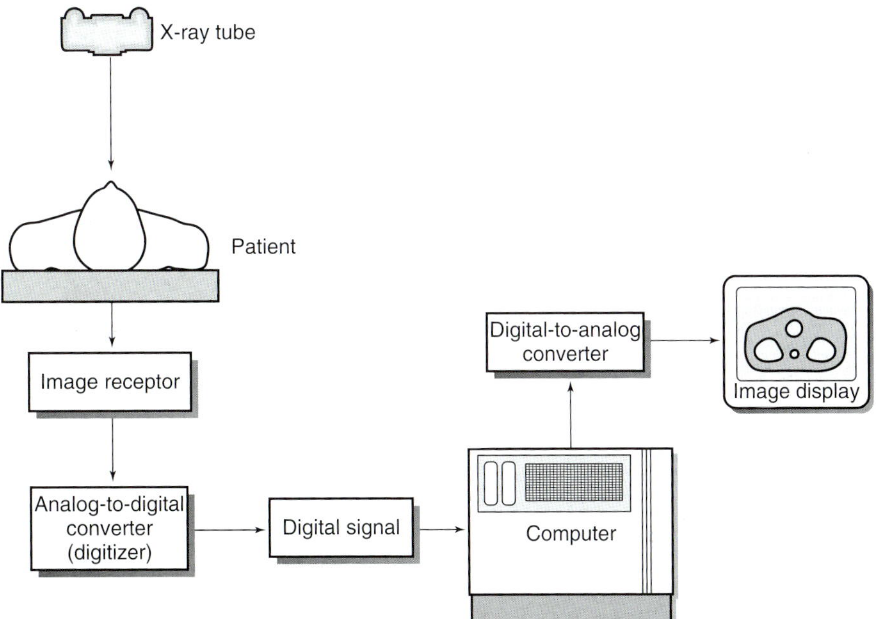


**FIGURE 2-4** The conversion of analog data into digital data for input to a digital computer.

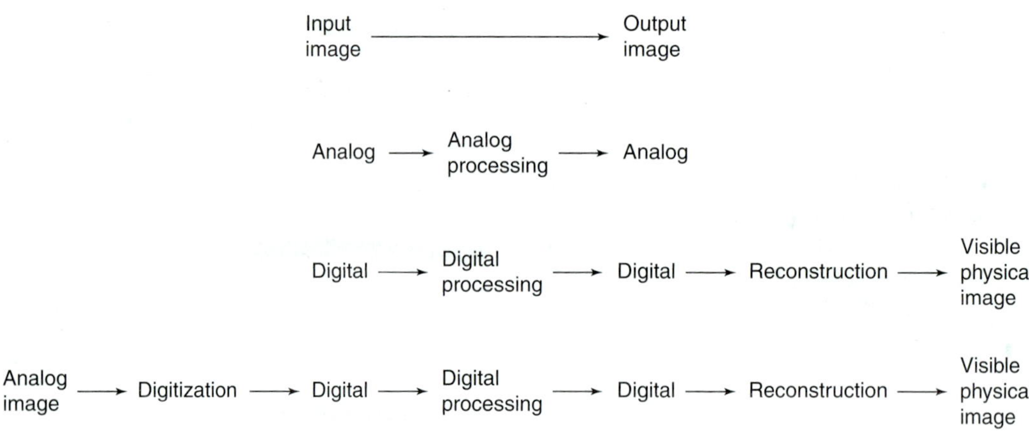


**FIGURE 2-6** Digital image processing.

**BOX 2-1 Image-Processing Operations**

- Image generation
- Image modification
  - Image enhancement
  - Image combination
  - Image restoration
- Image analysis
  - Pattern recognition
  - Image interpretation
  - Feature extraction

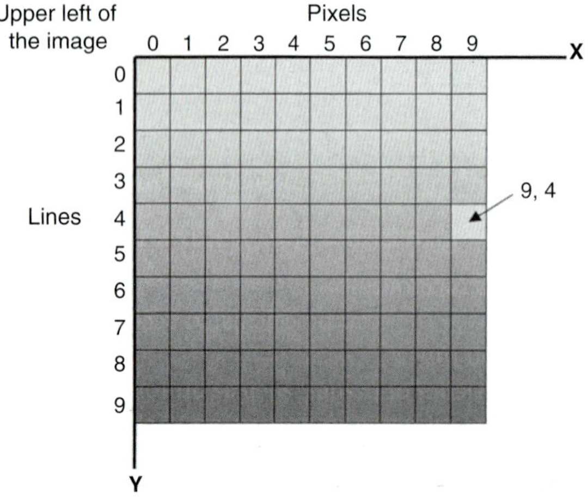


**FIGURE 2-7** A right-handed coordinate system used to describe digital images in the spatial location domain. The exact location of a pixel can be found using columns and rows. (See text for further explanation.)

certain features of the image. For example, Huang (2004) points out:

> One can use information appearing in the frequency domain and not easily available in the **spatial domain,** to detect some inherent characteristics of each type of radiological image. If the image has many edges, there would be many high-frequency components. On the other hand, if the image has only uniform materials, like water or plastic, then it has low-frequency components. On the basis of this frequency in the image, we can selectively change the frequency components to enhance the image. To obtain a smoother appearing image we can increase the amplitude of the low-frequency components, whereas to enhance the edges of bones in the hand x-ray image, we can magnify the amplitude of the high-frequency components.

## CHARACTERISTICS OF THE DIGITAL IMAGE

The structure of a digital image can be described with respect to several characteristics or fundamental parameters, including the **matrix,** pixels, voxels, and the bit depth (Bourne, 2010; Castleman, 1996; Dougherty, 2009; Pooley et al., 2001; Seeram & Seeram, 2008; Seibert, 1995).

### Matrix

Apart from being a numerical image, there are other elements of a digital image that are important to our understanding of digital image processing. A digital image is made up of a 2D array of numbers, called a matrix. The matrix consists of columns (M) and rows (N) that define small square regions called picture elements, or pixels. The dimension of the image can be described by M, N, and the size of the image is given by the following relationship:

$$M \times N \times k\text{bits.}$$

When M = N, the image is square. Generally, diagnostic digital images are rectangular in shape. When imaging a patient with a digital imaging modality, the operator selects the matrix size, sometimes referred to as the **field of view (FOV).** Typical matrix sizes

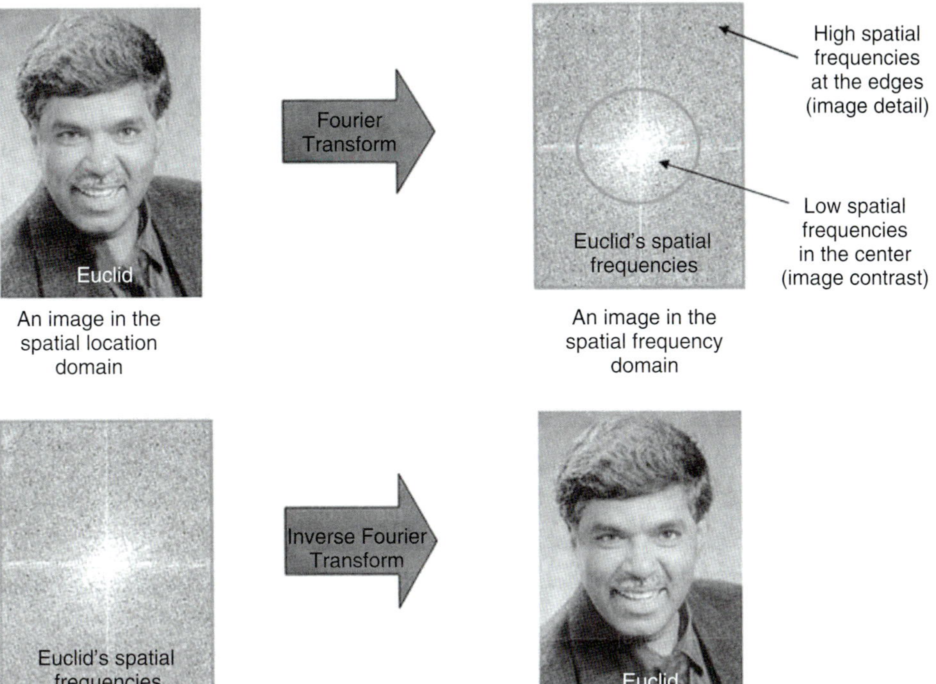


**FIGURE 2-8** The Fourier transform is used to convert an image in the spatial location domain into an image in the spatial frequency domain for processing by a computer. The inverse Fourier transform ($FT^{-1}$) is used to convert the spatial frequency domain image back into a spatial location image for viewing by humans. (From Seeram, E. (2004). *Radiologic Technology, 75*, 435-455. Reproduced by permission of the American Society of Radiologic Technologists.)

**TABLE 2-1 Typical Matrix Sizes for Different Types of Digital Diagnostic Images**

| Digital Imaging Modality | Matrix Size | Typical Bit Depth |
|---|---|---|
| Nuclear medicine | 128 × 128 | 12 |
| MRI | 256 × 256 | 12 |
| CT | 512 × 512 | 12 |
| Digital subtraction angiography | 1024 × 1024 | 10 |
| Computed radiography | 2048 × 2048 | 12 |
| Digital radiography | 2048 × 2048 | 12 |
| Digital angiography | 4096 × 4096 | 12 |

are shown in Table 2-1. It is important to note that as images become larger, they require more processing time and more storage space. Additionally, larger images will take more time to be transmitted to remote locations. In this regard, image compression is needed to facilitate storage and transmission requirements.

## Pixels

The pixels that make up the matrix are generally square. Each pixel contains a number (discrete value) that represents a brightness level. The numbers represent tissue characteristics being imaged. For example, in radiography and CT, these numbers are related to the atomic number and mass density of the tissues, and in MRI they represent other characteristics of tissues, such as proton density and relaxation times.

The **pixel size** can be calculated according to the following relationship:

$$\text{Pixel size} = \text{FOV/Matrix size}.$$

For digital imaging modalities, the larger the matrix size, the smaller the pixel size (for the same FOV) and the better the spatial resolution. The effect of the matrix size on picture clarity can be seen in Figure 2-9.

## Voxels

Pixels in a digital image represent the information contained in a volume of tissue in the patient. Such volume is referred to as a voxel (contraction for volume element). Voxel information is converted into numerical values contained in the pixels, and these numbers are assigned brightness levels, as illustrated in Figure 2-10.

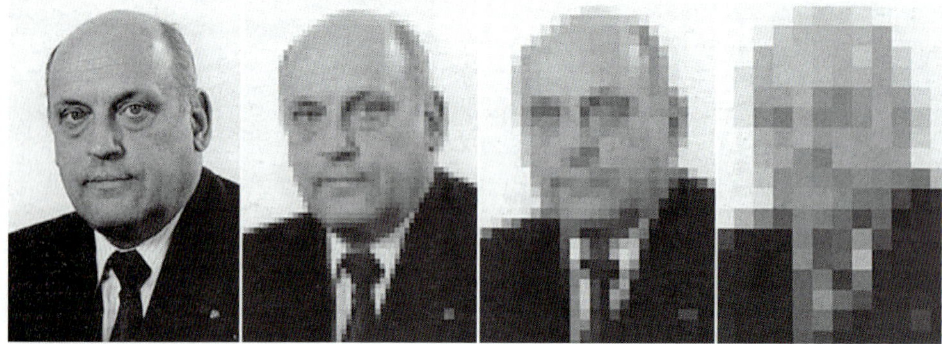

**FIGURE 2-9** An increased number of pixels in the image matrix improves the picture quality and enhances the perception of details in the image. (From Luiten, A.L. (1995). *Medicamundi, 40,* 95-100.)

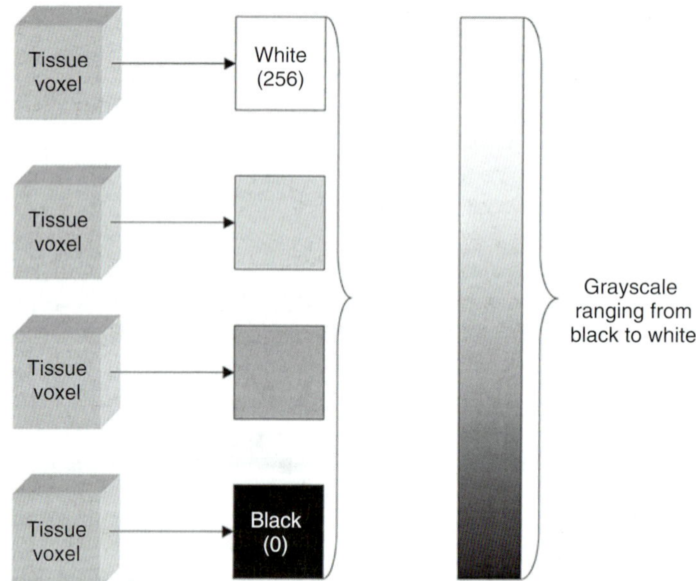


**FIGURE 2-10** Voxel information from the patient is converted into numerical values contained in the pixels, and these numbers are assigned brightness levels. The higher numbers represent high signal intensity (from the detectors) and are shaded white (bright) while the low numbers represent low signal intensity and are shaded dark (black).

## Bit Depth

In the relationship M × N × kbits, the term "kbits" implies that every pixel in the digital image matrix M × N is represented by k binary digits. The number of bits per pixel is the bit depth. Because the binary number system uses the base 2, kbits = $2^k$. Therefore each pixel will have $2^k$ gray levels. For example, in a digital image with a bit depth of 2, each pixel will have $2^2$ (4) gray levels (density). Similarly, a bit depth of 8 implies that each pixel will have $2^8$ (256) gray levels or shades of gray. The effect of bit depth is clearly seen in Figure 2-11. Table 2-1 also provides the typical bit depth for diagnostic digital images.

## Effect of Digital Image Parameters on the Appearance of Digital Images

The characteristics of a digital image, that is, the matrix size, the pixel size, and the bit depth, can affect the appearance of the digital image, particularly its spatial resolution and its density resolution.

Matrix size has an effect on the detail or spatial resolution of the image. The larger the matrix size (for the same FOV), the smaller pixel size, hence the better the appearance of detail. Additionally, as the FOV decreases without a change in matrix size, the size of the pixel decreases as well (recall the relationship pixel size = FOV/matrix size), thus improving detail.

The bit depth has an effect on the number of shades of gray, hence the contrast resolution of the image. This is clearly apparent in Figure 2-11.

## IMAGE DIGITIZATION

The primary objective during image digitization is to convert an analog image into numerical data for processing by the computer (Seibert, 1995). Digitization consists of three distinct steps: **scanning, sampling,** and **quantization**.

### Scanning

Consider an image (Fig. 2-12). The first step in digitization is the division of the picture into small regions, or scanning. Each small region of the picture is a picture element, or pixel. Scanning results in a grid characterized by rows and columns. The size of the grid usually depends on the number of pixels on each side of the grid. In Figure 2-12 the grid size is 9 × 9, which results in 81 pixels. The rows and columns identify a particular pixel by providing an address for that pixel. The rows and columns comprise a matrix; in this case, the matrix is 9 × 9. As the number of pixels in the image matrix increases, the image becomes more recognizable and facilitates better perception of image details.

### Sampling

The second step in image digitization is sampling, which measures the brightness of each pixel in the entire image (Fig. 2-12). A small spot of light is projected onto the transparency and the transmitted light is detected by a photomultiplier tube positioned behind the picture. The output of the photomultiplier tube is an electrical (analog) signal.

### Quantization

Quantization is the final step, in which the brightness value of each sampled pixel is assigned an integer (0, or a positive or negative number) called a *gray level*. The result is a range of numbers or gray levels, each of which has a precise location on the rectangular grid of pixels. The total number of gray levels is called the *grayscale*, such as eight-level grayscale (Fig. 2-12). The grayscale is based on the value of the gray levels; 0 represents black and 255 represents white. The numbers in between 0 and 255 represent shades of gray. In the case of two gray levels, the picture would show only black and white. An image can therefore be composed of any number of gray levels, depending on the bit depth.

In quantization, the electrical signal obtained from sampling is assigned an integer based on the

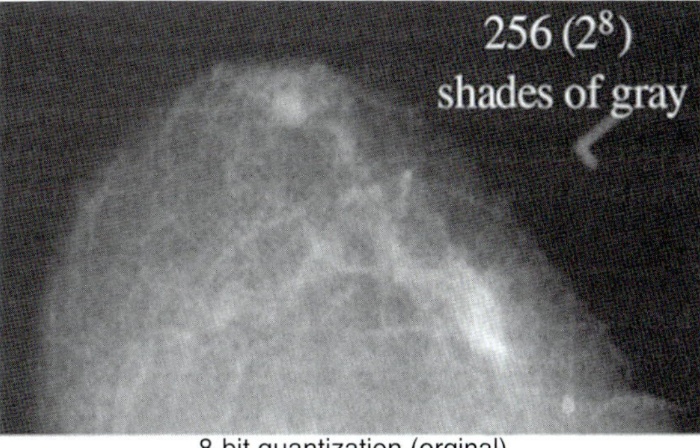


8-bit quantization (orginal)

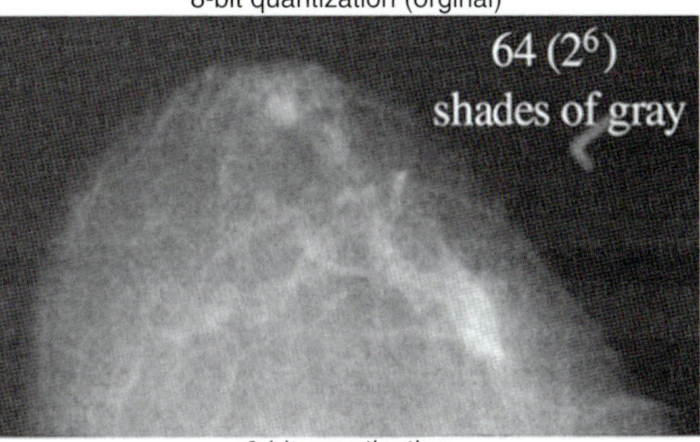


6-bit quantization

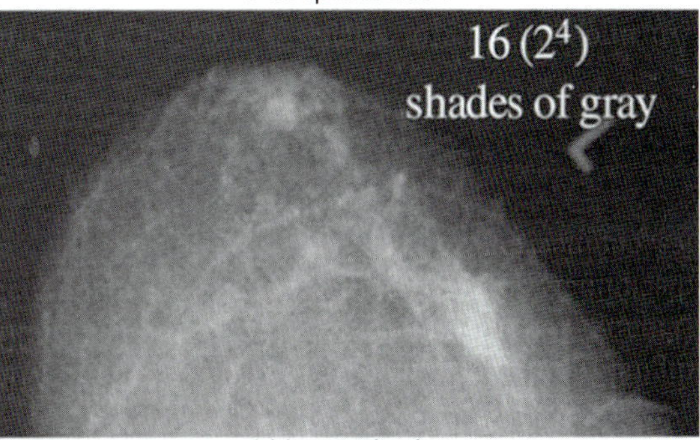


4-bit quantization

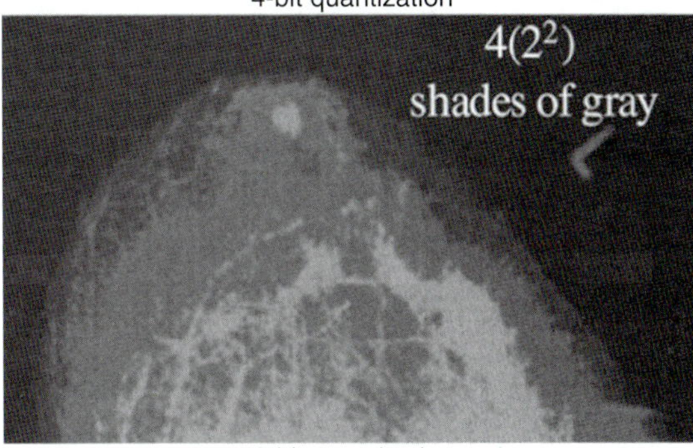


2-bit quantization

**FIGURE 2-11** The effect of bit depth on the quality of the digital image. Higher bit depths result in better image quality. (Images courtesy Bruno Jaagi, P.Eng-Biomedical Engineering Technology, British Columbia Institute of Technology.)

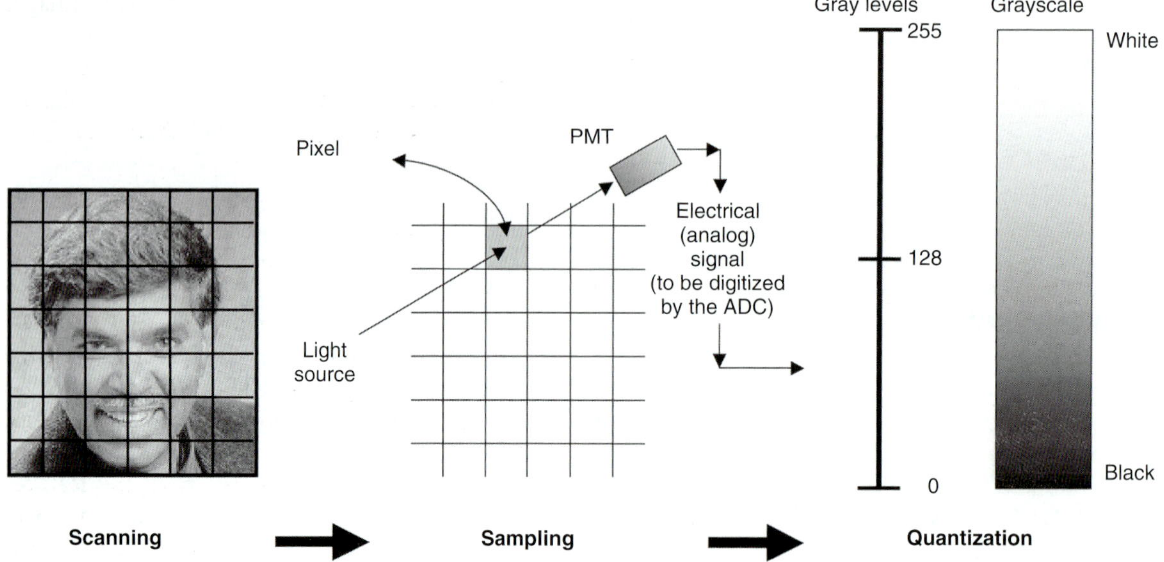


**FIGURE 2-12** Three general steps in digitizing an image: scanning, sampling, and quantization. (See text for further explanation.) Similar steps apply to digital diagnostic techniques. (From Seeram, E. (2004). *Radiologic Technology, 75,* 435-455. Reproduced by permission of the American Society of Radiologic Technologists.)

strength of the signal. In general, the value of the integer is proportional to the signal strength (Seibert, 1995).

The result of the quantization process is a digital image, an array of numbers representing the analog image that was scanned, sampled, and quantized. This array of numbers is sent to the computer for further processing.

## Analog-to-Digital Conversion

The conversion of analog signals to digital information is accomplished by the ADC. The ADC samples the analog signal at various times to measure its strength at different points. The more points sampled, the better the representation of the signal. This sampling process is followed by quantization.

Two important characteristics of the ADC are speed and accuracy. *Accuracy* refers to the sampling of the signal. The more samples taken, the more accurate the representation of the digital image (Fig. 2-13). If enough samples are not taken, the representation of the original signal will be inaccurate after computer processing (Fig. 2-14). This sampling error is referred to as *aliasing,* and it appears as an **artifact** on the image. Aliasing artifacts appear as Moiré patterns on the image (Baxes, 1994).

The sampling results in the division of the signal. The more parts to the signal, the greater the accuracy of the ADC. The measurement unit for these parts is

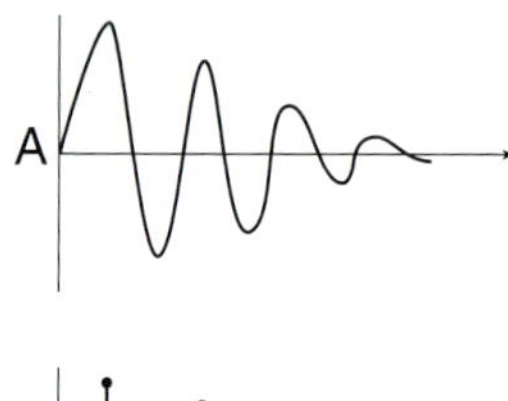


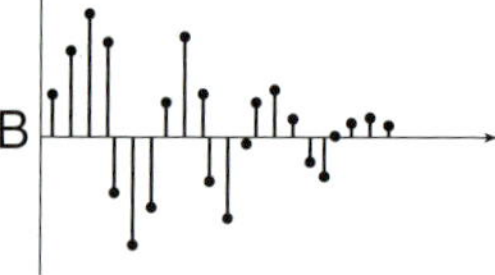


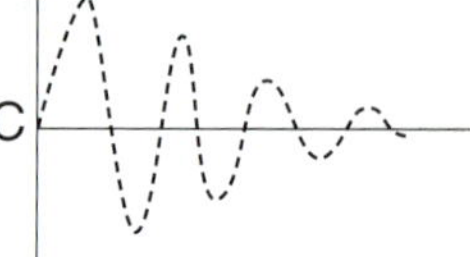


**FIGURE 2-13** Good sampling **(B)** of original analog signal **(A)** produces an accurate representation of the original signal **(C)** after computer processing.

the bit. Recall that a bit can be either 0 or 1. In a 1-bit ADC, the signal is divided in two parts ($2^1 = 2$). A 2-bit ADC generates four equal parts ($2^2 = 4$). An 8-bit ADC generates 256 equal parts ($2^8 = 256$). The higher the number of bits, the more accurate the ADC.

The ADC also determines the number of levels or shades of gray represented in the image. A 1-bit ADC results in two integers (0 and 1), which are represented as black and white. A 2-bit ADC results in four

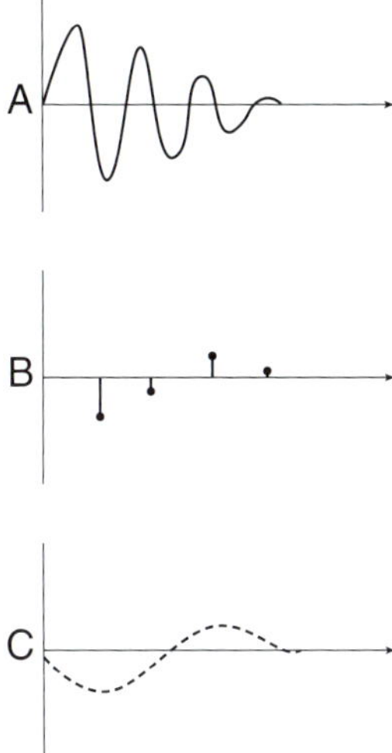


**FIGURE 2-14** Poor sampling **(B)** misrepresents the shape of the original **(A)** after computer processing **(C)**.

numbers, which produce a grayscale with four shades. An 8-bit ADC results in 256 integers ($2^8$), ranging from 0 to 255, with 256 shades of gray (Fig. 2-10).

The other characteristic of the ADC is *speed*, or the time taken to digitize the analog signal. In the ADC, speed and accuracy are inversely related—the greater the accuracy, the longer it takes to digitize the signal.

## Why Digitize Images?

Several operations are used in digital image processing to transform an input image into an output image to suit the needs of humans. Baxes (1994) identified at least five fundamental classes of operations: image enhancement, image restoration, image analysis, image compression, and image synthesis. Although it is not within the scope of this chapter to describe all of these in any great detail, it is noteworthy to mention the purpose of each of them and state their particular operations. For a more complete and thorough description of these classes, the interested reader should refer to the work of Baxes (1994). The following is a list of the five fundamental classes of operations.

1. *Image enhancement*: The purpose of this class of processing is to generate an image that is more pleasing to the observer. Certain characteristics such as contours and shapes can be enhanced to improve the overall quality of the image. The operations include contrast enhancement, edge enhancement, spatial and frequency filtering, image combining, and noise reduction.
2. *Image restoration*: The purpose of image restoration is to improve the quality of images that have distortions or degradations. Image restoration is commonplace in spacecraft imagery. Images sent to Earth from various camera systems on spacecrafts have distortions/degradations that must be corrected for proper viewing. Blurred images, for example, can be filtered to make them sharper.
3. *Image analysis*: This class of digital image processing allows measurements and statistics to be performed, as well as image **segmentation,** feature extraction, and classification of objects. Baxes (1994) indicated that "The process of analyzing objects in an image begins with image segmentation operations, such as image enhancement or restoration operations. These operations are used to isolate and highlight the objects of interest. Then the features of the objects are extracted resulting in object outlines or other object measures. These measures describe and characterize the objects in the image. Finally, the object measures are used to classify the objects into specific categories." Segmentation operations are used in 3D medical imaging (Seeram, 2001).
4. *Image compression*: The purpose of image compression of digital images is to reduce the size of the image to decrease transmission time and reduce storage space. In general, there are two forms of image compression, lossy and lossless compression (Fig. 2-15). In lossless compression there is no loss of any information in the image (detail is not compromised) when the image is decompressed. In lossy compression, there is some loss of image details when the image is decompressed. The latter has specific uses, especially in situations when it is unnecessary to have exact details of the original image. A more recent form of compression receiving attention in digital diagnostic imaging is wavelet (special waveforms) compression. The main advantage of this form of compression is that there is no loss in both spatial and frequency information. Compression has received a good deal of attention in the digital radiology department, including the PACS environment, because image datasets are becoming increasingly larger. For this reason it will be described further later in this chapter.
5. *Image synthesis*: These **processing operations** "create images from other images or non-image data. These operations are used when a desired image is either physically impossible or impractical to acquire, or does not exist in a physical form at all" (Baxes, 1994). Examples of operations are **image reconstruction** techniques that are the basis for the production of CT and MRI images

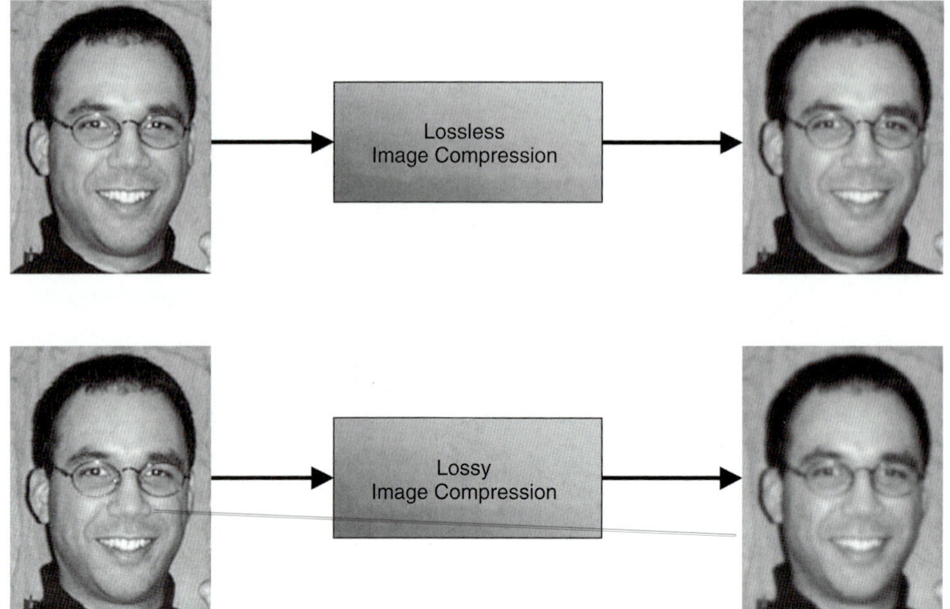


**FIGURE 2-15** The effects of two methods of image compression, lossless and lossy, on the quality of the image (visual appearance of the image) of Euclid's son David. (Images courtesy David Seeram.)

and 3D visualization techniques, which are based on computer graphics technology.

## Image-Processing Techniques

In general, image-processing techniques are based on three types of operations: **point operations** (point processes), **local operations** (area processes), and **global operations** (frame processes). The image-processing **algorithms** on which these operations are based alter the pixel intensity values (Baxes, 1994; Bourne, 2010; Dougherty, 2009; Lindley, 1991; Marion, 1991). The exception is the geometric-processing algorithm, which changes the position (spatial position or arrangement) of the pixel.

## Point Operations

**Point operations** are perhaps the least complicated and most frequently used image-processing technique. The value of the input image pixel is mapped on the corresponding output image pixel (Fig. 2-16). The algorithms for point operations enable the input image matrix to be scanned, pixel by pixel, until the entire image is transformed.

The most commonly used point-processing technique is called **gray-level mapping.** This is also referred to as "contrast enhancement," "contrast stretching," "histogram modification," "histogram stretching," or "**windowing.**" Gray-level mapping uses a **look-up table (LUT),** which plots the output and input gray levels against each other (Fig. 2-17).

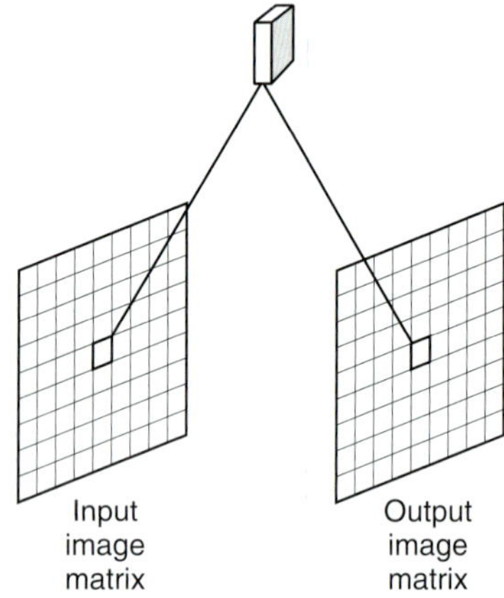


**FIGURE 2-16** In a point operation, the value of the input image pixel is mapped onto the corresponding output image pixel.

LUTs can be implemented with **hardware** or **software** for gray-level transformation. Figure 2-18 illustrates the transformation process. Gray-level mapping changes the brightness of the image and results in the enhancement of the display image.

Gray-level mapping results in a modification of the histogram of the pixel values. A **histogram** is a graph of the pixels in all or part of the image, plotted as a function of the gray level. A histogram can be created as follows:

1. Observe the image matrix (Fig. 2-19) and create a table of the number of pixels with a specific intensity value, as shown.

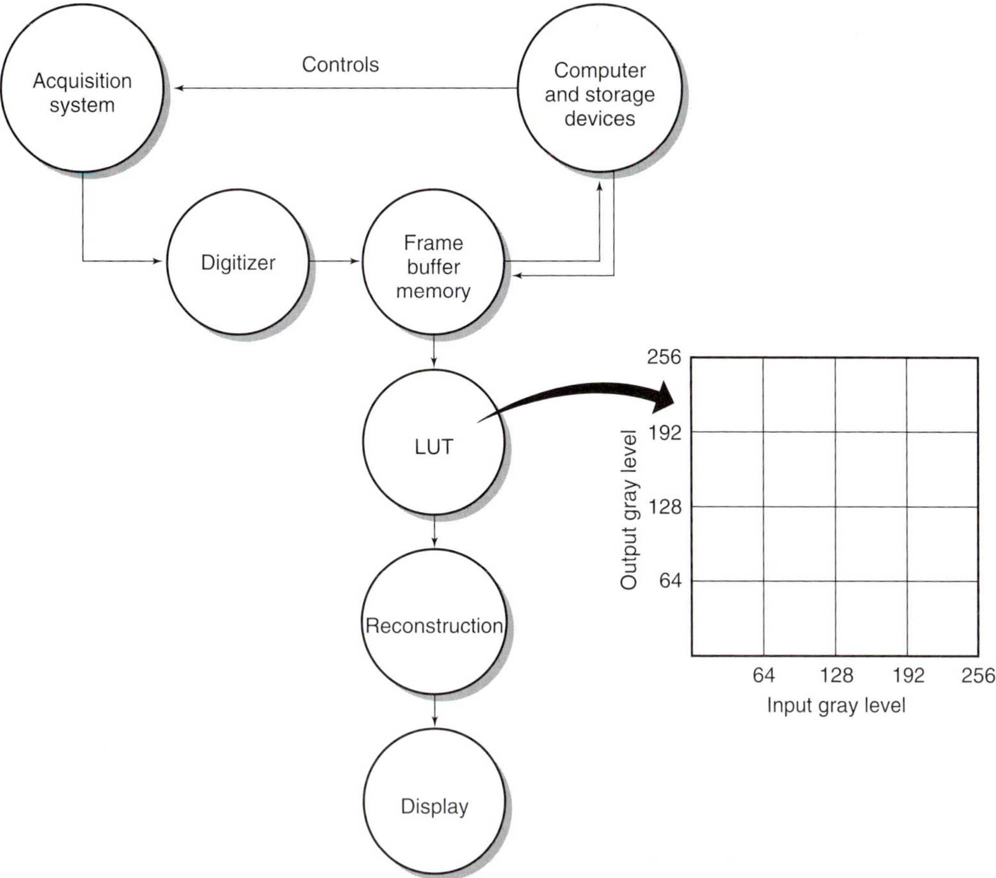


**FIGURE 2-17** Gray-level mapping. The LUT plots the input gray level against the output gray level.

2. Plot a graph of the number of pixels versus the gray levels (intensity or density values).

Histograms indicate the overall brightness and contrast of an image. If the histogram is modified or changed, the brightness and contrast of the image can be altered, a technique referred to as *histogram modification*, or histogram stretching. This is also an example of a point operation in digital image processing. If the histogram is wide, the resulting image has high contrast. If the histogram is narrow, the resulting image has low contrast. On the other hand, if the histogram values are closer to the lower end of the range of values, the image appears dark, as opposed to a bright image, in which the values are weighted toward the higher end of the range of values.

## Local Operations

A **local operation** is an image-processing operation in which the output image pixel value is determined from a small area of pixels around the corresponding input pixel (Fig. 2-20). These operations are also referred to as *area processes* or *group processes* because a group of pixels is used in the transformation calculation.

**Spatial frequency filtering** is an example of a local operation that concerns brightness information in an image. If the brightness of an image changes rapidly with **distance** in the horizontal or vertical direction, the image is said to have *high spatial frequency*. (An image with smaller pixels has higher frequency information than an image with larger pixels.) When the brightness changes slowly or at a constant rate, the image is said to have *low spatial frequency*. Spatial frequency filtering can alter images in several ways such as image sharpening, image smoothing, image blurring, noise reduction, and feature extraction (edge enhancement and detection).

There are two places to perform spatial frequency filtering: (1) in the frequency domain, which considers the FT or (2) in the spatial domain, which uses the pixel values (gray levels) themselves.

### Spatial Location Filtering: Convolution

**Convolution,** a general-purpose algorithm, is a technique of filtering in the space domain, as illustrated in Figure 2-21.

The value of the output pixel depends on a group of pixels in the input image that surrounds the input pixel of interest—pixel P5. The new value for P5 in the output image is calculated by obtaining its weighted average and that of its surrounding pixels. The average is computed by using a group of pixels called a **convolution kernel,** in which each pixel in the kernel is a weighting factor, or convolution coefficient. In general, the size of the kernel is a 3 × 3 matrix. Depending on the type of processing, different types of convolution kernels can be used, in which case the weighting factors are different.

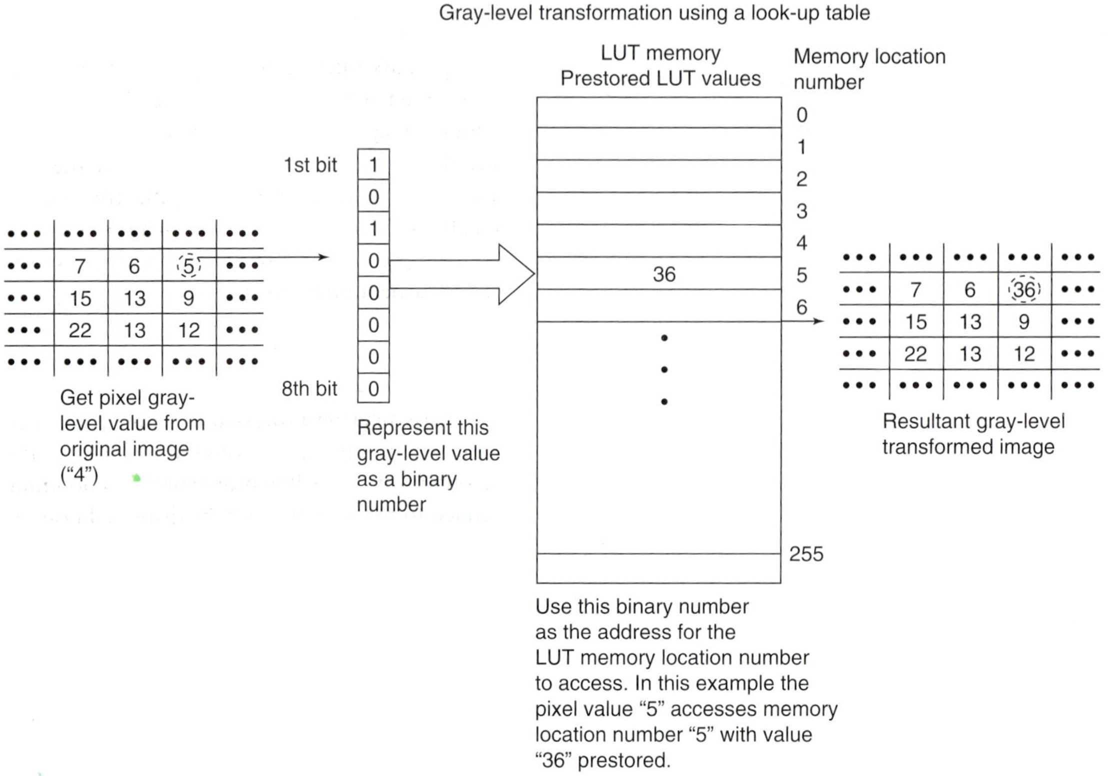

Gray-level transformation using a look-up table
LUT memory
Prestored LUT values
Memory location
number
0
1
2
3
4
5
6
255
36
1st bit
8th bit
1
0
1
0
0
0
0
0
7
6
5
15
13
9
22
13
12
Get pixel gray-
level value from
original image
("4")
Represent this
gray-level value
as a binary
number
36
Resultant gray-level
transformed image
Use this binary number
as the address for the
LUT memory location number
to access. In this example the
pixel value "5" accesses memory
location number "5" with value
"36" prestored.

**FIGURE 2-18** Gray-level transformation of an input image pixel. The algorithm uses the LUT to change the value of the input pixel (5) to 36, the new value of the output pixel. (From Huang, H. K. (2004). *PACS and imaging informatics: basic principles and applications.* Hoboken, NJ: John Wiley.)

2 6 7 5 4 1 3
8 7 3 4 6 1 2
8 8 7 6 1 3 8
5 6 1 2 7 3 4
6 1 2 5 6 7 8
2 6 8 6 7 1 6
4 3 5 6 8 1 4
No of
pixels
10
9
8
7
6
5
4
1 2 3 4 5 6 7 8
Relative density
1
2
3
4
5
6
7
8
7
5
5
5
4
10
6
7

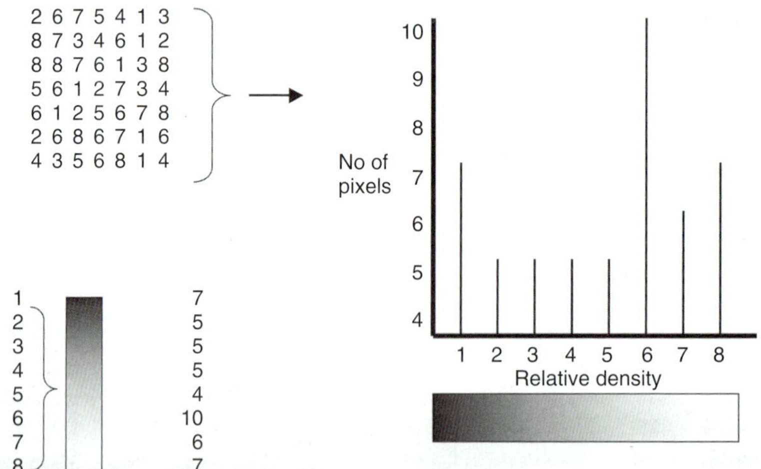

**FIGURE 2-19** The creation of a histogram. A histogram is a graph of the number of pixels in the entire image or part of the image having the same gray levels (density values), plotted as a function of the gray levels. (From Seeram, E. (2004). Digital image processing. *Radiologic Technology, 75,* 435-455. Reproduced by permission of the American Society of Radiologic Technologists.)

During convolution, the convolution kernel moves across the image, pixel by pixel. Each pixel in the input image, its surrounding neighbors, and the kernels are used to compute the value of the corresponding output pixel—each pixel is multiplied by its respective weighting factor and then summed. The resulting number is the value of the center output pixel. This process is applied to all pixels in the input image; each calculation requires nine multiplications and nine additions. This can be time-consuming, but special hardware can speed up the process.

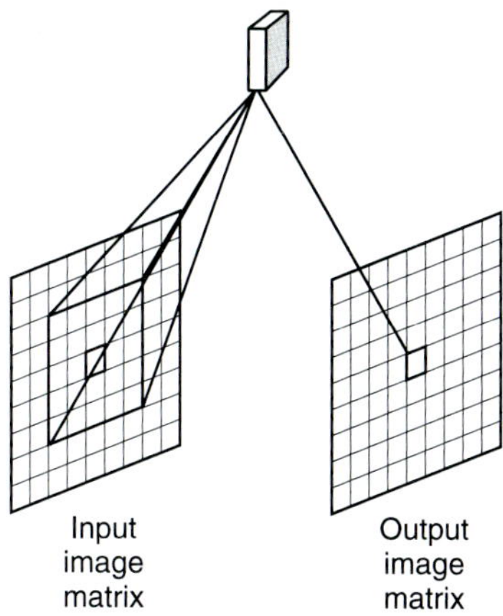


**FIGURE 2-20** In the local operation, the value is determined from a small area of pixels surrounding the corresponding input pixel.

### Spatial Frequency Filtering: High-Pass Filtering

The high-pass filtering process, also known as edge enhancement or sharpness, is intended to sharpen an input image in the spatial domain that appears blurred. The algorithm is such that first the spatial location image is converted into spatial frequencies by using the FT, followed by the use of a high-pass filter, which suppresses the low spatial frequencies to produce a sharper output image. This process is shown in Figure 2-22. The high-pass filter kernel is also shown.

### Spatial Frequency Filtering: Low-Pass Filtering

A low-pass filtering process uses a low-pass filter to operate on the input image with the goal of smoothing. The output image will appear blurred. Smoothing is intended to reduce noise and the displayed brightness

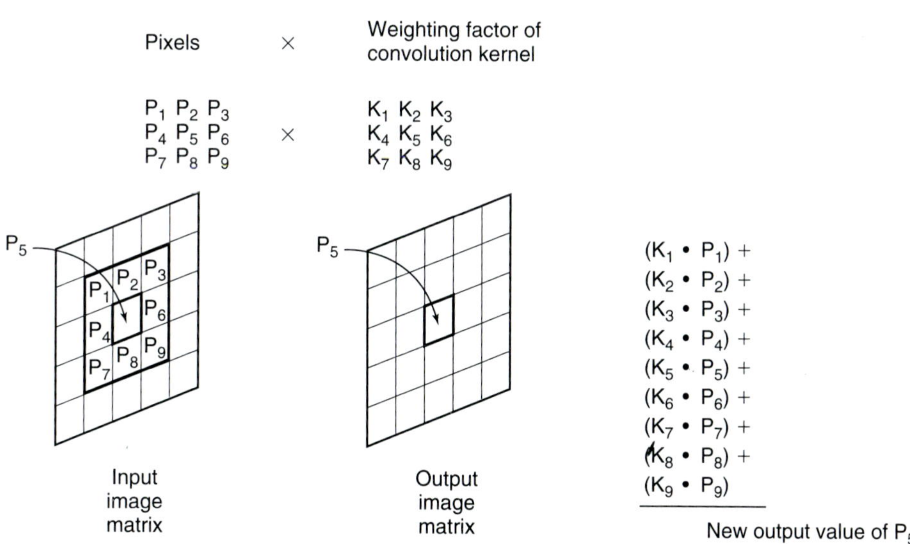


**FIGURE 2-21** In convolution, the value of the output pixel is calculated by multiplying each input pixel by its corresponding weighting factor of the convolution kernel (usually a 3 × 3 matrix). These products are then summed.

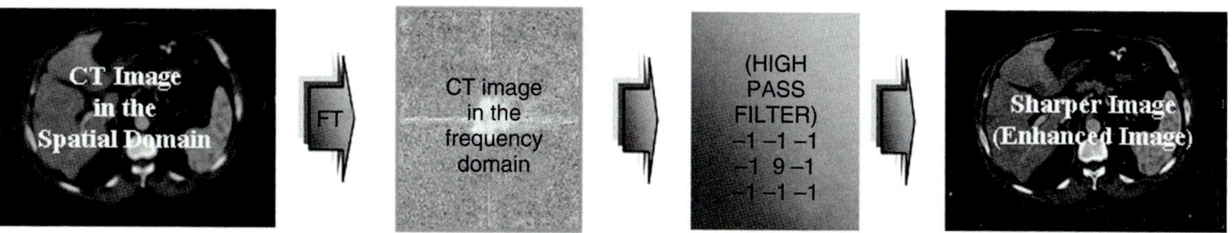


**FIGURE 2-22** The use of a high-pass filter to produce a sharper image. The filter is called a kernel and it suppresses the low spatial frequencies in the image.

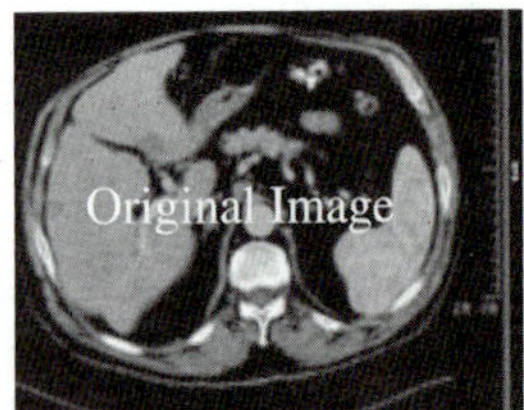

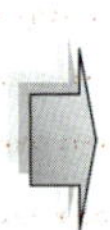
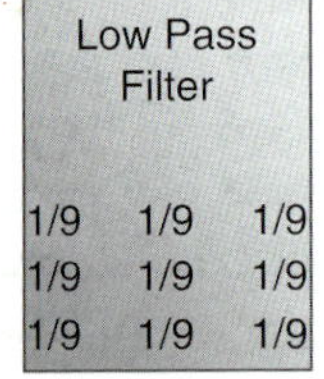

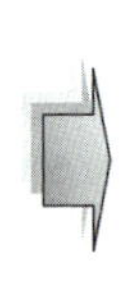
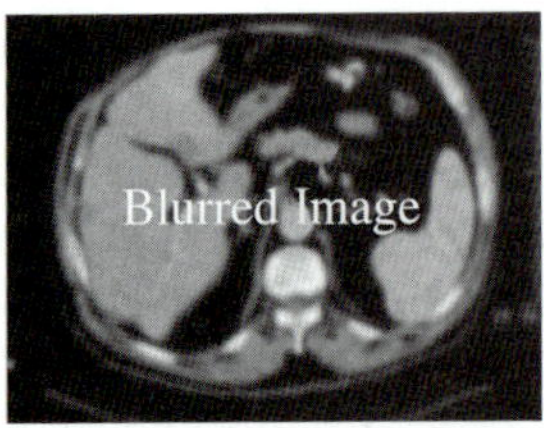


**FIGURE 2-23** The effect of a low-pass filter on picture quality. The low-pass filter kernel suppresses the high spatial frequencies in the image.

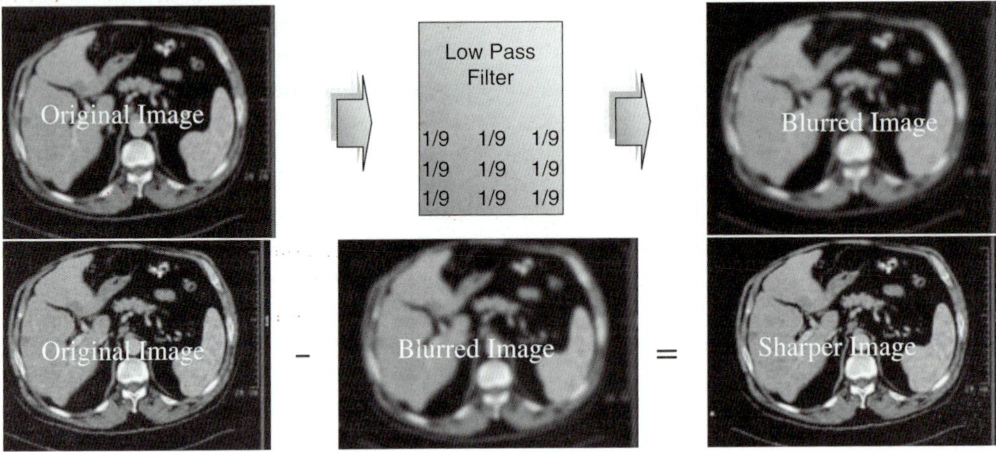


**FIGURE 2-24** The digital image-processing technique of unsharp (blurred) masking uses the blurred image produced from the low-pass filtering process and subtracts it from the original image to produce a sharp image.

levels of pixels; however, image detail is compromised (Fig. 2-23). The low-pass filter kernel is also shown.

### Spatial Frequency Processing: Unsharp (Blurred) Masking

The digital image-processing technique of unsharp (blurred) masking uses the blurred image produced from the low-pass filtering process and subtracts it from the original image to produce a sharp image (Fig. 2-24). It can be seen that the output image appears sharper.

## Global Operations

In **global operations,** the entire input image is used to compute the value of the pixel in the output image (Fig. 2-25). A common global operation is Fourier domain processing, or the FT, which uses filtering in the frequency domain rather than the space domain (Baxes, 1994). Fourier domain image-processing techniques can provide edge enhancement, image sharpening, and image restoration.

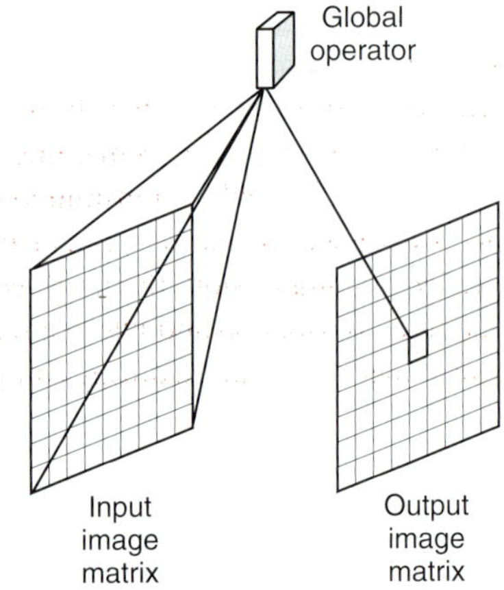


**FIGURE 2-25** In a global operation, the entire input image is used to compute the value of the pixel in the output image.

## Geometric Operations

**Geometric operations** are intended to modify the spatial position or orientation of the pixels in an image. These algorithms change the position rather than the intensity of the pixels, which is also a characteristic of point, local, and global operations. Geometric operations can result in the scaling and sizing of images and image rotation and translation (Castleman, 1996).

For a more detailed description of image-processing concepts, the interested reader should refer to Dougherty (2009) and Bourne (2010).

## IMAGE COMPRESSION OVERVIEW

The evolving nature of digital image acquisition, processing, display, storage, and **communications** in diagnostic radiology has resulted in an exponential increase in digital image files. For example, the number of images generated in a multislice CT examination can range from 40 to 3000. If the image size is 512 × 512 × 12, then one examination can generate 20 megabytes (MB) of data, and up. A CT examination consisting of two images per examination with an image size of 2048 × 2048 × 12 will result in 16 MB of data. A digital **mammography** examination can now generate 160 MB of data. Additionally, Huang (2004) points out that "the number of digital medical images captured per year in the US alone is over pentabytes that is, $10^{15}$, and is increasing rapidly every year." In this regard, it can safely be assumed that perhaps similar trends apply to Canada.

With this in mind, image compression can solve the problems of image data storage and improve communication speed requirements for huge amounts of digital data (Bourne, 2010; Dougherty, 2009; Seeram, 2004; Seeram & Seeram, 2008).

### What Is Image Compression?

The literature is replete with definitions of image compression; however, one that stands out in terms of clarity is offered by Alan Rowberg, MD, of the Department of Radiology, University of Washington: "Digital compression refers to using one or more of many software and/or hardware techniques to reduce information by removing unnecessary data. The remaining information is then encoded and either transmitted or stored in an archive or storage media, such as tape or disk. In a process called decompression, the user's equipment later decodes the information and fills in a representation of the data that was removed during compression."

This definition is the basis for understanding what image compression means.

### Types of Image Compression

As mentioned earlier in this chapter, there are two types of image data compression: lossless or reversible compression and lossy or irreversible compression. In the former, no information is lost when the image is decompressed or reconstructed; in the latter, there is some loss of information when the image is decompressed (Fig. 2-15).

Although it is not within the scope of this section to describe the technical details of the steps involved in image compression, the following points are noteworthy:

- In lossless or reversible compression, there is no loss of information in the compressed image data. Furthermore, lossless compression does not involve the process of quantization but makes use of image transformation and encoding to provide a compressed image.
- Lossy or irreversible compression involves at least three steps: image transformation, quantization, and encoding.

As noted by Erickson (2002), transformation is a step in which the image is transformed from grayscale values in the spatial domain to coefficients in some other domain. One familiar transformation is the FT used in reconstruction MRI. Other transforms such as the discrete cosine transform and the discrete wavelet transform are commonly used for image compression. No loss of information occurs in the transformation step. Quantization is the step in which the data integrity is lost. It attempts to minimize information loss by preferentially preserving the most important coefficients where less important coefficients are roughly approximated, often as zero. Quantization may be as simple as converting floating point values to integer values. Finally, these quantized coefficients are compactly represented for efficient storage or transmission of the image.

There are a number of other issues related to the use of irreversible compression in digital radiology, including the visual impact of compression (lossy compression) on diagnostic digital images and methods used to evaluate the effects of compression (Seeram, 2006a). It is also well established that the quality of digital images plays an important role in helping the radiologist to provide an accurate diagnosis. At low compression ratios (8:1 or less), the loss of image quality is such that the image is still "visually acceptable" (Huang, 2004). The concern now is related to what Erickson (2002) refers to as "compression tolerance," a term he defined as "the maximum compression in which the decompressed image is acceptable for interpretation and aesthetics."

Because lossy compression methods provide high to very high compression ratios compared with lossless methods, and keeping the term *compression tolerance* in mind, Huang, in 2004 pointed out that "currently lossy algorithms are not used by radiologists in primary diagnosis, because physicians and radiologists are concerned with the legal consequences of an incorrect diagnosis based on a lossy compressed image."

In a more recent study, examining the current status of irreversible compression use in radiology, Pinto do Santos et al., (2013) pointed out that "irreversible image compression allows markedly higher reduction of data volume in comparison with reversible compression algorithms but is, however, accompanied by a certain amount of mathematical and visual loss of information. Various national and international radiological societies have published recommendations for the use of irreversible image compression. The degree of acceptable compression varies across modalities and regions of interest.... Although mathematical loss due to rounding up errors and reduction of high frequency information occurs this results in relatively low visual degradation. It is still unclear where to implement irreversible compression in the radiological workflow as only few studies analyzed the impact of irreversible compression on specialized **image postprocessing.** As long as this is within the limits recommended... irreversible image compression could be implemented directly at the imaging modality ..."

### Visual Impact of Irreversible Compression on Digital Images

The goal of both lossless and lossy compression techniques is to reduce the size of the compressed image, to reduce storage requirements, and to increase image transmission speed. The size of the compressed image is influenced by the compression ratio (see definition of terms), with lossless compression methods yielding ratios of 2:1 to 3:1 (Huang, 2004), and lossy or irreversible compression having ratios ranging from 10:1 to 50:1 or more (Huang, 2004). It is well known that as the compression ratio increases, less storage space is required and faster transmission speeds are possible, but at the expense of image quality degradation.

A recent survey of the opinions of expert radiologists in the United States and Canada (Seeram, 2006b), on the use of irreversible compression in clinical practice showed that the opinions are wide and varied. This indicates that there is no consensus of opinion on the use of irreversible compression in primary diagnosis. Opinions are generally positive on the notion of image storage and image transmission advantages of image compression. Finally, almost all radiologists are concerned with the litigation potential of an incorrect diagnosis based on irreversible compressed images.

In providing a rationale for examining the tradeoffs between image quality and compression ratio, an interesting experiment is suggested by Huang (2004) using five compressed CT images (512 × 512 × 12) with compression ratios of 4:1, 8:1, 17:1, 26:1, and 37:1 together with the original image. Next, determine the order of quality of the images, and finally, determine which compression ratio provides an image quality that can be used to provide a diagnosis. In the generalized results of this simple experiment, Huang states that "reconstructed images with compression ratios ≤8:1 do not exhibit visible deterioration in image quality. In other words, a compression ratio of ≤8:1 is visually acceptable. But visually unacceptable does not necessarily mean that the ratio is not suitable for diagnosis because this depends on what diseases are under consideration."

## IMAGE SYNTHESIS OVERVIEW

One of the advantages of digital image processing is image synthesis, and examples of image synthesis are the image reconstruction methods used in CT and MRI, and 3D imaging operations. Although image reconstruction is based on mathematical procedures, 3D techniques are based on computer graphics technology. Both CT image reconstruction and 3D imaging will be described in detail in later chapters; therefore, only highlights will be mentioned here.

### Magnetic Resonance Imaging

The major system processes of MRI signal acquisition to image display are shown in Figure 2-26. First,

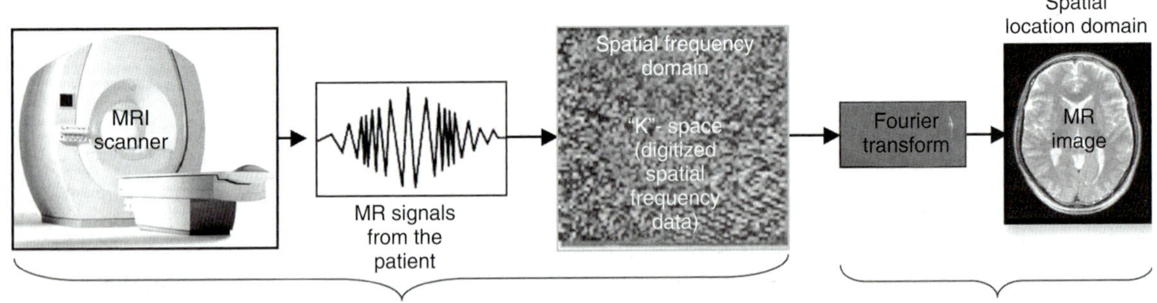


**FIGURE 2-26** The major processes of MRI signal acquisition to image display. First, MR signals are acquired from the patient, who is placed in the magnet during the imaging procedure. These signals are high and low frequencies collected from the patient. The signals are subsequently digitized and stored in what is referred to as k space, a frequency domain space. (Image courtesy Philips Medical Systems.)

magnetic resonance signals are acquired from the patient, who is placed in the magnet during the imaging procedure. These signals are high and low frequencies collected from the patient. The signals are subsequently digitized and stored in what is referred to as "k" space, which is a frequency domain space. Once k space is filled, the FT algorithm uses the data in k space to reconstruct magnetic resonance images, which are displayed on the monitor for viewing by a radiologist or technologist. Once displayed, images can be manipulated with special digital image-processing software to perform windowing and 3D image visualization.

## CT Imaging

A conceptual overview of CT imaging is shown in Figure 2-27. Attenuation data are collected from the patient by the detectors that send their electronic signals to the computer, having been digitized by the ADC. The computer then uses a special image reconstruction algorithm, referred to as the filtered **back-projection** algorithm, to build up a digital CT image. This image must be converted to a grayscale image to be displayed on a monitor for viewing by the radiologist and the technologist.

Displayed CT images can be manipulated with digital image-processing software to perform such processing as windowing, image reformatting, and 3D image visualization.

## Three-Dimensional Imaging in Radiology

3D imaging is gaining widespread attention in radiology (Beigelman-Aubry et al., 2005; Dalrymple et al., 2005; Neuman and Meyers, 2005; Seeram, 2004). Already it is used in CT, MRI, and other imaging modalities to provide both qualitative and **quantitative information** from images to facilitate and enhance diagnosis.

The general framework for 3D imaging is shown in Figure 2-28. Four major steps are shown: data acquisition, creation of what is referred to as 3D space (all voxel information is stored in the computer), processing for 3D image display, and finally, 3D image display. Digital processing can allow the observer to view all aspects of 3D space, a technique referred to as 3D visualization. The application of 3D

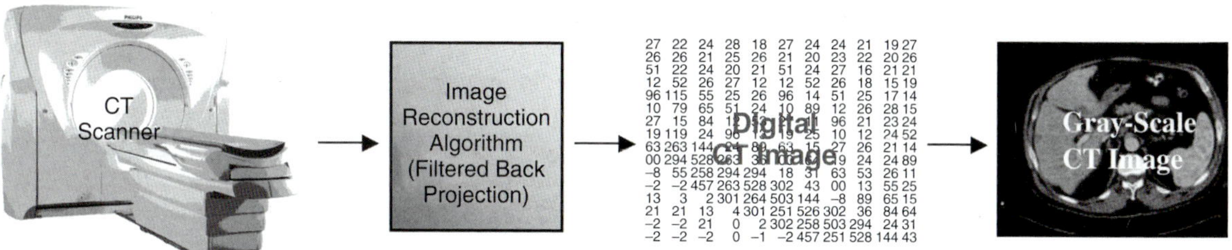


**FIGURE 2-27** A conceptual overview of CT imaging. Image reconstruction is performed by the filtered back-projection. (See text for further explanation.)

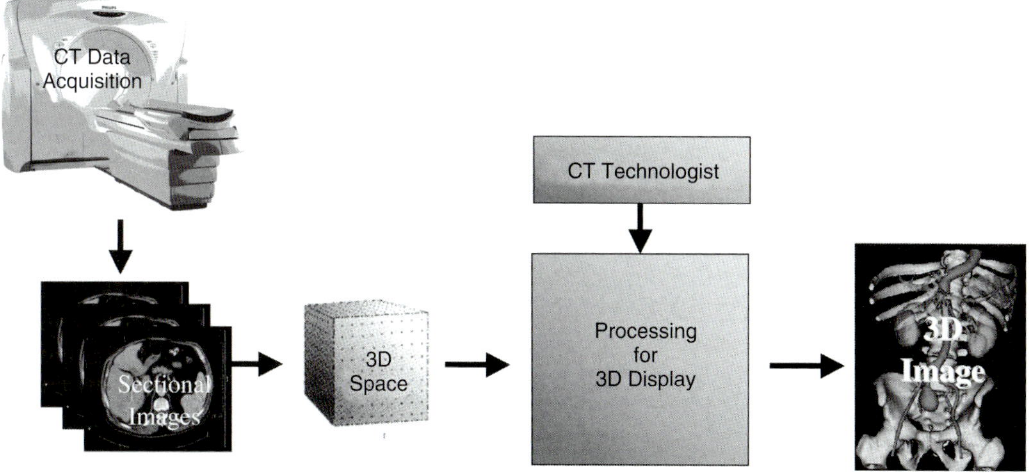


**FIGURE 2-28** The general framework for 3D imaging. Four major steps are shown: data acquisition, creation of what is referred to as 3D space, processing for 3D image display, and finally 3D image display. Digital processing can allow the observer to view all aspects of 3D space, a technique referred to as 3D visualization. (Image courtesy Philips Medical Systems.)

visualization techniques in radiology is referred to as 3D medical imaging.

Dr. Jayaram, from the Department of Radiology at the University of Pennsylvania, is a 3D imaging expert who notes that there are four classes of 3D imaging operations: preprocessing, visualization, manipulation, and analysis. Because the visualization operations are now quite popular in digital imaging departments using CT and MRI scanners, it is noteworthy to highlight the major ideas of at least two 3D visualization techniques—surface **rendering** and **volume rendering**. Rendering is the final step in 3D image production. It is a computer program used to transform 3D space into simulated 3D images to be displayed on a 2D computer screen.

Two classes of rendering techniques are used in radiology: surface and volume. *Surface rendering* is a simple procedure in which the surface of an object is created using contour data and shading the pixels to provide the illusion of depth. It uses only 10% of the data in 3D space and does not require a great deal of computation. *Volume rendering*, on the other hand, is a much more sophisticated technique. Volume rendering uses all the data in 3D space to provide additional information by allowing the observer to view more details inside the object, as is clearly illustrated in Figure 2-28. It also requires more computational power.

Applications of these rendering techniques are in several areas, including imaging the craniomaxillofacial complex; musculoskeletal system; the central nervous system; and cardiovascular, pulmonary, gastrointestinal, and genitourinary systems. 3D imaging is now popular in **CT angiography** (Fishman et al., 2006) and magnetic resonance angiography.

3D medical imaging uses stand-alone workstations featuring very powerful computers capable of a wide range of processing functions, including virtual reality imaging (VRI).

## Virtual Reality Imaging in Radiology

VRI requires sophisticated digital image-processing methods to facilitate the perception of 3D anatomy from a set of 2D images (Huang, 2004; Kalender, 2005; Seeram, 2004). The vast amount of data collected by multislice CT scanners, for example, provides the opportunity to develop VRI applications in radiology.

Virtual reality is a branch of computer science that immerses the users in a computer-generated environment and allows them to interact with 3D scenes. One common method that uses virtual reality concepts is virtual endoscopy, which is used to create inner views of tubular structures.

Virtual endoscopy involves a set of systematic procedures. These include data acquisition (careful selection of **scan parameters** in collecting data from the patient), image preprocessing (to optimize images before they are processed), 3D rendering, using both surface and volume rendering, and, finally, image display and analysis. Two software tools available for interactive image assessment include Philip's Voyager and General Electric's 3D Navigator (advanced visualization packages for the user to perform real-time navigation of structures using a "fly through" within and around tubular anatomy like a real endoscope. 3D imaging and VRI will be described in detail in a later chapter.

# IMAGE-PROCESSING HARDWARE

A basic image-processing system consists of several interconnected components (Fig. 2-29). The major components are the ADC, image storage,

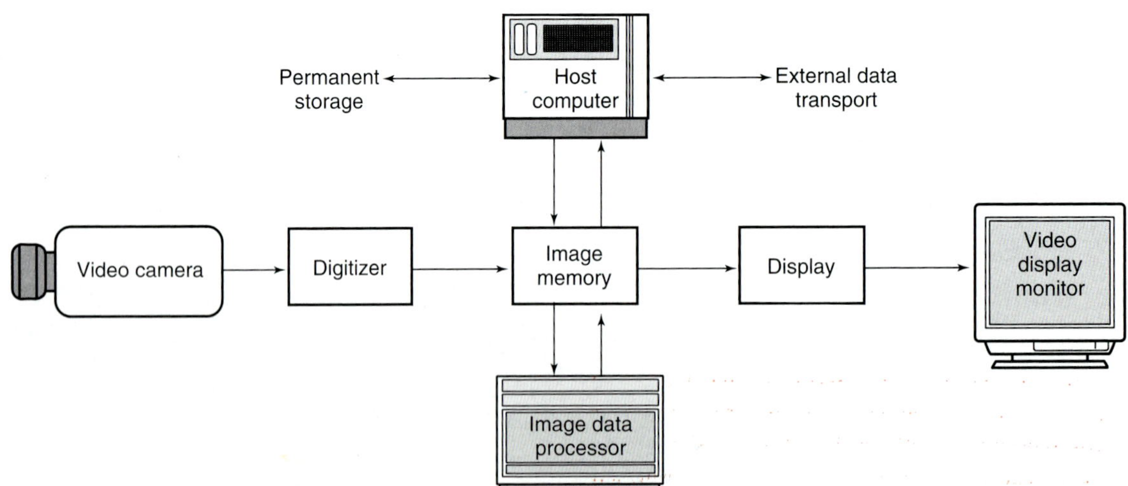


FIGURE 2-29 The essential hardware components of a generalized digital image-processing system.

image display, image processor, **host computer,** and DAC.

- *Data acquisition*: In Figure 2-29, the video camera is the data-acquisition device. In CT this would be represented by the x-ray tube and detectors and the detector electronics.
- *Digitizer*: As can be seen in Figure 2-29, the analog signal is converted into digital form by the digitizer, or ADC.
- *Image memory*: The digitized image is held in storage for further processing. Several components are connected to the image store and provide input and output. The size of this memory depends on the image. For example, a 512 × 512 × 8-bit image requires a memory of 2,097,152 bits.
- *DAC*: The digital image held in the memory can be displayed on a television monitor. However, because monitors work with analog signals, it is necessary to convert the digital data to analog signals with a DAC.
- *Internal image processor*: This processor is responsible for high-speed processing of the input digital data.
- *Host computer*: In digital image processing, the host computer is a primary component capable of performing several functions. For example, the host computer can read and write the data in the image store and provide archival storage on tape and disk storage systems. The host computer plays a significant role in applications that involve the transmission of images to another location, such as medical imaging.

## CT AS A DIGITAL IMAGE-PROCESSING SYSTEM

A number of imaging modalities in radiology use image-processing techniques, including digital radiography and fluoroscopy, nuclear medicine, MRI, ultrasonography, and CT. The future of digital imaging is promising in that a wide variety of applications have received increasing attention, such as 3D imaging (Seeram & Seeram, 2008). The major image-processing operations in medical imaging now common in the radiology department are presented in Table 2-2.

The basic components of a digital imaging system were illustrated in Figure 1-30. As a digital image-processing system, CT fits into this scheme. In addition, similar steps in image digitization can be applied to the CT process, as follows:

1. First, divide the picture into pixels. In CT, the slice of the patient is divided into small regions called voxels because the dimension of depth (**slice thickness**) is added to the pixel. The patient is scanned as the x-ray tube moves around the patient.
2. Next, sample the pixels. In CT, the voxels are sampled when x rays pass through them. This measurement is performed by detectors. The signal from the detector is in analog form and must be converted into digital form before it can be sent to the computer for processing.
3. The final step is quantization. In CT, the analog signal is also quantized and changed into a digital array for input into the computer. The digital data resulting from quantization are processed by the computer through a series of operations or techniques to modify the input image. In CT, the digital data are also subject to several processing algorithms so the output image can be displayed in a form suitable for human observation.

## IMAGE PROCESSING: AN ESSENTIAL TOOL FOR CT

Image postprocessing and its associated techniques such as data visualization, computer-aided detection,

**TABLE 2-2 Common Digital Image-Processing Operations Used in Diagnostic Digital Imaging Technologies**

| Digital Imaging Modality | Common Image-Processing Operations |
|---|---|
| CT | Image reformatting, windowing, region of interest, magnification, surface and volume rendering, profile, histogram, collage, image synthesis |
| MRI | Windowing, region of interest, magnification, surface and volume rendering, profile, histogram, collage, image synthesis |
| Digital subtraction angiography/digital fluoroscopy | Analytic processing, subtraction of images out of sequence, grayscale processing, temporal frame averaging, edge enhancement, pixel shifting |
| Computed radiography/digital radiography | Partitioned pattern recognition, exposure field recognition, histogram analysis, normalization of raw image data, grayscale processing (windowing), spatial filtering, dynamic range control, energy subtraction, etc. |

From Seeram, E. (2004). Digital image processing. *Radiologic Technology*, *75*, 435-455. Reproduced by permission.

and image dataset navigation have recently been identified as major research areas in the transformation of medical Imaging (Andriole and Morin, 2006). Image postprocessing methods in CT are intended to enhance the diagnostic interpretation skills of the radiologist. Several examples of these methods include image reformatting to display axial images in the coronal, sagittal, and oblique views; maximum intensity and minimum intensity projections; curved reformatting; shaded surface display; volume rendering; virtual reality; and physiologic imaging tools such as image fusion and CT perfusion. These methods will be described in detail in later chapters.

Digital image processing is now an essential tool in the CT and PACS environment, and already technologists and radiologists are actively involved in using the tools of image postprocessing, such as the digital image-processing operations and techniques outlined in this chapter. Training programs for both technologists and radiologists are also beginning to incorporate digital image processing as part of their curriculum (Seeram & Seeram, 2008). A suggested list of topics for a course on image processing in CT would be the chapter outline at the beginning of this chapter. These topics can be expanded beyond the content of this chapter.

## REVIEW QUESTIONS

Answer the following questions to check your understanding of the materials studied.

1. Digital image processing has its beginnings
   A. at NASA in their space program.
   B. at Siemens Healthcare.
   C. with Sir Godfrey Hounsfield at the EMI Labs in England.
   D. at the British Columbia Institute of Technology in Euclid's Lab.
2. Which of the following is not a visible image?
   A. a drawing
   B. a painting
   C. a mathematical image
   D. a photograph
3. Which of the following best describes a digital image?
   A. Discrete function
   B. Numerical representation of an object
   C. Cannot be processed by a computer
   D. A non-visible physical image
4. The logical steps in digitizing an image are:
   A. Scan, sample, and quantize.
   B. Sample, scan, and quantize.
   C. Quantize, sample, and scan.
   D. Sample, quantize, and scan.
5. Which of the following represents a picture element?
   A. Address
   B. Voxel
   C. Pixel
   D. Matrix
6. The process of measuring the brightness level of each pixel in an image is referred to as:
   A. Quantization.
   B. Sampling.
   C. Scanning.
   D. Analog-to-digital conversion.
7. A 10-bit ADC will divide up a signal into ___parts.
   A. 8
   B. 2
   C. 256
   D. 1024
8. Which of the following is an example of gray-level mapping?
   A. Local operation
   B. Point processing operation
   C. Geometric operation
   D. Global operation
9. Windowing in CT is an example of:
   A. Geometric operation.
   B. Local operation.
   C. Global operation.
   D. Point processing operation.
10. Poor sampling of the signal to be digitized by the ADC will result in which of the following artifacts?
    A. Beam hardening
    B. Partial volume
    C. Aliasing
    D. Streaking

## REFERENCES

Andriole, K. P., & Morin, R. (2006). Transforming medical imaging—the first SCAR TRIP Conference. *Journal of Digital Imaging, 19*, 6–16.

Baxes, G. A. (1994). *Digital image processing: principles and applications*. New York: John Wiley.

Beigelman-Aubry, D., Hill, C., Guibal, A., Savatovsky, J., & Grenier, P. A. (2005). Multi-detector row CT and post-processing techniques in the assessment of lung diseases. *Radiographics, 25*, 1639–1652.

Bourne, R. (2010). *Fundamentals of digital imaging in medicine*. London: Springer.

Castleman, K. R. (1996). *Digital image processing*. Upper Saddle, NJ: Prentice Hall.

Dalrymple, N. C., Prasad, S. R., Freckleton, M. W., et al. (2005). Introduction to the language of three-dimensional imaging with multi-detector CT. *Radiographics, 25*, 1409–1428.

Dougherty, G. (2009). *Digital image processing for medical applications*. Cambridge, UK: Cambridge University Press.

Erickson, B. J. (2002). Irreversible compression of medical images. *Journal of Digital Imaging, 15*, 5–14.

Fishman, E. K., Ney, D. R., Heath, D. G., Cori, F. M., Horton, K. M., & Johnson, P. T. (2006). Volume rendering versus maximum intensity projection in CT angiography: what works best, when, and why. *Radiographics, 26*, 905–922.

Green, W. B. (1989). *Digital image processing: a systems approach* (2nd ed.). New York: Van Nostrand Reinhold.

Huang, H. K. (2004). *PACS and imaging informatics: basic principles and applications*. Hoboken, NJ: John Wiley.

Kalender, W. A. (2005). *Computed tomography*. Munich: Publicis MCD Werbeagentur Verlag.

Lindley, C. A. (1991). *Practical image processing in C*. New York: John Wiley.

Luiten, A. L. (1995). Digital: discrete perfection. *Medicamundi, 40*, 95–100.

Marion, A. (1991). *Introduction to image processing*. London: Chapman and Hall.

Neuman, J., & Meyers, M. (2005). *Volume intensity projection: a new post-processing techniques for evaluating CTA*. The Netherlands: Philips Medical Systems.

Pinto dos Santos, D., et al. (2013). Irreversible image compression in radiology. Current status. *Radiologe, 53*(3), 257–260.

Pooley, R. A., McKinney, J. M., & Miller, D. A. (2001). The AAPM/RSNA physics tutorial for residents. Digital fluoroscopy. *Radiographics, 21*, 521–534.

Seeram, E. (2001). *Computed tomography—physical principles, clinical applications and quality control*. Philadelphia, PA: WB Saunders.

Seeram, E. (2004). Digital image processing. *Radiologic Technology, 75*, 435–455.

Seeram, E. (2006a). Irreversible compression in digital radiology. *Radiography, 12*, 45–59.

Seeram, E. (2006b). Using irreversible compression in digital radiology: a preliminary study of the opinions of radiologists. *Progress in biomedical optics and imaging—proceedings of the SPIE*, San Diego, Calif.

Seeram, E., & Seeram, D. (2008). Image postprocessing in digital radiology: a primer for technologists. *Journal of Medical Imaging and Radiation Sciences, 39*, 23–41.

Seibert, J. A. (1995). Digital image processing: basics. In S. Balter, & T. B. Shope (Eds.), *A categorical course in physics: physical and technical aspects of angiography and interventional radiology*. Oak Brook, IL: Radiological Society of North America.

# 3

# Physical Principles of Computed Tomography

## OUTLINE



## LEARNING OBJECTIVES

On completion of this chapter, you should be able to:

1. state the shortcomings of radiography and tomography and explain how these limitations are overcome by CT.
2. state what is meant by the term "data acquisition" and briefly explain two methods of data acquisition.
3. explain the meaning of:
   - relative transmission
   - penetration measurement
   - linear attenuation coefficient.
4. state Lambert–Beer law.
5. outline the principles of attenuation of a homogeneous and a heterogeneous beam of radiation.
6. explain what is meant by "data acquisition geometry" and "data processing."
7. describe the relationship between CT numbers and the linear attenuation coefficient ($\mu$).
8. state several reasons why a high kVp beam is used in CT.
9. describe the relationship between CT numbers and the gray scale of the CT image.
10. define window width (WW) and window level (WL).
11. discuss the characteristic features of the CT image.
12. explain the relationship between pixel size and the field of view (FOV) and matrix size.
13. draw and label the major equipment components of a CT scanner.
14. trace the flow of data in a CT scanner.
15. describe each of the following:
    - raw data
    - convolved data
    - reconstructed data
    - image data.
16. list the advantages and limitations of CT.

## KEY TERMS TO WATCH FOR AND REMEMBER

The following key terms/concepts are important to your understanding of this chapter.

**array processor**
**attenuation**
**contrast factor**
**CT numbers**
**data acquisition**
**data acquisition geometry**
**data processing**
**energy dependence**
**field of view (FOV)**
**heterogeneous beam**
**homogeneous beam**
**host computer**
**Lambert–Beer's Law**
**linear attenuation coefficient**
**matrix**
**pixel size**
**preprocessor**
**raw data**
**relative transmission**
**slice-by-slice data acquisition**
**volume data acquisition**
**windowing**
**window width (WW)**
**window level (WL)**

The information presented in a computed **tomography (CT)** image differs from a conventional radiographic image because it shows cross-sectional (transaxial) views of patient anatomy. In addition, CT produces 3D images that are computer generated (digital image after processing) with the use of the transaxial dataset (Fig. 3-1). Other significant differences in CT imaging are detailed in the following chapters. This chapter presents the physical principles of CT, a review of conventional tomography, and the limitations of radiography, which are helpful in understanding the CT image.

## LIMITATIONS OF RADIOGRAPHY AND TOMOGRAPHY

In both radiography and tomography, x-rays pass through the patient and are absorbed in different ways by the body's tissues. For example, because bone is denser, it absorbs more x rays than less dense soft tissues. This differential absorption is contained in the x-ray beam that passes through the patient and is recorded on radiographic film or a radiographic digital detector, such as a computed radiography imaging plate, for example.

### Limitations of Film-Based Radiography

The major shortcoming of radiography is the superimposition of all structures on the film, which makes it difficult and sometimes impossible to distinguish a particular detail (Fig. 3-2). This is especially true when structures differ only slightly in density, as is often the case with some tumors and their surrounding tissues. Although multiple views such as laterals and obliques can be taken to localize a structure, the problem of superimposition in radiography still persists.

A second limitation is that radiography is a qualitative rather than quantitative process (Fig. 3-3). It is difficult to distinguish between a homogeneous object of nonuniform thickness and a heterogeneous object (Fig. 3-3) (includes bone, soft tissue, and air) of uniform thickness (Marshall, 1976).

### Limitations of Conventional Tomography

The problem of superimposition in radiography can be somewhat overcome by conventional tomography (Bocage, 1974; Vallebona, 1931). The most common method of conventional tomography is sometimes referred to as *geometric tomography* to distinguish it from CT (Fig. 3-4). When the **x-ray tube** and film are moved simultaneously in opposite directions, unwanted sections can be blurred while the desired layer or section is kept in focus.

The immediate goal of tomography is to eliminate structures above and below the focused section, or the focal plane. However, this is difficult to achieve, and under no circumstances can all unwanted planes be removed. The limitations of tomography include persistent image blurring that cannot be completely

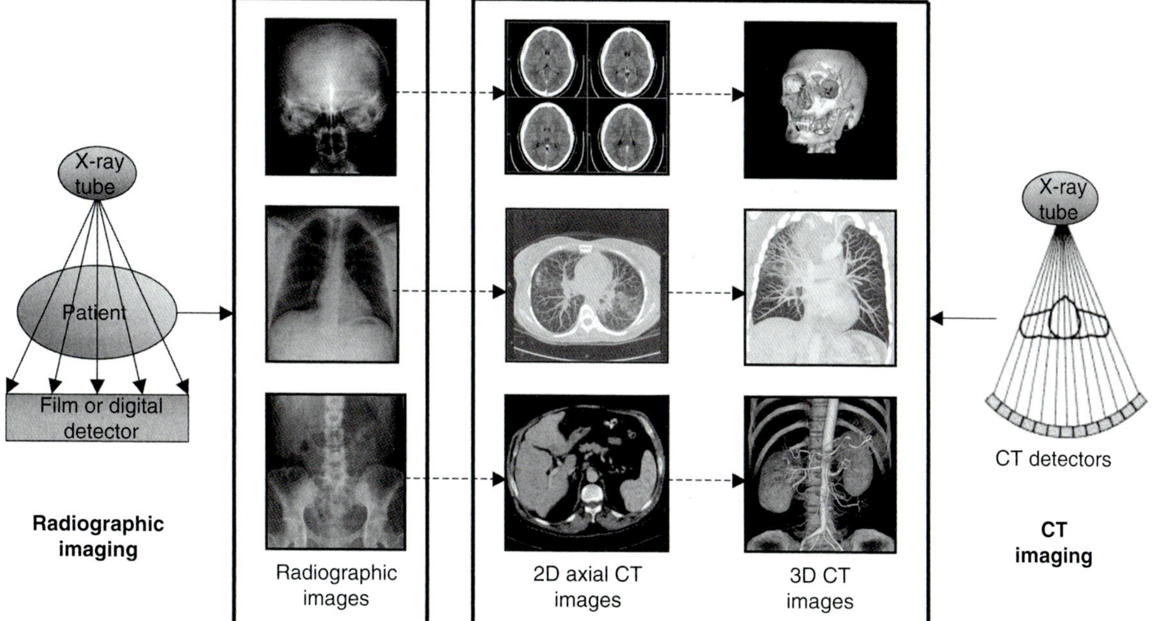


**FIGURE 3-1** The most conspicuous difference between conventional radiographic imaging and CT imaging is that CT shows cross-sectional or transaxial anatomy, which can be subject to digital post-processing operations to produce 3D images. (3D CT images courtesy Philips Medical Systems.)

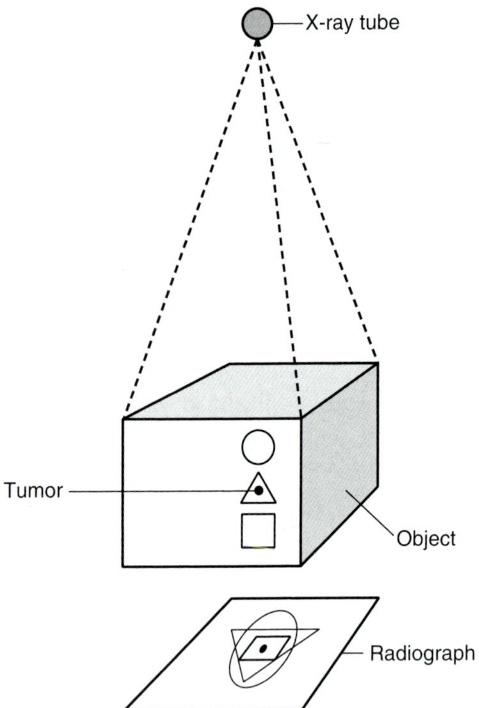


**FIGURE 3-2** The major shortcoming of radiography is that the superimposition of all structures on the radiograph makes it difficult to discriminate whether the tumor is in the circle, triangle, or square.

removed, degradation of image contrast because of the presence of scattered radiation created by the open geometry of the x-ray beam, and other problems resulting from film-screen combinations.

In addition, both radiography and tomography fail to adequately demonstrate slight differences in subject contrast, which are characteristic of soft tissue. The differences for soft tissues such as human fat, water, human cerebrospinal fluid, human plasma, monkey pancreas, monkey white matter, monkey gray matter, monkey liver, monkey muscle, and human red blood cells are 0.194, 0.222, 0.227, 0.227, 0.230, 0.230, 0.235, 0.236, 0.238, and 0.246, respectively (Ter-Pogossian et al., 1974). Radiographic film is not sensitive enough to resolve these small differences because typical film-screen combinations used today can only discriminate x-ray intensity differences of 5% to 10%.

The limitations of radiography and tomography result in the inability of film to image very small differences in tissue contrast. In addition, contrast cannot be adjusted after it has been recorded on the film. Digital imaging modalities such as CT, for example, can alter the contrast to suit the needs of the human observer (radiologists and technologists) by use of various digital **image postprocessing** techniques (see Chapter 2).

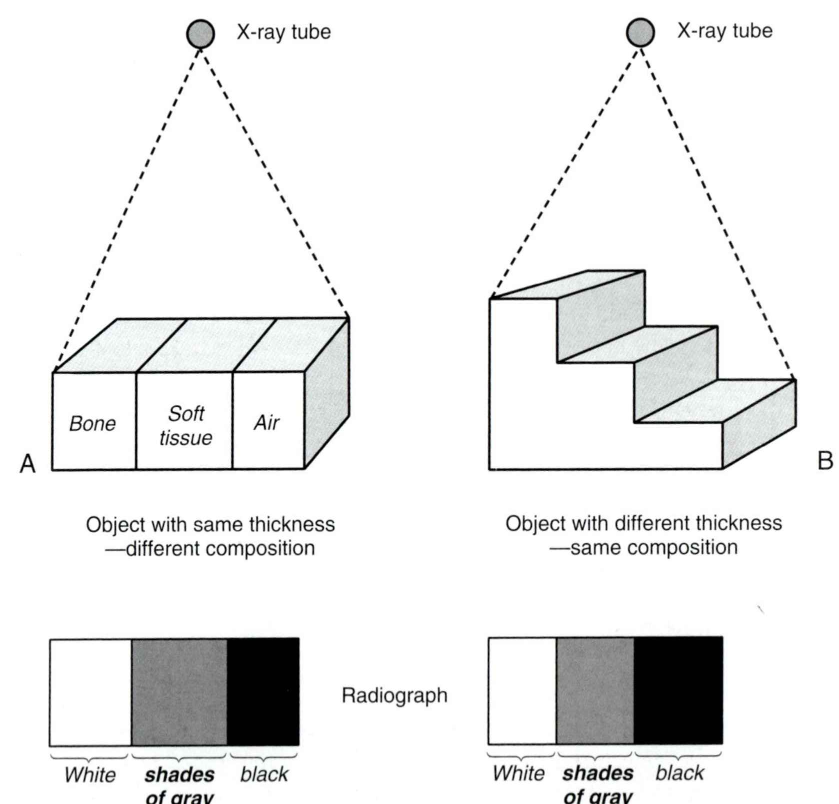


**FIGURE 3-3** Radiography is a qualitative rather than quantitative procedure. Two radiographs can appear the same although the two objects, **A** and **B**, are entirely different. (From Seeram, E. (1982). *Computed tomography technology*. Philadelphia, PA: WB Saunders.)

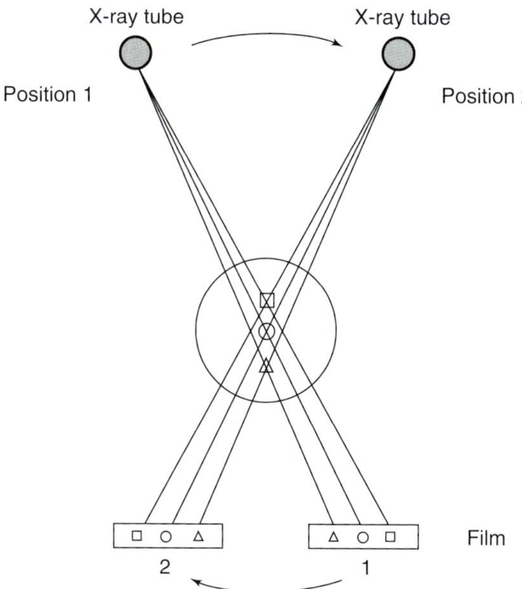


**FIGURE 3-4** Basic principles of conventional tomography. The x-ray tube and film move simultaneously and in opposite directions to ensure that the desired section (O) of the patient is imaged by blurring out structures above (□) and below (Δ) the plane of interest (O). (From Seeram, E. (1982). *Computed tomography technology*. Philadelphia, PA: WB Saunders.)

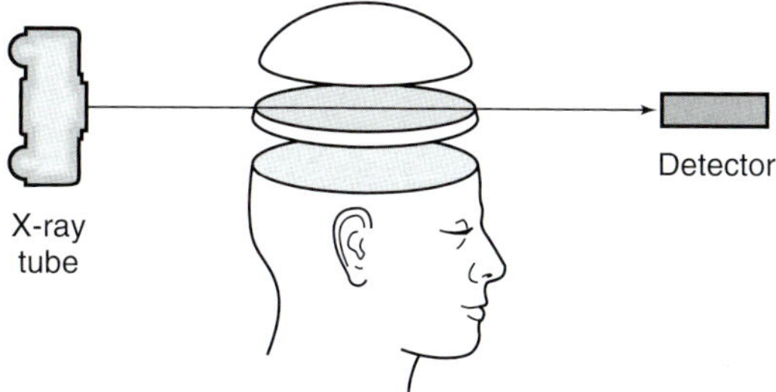


**FIGURE 3-5** In CT a thin beam is transmitted through a specific cross section, striking special detectors opposite the x-ray tube.

## Enter CT

The goal of CT is to overcome the limitations of radiography and tomography by achieving the following (Hounsfield, 1973):

1. Minimal superimposition
2. Improved image contrast
3. The recording of very small differences in tissue contrast

The basic methodological approach to these three tasks is shown in Figure 3-5. A few important points can be noted from this figure, as follows:

1. A beam of x rays is transmitted through a specific cross section of the patient. This procedure removes the problem of superimposition of structures above and below the specific cross section or slice of tissue.
2. The beam of x rays is highly collimated into a thin beam (a very narrow beam) that only passes through the cross section of tissue to be imaged. This procedure is intended to minimize scatter production and improve the contrast of the image.
3. When the x-ray beam passes through the patient, it strikes special electronic detectors positioned opposite the x-ray tube. These detectors are quantitative and can measure very small differences in tissue contrast. (However, the film-screen detector in radiography is considered a qualitative detector and cannot record these small differences.) In addition, the **analog signals** from the electronic detectors are first converted into digital data and are subsequently processed by a digital computer that uses special **algorithms** to reconstruct an image of the cross section.

# PHYSICAL PRINCIPLES

CT can be described in terms of physical principles and technological considerations. The physical principles involve physics and mathematical concepts to understand the way the image is produced, and the technological considerations involve the practical implementation of scientific and engineering principles such as computer science and technology. The physical principles and technology of CT include the three processes referred to in Chapter 1: data acquisition; data processing; and image display, storage, and communication. This section discusses each process in basic terms; they are described in more detail in later chapters.

## Data Acquisition

**Data acquisition** refers to the systematic collection of information from the patient to produce the CT image. The two methods of data acquisition are **slice-by-slice data acquisition** and **volume data acquisition** (Fig. 3-6).

In conventional slice-by-slice data acquisition, data are collected through different beam geometries to scan the patient. Essentially, the x-ray tube rotates around the patient and collects data from the first slice. The tube stops, and the patient moves into position to scan the next slice. This process continues until all slices have been individually scanned.

In volume data acquisition, a special **beam geometry** referred to as *spiral* or *helical geometry* is used to scan a volume of tissue rather than one slice at a time (Fig. 3-6). In spiral/helical CT, the x-ray tube rotates around the patient and traces a spiral/helical path to scan an entire volume of tissue while

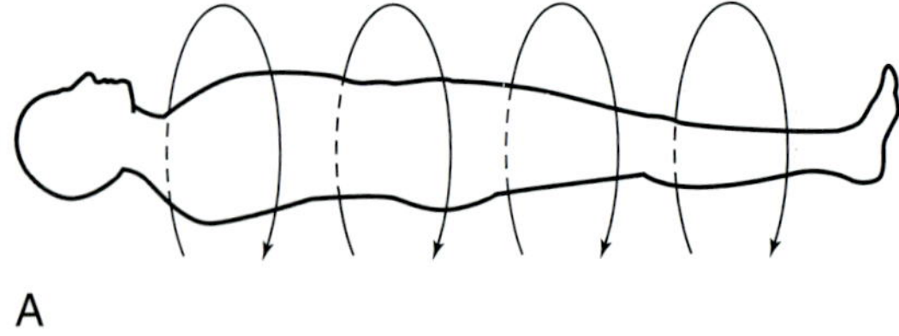
A

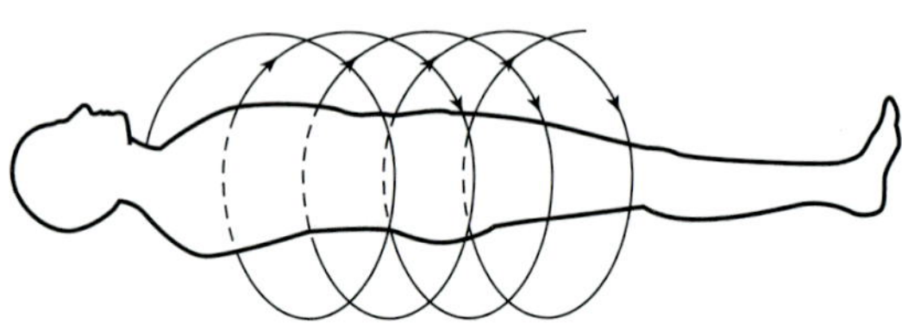
B

**FIGURE 3-6** **A,** Conventional slice-by-slice CT data acquisition. **B,** Volume CT data acquisition.

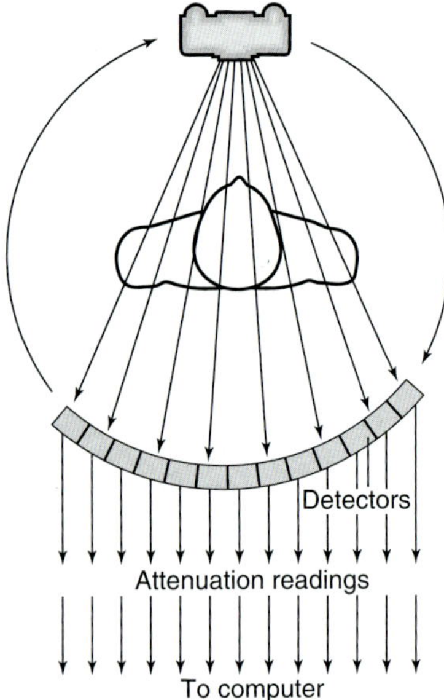


**FIGURE 3-7** During scanning, the x-ray tube and detectors rotate around the patient to collect views.

the patient holds a single breath. This method generates a single slice per one revolution of the x-ray tube and is often referred to as a single-slice spiral/helical CT (SSCT). To improve the volume coverage speed performance of SSCT, multislice spiral/helical CT (MSCT) has become available for faster imaging of patients. MSCT scanners generate multiple slices per one revolution of the x-ray tube. For example, MSCT scanners can now generate 4, 8, 16, 32, 40, 64, or 320 slices per revolution of the x-ray tube. Additionally, in 2007, an MSCT scanner that can produce 320 slices per revolution of the x-ray tube became commercially available. Furthermore, Dual Source (two x-ray tubes) CT scanners are now available in clinical CT practice. The 320-slice dynamic volume scanner and Dual Source CT scanner are described in Chapter 11.

The first step in data acquisition is **scanning** (Fig. 3-7). During scanning, the x-ray tube and detectors rotate around the patient to collect views (intensity readings). The detectors measure the radiation transmitted through the patient from various locations. As a result, **relative transmission** values (Hounsfield, 1973) or attenuation measurements (Sprawls, 1995) can be calculated as follows:

$$\text{Relative transmission} = \text{Log}\,\frac{\text{Intensity of x rays at the source } (I_0)}{\text{Intensity of x rays at the detector } (I)}$$

The relative transmission values are sent to the computer and stored as raw data.

A large number of transmission measurements are needed to reconstruct the CT image. In general, several hundred views are obtained. Each view is composed of a number of rays, and the total transmission measurements for each scan are given by the following relationship (Sprawls, 1995):

Total number of transmission measurements = Number of views × Number of rays in each view

## Radiation Attenuation-Basic Physics

The problem with CT is determining the attenuation in the tissues and using this information to reconstruct an image of the slice of tissue. The solution to this problem is complex and involves physics, mathematics, and computer science. This book takes a fundamental approach to the problem and its solution. The study begins with an understanding of attenuation of radiation in general and attenuation in CT in particular.

**Attenuation** is the reduction of the intensity of a beam of radiation as it passes through an object—some photons are absorbed, but others are scattered. Attenuation depends on the electrons per gram, atomic number, tissue density, and radiation energy used. In addition, because there are two types of radiation beams (homogeneous and heterogeneous), a study of how each of these beams is attenuated is important to understand the problem in CT. Attenuation in CT depends on the effective atomic density (atoms/volume), the atomic number ($Z$) of the absorber, and the photon energy.

In a **homogeneous beam,** all the photons have the same energy, whereas in a **heterogeneous beam** the photons have different energies. A homogeneous beam is also referred to as a *monochromatic* or *monoenergetic* beam, and a heterogeneous beam is referred to as a *polychromatic* beam.

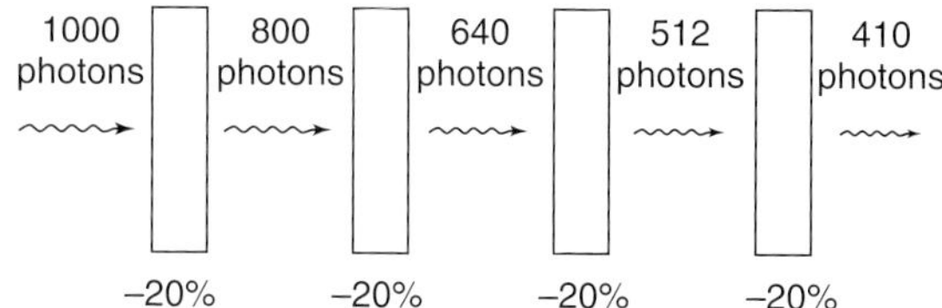


**FIGURE 3-8** Attenuation of a homogeneous beam of radiation through water. The absorber is 1 cm of water.

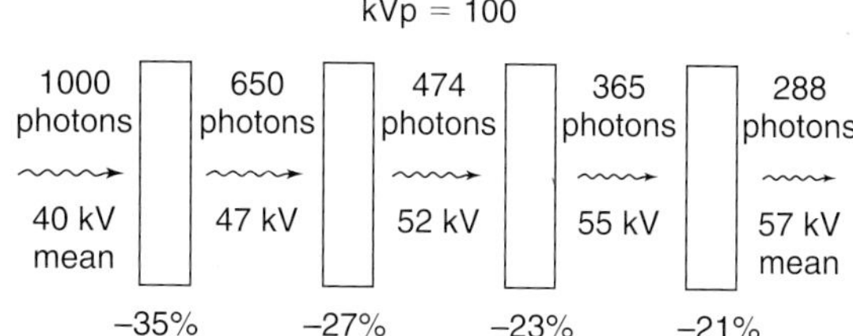


**FIGURE 3-9** Attenuation of a heterogeneous beam of radiation through water.

When Hounsfield invented the CT scanner, he used a homogeneous beam (Fig. 3-8) in his initial experiments because such a beam satisfies the requirements of the **Lambert–Beer law,** an exponential relationship that describes what happens to the photons as they travel through the tissues according to the following attenuation:

$$I = I_0 e^{-\mu x}, \quad \textbf{(3-1)}$$

where $I$ is the transmitted intensity, $I_0$ is the original intensity, $x$ is the thickness of the object, $e$ is Euler's constant (2.718), and $\mu$ is the linear attenuation coefficient.

The goal of CT is to calculate the **linear attenuation coefficient** ($\mu$), which indicates the amount of attenuation that has occurred. Therefore it is a quantitative measurement with a unit of per centimeter ($cm^{-1}$)—hence the term *linear* (Kalender, 2005).

The equation $I = I_0 e^{-\mu x}$ can be solved to find the value of $\mu$:

$$\begin{aligned} I &= I_0 e^{-\mu x} \\ I/I_0 &= e^{-\mu x} \\ \ln I/I_0 &= {}^{-\mu x} \\ \ln I/I_0 &= \mu x \\ \mu &= (1/x) \cdot (I_0/I) \end{aligned} \quad \textbf{(3-2)}$$

where *ln* is the natural logarithm. In CT, the values of $I$ and $I_0$ are known (these are measured by the detectors), and $x$ is also known. Hence $\mu$ can be calculated.

Figure 3-8 shows the attenuation of a homogeneous beam of radiation. Each section of the absorber attenuates the beam by equal amounts; that is, each 1-cm section removes 20% of the photons remaining in the beam. The initial beam intensity of 1000 photons is reduced to 410 photons; in other words, the quantity of photons is reduced. In a homogeneous beam the quality of the beam, or beam energy, does not change. If the starting beam energy is 88 kiloelectron volts (keV), the transmitted photons all have an energy of 88 keV.

In the early experiments conducted by Hounsfield, the radiation was from a gamma source and the attenuation was that of a homogeneous beam. One problem he encountered was that it took too long to scan and produce an image, and therefore he substituted a beam produced by a conventional x-ray tube. This beam is a heterogeneous beam of radiation that consists of a range of energies. The attenuation of a heterogeneous or polychromatic beam is somewhat different from that of a homogeneous beam; therefore Hounsfield had to make several assumptions and adjustments to determine the linear attenuation coefficients.

During the attenuation of a heterogeneous beam (Fig. 3-9), as the beam passes through equal thicknesses of material, the attenuation is not exponential; rather both the quantity and quality of the photons change. In Figure 3-9, the initial quantity of photons is 1000 with a mean beam quality (energy) of 40 kilovolts (kV). Each block of water removes different quantities of photons, and the mean energy of the transmitted photons increases to 57 kV. The first centimeter of water attenuates more photons than subsequent 1-cm blocks of water. Also, the lower energy photons are absorbed, which allows the higher energy photons to pass through. As a result, the penetrating power of the photons increases and the beam becomes harder.

The equation $I = I_0 e^{-\mu x}$ applies only to a homogeneous beam. It then follows that in CT, which is based on the use of a heterogeneous beam, it is necessary to make the heterogeneous beam approximate a homogeneous beam to satisfy the equation.

It was stated earlier that attenuation is the result of absorption and scattering. X rays can be attenuated because of the photoelectric effect, or they can be attenuated and scattered by the Compton effect. The total attenuation is then given by the following:

$$I = I_0 e^{-(\mu_p + \mu_c)x} \quad \textbf{(3-3)}$$

where $\mu_p$ is the linear attenuation coefficient that results from photoelectric absorption, and $\mu_c$ is the linear attenuation coefficient that results from the Compton effect.

The photoelectric effect occurs mainly in tissues with a high atomic number, $Z$ (such as bone and contrast medium), and occurs minimally in some soft tissues and substances with a lower *Z*. The Compton effect occurs in soft tissues, and differences in density result in differences in Compton interactions. In addition, the photoelectric effect depends on the beam energy (kVs); however, the Compton effect is less likely to dominate as the beam energy increases and "the **energy dependence** is not nearly as dramatic as it is with the photoelectric effect" (Morgan, 1983).

Equation 3-2, like Equation 3-1, holds true only for a homogeneous beam of radiation. If a heterogeneous beam is used in CT, how is the linear attenuation coefficient determined in CT? The concern is with the number of photons, *N*, which pass through the tissue during scanning, rather than with the intensity, *I*. Equation 3-1 can therefore be expressed as

$$N = N_0 e^{-\mu x} \quad \textbf{(3-4)}$$

where *N* is the number of transmitted photons, $N_0$ is the number of photons entering the tissue (incident photons), *x* is the thickness of the tissue, $\mu$ is $\mu_p + \mu_c$ (linear attenuation coefficients of the tissue), and e is the base of the natural logarithm.

Equation 3-3 applies to a homogeneous block of tissue. However, a slice of tissue in the patient through which the radiation passes is not homogeneous because the tissue is composed of several different substances. In this case, the slice is divided into a number of small regions, "each characterized by its own linear attenuation coefficient" (Morgan, 1983). This can be shown as

$$N_0 \rightarrow \boxed{\mu_1 \,|\, \mu_2 \,|\, \mu_3 \,|\, \mu_4 \,|\, \mu_5} \,//\, \boxed{\mu_n} \rightarrow N$$

In this situation, the linear attenuation coefficients can be determined as follows:

$$N = N_0 e^{-(\mu_1 + \mu_2 + \mu_3 + \mu_4 + \mu_5 \cdots + \mu_n)x} \quad \textbf{(3-5)}$$

## Data Acquisition Geometries

The way that the x-ray tube and detectors are arranged to collect transmission measurements describes the **data acquisition geometry** of the CT system. Two types of geometries are illustrated in Figure 3-10. In Figure 3-10, *A*, the x-ray tube and detectors are coupled and rotated 360 degrees around the patient to collect transmission measurements by using a fan beam of radiation. In Figure 3-10, *B*, the x-ray tube rotates 360 degrees around the patient and is positioned inside a stationary ring of detectors. The radiation beam also describes a fan. It is interesting to note that the geometry shown in Figure 3-10, *A*, has become commonplace in modern CT scanners.

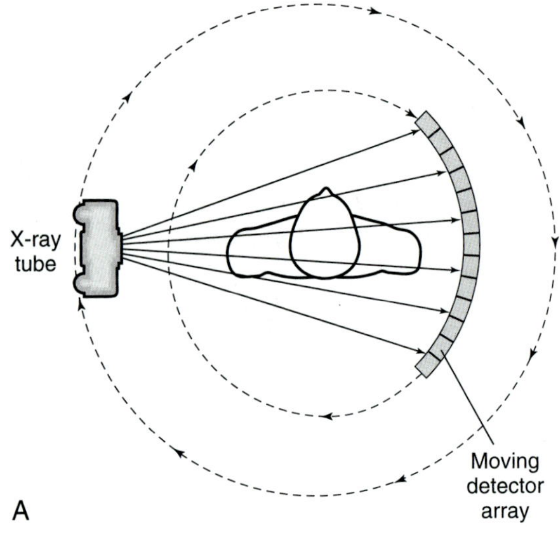


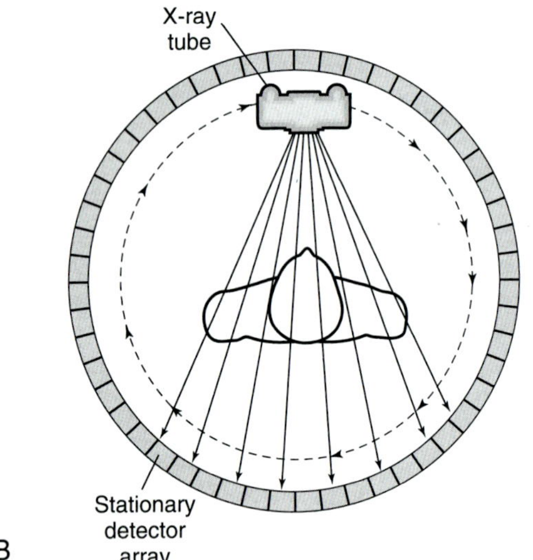


**FIGURE 3-10** Two data acquisition geometries. **A,** Continuous rotation. **B,** Stationary detectors.

## Data Processing

**Data processing** essentially constitutes the mathematical principles involved in CT. Data processing is basically a two-step process (Fig. 3-11). First, the **raw data** (data received from the detectors) undergo some form of preprocessing, in which corrections are made and some reformatting of the data occurs. This is necessary to facilitate the next step in data processing, which is **image reconstruction.** In this step, the scan data, which represent attenuation readings, are converted into a digital image characterized by **CT numbers** (Fig. 3-12).

Conversion of the attenuation readings into a CT image is accomplished by mathematical procedures referred to as *reconstruction algorithms*. These algorithms include simple **back-projection,** iterative methods, and analytic methods. For MSCT scanners

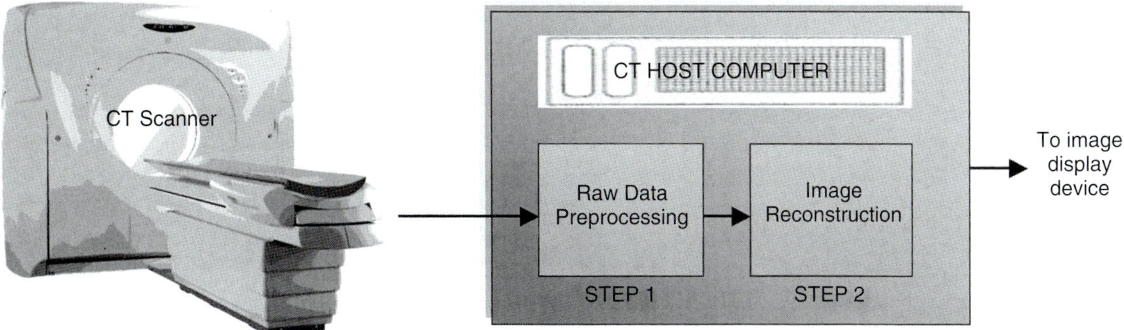


**FIGURE 3-11** The two major data processing steps in CT.

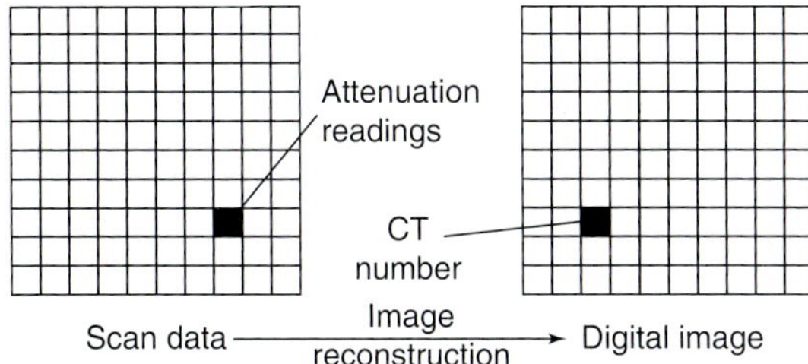


**FIGURE 3-12** Data acquired by scanning an object measures beam penetration. A digital image is created by converting these data into CT numbers.

that offer 16, 64, and 320 slices per revolution of the x-ray tube and detectors, other reconstruction algorithms referred to as **cone-beam** algorithms are used (Kalender, 2005). These algorithms are described further in Chapters 5 and 6. After data processing, the reconstructed image is displayed for viewing and subsequently sent for storage or communicated through the picture archiving and communication system (PACS) to remote sites for review by other physicians (Fig. 3-13).

## CT Numbers

As shown in Figure 3-12, each **pixel** in the reconstructed image is assigned a CT number. CT numbers are related to the linear attenuation coefficients (μ) of the tissues that comprise the slice (Table 3-1) and can be calculated as follows:

$$\text{CT number} = \frac{\mu_t - \mu_w}{\mu_w} \cdot K \qquad \textbf{(3-6)}$$

where $\mu_t$ is the attenuation coefficient of the measured tissue, $\mu_w$ is the attenuation coefficient of water, and $K$ is a constant or contrast factor.

The value of $K$ determines the **contrast factor,** or scaling factor. In the first EMI scanner, the value of $K$ was 500, which resulted in a contrast scale of 0.2% per CT number. The CT numbers obtained with a contrast factor of 500 were referred to as *EMI numbers.* Later, the contrast factor was doubled to give a factor of 1000, and the CT numbers obtained with this factor are referred to as the *Hounsfield (H) scale.* The H scale expresses μ more precisely because the contrast scale is now 0.1% per CT number. (Both the H and EMI scales are shown in Fig. 3-14). CT numbers are established on a relative basis with the attenuation of water as a reference. Thus the CT number for water is always 0, whereas those for bone and air are +1000 and −1000, respectively, on the H scale. An elaboration of the H scale for several tissues is illustrated in Figure 3-15. Note the range of CT numbers for water, air, fat, kidney, pancreas, blood, and liver.

The computer calculates the CT numbers, which can be printed as a numerical image (Fig. 3-16). This image must be converted into a grayscale image because it is more useful to the radiologist than a numerical printout. To facilitate this conversion, brightness levels that correspond with the CT numbers must be established (Fig. 3-17). In Figure 3-17, the upper (+1000) and lower (−1000) limits of the scale represent white and black, respectively. All other values represent various shades of gray.

## CT and Energy Dependence

The linear attenuation coefficient (μ) is affected by several factors, including the energy of the radiation or energy dependence. For example, the linear attenuation coefficients for water at 60, 84, and 122 keV are 0.206, 0.180, and 0.166, respectively. It then follows that photon energy also affects CT numbers because they can be calculated on the basis of the attenuation coefficients by the equation

$$\ln I_0/I = \int \mu\,(E,x)\,dx \qquad \textbf{(3-7)}$$

In this summation equation, $E$ represents the photon energy and demonstrates that the attenuation coefficient changes with the beam energy.

In the original CT scanner, CT numbers were calculated on the basis of 73 keV, which is the effective

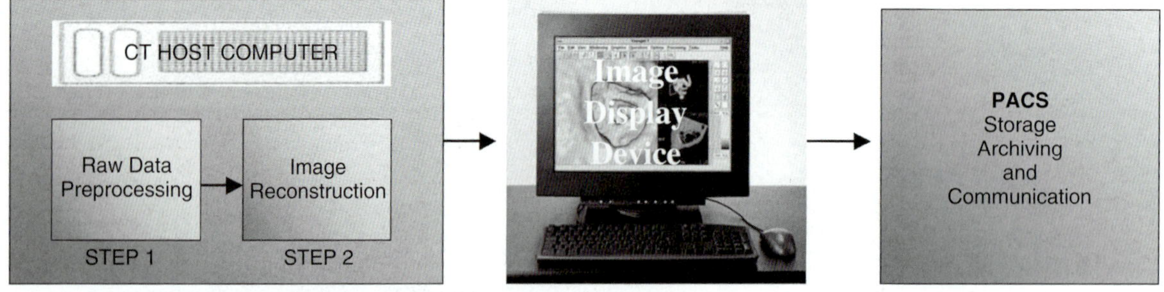


**FIGURE 3-13** The reconstructed CT image is displayed for viewing and subsequently sent for storage or communicated by the PACS to physicians at remote sites.

**TABLE 3-1 Linear Attenuation Coefficients for Various Body Tissues***

| Tissues | Linear Attenuation Coefficient ($cm^{-1}$) |
|---|---|
| Bone | 0.528 |
| Blood | 0.208 |
| Gray matter | 0.212 |
| White matter | 0.213 |
| Cerebrospinal fluid | 0.207 |
| Water | 0.206 |
| Fat | 0.185 |
| Air | 0.0004 |

*At 60 keV.

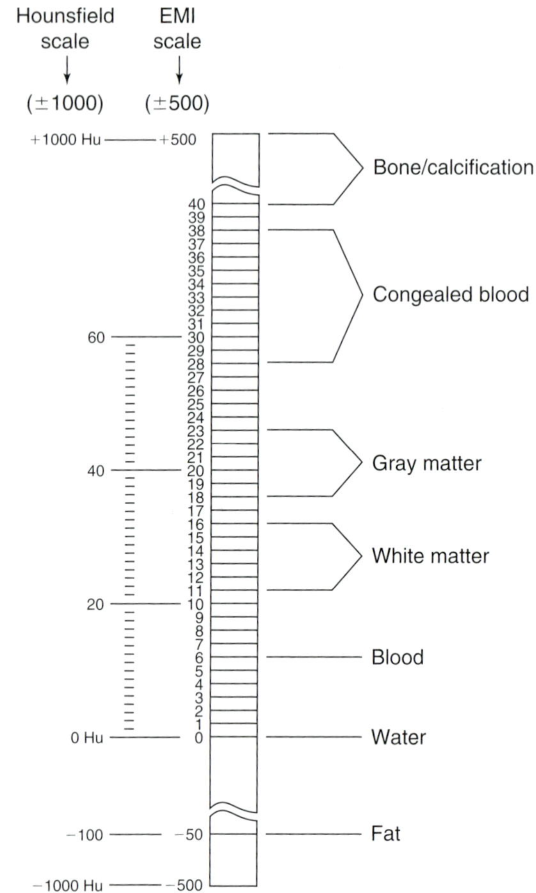


**FIGURE 3-14** Distribution of CT numbers on the Hounsfield and EMI scales. (From Seeram, E. (2001). *Computed tomography technology*. Philadelphia, PA: WB Saunders.)

energy of a 230 peak kilovolt beam after passing through 27 cm of water (Zatz, 1981). At 73 keV, the linear attenuation coefficient for water is 0.19 $cm^{-1}$. For example, if the linear attenuation coefficients for bone and water are 0.38 and 0.19 $cm^{-1}$, respectively, and the scaling factor (K) of the scanner is 1000, the CT numbers for bone and water can be calculated:

$$CT_{bone} = \frac{\mu_{bone} - \mu_{water}}{\mu_{water}} \cdot K$$
$$= \frac{0.38-0.19}{0.19} \cdot 1000$$
$$= \frac{0.19}{0.19} \cdot 1000$$
$$= 1000$$

Thus the CT number for bone is 1000. Thus the CT number for water is 0.

In CT, a high-kilovolt technique (about 120 kV) is generally used for the following reasons:

1. To reduce the dependence of attenuation coefficients on photon energy
2. To reduce the contrast of bone relative to soft tissues
3. To produce a high radiation flux at the detector

These reasons are important to ensure optimum detector response (e.g., to reduce **artifacts** caused by changes in skull thickness, which can conceal small changes in attenuation in soft tissues, and to minimize artifacts resulting from **beam-hardening** effects).

CT numbers may vary because of their energy dependence. It is therefore essential that the CT system ensure the accuracy and reliability of these numbers because the consequences can be disastrous and might lead to a misdiagnosis. The system

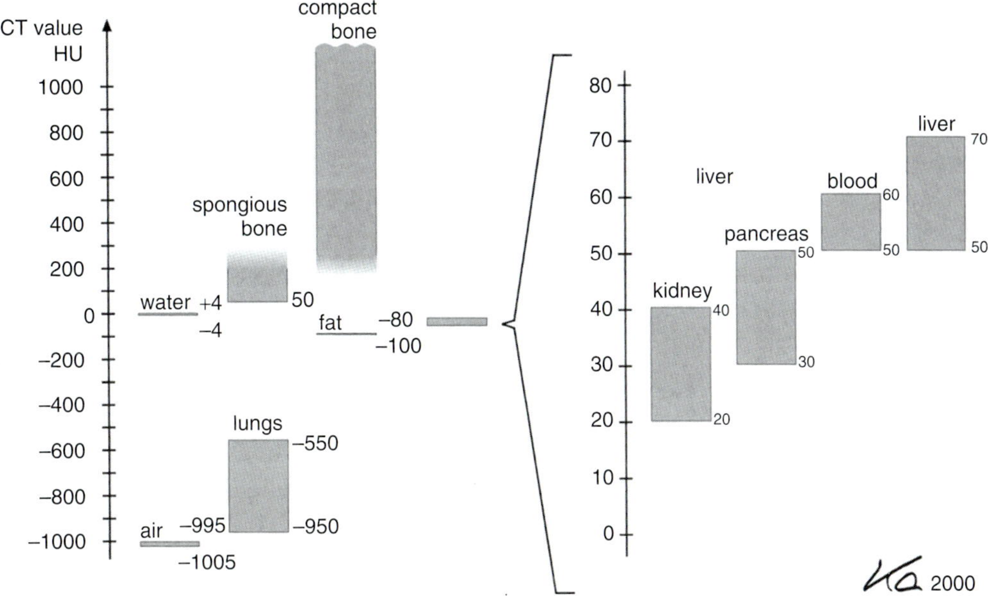


**FIGURE 3-15** An elaboration of the Hounsfield scale for several tissues not shown in Figure 3-14. (From Kalender, W. A. (2005). *Computed tomography* (2nd ed.). Erlangen, Germany: Publicis Kommunikations Agentur Gmbh; © 2005 by Publicis Kommunikations Agentur GmbH, GWA, Erlangen, Germany. Reproduced by permission.)

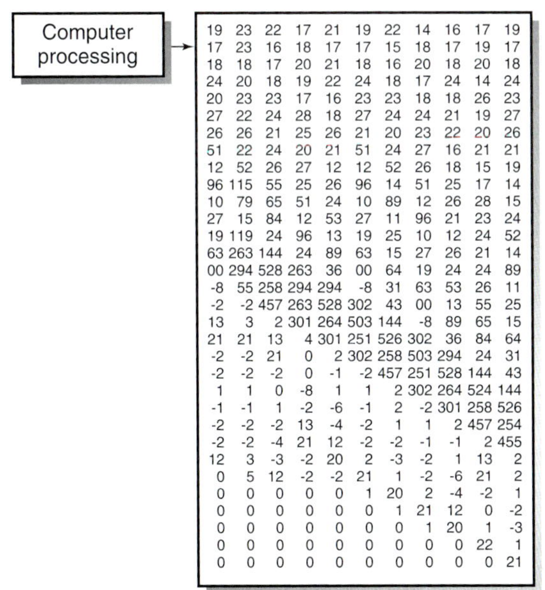


**FIGURE 3-16** Appearance of the CT image after computer processing. This is a numerical printout of the processed image.

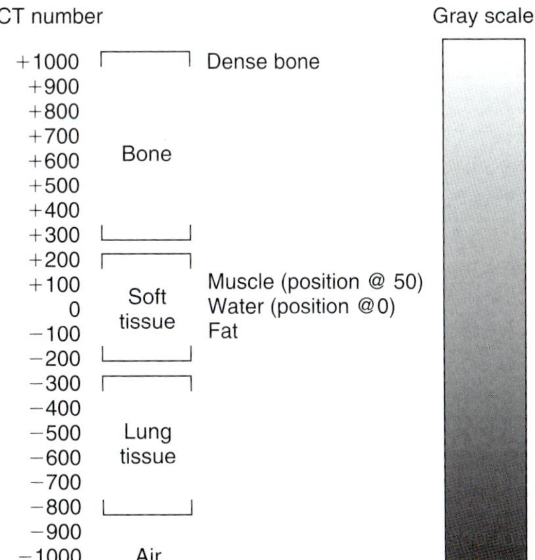


**FIGURE 3-17** The relationship between CT number and the brightness level.

incorporates a number of correction schemes to maintain the precision of the CT numbers.

## Image Display, Storage, and Communication

The third and final step in the CT process involves image display, storage, and communication. After the CT image has been reconstructed, it exits the computer in digital form (Figs. 3-12 and 3-16). This must be converted to a form that is suitable for viewing and meaningful to the observer (Seeram & Seeram, 2008).

***Display device.*** The grayscale image is displayed on a television monitor (Cathode ray tube [CRT]) or liquid crystal display, which is an essential component of the control or viewing console (Fig. 3-13).

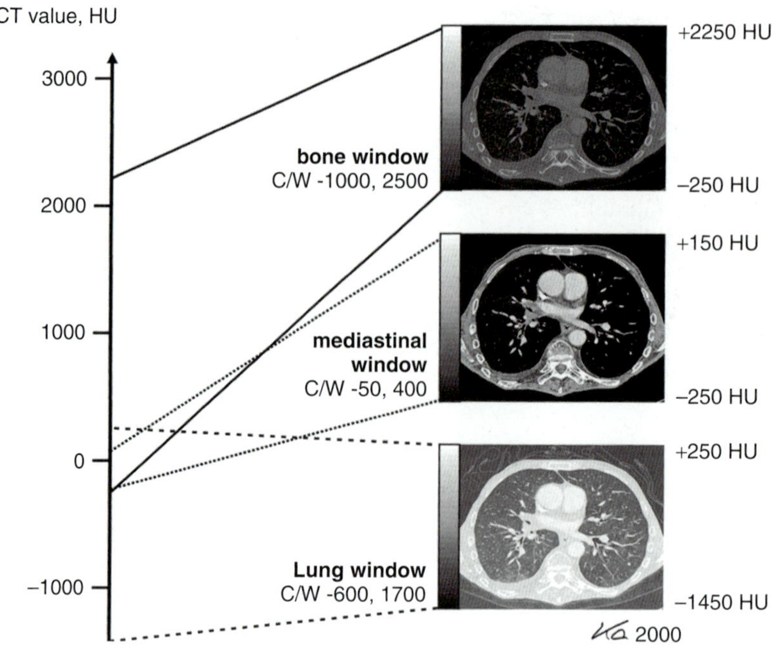


**FIGURE 3-18** Windowing is a digital image postprocessing operation intended to alter the image contrast (a function of the WW) and the image brightness (a function of the window center, C, or WL, as it is often referred). (From Kalender, W. A. (2005). *Computed tomography* (2nd ed.). Erlangen, Germany: Publicis Kommunikations Agentur GmbH; 2005 by Publicis Kommunikations Agentur GmbH, GWA, Erlangen, Germany. Reproduced by permission.)

In the display and manipulation of grayscale images for diagnosis, it is important to optimize image fidelity (i.e., the faithfulness with which the device can display the image). This is influenced by physical characteristics such as luminance, resolution, **noise,** and **dynamic range.** These topics are beyond the scope of this chapter.

Resolution, however, is an important physical parameter of the grayscale display monitor and is related to the size of the pixel **matrix,** or matrix size. The display matrix can range from 64 × 64 to 1024 × 1024, but high-performance monitors can display an image with a 2048 × 2048 matrix (Dwyer et al., 1992).

***Windowing.*** The CT image is composed of a range of CT numbers (e.g., +1000 to −1000, for a total of 2000 numbers) that represent varying shades of gray (Fig. 3-17). The range of numbers is referred to as the **window width (WW),** and the center of the range is the **window level (WL)** or *window center* (C). Both the WW and WL are located on the control console. These controls can alter the image contrast and brightness. With a WW of 2000 and a WL of 0, the entire grayscale is displayed and the ability of the observer to perceive small differences in soft tissue attenuation will be lost, because the human eye can perceive only about 40 shades of gray (Castleman, 1994).

The process of changing the CT image grayscale in this way is referred to as **windowing** (Fig. 3-18). Although the WW controls the image contrast, the WL or C controls the image brightness. As can be seen in Figure 3-18, as the WL or C increases the image goes from white (bright) to dark (less bright) and the image contrast changes for different values of WWs. The image contrast is optimized for the anatomy under study; therefore, specified values of WW and WL or C must be used during the initial scanning of the patient. Note that in Figure 3-18 three windows are shown: the bone window (optimized for imaging bone), the **mediastinal** window (optimized for imaging the mediastinal structures), and the lung window (optimized for imaging the lungs). Windowing is described in detail in a later chapter.

## Format of the CT Image

The original clinical CT images were composed of an 80 × 80 matrix for a total of 6400 pixels. The size of the matrix is chosen by the technologist before the CT examination and depends on the anatomy under study. The technologist must select the **field of view (FOV)** or reconstruction circle, which is a circular region from which the transmission measurements are recorded during scanning. This region is specifically referred to as the *scan FOV.*

During data collection and image reconstruction, a matrix is placed over the scan FOV to cover the slice to be imaged. In general, a technologist can

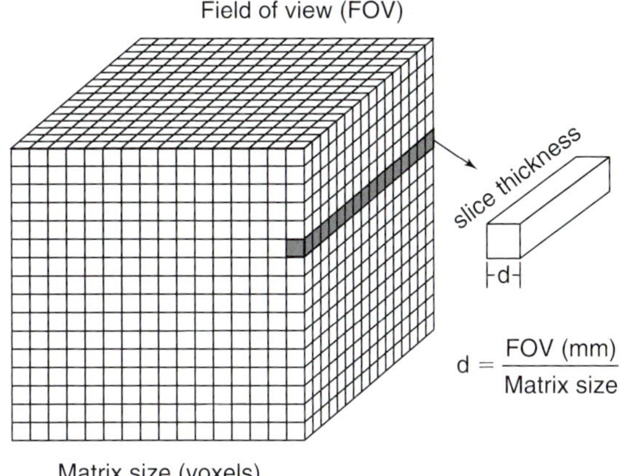


**FIGURE 3-19** Voxel size depends on slice thickness, matrix size, and FOV.

select the FOV appropriate to the examination within three to four scan FOVs.

Because the slice to be scanned has the dimension of depth, the pixel is transformed into a voxel, or volume element. The radiation beam passes through each voxel and a CT number is then generated for each pixel in the displayed image. The display FOV can be equal to or less than the scan FOV.

The **pixel size** can be computed from the FOV and the matrix size through the following relationship:

$$\text{Pixel size},\ d = \text{field of view/matrix size}$$

For example, if the reconstruction circle (FOV) is 25 cm and the matrix size is $512^2$, the pixel size can be determined as follows:

$$\begin{aligned} \textit{Pixel size} &= 25.10\ \text{mm} / 512 \\ &= 25.10\ \text{mm} / 512 \\ &= 0.488\ \text{mm} \\ &= 0.49\ \text{mm} \\ &= 0.5\ \text{mm} \end{aligned}$$

The pixel size generally ranges from 1 mm to 10 mm on most scanners. Thus voxel size depends not only on the thickness of the slice but also on the matrix size and the FOV (Fig. 3-19). When the voxel dimensions of length, width, and height are equal, that is, describe a perfect cube, the imaging process is referred to as *isotropic imaging* (see Chapters 1 and 11).

Finally, each pixel in the CT image can have a range of gray shades. The image can have 256 ($2^8$), 512 ($2^9$), 1024 ($2^{10}$), or 2048 ($2^{11}$) different grayscale values. Because these numbers are represented as bits, a CT image can be characterized by the number of bits per pixel. CT images can have 8, 9, 10, 11, or 12

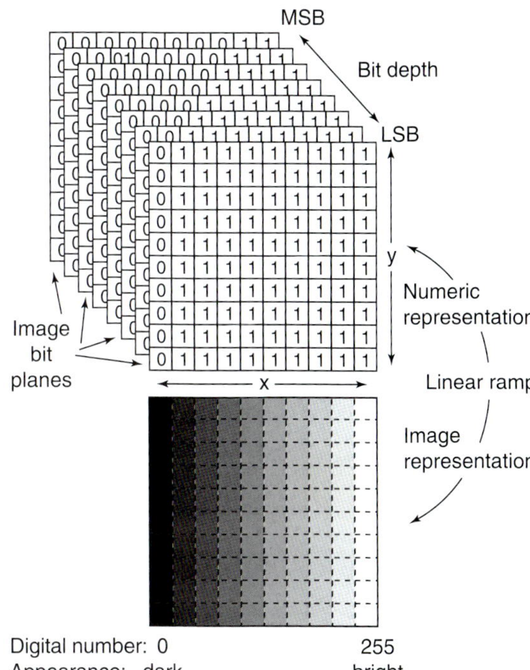


**FIGURE 3-20** Representation of the digital image as a stack of bit planes. Encoding of the least significant bit (LSB) to the most significant bit (MSB) as bit planes is shown. The corresponding grayscale image indicates digital value and brightness relationships. (From Seibert, J. A. (1995). Digital image processing basics. In S. Balter, & T. B. Shope (Eds.), *RSNA categorical course in physics: physical and technical aspects of angiography and interventional radiology*. Oak Brook, IL: RSNA.)

bits per pixel. The image therefore consists of a series of **bit** planes referred to as the *bit depth* (Fig. 3-20; Seibert, 1995). The numerical value of the pixel represents the brightness of the image at that pixel position. A 12-bits-per-pixel CT image would represent numbers ranging from −1000 to 3095 for a total of 4096 ($2^{12}$) different shades of gray (Barnes & Lakshminarayanan, 1989).

## TECHNOLOGICAL CONSIDERATIONS

The ultimate goal of a CT scanner is to produce high-quality CT images with minimal radiation dose and physical discomfort to the patient. Whether this is achieved depends on the design of the CT system, which influences the performance of the system's components. In this section, *design* refers to the technology necessary to produce a CT image.

The technology of a CT scanner encompasses a number of subsystems (Fig. 3-21). The major subsystems are described briefly to demonstrate the flow of data through the system.

## Data Flow in a CT Scanner

The subsystems shown in Figure 3-21 include the x-ray tube, power supply, and cooling system; beam geometry, defined by collimators and characterized by tube scanning motion; and detectors, detector electronics, **preprocessors, host computer** with fast-access memory, **high-speed array processors,** digital image processor, storage, display, and system control.

The flow of data from Figure 3-21 is summarized in Figure 3-22. The language that describes some of the events (e.g., **convolution** and *back-projection*) is explained further in subsequent chapters.

## Sequence of Events

The events represented in the data flow are as follows:

1. The x-ray tube and detectors rotate around the patient, who is positioned in the **gantry** aperture for the CT examination. This step is characterized by the beam geometry and method of scanning and involves the passage of x rays through the patient. The x-ray beam is highly collimated by prepatient collimators.
2. The radiation is attenuated as it passes through the patient. The transmitted photons are measured by two sets of detectors; a reference detector, which measures the intensity of radiation from the x-ray tube; and another set that records x-ray transmission through the patient.
3. The transmitted beam and reference beam are both converted into electrical current signals that are amplified by special circuits. This is followed by logarithmic amplification, in which the relative transmission readings ($I_0/I$) are changed into **attenuation** ($\mu$) and thickness ($x$) data through the use of Equation 3-2:

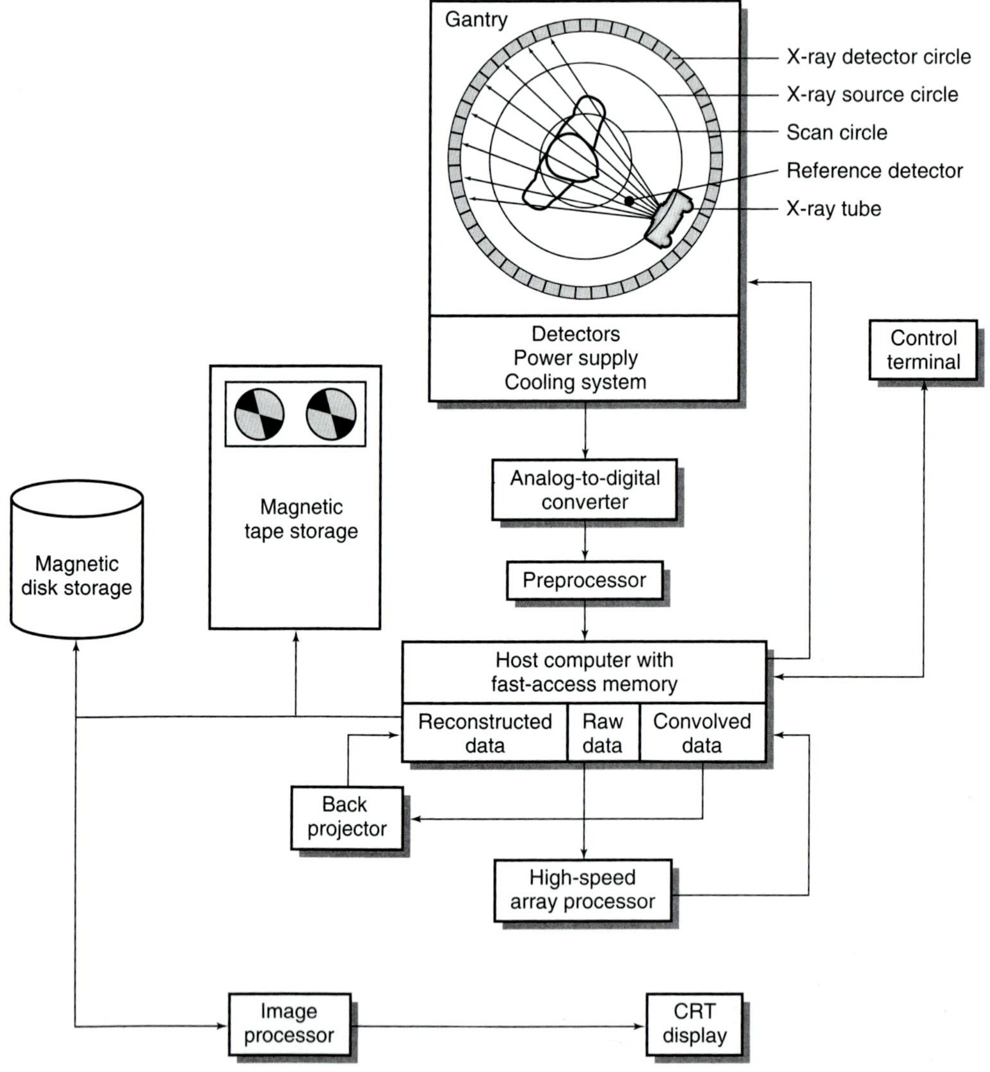


**FIGURE 3-21** Fourth-generation CT scanner configuration with major subsystems. (From Huang, H. K. (2004). *PACS and imaging informatics.* Hoboken, NJ: John Wiley.)

$$\mu = \frac{1}{x} \ln I_0/I$$

4. Before the data are sent to the computer, they must be converted into digital form. This is done by the **analog-to-digital converters,** or *digitizers.* Steps 2, 3, and 4 constitute the second step in the data acquisition process.
5. Data processing begins. The digital data undergo some form of preprocessing, which includes corrections and reformatting. "Some of the corrections to the data will include subtraction of the air reference detector signal to normalize the attenuation data, obtaining local averages of detectors to determine if any detectors are outside a predetermined standard deviation which help locate bad detectors, and corrections due to dead time losses (i.e., detection **response time** losses) by the individual detectors" (Huang, 2004). The data are now referred to as *reformatted raw data.* Additional data corrections are performed on the data by using computer software.
6. As shown in Figure 3-22, convolution is performed on the data by the array processors.
7. The specific reconstruction algorithm then reconstructs an image of the internal anatomic structures under examination.
8. The reconstructed image can then be displayed or stored on magnetic or optical tape or disks.
9. The image processor shown in Figure 3-21 allows the performance of various digital image **post-processing operations** on the displayed image (Seeram & Seeram, 2008). Figure 3-21 does not show the **digital-to-analog converter,** a component positioned between the image processor and the CRT display or between the host computer and control terminal, which has a CRT display unit.
10. The control terminal is usually an operator's control console, which completely controls the CT system.

## ADVANTAGES AND LIMITATIONS OF CT

### Advantages

The main advantages of CT stem from the fact that the technique overcomes the limitations of radiography and conventional tomography. Compared with radiography and conventional tomography, CT offers the following advantages:

1. Excellent **low-contrast resolution** is possible because (1) a highly collimated beam is used to take an image of a cross-sectional slice of the patient and (2) more sensitive radiation detectors (compared with film-screen or digital radiography detectors) are used to measure the radiation transmitted through the slice. CT offers the best low-contrast resolution compared with radiography, nuclear medicine, and ultrasonography. For example, the contrast resolution (in millimeters at 0.5% difference) for CT is 4 compared to 10, 10, and 20 for radiography, ultrasonography, and nuclear medicine, respectively. It is interesting to note here that the contrast resolution (mm at 0.5% difference) for **magnetic resonance imaging (MRI)** is 1 (Bushong, 2013).

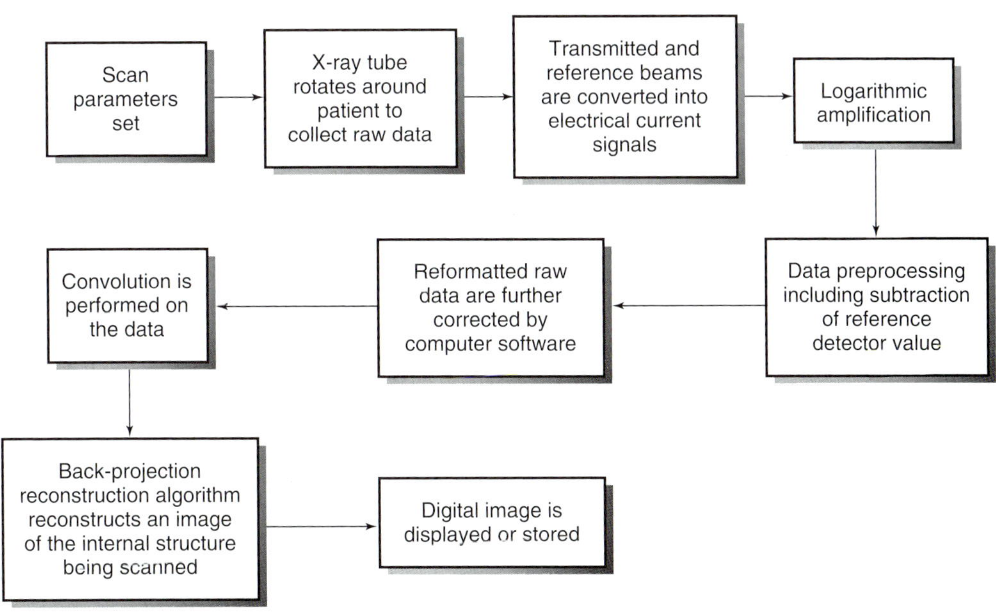


**FIGURE 3-22** Data flow in a CT system.

2. By changing the WW and WL settings in image windowing, the contrast scale of the image can be varied to suit the needs of the observer (Seeram, 2004; Seeram & Seeram, 2008).
3. With spiral/helical volume data acquisition, CT scanning in spiral/helical geometry has overcome several limitations of conventional start–stop acquisition. Its advantages include volume data acquisition in a single breath rather than slice-by-slice acquisition, improvements in 3D imaging, multiplanar image reformatting, and other applications, such as continuous imaging, **CT angiography,** and virtual reality imaging, or CT endoscopy.
4. CT has made available a variety of techniques intended to facilitate the diagnostic process such as xenon CT (the use of inhaled stable xenon to study blood flow), quantitative CT (determination of bone mineral content), dynamic CT (rapid-sequence CT scanning to study physiology), perfusion CT, and high **spatial resolution** CT scanning to optimize the spatial resolution. In addition, CT can assist in radiation treatment planning. Additionally, CT can be coupled to single-photon **emission CT** (SPECT) and **positron emission tomography (PET) scanners** to produce fused SPECT/CT (Jones et al., 2013) and PET/CT images, in an effort to provide more information about the patient's medical condition.
5. Regarding image manipulation and analysis, the digital nature of the CT image makes it a candidate for digital **image processing.** Through the application of certain image-processing algorithms, the image can be modified to enhance its information content or analyzed to obtain information about the shape and texture of lesions.
6. CT now produces 3D images routinely. These images are intended to enhance image information content and improve the diagnostic interpretation skills of the radiologist. 3D imaging is described in detail in Chapter 13.

### Limitations

CT is not without its limitations. Compared with radiography and tomography, the following disadvantages can be noted:

1. The spatial resolution (line pairs per millimeter) of CT is "notably poorer" (Hendee & Ritenour, 1992) compared with radiography. For example, the spatial resolution for CT is 2. For nuclear medicine, ultrasonography, and MRI, the spatial resolution is 0.1, 0.25, and 2, respectively.
2. The dose in CT is generally higher for similar anatomic regions, although significant efforts have been made to reduce and optimize the dose to the patient (see Chapter 10).
3. In CT, it is difficult to image anatomic regions in which soft tissues are surrounded by large amounts of bone, such as the posterior fossa, spinal cord, pituitary, and the interpetrous space (Oldendorf & Oldendorf, 1991). The imaging process may create artifacts that may obscure diagnosis.
4. The presence of metallic objects on the patient produces streak artifacts on CT images. CT also creates other artifacts not common to radiography, and several efforts have recently been made to reduce these artifacts.

These limitations have not hindered the development of CT or restricted its use. Instead, they have opened avenues for problem solving and research. At present, CT continues to be a useful diagnostic tool in medicine, and more and more research is under way to improve the performance of CT scanners (Kalender, 2005; Mori et al., 2006; Mutic et al., 2004; Seeram, 2014).

## REVIEW QUESTIONS

Answer the following questions to check your understanding of the materials studied.

1. Which of the following is a shortcoming of radiography?
   A. image blur due to tube motion
   B. contrast degradation since low kVP techniques are used
   C. superimposition of structures
   D. the presence of ghost images due to tube movement
2. CT overcomes the limitations of radiography and tomography by:
   A. reducing the problem of superimposition.
   B. improving the contrast of the image.
   C. using quantitative detectors.
   D. all are correct.
3. Data acquisition in CT refers to:
   A. acquiring information from the CT detectors.
   B. acquiring information from the computer.
   C. acquiring data from the patient through a systematic motion of the x-ray tube and detectors.
   D. all are correct.
4. Which of the following is used to calculate relative transmission or penetration measurements?
   A. log of the ratio of intensity of x rays at the x-ray tube ($I_o$) to the intensity of the detector (I)
   B. log of $I/I_o$
   C. log of $I \times I_o$
   D. $I/I_o$

## REVIEW QUESTIONS—cont'd

5. Attenuation of a beam of radiation depends on:
   A. atomic number.
   B. density and electrons/gm of tissue.
   C. the energy of the radiation.
   D. all are correct.
6. Which of the following represents Lambert–Beer law?
   A. $I = I_o e^{-\mu x}$
   B. $I = I_o^{-\mu x}$
   C. $I_o = I_e^{-\mu x}$
   D. $I = I_o / e^{-\mu x}$
7. Which of the following represents Lambert–Beer law?
   A. CT number = $\mu_{water} + \mu_{tissue} \times k$
   B. CT number = $\mu_{tissue} - \mu_{water} \times k / \mu_{tissue}$
   C. CT number = $\mu_{water} - \mu_{tissue} \times k / \mu_{water}$
   D. CT number = $\mu_{tissue} - \mu_{water} \times k / \mu_{water}$
8. The range of CT numbers is called the:
   A. window width.
   B. window level.
   C. field of view.
   D. dynamic range.
9. Convolved data are:
   A. reformatted raw data.
   B. data that have been filtered.
   C. data from the preprocessor.
   D. data from the back projector.
10. Data from the CT detectors are first sent to the:
    A. array processor.
    B. host computer.
    C. back projector.
    D. preprocessor.

## REFERENCES


Barnes, G. T., & Lakshminarayanan, A. V. (1989). Computed tomography: physical principles and image quality considerations. In J. T. Lee, et al. (Ed.), *Computed tomography with MRI correlation* (2nd ed.). New York: Raven Press.

Bocage, E. M. (1974). Patent No. 536, 464, Paris. Quoted in Massiot J: History of tomography. *Medicamundi, 19*, 106–115.

Bushong, S. (2013). *Magnetic resonance imaging—physical and biological principles* (3rd ed.). St. Louis, MO: Mosby.

Castleman, K. R. (1994). *Digital image processing* (2nd ed.). Upper Saddle, NJ: Prentice Hall.

Dwyer, S. J., Stewart, B. K., Sayre, J. W., et al. (1992). Performance characteristics and image fidelity of gray-scale monitors. *Radiographics, 12*, 765–772.

Hendee, W. R., & Ritenour, E. R. (1992). *Medical imaging physics* (3rd ed.). St. Louis, MO: Mosby.

Hounsfield, G. H. (1973). Computerized transverse axial scanning (tomography), I: description of the system. *British Journal of Radiology, 46*, 1016–1022.

Huang, H. K. (2004). *PACS and imaging informatics.* Hoboken, NJ: John Wiley.

Jones, D. W., Hogg, P., & Seeram, E. (Eds.). (2013). *Practical SPECT/CT in nuclear medicine.* London: Springer.

Kalender, W. (2005). *Computed tomography—fundamentals, system technology, image quality, applications.* Erlangen, Germany: Publicis Corporate Publishing.

Marshall, C. H. (1976). Principles of computed tomography. *Postgraduate Medicine, 59*, 105–109.

Morgan, C. L. (1983). *Basic principles of computed tomography.* Baltimore, MD: University Park Press.

Mori, S., Endo, M., Nishizawa, K., Murase, K., Fujiwara, H., & Tanada, S. (2006). Comparison of patient doses in 256-slice CT and 16-slice CT scanners. *British Journal of Radiology, 79*, 56–61.

Mutic, S., Palta, J. R., Butker, E. K., et al. (2004). Quality assurance for computed tomography simulators and computed tomography simulation process: report of the AAPM Radiation Therapy Committee Task Group No 66. *Medica Physica, 30*, 2762–2792.

Oldendorf, W., & Oldendorf, W., Jr. (1991). *MRI primer.* New York: Raven Press.

Seeram, E. (1982). *Computed tomography technology.* Philadelphia, PA: WB Saunders.

Seeram, E. (2001). *Computed tomography technology.* Philadelphia, PA: WB Saunders.

Seeram, E. (2004). Digital image processing. *Radiologic Technology, 75*, 435–455.

Seeram, E. (2014). CT dose optimization. *Radiologic Technology, 85*, 655–675.

Seeram, E., & Seeram, D. (2008). Image postprocessing in digital radiology: a primer for technologists. *Journal of Medical Imaging and Radiation Sciences, 39*, 23–41.

Seibert, J. A. (1995). Digital image processing basics. In S. Balter, & T. B. Shope (Eds.), *RSNA categorical course in physics: physical and technical aspects of angiography and interventional radiology.* Oak Brook, IL: Radiological Society of North America.

Sprawls, P. (1995). *Physical principles of medical imaging* (2nd ed.). Rockville, MD: Aspen.

Ter-Pogossian, M. M., Phelps, M. E., Hoffman, E. J., & Eichling, J. O. (1974). The extraction of the yet unused wealth of information in diagnostic radiology. *Radiology, 113*, 515–520.

Vallebona, A. (1931). Radiography with great enlargement (microradiography) and a technical method for radiographic dissociation of the shadow. *Radiology, 17*, 340–341.

Zatz, L. M. (1981). Basic principles of computed tomography scanning. In T. H. Newton, & D. G. Potts (Eds.), *Radiology of the skull and brain.* St. Louis, MO: Mosby.

# 4

# Data Acquisition Concepts

## OUTLINE



## LEARNING OBJECTIVES

On completion of this chapter, you should be able to:

1. identify the basic components of a typical data acquisition scheme used in CT scanning.
2. explain each of the following:
   - scanning
   - ray
   - view
   - projection profile
   - data sample.
3. describe the essential characteristics of five generations of CT data acquisition geometries.
4. compare and contrast two types of slip-ring systems for use in CT scanners.
5. describe the elements of an x-ray generator used in CT.
6. outline the main features of x-ray tubes, filtration, and collimation in CT.
7. describe recent design innovations in CT x-ray tubes.
8. describe briefly what is meant by each of the following characteristics of CT detectors:
   - efficiency
   - stability
   - response time
   - dynamic range.
9. outline the principles of each of the following types of detectors:
   - scintillation detectors
   - gas-ionization detectors.
10. outline the essential design innovations in CT detectors and detector electronics.
11. state the purpose of the DAS and explain how it works.
12. outline briefly the essential elements of three methods of increasing the number of samples (transmission measurements) needed for image reconstruction in CT.

## KEY TERMS TO WATCH FOR AND REMEMBER

The following key terms/concepts are important to your understanding of this chapter.

**absorption efficiency**
**adaptive section collimation**
**afterglow**
**beam geometry**
**capture efficiency**
**collimation**
**continuous rotation**
**data acquisition system (DAS)**
**data sample**
**dynamic range**
**efficiency**
**electron beam CT scanner (EBCT scanner)**
**filtration**
**gas-ionization detectors**
**high-frequency generator**
**high-voltage slip-ring system**
**low-voltage slip-ring system**
**projection profile**
**ray**
**response time**
**scintillation detectors**
**spiral-helical scanning**
**stability**
**view**
**x-ray tube**
**z-flying focal spot technique**

## BASIC SCHEME FOR DATA ACQUISITION

In computed tomography (CT), transmission measurements, or projection data, are systematically collected from the patient. Several schemes are available for such data collection, each based on a specific "geometrical pattern of scanning" (Villafana, 1987).

Data acquisition refers to the method by which the patient is scanned to obtain enough data for image reconstruction. *Scanning* is defined by the beam geometry, which characterizes the particular CT system and also plays a central role in spatial resolution and artifact production.

Two elements in a basic scheme for data acquisition (Fig. 4-1) are the beam geometry and the components comprising the scheme. Beam geometry refers to the size, shape, and motion of the beam and its path, and *components* refer to those physical devices that shape and define the beam, measure its transmission through the patient, and convert this information into digital data for input into the computer.

The following points should be noted from Figure 4-1:

1. The x-ray tube and detector are in perfect alignment.
2. The tube and detector scan the patient to collect a large number of transmission measurements.
3. The beam is shaped by a special filter as it leaves the tube.
4. The beam is collimated to pass through only the slice of interest.
5. The beam is attenuated by the patient and the transmitted photons are then measured by the detector.
6. The detector converts the x-ray photons into an electrical signal (analog data).
7. These signals are converted by the analog-to-digital converter (ADC) into digital data.
8. The digital data are sent to the computer for image reconstruction.

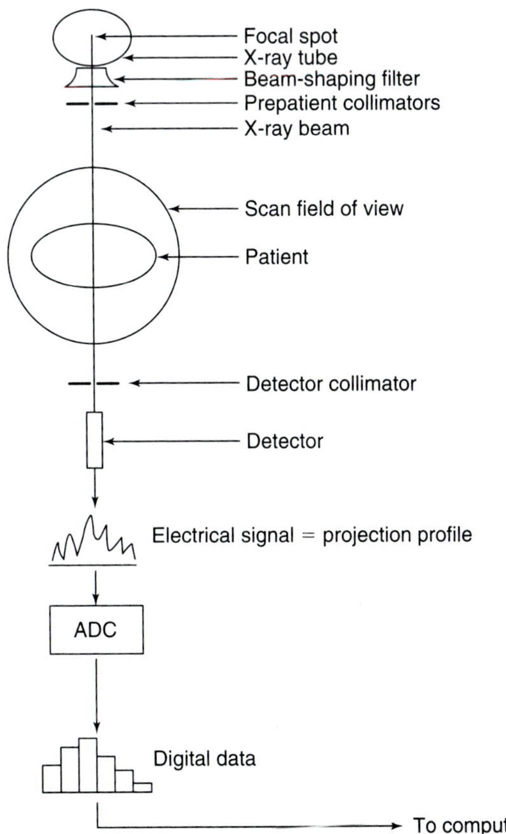


**FIGURE 4-1** Basic data acquisition scheme in CT.

## Terminology

Consider the first data acquisition scheme used by Hounsfield (1973) and others early in the development of CT (Fig. 4-2). The **x-ray tube** and detector move across the object or patient in a straight line, or translate, to collect several transmission measurements. After the first translation, the tube and detector rotate by 1 degree to collect more measurements. This sequence is repeated until data are collected for at least 180 degrees for one slice of the anatomy. Scanning also includes the movement of the patient through the **gantry** to scan the next slice. This sequence is repeated until all slices have been scanned.

The x-ray beam that emanates from the tube consists of several rays. In CT, a **ray** is the part of the beam that falls on one detector. In Figure 4-2, the line from the x-ray tube to the detector is considered a single ray, and a collection of these rays for one translation across the object constitutes a **view**.

Projection data are collected by the detector because each ray is attenuated by the patient and subsequently transmitted and projected on the detector. The detector in turn generates an electrical signal, which represents a signature of the **attenuation** as the ray moves across the slice. This signal represents a profile. Although a view generates a profile, a ray generates only a small part of the profile. In addition, each transmission measurement is referred to as a **data sample**.

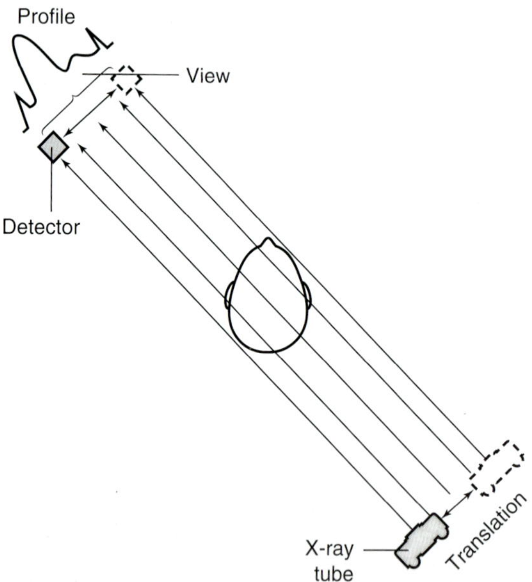


**FIGURE 4-2** In CT, a *ray* is the part of the x-ray beam that falls onto one detector. A *view* is a collection of these rays for one translation across the object. The view generates what is called a *profile*.

The production of a CT image of one slice of the anatomy requires a large set of data samples taken at different locations to satisfy the image reconstruction process. The total number of data samples ($DS_{total}$) per scan is given by the following expression:

$$DS_{total} = \text{number of detectors} \cdot \text{number of data samples per detector} \quad (4\text{-}1)$$

or

$$DS_{total} = \text{number of data samples per view} \cdot \text{number of views} \quad (4\text{-}2)$$

## DATA ACQUISITION GEOMETRIES

Three primary types of acquisition geometries are *parallel beam geometry*, *fan beam geometry*, and CT scanning in *spiral or helical geometry*, which is the most recently developed geometry. As a result, a simple categorization of CT equipment has evolved based on the scanning geometry, scanning motion, and number of detectors, as follows (Fig. 4-3):

1. *First-generation* scanners were based on the parallel beam geometry and translate-rotate scanning motion.

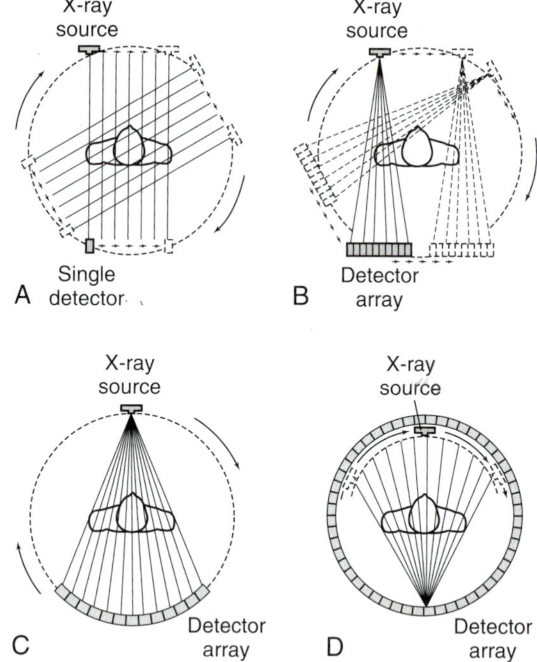


**FIGURE 4-3** The geometries of the first four generations of CT scanners. **A,** First generation, parallel beam, translate, and rotate. **B,** Second generation, fan beam, translate, and rotate. **C,** Third generation, fan beam and rotate only. **D,** Fourth generation, fan beam and stationary circular detector.

2. *Second-generation* scanners were based on the fan beam geometry and translate-rotate motion.
3. *Third-generation* scanners were based on fan beam geometry and complete rotation of the tube and detectors.
4. *Fourth-generation* scanners were based on fan beam geometry and complete rotation of the x-ray tube around a stationary ring of detectors.
5. *Fifth-generation* scanners were developed primarily for **high-speed CT** scanning. These scanners are based on special configurations intended to facilitate very fast scanning.
6. *Sixth-generation* scanners have multiple x-ray tubes and detectors. These scanners are intended specifically to image moving structures, such as the heart. One such recent scanner is the dual-source CT (DSCT) scanner (McCollough et al., 2007).
7. *Seventh-generation* scanners use flat-panel digital area detectors similar to the ones used in digital radiography (Flohr et al., 2005; Kalender, 2005).

## First-Generation Scanners

Parallel beam geometry was first used by Hounsfield (1973). The first EMI brain scanner and other earlier scanners were based on this concept.

Parallel beam geometry is defined by a set of parallel rays that generates a **projection profile** (Fig. 4-2). The data acquisition process is based on a translate-rotate principle, in which a single, highly collimated x-ray beam and one or two detectors first translate across the patient to collect transmission readings. After one translation, the tube and detector rotate by 1 degree and translate again to collect readings from a different direction. This is repeated for 180 degrees around the patient. This method of scanning is referred to as *rectilinear pencil beam scanning*.

First-generation CT scanners took at least 4.5 to 5.5 minutes to produce a complete scan of the patient, which restricted patient throughput. The image reconstruction **algorithm** for first-generation CT scanners was based on the parallel beam geometry of the image reconstruction space (a square or circle in which the slice to be reconstructed must be **positioned**).

## Second-Generation Scanners

Second-generation scanners were based on the translate-rotate principle of first-generation scanners with a few fundamental differences, such as a linear detector array (about 30 detectors) coupled to the x-ray tube and multiple pencil beams. The result is a beam geometry that describes a small fan whose apex originates at the x-ray tube. This is the fan beam geometry shown in Figure 4-3, *B*, *C*, and *D*.

Also, the rays are divergent instead of parallel, resulting in a significant change in the image reconstruction algorithm, which must be capable of handling projection data from the fan beam geometry.

In second-generation scanners, the fan beam translates across the patient to collect a set of transmission readings. After one translation, the tube and detector array rotate by larger increments (compared with first-generation scanners) and translate again. This process is repeated for 180 degrees and is referred to as *rectilinear multiple pencil beam scanning*. The x-ray tube traces a semicircular path during scanning.

The larger rotational increments and increased number of detectors result in shorter scan times that range from 20 seconds to 3.5 minutes. In general, the time decrease is inversely proportional to the number of detectors. The more detectors, the shorter is the total scan time.

## Third-Generation Scanners

Third-generation CT scanners were based on a fan beam geometry that rotates continuously around the patient for 360 degrees (Fig. 4-3). The x-ray tube is coupled to a curved detector array that subtends an arc of 30 to 40 degrees or greater from the apex of the fan. As the x-ray tube and detectors rotate, projection profiles are collected and a view is obtained for every fixed point of the tube and detector. This motion is referred to as *continuously rotating fan beam scanning*. The path traced by the tube describes a circle rather than the semicircle characteristic of first- and second-generation CT scanners. Third-generation CT scanners collect data faster than the previous units (generally within a few seconds). This scan time increases patient throughput and limits the production of artifacts caused by respiratory motion.

## Fourth-Generation Scanners

Essentially, fourth-generation CT scanners feature two types of beam geometries: a rotating fan beam within a stationary ring of detectors and a nutating fan beam in which the apex of the fan (x-ray tube) is located outside a nutating ring of detectors.

### Rotating Fan Beam Within a Circular Detector Array

The main data acquisition features of a fourth-generation CT scanner are as follows:

1. The x-ray tube is positioned within a stationary, circular detector array (Fig. 4-4).

2. The beam geometry describes a wide fan.
3. The apex of the fan now originates at each detector. Figure 4-4 shows two fans that describe two sets of views.
4. As the tube moves from point to point within the circle, single rays strike a detector. These rays are produced sequentially during the point's circular travel.
5. Scan times are very short and vary from scanner to scanner, depending on the manufacturer.
6. The x-ray tube traces a circular path.
7. The image reconstruction algorithm is for a fan beam geometry in which the apex of the fan is now at the detector, as opposed to the x-ray tube in the third-generation systems.

### Rotating Fan Beam Outside a Nutating Detector Ring

In this scheme, the x-ray tube rotates outside the detector ring (Fig. 4-5). As it rotates, the detector ring tilts so that the fan beam strikes an array of detectors located at the far side of the x-ray tube while the detectors closest to the x-ray tube move out of the path of the x-ray beam. The term *nutating* describes the tilting action of the detector ring during data collection. Scanners with this type of scanning motion eliminate the poor geometry of other schemes, in which the tube rotates inside its detector ring, near the object. However, nutate-rotate systems are not currently manufactured.

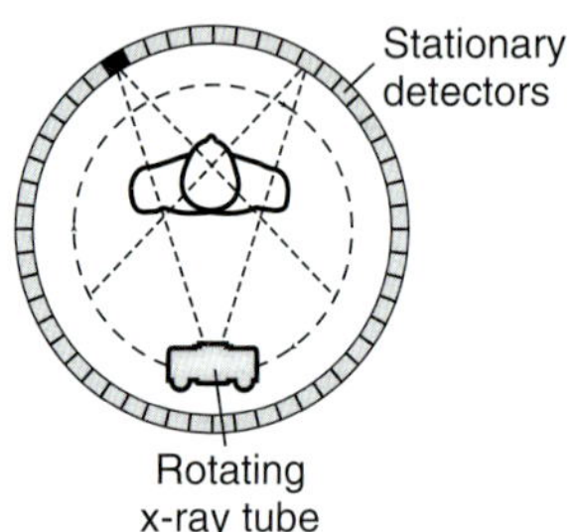


**FIGURE 4-4** In a fourth-generation scanner, each detector position gives rise to a fan.

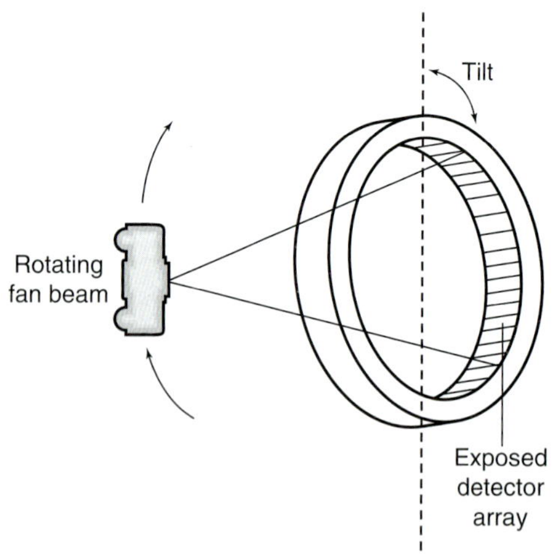


**FIGURE 4-5** Rotating fan beam outside a nutating detector ring. *Nutating* refers to how the detector ring tilts to expose an array of detectors to the x-ray beam. Nutate-rotate systems are no longer manufactured.

## Multislice CT Scanners: CT Scanning in Spiral-Helical Geometry

Scanning in **spiral-helical geometry** is the most recent development in CT data acquisition. The need for faster scan times and improvements in 3D and multiplanar reconstruction have encouraged the development of **continuous rotation** scanners, or volume scanners, in which the data are collected in volumes rather than individual slices. CT scanning in spiral/helical geometry is based on slip-ring technology, which shortens the high-tension cables to the x-ray tube to allow continuous rotation of the gantry. The path traced by the x-ray tube, or fan beam, during the scanning process describes a spiral (Fig. 4-6) or a helix. The terms *spiral geometry* (Siemens) and *helical geometry* (Toshiba) are commonly and synonymously used to describe the **data acquisition geometry** of continuous rotation scanners (see Appendix A). This geometry is obtained during the scanning process. As the tube rotates, the patient is transported through the gantry aperture for a single breath-hold. Because this results in a volume of the patient being scanned, the term **volume CT** is also used.

### Spiral/Helical Geometry Scanners

These systems have evolved through the years from two to eight slices per revolution of the x-ray tube and detectors (360-degree rotation) to 16, 32, 40, 64, and 320 slices per 360-degree rotation. In 2007, a prototype scanner featuring 256 slices per 360-degree rotation was developed by Toshiba Medical Systems (Japan) for imaging moving structures such as the heart and lungs. One striking feature of this scanner compared with other multislice scanners is that it

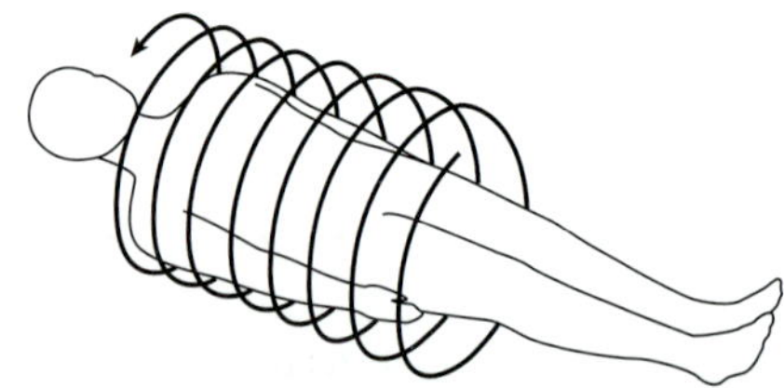

**FIGURE 4-6** The path traced by the x-ray tube in CT scanning describes a spiral or helix. These terms are used interchangeably.

covers the entire heart in a single rotation (Fig. 4-7). The lessons learned from this scanner subsequently led to the 320 CT scanner popularly known as the Aquilion family of CT scanners (examples include the Aquilion ONE and the Aquilion PRIME family of scanners [40, 80, and 160 slices per revolution] commercially available from Toshiba Medical Systems).

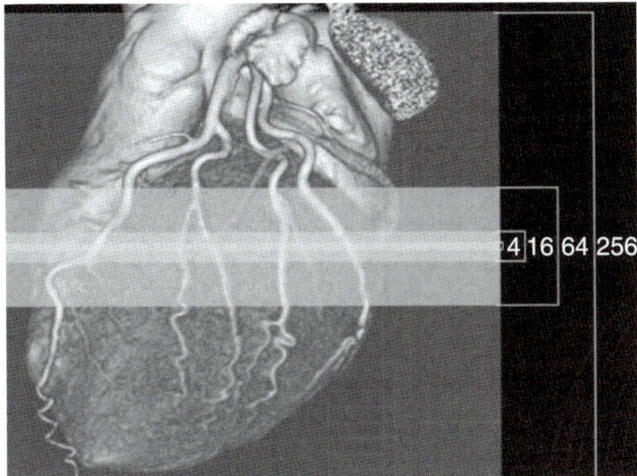


**FIGURE 4-7** The 256 prototype CT scanner featuring 256 slices per 360-degree rotation was developed by Toshiba Medical Systems (Japan) to image moving structures such as the heart and lungs. One striking feature of this scanner compared with other multislice scanners is that it covers the entire heart in a single rotation. (Courtesy Toshiba America Medical Systems.)

An interesting point with respect to scanners capable of imaging 16 or greater slices per 360-degree rotation is that the beam becomes a cone. These systems are therefore based on *cone-beam geometries* (as opposed to *fan beam geometries*) because the detectors are 2D detectors. This means that cone-beam algorithms (as opposed to fan beam algorithms) are used to reconstruct images. **Multislice CT (MSCT)** scanner principles and concepts are described in detail in Chapter 11.

## Fifth-Generation Scanners

Fifth-generation scanners are classified as high-speed CT scanners because they can acquire scan data in milliseconds. Two such scanners are the **electron-beam CT scanner (EBCT;** Fig. 4-8) and the dynamic spatial reconstructor (DSR) scanner. In the EBCT scanner, the data acquisition geometry is a fan beam of x rays produced by a beam of electrons that scans several stationary tungsten target rings. The fan beam passes through the patient, and the x-ray transmission readings are collected for image reconstruction. The DSR scanner was labeled a high-speed CT scanner capable of producing dynamic 3D images of volumes of the patient. The DSR is now obsolete and is not described further in this book.

The principles and operation of the EBCT scanner were first described by Boyd et al. (1979) as a result of research done at the University of California at San Francisco during the late 1970s. In 1983, Imatron

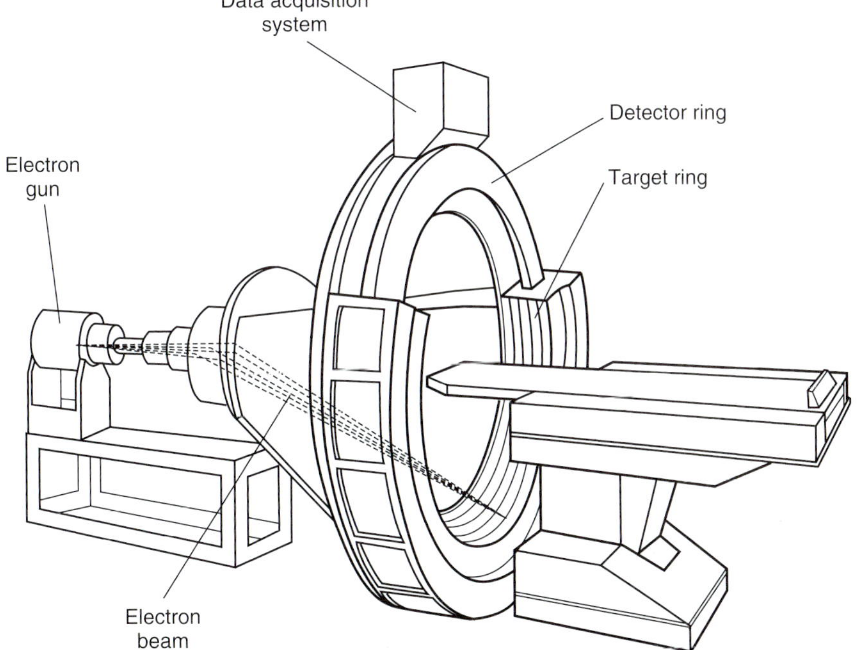


**FIGURE 4-8** The essential components of an EBCT scanner. The data acquisition geometry is a fan beam of x rays produced by the electron beam striking the tungsten targets.

developed Boyd's high-speed CT scanner for imaging the heart and circulation (Boyd & Lipton, 1983). At that time, the machine was referred to by such names as the *cardiovascular computed tomography* scanner and the *cine CT* scanner. Today, the machine is known as the *EBCT scanner* (McCollough, 1995). It is expected that more of these machines will be distributed worldwide in the near future. (Siemens Medical Systems will distribute the EBCT scanner under the name "Evolution.")

The overall goal of the EBCT scanner is to produce high-resolution images of moving organs (e.g., the heart) that are free of artifacts caused by motion. In this respect, the scanner can be used for imaging the heart and other body parts in both adults and children. The scanner performs this task well because its design enables it to acquire CT data 10 times faster than conventional CT scanners.

The design configuration of the EBCT scanner (Fig. 4-8) is different from that of conventional CT systems in the following respects:

1. The EBCT scanner is based on electron-beam technology and no x-ray tube is used.
2. There is no mechanical motion of the components.
3. The acquisition geometry of the EBCT scanner is fundamentally different compared with those of conventional systems.

The basic configuration of an EBCT scanner is shown in Figure 4-8. At one end of the scanner is an electron gun that generates a 130-kilovolt (kV) electron beam. This beam is accelerated, focused, and deflected at a prescribed angle by electromagnetic coils to strike one of the four adjacent tungsten target rings. These stationary rings span an arc of 210 degrees. The electron beam is steered along the rings, which can be used individually or in any sequence. As a result, heat dissipation does not pose a problem as it does in conventional CT systems.

When the electron beam collides with the tungsten target, x rays are produced. Collimators shape the x rays into a fan beam that passes through the patient, who is positioned in a 47-cm scan field, to strike a curved, stationary array of detectors positioned opposite the target rings.

The detector array consists of two separate rings holding a 216-degree arc of detectors. The first ring holds 864 detectors, each half the size of those in the second ring, which holds 432 detectors (McCollough, 1995). This arrangement allows for the acquisition of either two image slices when one target ring is used or eight image slices when all four target rings are used in sequence.

Each solid-state detector consists of a luminescent crystal and cadmium tungstate (which converts x rays to light) coupled optically with silicon photodiodes (which convert light into current) connected to a preamplifier. The **output** from the detectors is sent to the **data acquisition system (DAS;** Fig. 4-8).

The DAS consists of ADCs, or digitizers, that sample and digitize the output signals from the detectors. In addition, the digitized data are stored in bulk in random access memory, which can hold data for hundreds of scans in the multislice and single-slice modes. This information is subsequently sent to the computer for processing.

The computer for the EBCT scanner is capable of very fast reconstruction speeds, and image reconstruction is based on the filtered **back-projection** algorithm used in conventional CT systems.

The EBCT scanner does not have any moving physical parts and, as noted by Flohr et al. (2005), "the EBCT principle is currently not considered adequate for state-of-the-art cardiac imaging or for general radiology applications."

## Sixth-Generation Scanners: The Dual-Source CT Scanner

The overall goal of the MSCT scanners mentioned previously is to improve the volume coverage speed while providing improved spatial and **temporal resolution** compared with the older four slices per 360-degree rotation scanner. Although the current 64-slice volume scanners produce better spatial resolution in the order of 0.4 mm **isotropic** voxels (Flohr et al., 2006; McCollough et al., 2007) and temporal resolution compared with the 16-slice volume CT scanner, they fail to deal effectively with artifacts created in **CT angiography** (CTA) and the problem of the mechanical forces that need to be addressed in attempting to decrease the rotation time of the x-ray tube and detectors (Flohr et al., 2006). To solve these problems, for example, a new-generation scanner has been introduced. This is the DSCT scanner.

This scanner consists of two x-ray tubes and two sets of detectors that are offset by 90 degrees (Fig. 4-9). The DSCT scanner is designed for cardiac CT imaging because it provides the temporal resolution needed to image moving structures such as the heart. The DSCT scanner will be described further in Chapter 11.

## Seventh-Generation Scanners: Flat-Panel CT Scanners

**Flat-panel digital detectors** similar to the ones used in digital radiography are now being considered for use in CT; however, these scanners are still in the prototype development and are not available for use in clinical imaging. Perhaps they may be labeled seventh-generation CT scanners on the basis of the simple categorization mentioned above.

A flat-panel CT scanner prototype is shown in Figure 4-10. The x-ray tube and detectors are coupled and positioned in the CT gantry. The detector consists of a cesium iodide (CsI) scintillator coupled to an amorphous, silicon thin-film transistor array. These flat-panel detectors produce excellent spatial resolution but lack good contrast resolution; therefore, they are also used in angiography to image blood vessels, for example, where the image sharpness is of primary importance. As noted by Flohr et al. (2005),

> the combination of area detectors that provide sufficient image quality with fast gantry rotation speed will be a promising technical concept for medical CT systems. The vast spectrum of potential applications may bring about another quantum leap in the evolution of medical CT imaging.

In addition, flat-panel detectors are also being investigated for use in CT of the breast, and currently several dedicated breast CT prototypes are being developed (Glick et al., 2007; Kwan et al., 2007). Breast CT is described further in Chapter 12.

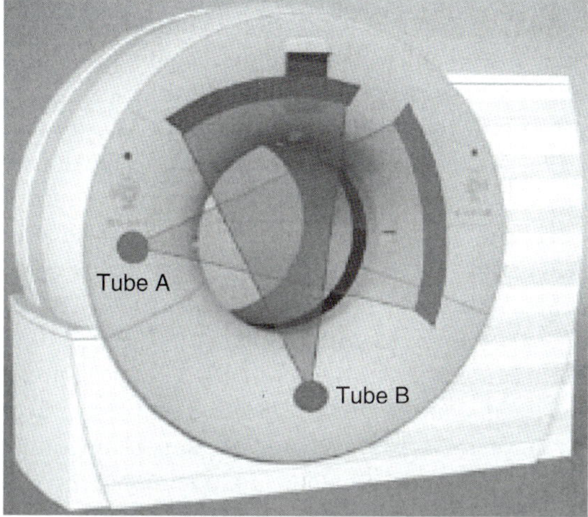


**FIGURE 4-9** The DSCT scanner. This scanner consists of two x-ray tubes and two sets of detectors that are offset by 90 degrees and it is particularly designed for cardiac CT imaging. (From Flohr, T. G., McCollough, C. H., Bruder, H., et al. (2006). *European Radiology, 16*, 256-268. With kind permission of Springer Science and Business Media.)

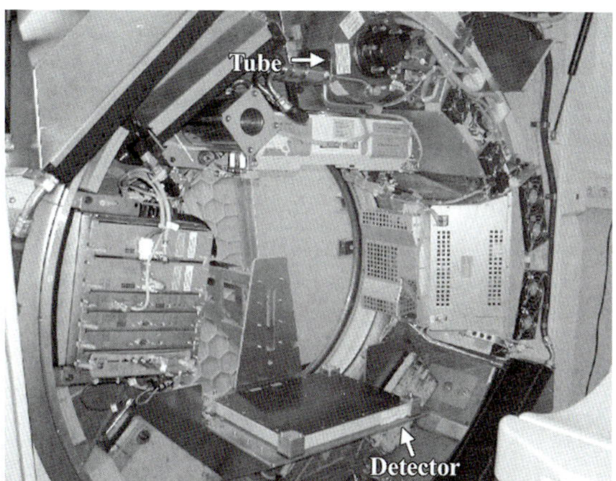


**FIGURE 4-10** A flat-panel CT scanner prototype. The x-ray tube and detectors are coupled and positioned in the CT gantry. The detector consists of a CsI scintillator coupled to an amorphous silicon TFT array. (From Flohr, T. G., Schaller, S., Stierstorfer, K., et al. (2005). *Radiology, 235*, 756-773. Reproduced by permission.)

## SLIP-RING TECHNOLOGY

Spiral-helical CT is made possible through the use of slip-ring technology, which allows for continuous gantry rotation. Slip rings (Fig. 4-11) are "electromechanical devices consisting of circular electrical conductive rings and brushes that transmit electrical energy across a rotating interface" (Brunnett et al., 1990). Today, CT scanners incorporate slip-ring design and are referred to as *continuous rotation, volume CT*, or *slip-ring*

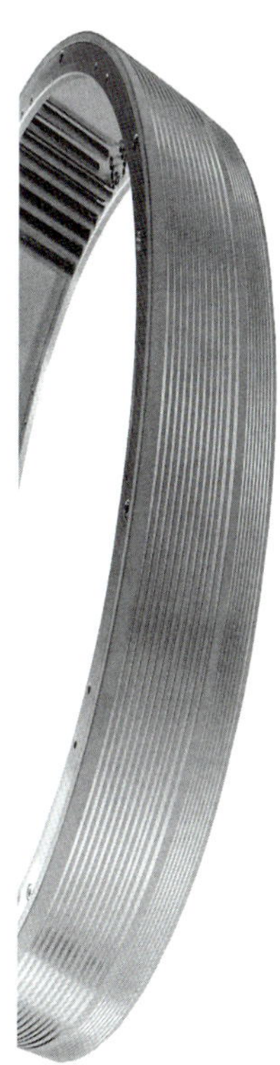

**FIGURE 4-11** Conductive rings (*upper strips*) of one slip-ring system. Each strip carries voltage to components such as the generator, x-ray tube, and collimators. (Courtesy Elscint, Hackensack, NJ.)

scanners. Slip-ring technology is not a new idea and has been applied previously in CT. For example, the Varian V-360-3 CT scanner (an old model CT scanner) was based on slip-ring design to achieve continuous rotation of the gantry. Such rotation results in very fast data collection, which is mandatory for certain clinical procedures such as dynamic CT scanning and CTA.

In addition, slip rings not only provide the electrical power to operate the x-ray tube but also transfer the signals from the detectors for input into the image reconstruction computer.

## Design and Power Supply

Two slip-ring designs are the disk (Fig 4-12, *A*) or pancake type (Fig. 4-12, *B*) and cylinder. In the disk design, the conductive rings form concentric circles in the plane of rotation. The cylindrical design includes conductive rings positioned along the axis of rotation to form a cylinder (Fig. 4-13, *A*). The brushes that transmit electrical power to the CT components glide in contact grooves on the stationary slip ring (Fig. 4-13, *A*).

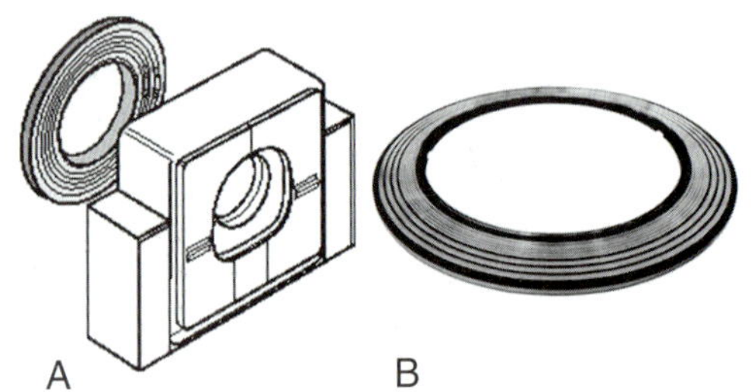


**FIGURE 4-12** Slip rings based on the disk design concept **(A)** or the pancake type **(B)**. The rings are positioned as concentric circles within the plane of rotation. This is a characteristic design of the Siemens Somatom Plus CT scanner. (**A,** Courtesy Siemens Medical Systems; **B,** Courtesy Venturetec Mechatronics, Germany.)

Two common brush designs are the wire brush and the composite brush. The wire brush uses conductive wire as a sliding contact. "A brush consists of one or more wires arranged such that they function as a cantilever spring with a free end against the conductive ring. Two brushes per ring are often used to increase either communication reliability or current carrying capacity" (Brunnett et al., 1990). The composite brush uses a block of some conductive material (e.g., a silver-graphite alloy) as a sliding contact. A variety of different spring designs are commonly used to maintain contact between the brush and ring including cantilever, compression, or constant force. Examples of brush blocks are shown in Figure 4-13, *B* and *C*.

The most recent advance in the design of slip rings is the *contactless slip ring* as shown in Figure 4-14. This design makes it possible to transfer electrical energy across a rotating interface without the use of electrical contacts.

Slip-ring scanners provide continuous rotation of the gantry through the elimination of the long high-tension cables to the x-ray tube used in conventional start–stop scanners, which must be unwound after a complete rotation. In conventional scanners, these cables originate from the high-voltage generator, usually located in the x-ray room. The high-voltage generators of slip-ring scanners are located in the gantry. Scanners with either low-voltage or high-voltage slip rings, based on the power supply to the slip ring, are available (Fig. 4-15).

### Low-Voltage Slip Ring

In a **low-voltage slip-ring system,** 480 alternating (AC) power and x-ray control signals are transmitted to slip rings by means of low-voltage brushes that glide in contact grooves on the stationary slip ring. The slip ring then provides power to the high-voltage transformer, which subsequently transmits high

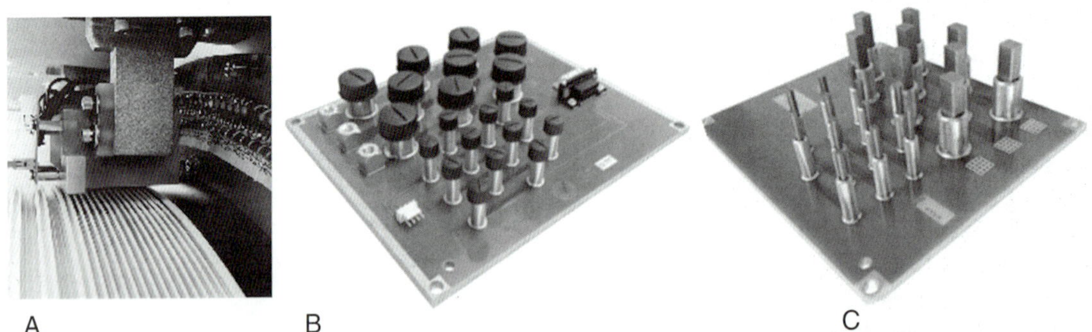


**FIGURE 4-13** Slip ring based on the cylindrical design characteristic of the Picker PQ-2000 CT scanner. The brushes glide in contact grooves on the stationary slip ring **(A)**. Examples of two types of block brushes are shown in **B** and **C**. (**A,** Courtesy Picker International, Cleveland, Ohio; **B** and **C,** Courtesy Venturetec Mechatronics, Germany.)

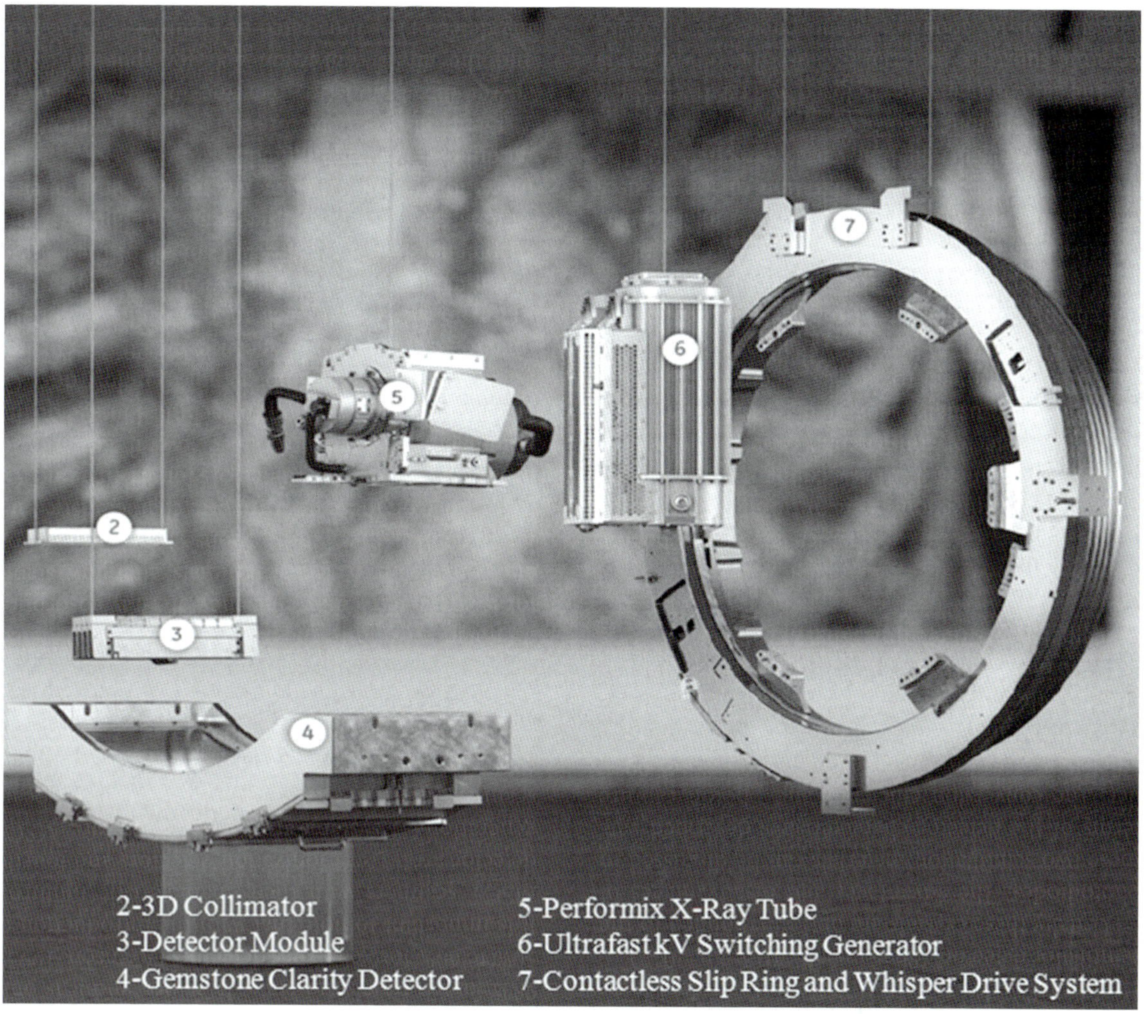

**FIGURE 4-14** A contactless slip ring (7) together with several data acquisition components, such as the x-ray tube and generator and the collimator and detector module. (Courtesy GE Healthcare.)

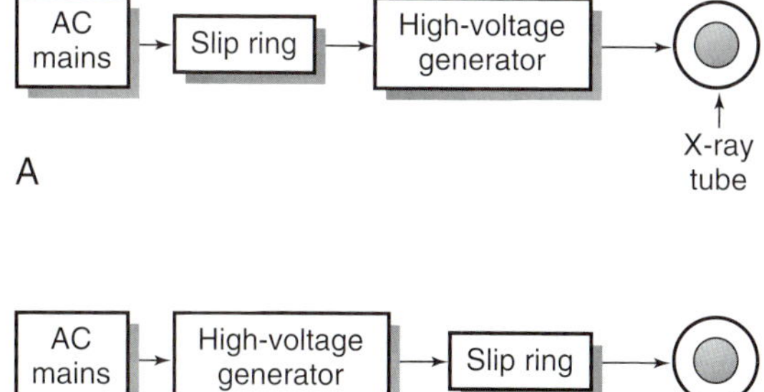


**FIGURE 4-15** Basic differences between low-voltage **(A)** and high-voltage **(B)** slip-ring CT scanners in terms of high-voltage power to the x-ray tube.

voltage to the x-ray tube (Fig. 4-15, *A*). In this case, the x-ray generator, x-ray tube, and other controls are positioned on the orbital scan frame.

### High-Voltage Slip Ring

In a **high-voltage slip-ring system** (Fig. 4-15, *B*), the AC delivers power to the high-voltage generator, which subsequently supplies high voltage to the slip ring. The high voltage from the slip ring is transferred to the x-ray tube. In this case, the high-voltage generator does not rotate with the x-ray tube.

## Advantages

The major advantage of slip-ring technology is that it facilitates continuous rotation of the x-ray tube so that volume data can be acquired quickly from the patient. As the tube rotates continuously, the patient is translated continuously through the gantry aperture. This results in CT scanning in spiral geometry. Other advantages are as follows:

1. Faster scan times and minimal interscan delays
2. Capacity for continuous acquisition protocols
3. Elimination of the start–stop process characteristic of conventional CT scanners
4. Removal of the cable wraparound process

## X-RAY SYSTEM

In his initial experiments, Hounsfield (1973) used low-energy, monochromatic **gamma-ray** radiation. He later conducted experiments with an x-ray tube because of several limitations imposed by the monochromatic radiation source, such as the low radiation intensity rate, large source size, low source strength, and high cost. Subsequently, CT scanners were manufactured to function with x-ray tubes to provide the high radiation intensities necessary for clinical high-contrast CT scanning. However, the **heterogeneous beam** was problematic because it did not obey the Lambert–Beer exponential law (see Equation 3-1).

The components of the x-ray system include the x-ray generator, x-ray tube, x-ray beam filter, and collimators (Figs. 4-1 and 4-14).

### X-Ray Generator

CT scanners use three-phase power for the efficient production of x rays. In the past, generators for CT scanners were based on the 60-Hertz (Hz) voltage frequency, so the high-voltage generator was a bulky piece of equipment located in a corner of the x-ray room. A long high-tension cable ran from the generator to the x-ray tube in the gantry.

CT scanners now use **high-frequency generators,** which are small, compact, and more efficient than conventional generators. These generators are located inside the CT gantry. In some scanners, the high-frequency generator is mounted on the rotating frame with the x-ray tube; in others it is located in a corner of the gantry and does not rotate with the tube.

In a high-frequency generator (Fig. 4-16), the circuit is usually referred to as a *high-frequency inverter circuit.* The low-voltage, low-frequency current (60 Hz) from the main power supply is converted to high-voltage, high-frequency current (500 to 25,000 Hz) as it passes through the components, as shown in Figure 4-16. Each component changes the low-voltage, low-frequency AC waveform to supply the x-ray tube with high-voltage, high-frequency direct current of almost constant potential. After high-voltage rectification and smoothing, the voltage ripple from a high-frequency generator is less than 1%, compared with 4% from a three-phase, 12-pulse generator. This makes the high-frequency generator more efficient at x-ray production than its predecessor. The x-ray **exposure** technique obtained from these generators depends on the generator power output. The power ratings of CT generators vary and depend on the CT vendor; however, typical ratings can range from 20 to 100 kilowatts (kW; Kalender, 2005). More recently CT manufacturers have generators capable of 120 kW. The interested student should refer to CT manufacturers' website descriptions for up-to-date specifications on CT x-ray generators. An output capacity of, say, 60 kW will provide a range of kilovolt and milliampere settings, where 80 and 120 to 140 kV and 20 to 500 milliamperes (mA) with 1-mA increments are typical.

### X-Ray Tubes

The radiation source requirement in CT depends on two factors: (1) radiation attenuation, which is a function of radiation beam energy, the atomic number and density of the absorber, and the thickness of the object and (2) the quantity of radiation required for transmission. X-ray tubes satisfy this requirement.

First- and second-generation scanners used *fixed-anode, oil-cooled x-ray tubes*, but *rotating anode x-ray tubes* have become common in CT because of the demand for increased output. These rotating anode tubes, an example of which is shown in Figure 4-17, produce a heterogeneous beam of radiation from a

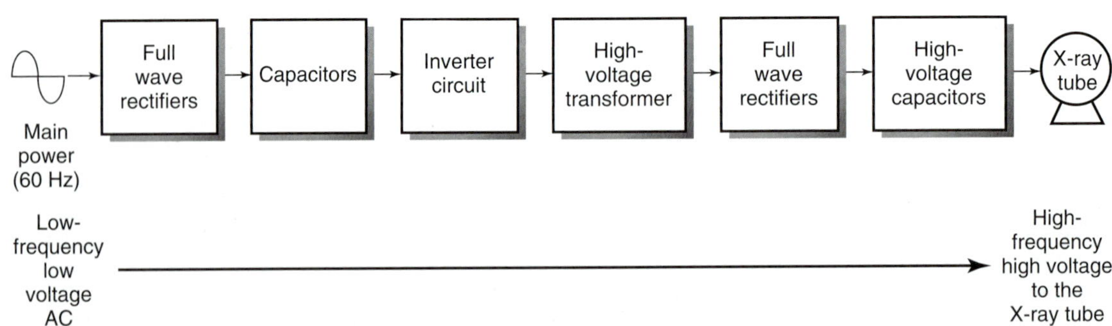


**FIGURE 4-16** The basic components of a high-frequency generator used in modern CT scanners.

large-diameter anode disk with focal spot sizes to facilitate the spatial resolution requirements of the scanner. The disk is usually made of a rhenium, tungsten, and molybdenum (RTM) alloy and other materials with a small target angle (usually 12 degrees) and a rotation speed of 3600 revolutions per minute (rpm) to 10,000 rpm (high-speed rotation). Figure 4-17, *B*, shows an upgraded tube based on the technology used in the tube shown in Figure 4-17, *A*.

The introduction of spiral/helical CT with continuous rotation scanners has placed new demands on x-ray tubes. Because the tube rotates continually for a longer period compared with conventional scanners, the tube must be able to sustain higher power levels. Several technical advances in component design have been made to achieve these power levels and deal with the problems of heat generation, heat storage, and heat dissipation. For example, the tube envelope, cathode assembly, anode assembly including anode rotation, and target design have been redesigned (Fox, 1995; Homberg & Koppel, 1997).

The glass envelope ensures a vacuum, provides structural support of anode and cathode structures, and provides high-voltage insulation between the anode and cathode. Internal getters (ion pumps) remove air molecules to ensure a vacuum. Although the borosilicate glass provides good thermal and electrical insulation, electrical arcing results from tungsten deposits on the glass caused by vaporization. Tubes with metal envelopes, which are now common, solve this problem. Ceramic insulators (Fig. 4-17, *A*) isolate the metal envelope from the anode and cathode voltage. Metal envelope tubes have larger anode disks; for example, the tube shown in Figure 4-17 has a disk with a 200-mm diameter compared with the 120- to 160-mm diameter typical of conventional tubes. This feature allows the technologist to use higher tube currents. Heat-storage capacity is also increased with an improvement in heat dissipation rates.

The cathode assembly consists of one or more tungsten filaments positioned in a focusing cup. The getter is usually made of barium to ensure a vacuum by the absorption of air molecules released from the target during operation.

The anode assembly consists of the disk, rotor stud and hub, rotor, and bearing assembly. The large anode disk is thicker than conventional disks; the three basic designs are the conventional all-metal disk (Fig. 4-18), the brazed graphite disk, and the chemical vapor deposition (CVD) graphite disk. In conventional tubes, the all-metal disk (Fig. 4-18, *A*) consists of a base body made of titanium, zirconium, and molybdenum with a focal track layer of 10% rhenium and 90% tungsten. It can transfer heat from the focal track very quickly. Unfortunately, tubes with this all-metal design cannot meet the needs of spiral/helical CT imaging because of their weight.

The brazed graphite anode disk (Fig. 4-18, *B*) consists of a tungsten-rhenium focal track brazed to a graphite base body. Graphite increases the heat-storage capacity because of its high thermal capacity, which is about 10 times that of tungsten. As noted by Fox (1995), the material used in the brazing process influences the operating temperature of the tube, and the higher temperatures result in higher heat-storage capacities and faster cooling of the anode. Tubes for spiral/helical CT scanning are based mostly on this type of design.

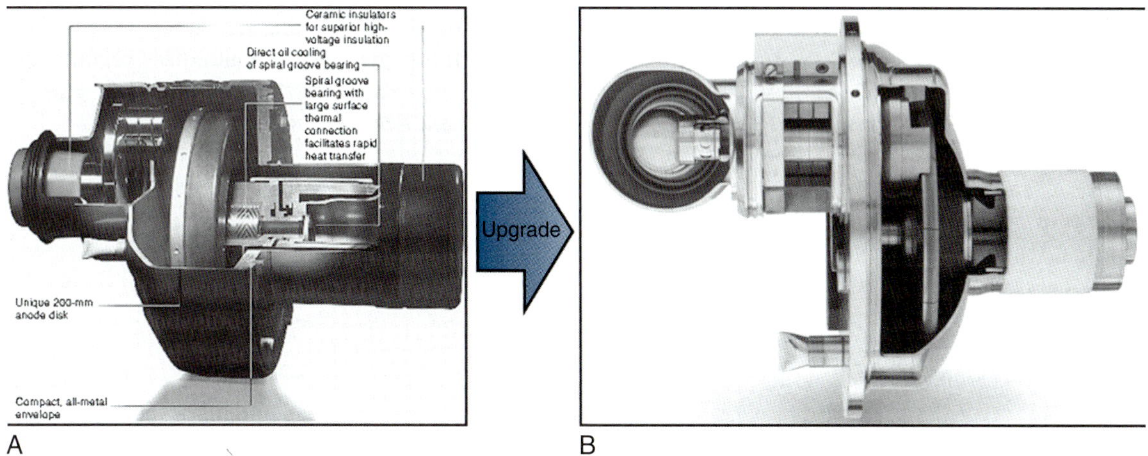


**FIGURE 4-17** A modern rotating anode x-ray tube used in CT scanners. The tube shown in **(B)** is an upgraded tube based on the technology used in the tube shown in **(A)**. (**A,** Courtesy Philips Medical Systems, Shelton, Conn; **B,** Courtesy Philips Healthcare.)

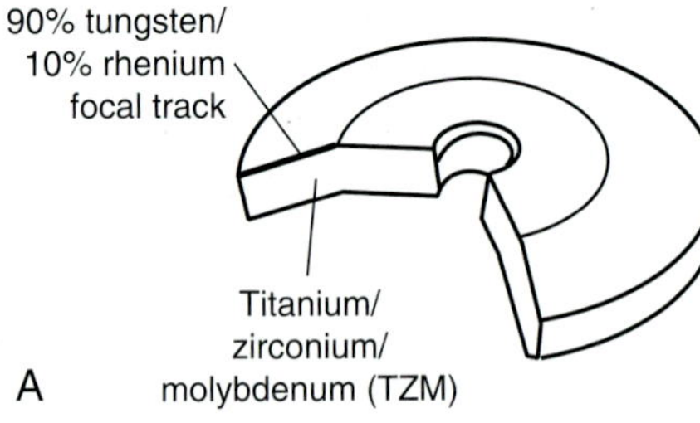


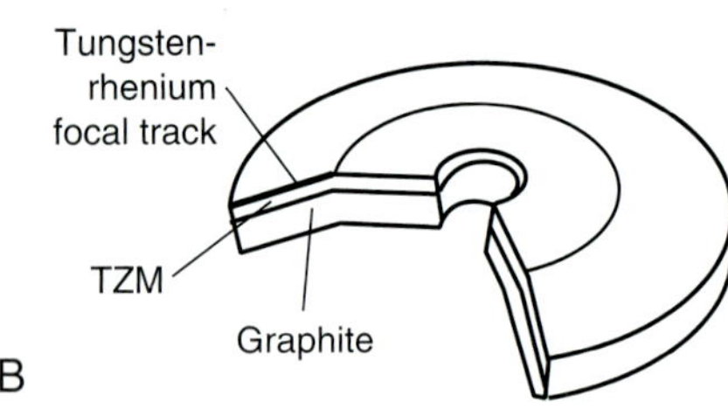


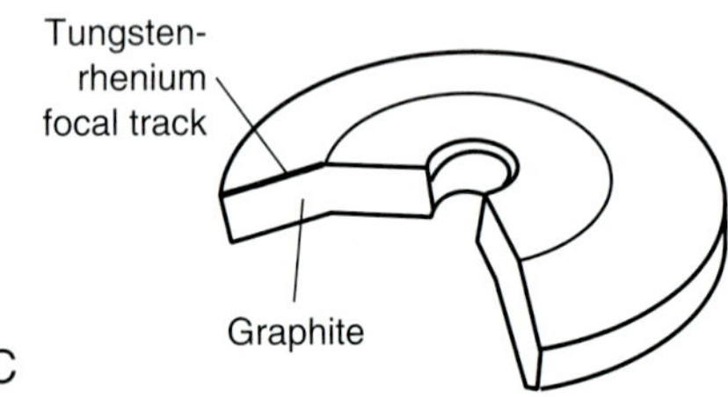


**FIGURE 4-18** Three types of disk designs for modern x-ray tubes used in CT scanners: **(A)** conventional all-metal disk; **(B)** brazed graphite anode disk; and **(C)** CVD graphite anode disk.

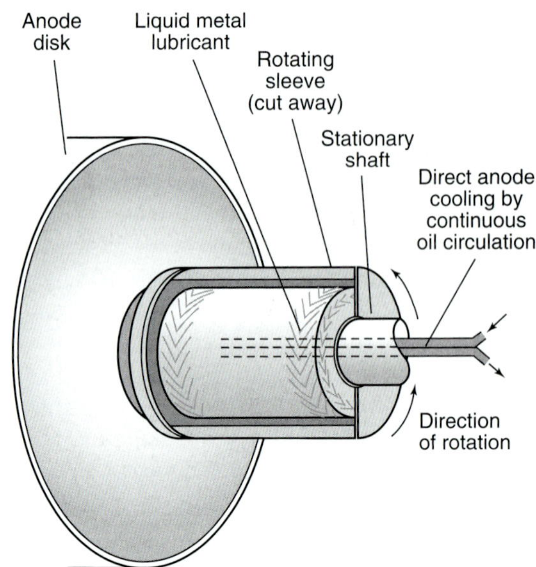


**FIGURE 4-19** The anode assembly of a modern x-ray tube used in CT imaging. The main parts of the assembly are the disk, rotor, and bearing assembly that contains liquid metal lubricant.

The final type of anode design (Fig. 4-18, *C*) is also intended for use in spiral/helical CT x-ray tubes. The disk consists of a graphite base body with a tungsten-rhenium layer deposited on the focal track by a chemical vapor process. This design can accommodate large, lightweight disks with large heat-storage capacity and fast cooling rates (Fox, 1995).

The purpose of the bearing assembly is to provide and ensure smooth rotation of the anode disk. In CT, high-speed anode rotation allows the use of higher loadability. Rotation speeds of 10,000 rpm are possible with increased frequency to the stator windings. Smooth rotation of the disk is possible because of the ball bearings lubricated with silver; however, because ball-bearing technology results in mechanical problems and limits x-ray tube performance, a liquid-bearing method to improve anode disk rotation was introduced (Fig. 4-19).

The stationary shaft of the anode assembly consists of grooves that contain gallium-based liquid metal alloy. During anode rotation, the liquid is forced into the grooves and results in a hydroplaning effect between the anode sleeve and liquid (Homberg & Koppel, 1997). The purpose of this bearing technology is to conduct heat away from the x-ray tube more efficiently than conventional ball bearings with improved tube cooling. Additionally, the liquid-bearing technology is free of vibrations and **noise.**

As noted by Fox (1995), the rotor hub and rotor stud also prevent the transmission of heat from the disk to the bearings. The rotor is a copper cylinder "brazed to an inner steel cylinder with a ceramic coating around the outside to enhance heat radiation" (Fox, 1995).

The working life of the tubes can range from about 10,000 to 40,000 hours, compared with 1000 hours, which is typical of conventional tubes with conventional bearing technology.

### Straton X-Ray Tube: A New X-Ray Tube for MSCT Scanning

As noted above, the fundamental problem with conventional x-ray tubes is that of heat dissipation and slow cooling rates. Efforts have been made to deal with these problems by introducing various designs, such as large anode disks and the introduction of the compound anode design (RTM disk), which has higher heat-storage capacities and cooling rates. Additionally, as gantry rotation times increase, higher milliampere values are needed to provide the same milliamperes per rotation. As the electrical load

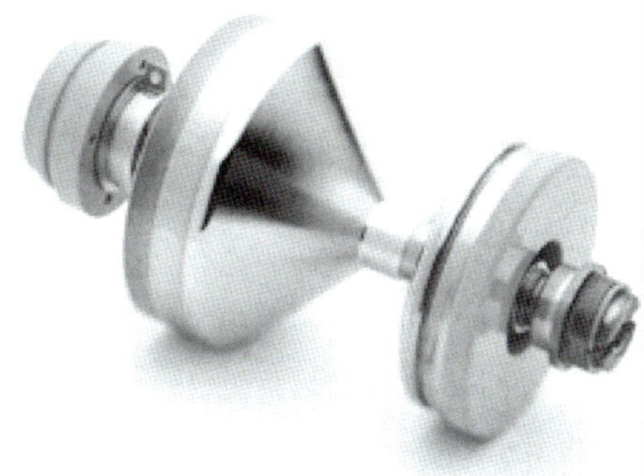

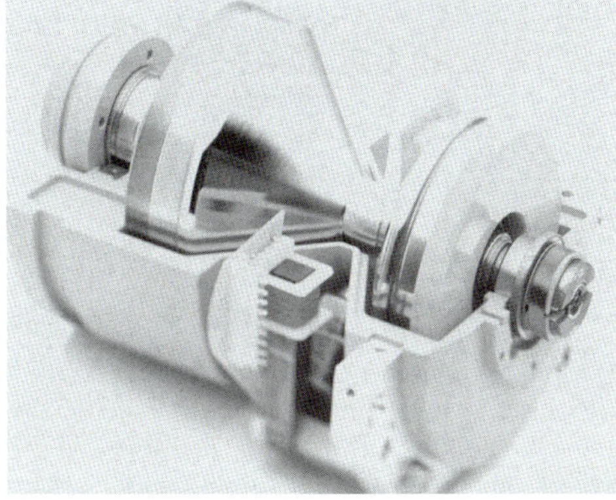

**FIGURE 4-20** The Straton x-ray tube, a new x-ray tube for MSCT scanning. (See text for further description.) (Courtesy Siemens Medical Solutions, Germany.)

(milliamperes and kilovolts) increases, faster anode cooling rates are needed. Despite these efforts, the problems of heat transfer and slow cooling rates still persist with MSCT scanners, especially for multiple longer scan times and cardiac CT imaging.

To overcome these problems, a new type of x-ray tube has been introduced for use with MSCT scanners. This unique and revolutionary tube was designed by Siemens Medical Solutions (Siemens AG Medical Solutions, Erlangen, Germany). Because this tube represents a new technology for dealing with the problem of x-ray tube heat in MSCT scanning and leads to an innovative method of improving image quality in CT, it is described here.

A photograph of the Straton x-ray tube is shown in Figure 4-20. As can be seen, it is encased in a protective housing that contains oil for cooling. The tube is compact in design and is much smaller than conventional x-ray tubes described earlier. This size ensures a fast gantry rotation of 0.37 seconds (Kalender, 2005).

The Straton x-ray tube, illustrated in Figure 4-21, has anode and cathode structures, deflection coils, an electron beam, and a motor. The electron beam produced by the filament housed in the cathode assembly is deflected to strike the anode (120-mm diameter) to produce x rays used for imaging. The motor provides the rotation of the

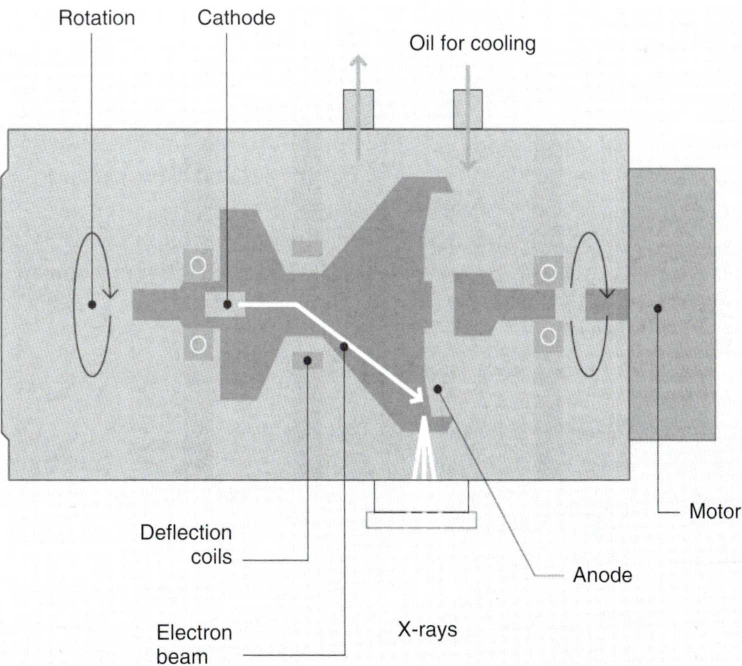


**FIGURE 4-21** The Straton x-ray tube. This diagram shows the anode and cathode structures, deflection coils, an electron beam, and a motor. (See text for further explanation.) (Courtesy Siemens Medical Solutions, Germany.)

entire tube, which is immersed in oil. It is important to note that the anode is in direct contact with the oil (directly cooled tube), which is forced out of the housing for cooling and subsequently circulates back into the housing. Because the anode is in direct contact with the circulating oil, very high cooling rates of 5.0 MHU/min result in about 0 MHU anode heat-storage capacity. The advantage of this is that high-speed **volume scanning** is possible with high milliamperes and long exposure times for increasing length of anatomic coverage. A comparison of the design structures of both conventional and the Straton x-ray tubes is illustrated in Figure 4-22. Another important feature of the Straton x-ray tube relates to the electron beam from the cathode. This beam is deflected to strike the anode at two precisely located focal spots (Fig. 4-23) that vary in size. Kalender (2005) reported that the sizes can be 0.6 mm × 0.17 mm, 0.8 mm × 1.1 mm, and 0.7 mm × 0.7 mm. The electron beam alternates at about 4640 times per second to create two separate x-ray beams that pass through the patient and fall on the detectors. This is described later in the chapter.

## Alternative X-Ray Tube Designs for Multislice CT

Two alternative designs in x-ray tube technology for use in MSCT are shown in Figure 4-24, one from Philips Healthcare (2005; Fig 4-24, *A*) and the other from Siemens Healthcare (Fig 4-24, *B*). Both of these

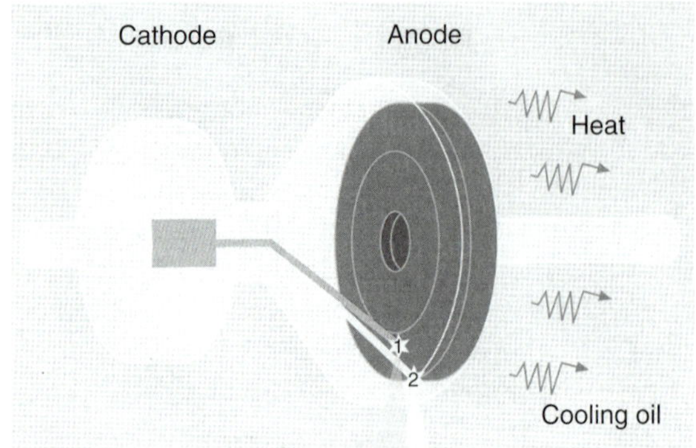


**FIGURE 4-23** An important feature of the Straton x-ray tube is that the electron beam from the cathode is deflected to strike the anode at two precisely located focal spots that vary in size. (Courtesy Siemens Medical Solutions, Germany.)

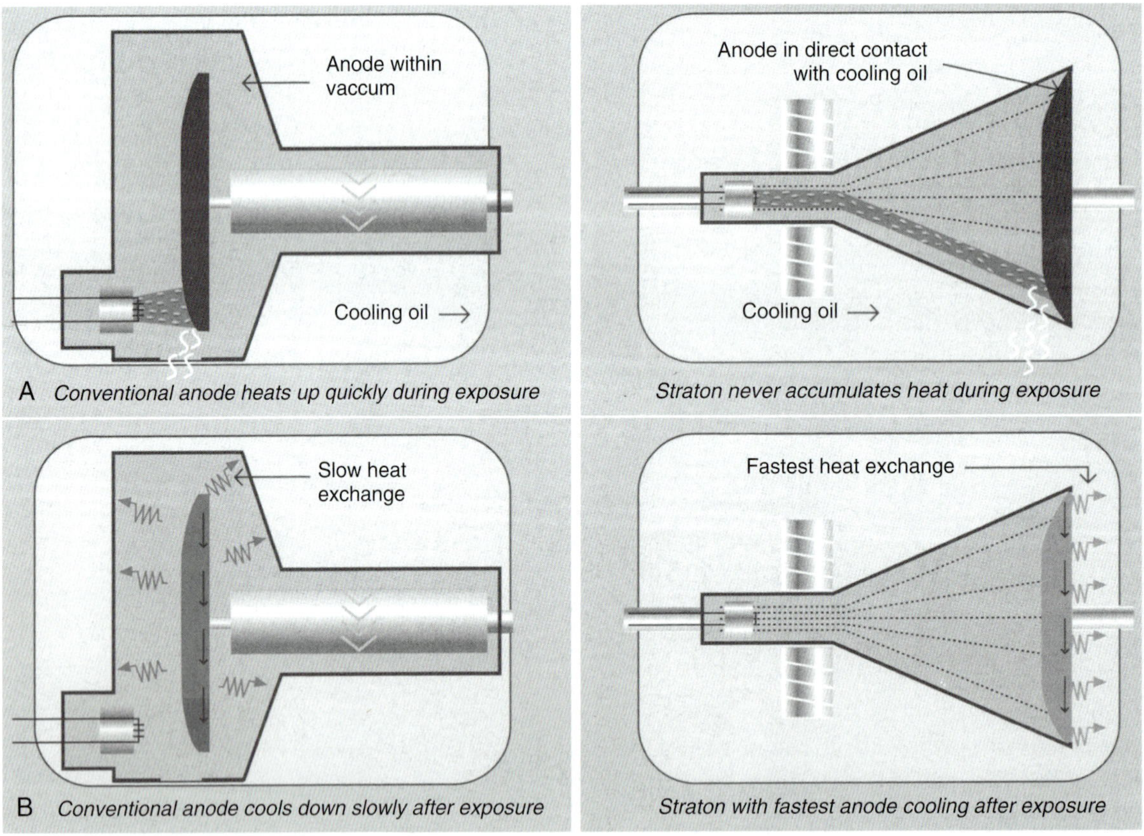

**FIGURE 4-22** A comparison of the design structures of both conventional and the Straton x-ray tubes. (Courtesy Siemens Medical Solutions, Germany.)

x-ray tubes are *directly cooled x-ray tubes* (direct anode cooling).

The Philips Healthcare x-ray tube is an upgraded Maximus Rotalix Ceramic (iMRC) x-ray tube technology (second-generation technology) based on metal/ceramic technology and a noiseless wear-free spiral groove bearing with a large area liquid metal contact and a 200-mm graphite-backed, dual-suspended hydrodynamic bearing with a segmented all-metal (Shefer et al., 2013) anode disk, which facilitates very high heat loading capacity and rapid heat dissipation. The upgraded tube also features what has been referred to as the dynamic focal spot (DFS), which increases the data **sampling** and generates artifact-free ultra-high spatial resolution. The updated technical data for the iMRC 800 x-ray tube are listed in Table 4-1.

Another alternative design in MSCT x-ray tubes is the Vectron x-ray tube (Fig 4-24, *B*), a direct anode cooling x-ray tube based on the Straton x-ray tube direct anode cooling technology. This tube is available from Siemens Healthcare and it operates with tube voltages ranging from 70 to 150 kV in increments of 10 kV. Based on the flying focal spot approach of z-Sharp, the electron beam is now accurately and rapidly deflected, creating two focal spots alternating at 4480 times/s. This feature significantly increases in-plane resolution. The Vectron tube also uses a small focal point of 0.4 mm × 0.5 mm and is capable of up to 0.22 line pairs per centimeter in routine CT scanning without increasing the dose to the patient (Siemens Healthcare, personal **communications,** 2015).

## Filtration

Radiation from x-ray tubes consists of long and short wavelengths. The original experiments in the development of a practical CT scanner used monochromatic radiation to satisfy the Lambert–Beer exponential attenuation law. However, in clinical CT, the beam is polychromatic. Because it is essential that the polychromatic beam has the appearance of a monochromatic beam to satisfy the requirements of the reconstruction process, a special filter must be used.

In CT, **filtration** serves a dual purpose:

1. Filtration removes long-wavelength x rays because they do not play a role in CT image formation; instead they contribute to patient dose. As a result of filtration, the mean energy of the beam increases and the beam becomes "harder," which may cause **beam-hardening** artifacts.

**TABLE 4-1 Specifications for the Philips MRC X-Ray Tube**

| Features | Values |
|---|---|
| Maximum tube power | 60 kW |
| Nominal anode input power (IEC 60613) | 85 kW (small) and 120 kW (large) |
| Effective heat-storage capacity | 26 MHUeff |
| Anode heat-storage capacity (IEC 60613) | 8 MHU |
| Maximum heat content of assembly | 12 MHU |
| Maximum continuous heat dissipation | 6.1 kW |
| Anode disk diameter | 200 mm |
| Anode angle | 7 degrees |
| Focal spot size (IEC 60336/93) | 0.5 × 1.0 (small) and 1.0 × 1.0 (large) |
| Tube voltages | 90, 120, 140 kV |
| Tube current | 20 to 500 mA |
| High g forces spiral groove bearing, directly cooled anode | |

Courtesy Philips Medical System.

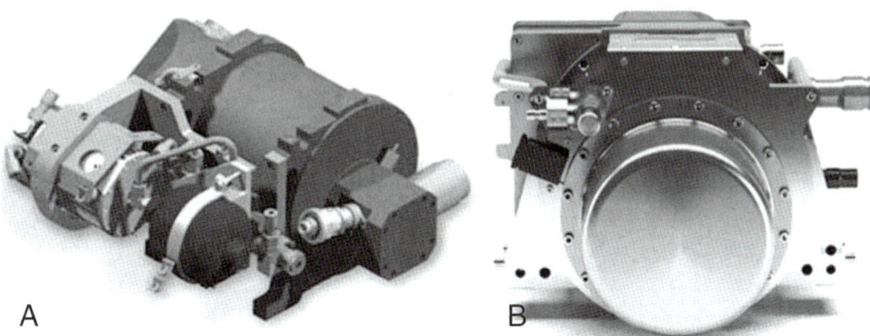


**FIGURE 4-24** Two alternative designs of directly cooled x-ray tubes (direct anode cooling) for use specifically in CT scanning. **A,** The Philips Healthcare upgraded x-ray tube is installed in the x-ray tube housing and is available as a complete tube housing assembly. **B,** The other design of a directly cooled x-ray tube from Siemens Healthcare. (**A,** Courtesy Philips Healthcare; **B,** Courtesy Siemens Healthcare.)

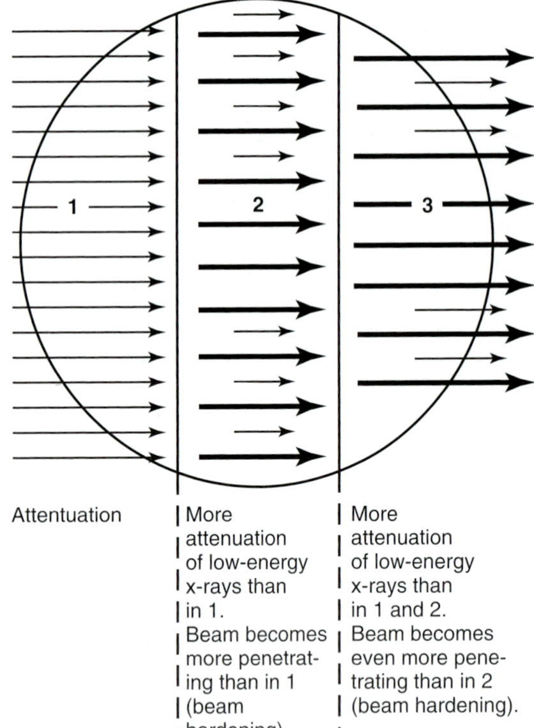


**FIGURE 4-25** Attenuation of radiation through a circular object. The beam becomes more penetrating (harder) in section 3 because of differences in attenuation in sections 1 and 2. The heavier arrows indicate less attenuation and more penetrating rays.

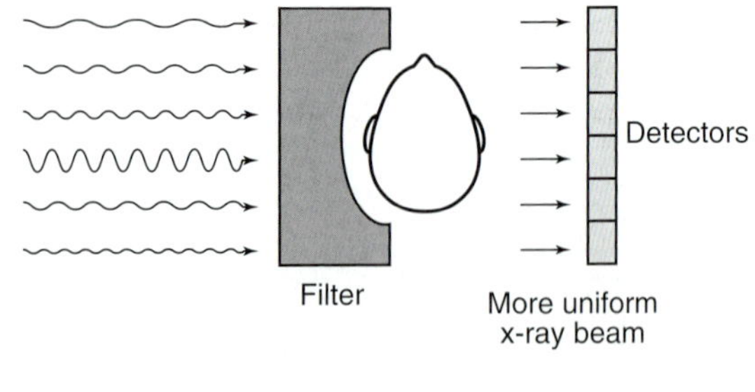


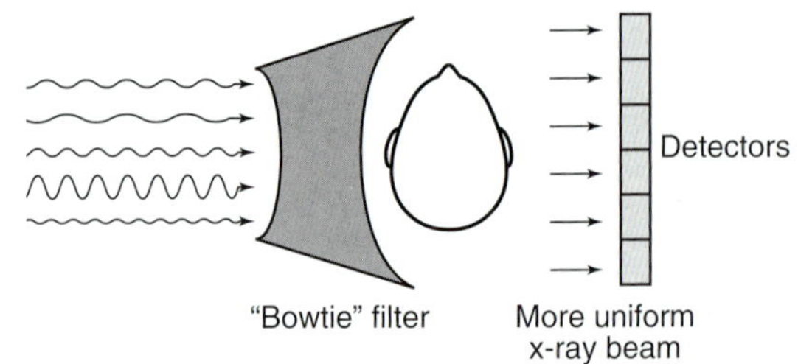


**FIGURE 4-26** Two types of beam-shaping filters for use in CT. These filters attenuate the beam so that a more uniform (monochromatic) beam falls onto the detectors. This uniform beam reduces the dynamic range of the electronics (analog-to-digital converters).

Recall that the total filtration is equal to the sum of the inherent filtration and the added filtration. In CT the inherent filtration has a thickness of about 3 mm Al-equivalent. The added filtration, on the other hand, consists of filters that are flat or shaped filters made of copper sheets, for example, the thickness of which can range from 0.1 to 0.4 mm (Kalender, 2005).

2. Filtration shapes the energy distribution across the radiation beam to produce uniform beam hardening when x rays pass through the filter and the object.

In Figure 4-25, the attenuation differs in sections 1, 2, and 3 and the penetration increases in sections 2 and 3. This results from the absorption of the soft radiation in sections 1 and 2, which is referred to as *hardening of the beam*. Because the detector system does not respond to beam-hardening effects for the circular object shown, "the problem can be solved by introducing additional filtration into the beam" (Seeram, 2009). In the original EMI scanner, this problem was solved with a water bath around the patient's head. Today, specially shaped filters conform to the shape of the object and are positioned between the x-ray tube and the patient (Fig. 4-26). These filters are called shaped filters, such as the "bowtie" filter, and are usually made of Teflon, a material that has low atomic number and high density, so as not to have a significant impact on beam hardening. "The term 'bowtie' applies to a class of filter shapes featuring bilateral symmetry with a thickness that increases with the **distance** from the centre. Bowtie filters compensate for the difference in beam path length through the axial plane of the object such that a more uniform fluence can be delivered to the detector" (Zhang et al., 2013).

## Collimation

The purpose of **collimation** in conventional radiography and fluoroscopy is to protect the patient by restricting the beam to the anatomy of interest only. In CT, collimation is equally important because it affects patient dose and image quality (Fig. 4-27). The basic collimation scheme in CT is shown in Figure 4-27, *A*, with adjustable prepatient, postpatient, and predetector collimators. These detectors must be perfectly aligned to optimize the imaging process. This alignment is accomplished with the fixed collimators, not shown in Fig 4-27, *A*.

Prepatient collimation design is influenced by the size of the focal spot of the x-ray tube because of the penumbra effect associated with focal spots. The larger the focal spot, the greater the penumbra and the more complicated is the design of the collimators.

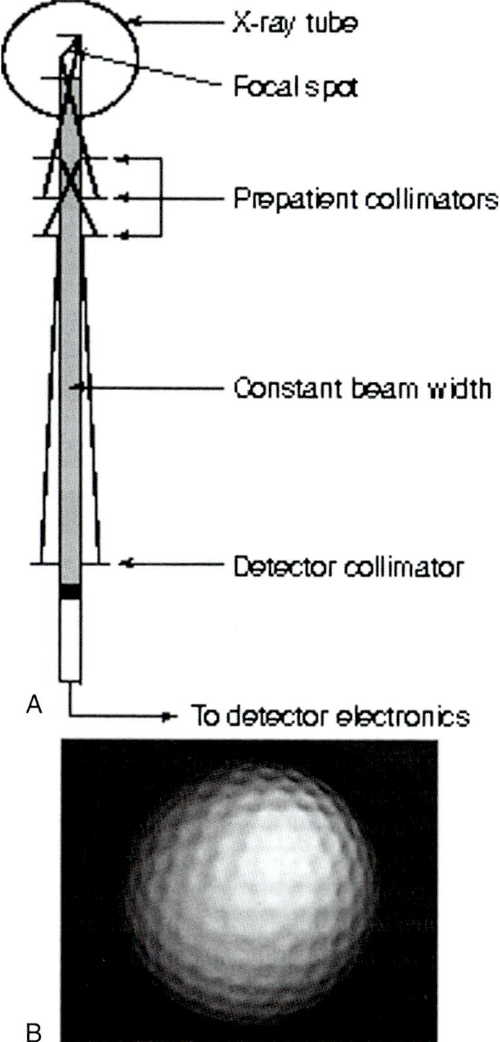


**FIGURE 4-27 A,** Collimation scheme typical of CT scanning. **B,** The removal of scattered radiation by the two sets of collimators improves the resolution of the golf ball dimples. (Courtesy Shimadzu Medical Systems, Seattle, Wash.)

In general, a set of collimator sections is carefully arranged to shape the beam, which is proximal to the focal spot. Both proximal and distal (predetector) collimators are arranged to ensure a constant beam width at the detector. Detector collimators also shape the beam and remove scattered radiation. Such removal improves axial resolution as illustrated in Figure 4-27, *B*, in which the golf ball dimples are apparent. The collimator section at the distal end of the collimator assembly also helps define the thickness of the slice to be imaged. Various **slice thicknesses** are available depending on the type of scanner.

Some scanners incorporate an antiscatter grid to remove radiation scattered from the patient. This grid is placed just in front of the detectors and it is intended to improve image quality.

### Adaptive Section Collimation

The introduction of MSCT scanners posed some challenges with the design of the collimation scheme especially as the detectors become wider. The problems are related to what has been referred to as overscanning and overbeaming (Goo, 2012). While overbeaming "relates to x-ray beams being slightly wider than the detector which means that patients are exposed over a small area without the signal being detected" (Kalender, 2014), overscanning "refers to exposure of the patient outside the imaged range which occurs for spiral CT with multi-row detectors at the start and the end of the scan" (Kalender, 2014). These two problems result in increased dose to the patient. For example, overscanning may result in an increase of 5% to 30% in dose keeping the length of the scan in mind (Kalender, 2014).

The problems of overscanning and overbeaming can be solved using a technique called **adaptive section collimation** (Deak et al., 2009). With adaptive section collimation (see Fig. 10-13) "parts of the x-ray beam exposing tissue outside of the volume to be imaged are blocked in the z-direction by dynamically adjusted collimators at the beginning and at the end of the CT scan" (Deak et al., 2009). These two concepts, overbeaming and overscanning, are discussed in more detail in Chapter 10.

## CT DETECTOR TECHNOLOGY

The position of the CT detection system is shown in Figure 4-28. CT detectors capture the radiation beam from the patient and convert it into electrical signals, which are subsequently converted into binary coded information.

### Detector Characteristics

Detectors exhibit several characteristics essential for CT image production affecting good image quality, such as efficiency, response time (speed of response), dynamic range, accuracy, stability, resolution, cross talk, and afterglow (Shefer et al., 2013).

**Efficiency** refers to the ability to capture, absorb, and convert x-ray photons to electrical signals. CT detectors must possess high capture efficiency, absorption efficiency, and conversion efficiency. **Capture efficiency** refers to the efficiency with which the detectors can obtain photons transmitted from the patient; the size of the detector area facing the beam and distance between two detectors determines capture efficiency. **Absorption efficiency** refers to

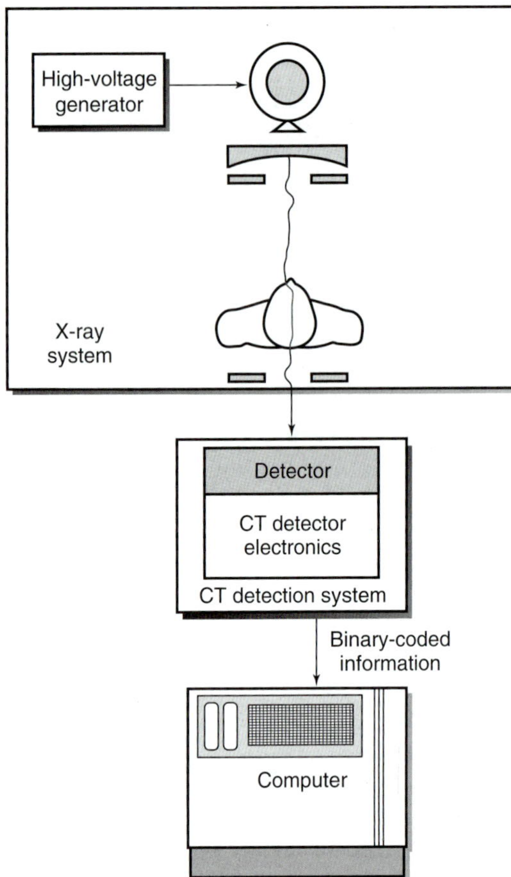


**FIGURE 4-28** Relationship of the CT detection system to the x-ray system and computer.

the number of photons absorbed by the detector and depends on the atomic number, physical density, size, and thickness of the detector face (Seeram, 2009; Villafana, 1987).

**Stability** refers to the steadiness of the detector response. If the system is not stable, frequent calibrations are required to render the signals useful.

The **response time** of the detector refers to the speed with which the detector can detect an x-ray event and recover to detect another event. Response times should be very short (i.e., microseconds) to avoid problems such as afterglow and detector "pile-up."

The **dynamic range** of a CT detector is the "ratio of the largest signal to be measured to the precision of the smallest signal to be discriminated (i.e., if the largest signal is 1 μA and the smallest signal is 1 nA, the dynamic range is 1 million to 1)" (Parker & Stanley, 1981). The dynamic range for most CT scanners is about 1 million to 1. The total detector efficiency, or dose efficiency, is the product of the capture efficiency, absorption efficiency, and conversion efficiency (Seeram, 2009; Villafana, 1987).

**Afterglow** refers to the persistence of the image even after the radiation has been turned off. CT detectors should have low afterglow values, such as <0.01%, 100 milliseconds after the radiation has been terminated (Kalender, 2005).

Finally, while *resolution* is influenced by several factors such as the detector element size, focal spot size, and sampling size (detector **pitch**), *cross talk* refers to the amount of signal from one detector element that may leak over into an adjacent detector (Goldman, 2000).

## Types

The conversion of x-rays to electrical energy in a detector is based on two fundamental principles (Fig. 4-29). Scintillation detectors (luminescent materials) convert x-ray energy into light, after which the light is converted into electrical energy by a photodetector (Fig. 4-29, *A*). Figure 4-29, *B*, shows the corresponding electronic symbol. This type of photodetector is referred to as a photovoltaic detector array (PDA) and it is based on front illumination. Current CT scanners now make use of back-illuminated PDA. For a discussion of back-illuminated PDA, the interested reader should refer to Shefer et al. (2013). Gas-ionization detectors, on the other hand, convert x-ray energy directly to electrical energy.

### Scintillation Detectors

**Scintillation detectors** are solid-state detectors that consist of a scintillation crystal coupled to a photodiode tube. When x rays fall onto the crystal, flashes of light, or scintillations, are produced. The light is then directed to the photomultiplier, or PM tube. As illustrated in Figure 4-30, the light from the crystal strikes the photocathode of the PM tube, which then releases electrons. These electrons cascade through a series of dynodes that are carefully arranged and maintained at different potentials to result in a small output signal.

In CT, scintillation detectors must exhibit a

> high light output, high x-ray stopping power, good spectral match with the photo-detector, short primary decay time (up to tens of μs), low afterglow, radiation damage resistance, light-output stability (time, temperature), compact packaging, and easy machining. In many cases it is uniformity of a certain property that is more important and more challenging to achieve, rather than meeting a required absolute value (Shefer et al., 2013).

As a result, single crystals and polycrystalline ceramics have become popular scintillators for use in CT imaging. Scintillation detectors have experienced

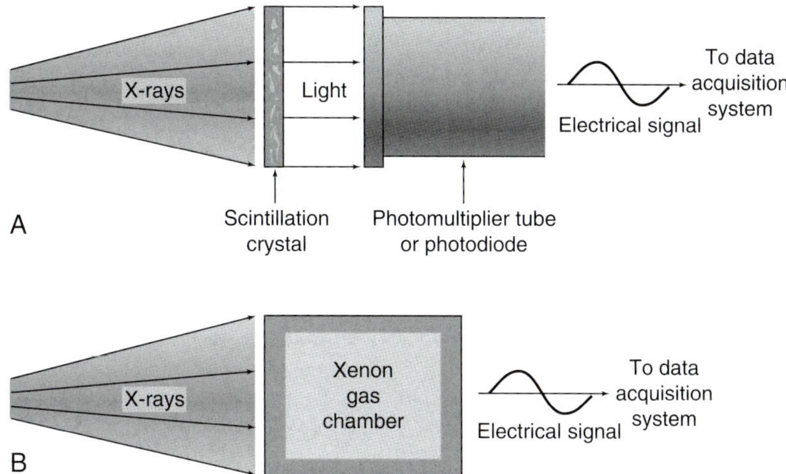


**FIGURE 4-29** Two methods for converting x-ray photons into electrical energy. **A,** Scintillation crystal detection and conversion scheme. **B,** Conversion of x rays into electrical energy through gas ionization.

significant changes through the years and a few of the highlights of these developments will be described later in this section.

In the past, early scanners used sodium iodide crystals coupled to PM tubes. Because of afterglow problems and the limited dynamic range of sodium iodide, other crystals such as calcium fluoride and bismuth germanate were used in later scanners. Furthermore, solid-state photodiode multiplier scintillation crystal detectors are used (Fig. 4-31). The photodiode is a semiconductor (silicon) whose *p-n* junction allows current flow when exposed to light. A lens is an essential part of the photodiode and is used to focus light from the scintillation crystal to the *p-n* junction, or semiconductor junction. When light falls on the junction, electron hole pairs are generated and the electrons move to the *n* side of the junction while the holes move to the *p* side. The amount of current is proportional to the amount of light. Photodiodes are normally used with amplifiers because of the low output from the diode. In addition, the response time of a photodiode is extremely fast (about 0.5 to 250 nanoseconds, depending on its design).

Scintillation materials currently used with photodiodes are *cadmium tungstate* ($CdWO_4$) and a *ceramic material* made of high-purity, rare earth oxides based on doped rare earth compounds such as yttria $(Y,Gd)_2O_3$:Eu, and gadolinium oxysulfide ultrafast ceramic (UFC) ($Gd_2O_2S$:Pr,Ce[GOS]; Kalender, 2005; Shefer et al., 2013). More recently GE Healthcare (GE) has made use of what they refer to as the GE Gemstone, a garnet of the type $(Lu,Gd,Y,Tb)_3(Ga,Al)_5O_{12}$ detector. This is the first garnet scintillator for use in CT (Shefer et al., 2013). Furthermore, Philips

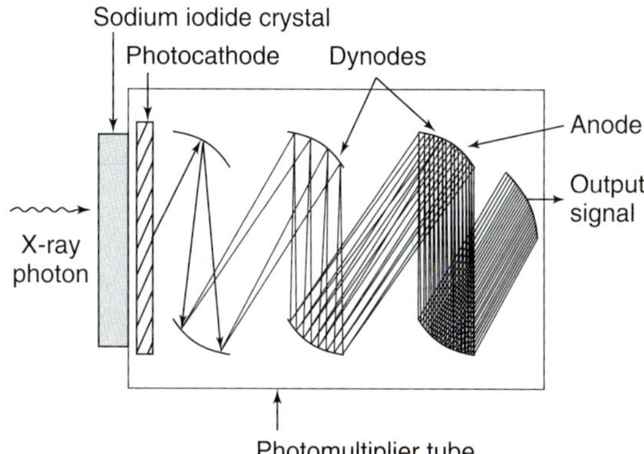


**FIGURE 4-30** Schematic representation of a scintillation detector based on the photomultiplier tube.

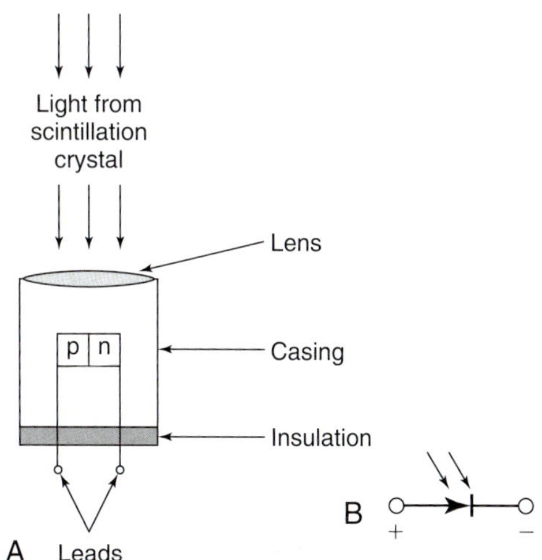


**FIGURE 4-31** **A,** Basic structure of a photodiode. **B,** The electronic symbol of a photodiode.

Healthcare makes use of ZnSe:Te in their dual-layer scintillator detectors (Shefer et al., 2013; Xu, 2012).

Usually these crystals are optically bonded to the photodiodes. The advantages and disadvantages of these two scintillation materials can be discussed in terms of the detector characteristics described earlier. The conversion efficiency and photon capture efficiency of cadmium tungstate are 99% and 99%, respectively, and the dynamic range is 1 million to 1. On the other hand, the absorption efficiency of the ceramic rare earth oxide is 99%, whereas its scintillation efficiency is three times that of $CdWO_4$.

### Gas-Ionization Detectors

**Gas-ionization detectors,** which are based on the principle of ionization, were introduced in third-generation scanners. The basic configuration of a gas-ionization detector consists of a series of individual gas chambers, usually separated by tungsten plates carefully positioned to act as electron collection plates (Fig. 4-32). When x rays fall on the individual chambers, ionization of the gas (usually xenon) results and produces positive and negative ions. The positive ions migrate to the negatively charged plate, whereas the negative ions are attracted to the positively charged plate. This migration of ions causes a small signal current that varies directly with the number of photons absorbed.

The gas chambers are enclosed by a relatively thick ceramic substrate material because the xenon gas is pressurized to about 30 atmospheres to increase the number of gas molecules available for ionization. Xenon detectors have excellent stability and fast response times and exhibit no afterglow problems. However, their quantum detection efficiency (QDE) is less than that of solid-state detectors. As reported in the past, the QDE is 95% to 100% for crystal solid-state scintillation detectors and 94% to 98% for ceramic solid-state detectors, and it is only 50% to 60% for xenon gas detectors (Arenson, 1995). It is important to note that with the introduction of MSCT scanners with their characteristic multirow detector arrays, gas-ionization detectors and fourth-generation CT systems are not used anymore. MSCT scanners are all based on the third-generation beam geometry (rotate-rotate principle) and use solid-state detector arrays (Kalender, 2005).

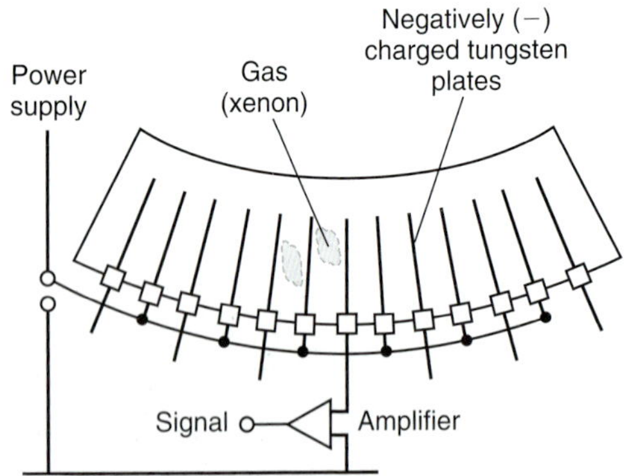


FIGURE 4-32 The basic configuration of a gas ionization detector consists of a series of individual gas chambers separated by tungsten plates.

## Design Innovations

As noted previously, the performance of a CT detector is characterized by efficiency of x-ray absorption and conversion to electrical signals, afterglow, stability, dynamic range, and response time. In an effort to improve on these performance characteristics and produce more efficient detectors for CT imaging, CT manufacturers have introduced several design innovations in an effort to improve clinical image quality (spatial resolution and image noise) in low-dose CT imaging (reduced dose; Shefer et al., 2013). Furthermore, artifact-free images are one of the advantages of these innovations. It is not within the scope of this chapter to describe the details of all of these innovations; however, a few, such as scintillators, miniaturization of the detector electronics, and detector module, will be highlighted.

Generally, CT detectors can be of the *conventional energy integration (EI) detector, dual-layer detector,* and the *direct conversion detector* (photon counting detector) as illustrated in Figure 4-33. The more commonplace CT detectors are of the first type, that is, the EI detector. Innovations involving the first two types will be briefly described next. The photon counting detector will not be described; however, semiconductors such as cadmium telluride (CdTe) and cadmium zinc telluride (CZT) have been used (Xu, 2012) because they can convert x-ray photons directly into electron hole pairs (electric charge)

> thereby avoiding the signal spread encountered with the light emitted by the commonly used scintillators. In consequence, no optical separation of detector elements is required, and geometric efficiency approaches the desired 100%. The charges generated can be collected within nanoseconds which makes it possible to count single photons and to determine the energy of each photon. Instead of analogue integration of intensities, digital counts of photons result with little or no influence of electronic noise (Kalender, 2014).

The innovations in CT detector technology have resulted in propriety detectors from four CT manufacturers, listed in Table 4-2, which lists five different types of current CT detectors, including the scintillators used. These propriety detectors are the Gemstone

Clarity Detector (GE Healthcare), the NanoPanel Prism Detector (Philips Healthcare), the PURE Vision CT Detector (Toshiba Medical Systems), the Stellar Detector (Siemens Healthcare), and the Quantum Vi Detector (Toshiba Medical Systems). The first four detector modules are shown in Figure 4-34, which shows the scintillators coupled to the detector modules (which contain the detector electronics). The details of these five detectors are not within the scope of this chapter; however, a brief overview of two of them will be highlighted for the purpose of illustrating the innovations in detector technology that lead to improved image quality in low dose CT imaging.

## The Stellar Detector

The Siemens Healthcare Stellar Detector falls in the category of the first *third-generation CT detectors* developed by Siemens Healthcare and is a fully integrated detector for CT imaging. Figure 4-35, *A* illustrates the major components of the Stellar Detector, which include the UFC scintillator, the back-illuminated photodiode, and the metal oxide semiconductor (CMOS) wafer that includes the ADC, and a ceramics substrate. The principle of operation is as follows: the light emitted from the UFC scintillator reaches the backside-illuminated photodiode, and as described by Ulzheimer and Freund (2012), "a **digital signal** is then produced on the other side of the wafer. This geometry consists of a 3D package of electronic circuits in a through-silicon via (TSV)—a

**TABLE 4-2 Names of the Most Recent Propriety Detectors from CT Manufacturers**

| Detector Name | Scintillator | CT Manufacturer |
|---|---|---|
| Gemstone Clarity Detector | Lutetium (Lu)-based garnet (gemstone-rare earth-based oxide) | General Electric Healthcare |
| NanoPanel Prism Detector | Top layer: yttrium-based garnet scintillator<br>Bottom layer: GOS | Philips Healthcare |
| Stellar Detector | UFC | Siemens Healthcare |
| Quantum Vi Detector | Pr GOS | Toshiba Medical Systems |
| PURE Vision CT Detector | Pr is an active additive of Toshiba GOS | Toshiba Medical Systems |

*Pr*, praesodynium-doped.

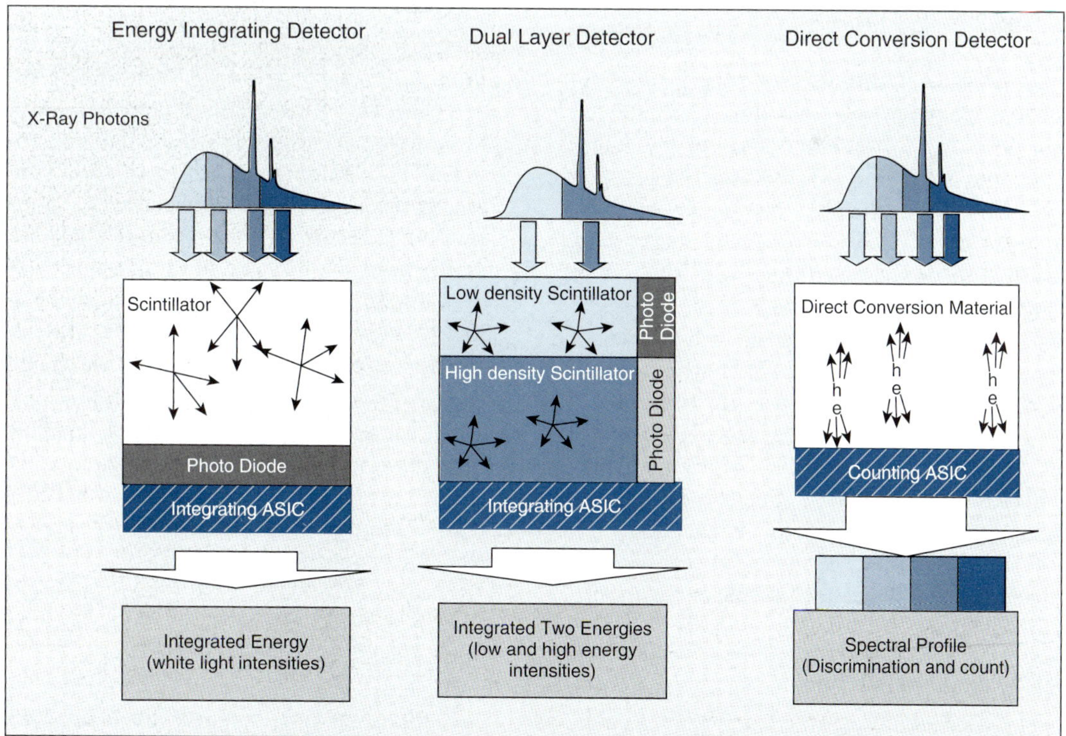


**FIGURE 4-33** Three types of detectors used in CT. While the conventional EI detector is illustrated on the left, the dual-layer (DL) detector is shown in the middle, and the direct-conversion (DiCo) detector is schematically shown on the right. (From Shefer, E., Altman, A., Behling, R., et al. (2013). *Current Radiology Reports*, *1*, 76-91. Reproduced by permission.)

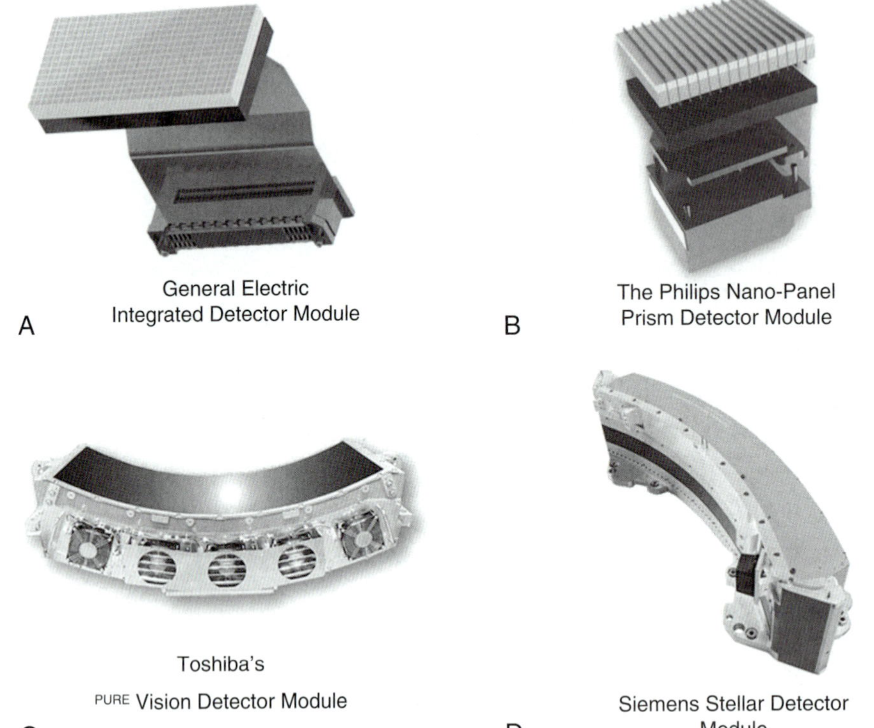


**FIGURE 4-34 A-D,** Four detector modules including recent innovations show the scintillators coupled to the detector modules, which contain the detector electronics. (**A,** Courtesy GE Healthcare; **B,** Courtesy Philips Healthcare; **C,** Courtesy Toshiba Medical Systems; **D,** Courtesy Siemens Healthcare.)

high performance technique for creating vertical connections that pass completely through the silicon wafer." Figure 4-35, *B*, shows a photo of the Stellar Detector array and, although it is not obvious, the ADC is located below the photodiode array.

By virtue of its design innovations such as the miniaturization of the electronics with the aid of nanotechnology, the electronics are totally integrated in the photodiode (Siemens TrueSignal Technology): "Stellar detectors can measure smaller signals over a wide dynamic range which reduces the noise in CT images and enhances CT image quality" (Ulzheimer & Freund, 2012). Figure 4-36, shows a visual comparison of the image quality obtained when using the Stellar Detector compared to a conventional CT detector. Miniaturization of the electronics will be described briefly in the section on Detector Electronics in this chapter.

## The NanoPanel Prism Detector

The NanoPanel Prism detector is a Philips Healthcare dual-layer detector based on technology that was first proposed by Brooks and Di Chiro (1978) who published an article titled "Split Detector Computed Tomography: A Preliminary Report" in the journal *Radiology*. A few years later, Philips Healthcare researchers (Altman et al., 2006; Carmi et al., 2005) developed another approach to detector-based **spectral CT imaging** using a dual-layer detector, "through two attached scintillator layers, optically separated, and read by a side-looking, edge-on, silicon photodiode, thin enough to maintain the same detector pitch and geometrical efficiency as a conventional CT detector" (Shefer et al., 2013), as illustrated in Figure 4-37. The configuration of the dual-layer detector allows for acquisition of both low and high energies for every exposure used in CT imaging.

The dual-layer detector is configured as a 3D tile-patterned arrangement featuring a number of modules in which each module is made up of three highly integrated components (Shefer et al., 2013) as follows:

1. A top layer of low-density scintillator (ZnSe), which absorbs low-energy x-ray photons that are subsequently converted to light photons
2. A bottom layer of high-density scintillator (GOS), which absorbs high-energy x-ray photons that are subsequently converted to light photons
3. Both top and bottom scintillators are coupled to a vertically positioned (edge-on) thin front-illuminated photodiode (FIP), which converts light into

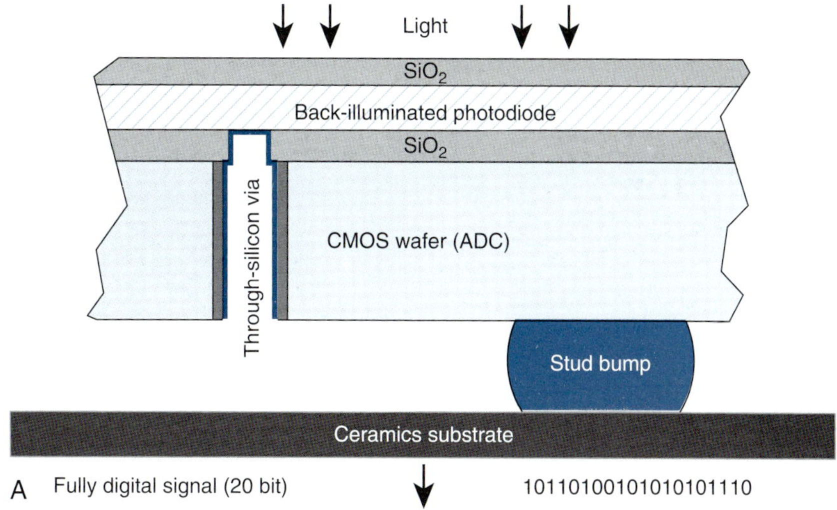


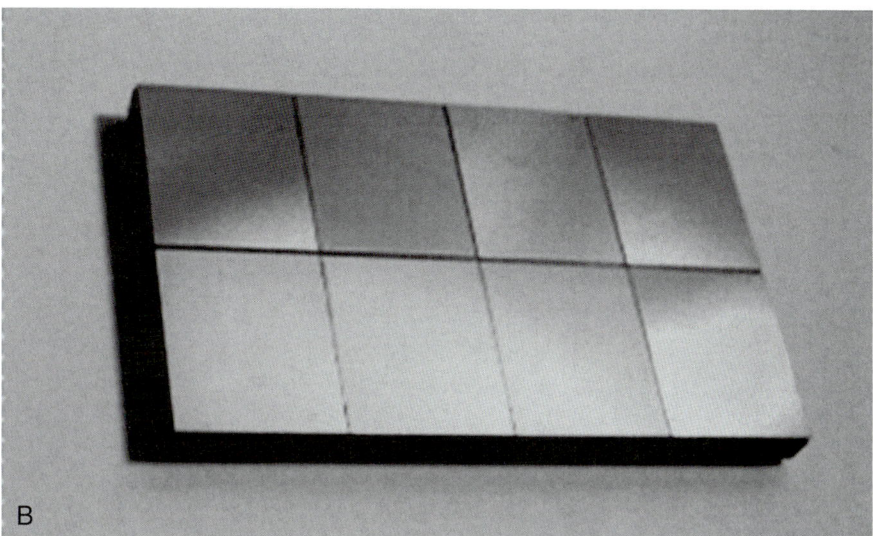


**FIGURE 4-35** Major components of the Siemens Healthcare Stellar Detector **(A)** and a photograph of the detector array **(B)**. (See text for further explanation.) (Courtesy Siemens Healthcare.)

electrical signals; the FIP is placed under the scattered radiation grid, so it will not compromise the detector's geometric efficiency

4. An application-specific integrated circuit (ASIC) designed for the purpose of ADC, and integration of the two energies, that is, low- and high-energy spectra

The materials used in the construction of the NanoPanel Prism dual-layer detector has been carefully selected and machined to ensure optimum performance in characteristics such as photon conversion efficiency, geometric efficiency, dynamic range, stability, **linearity,** uniformity, noise, and cross talk, all of which influence the final CT image quality (Gabbai et al., 2013)

## Detector-Based Spectral CT

*Spectral CT* involves exploiting the transmitted x-ray photons through the patient. Essentially there are two approaches to doing this: energy weighting and material decomposition (Xu, 2012).

While *energy weighting*

> requires a photon-counting energy-resolving detector which is capable of detecting the individual photons and measuring the correct photon energies accordingly……..material decomposition is to differentiate and characterize different materials and tissues in an examined object by decomposing the energy-dependent **linear attenuation coefficients** into a linear combination of energy-dependent basis functions and the corresponding basis set coefficients (Xu, 2012).

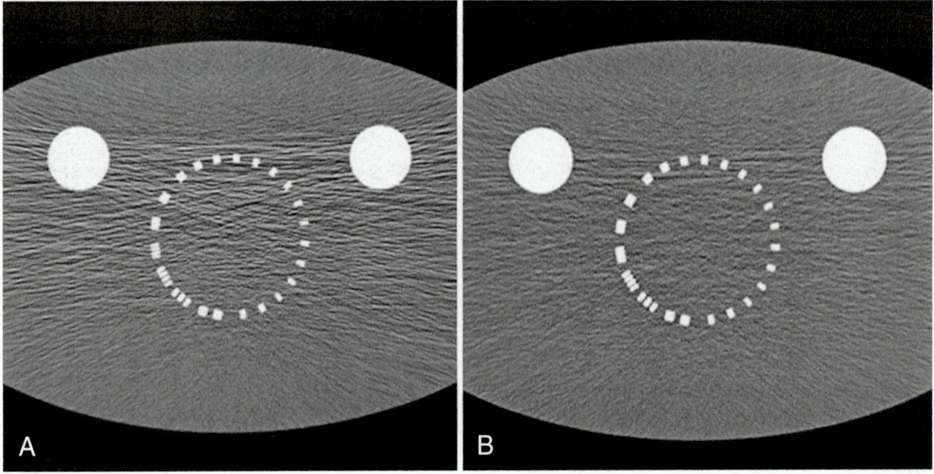


**FIGURE 4-36** Two images of a hip phantom with a resolution insert that shows the improvement in image quality using the Stellar Detector and a conventional CT detector. It is clear that the noise patterns seen on the image obtained with the conventional CT detector **(A)** are substantially reduced on the image obtained with the Stellar Detector **(B)**. (Courtesy Siemens Healthcare.)

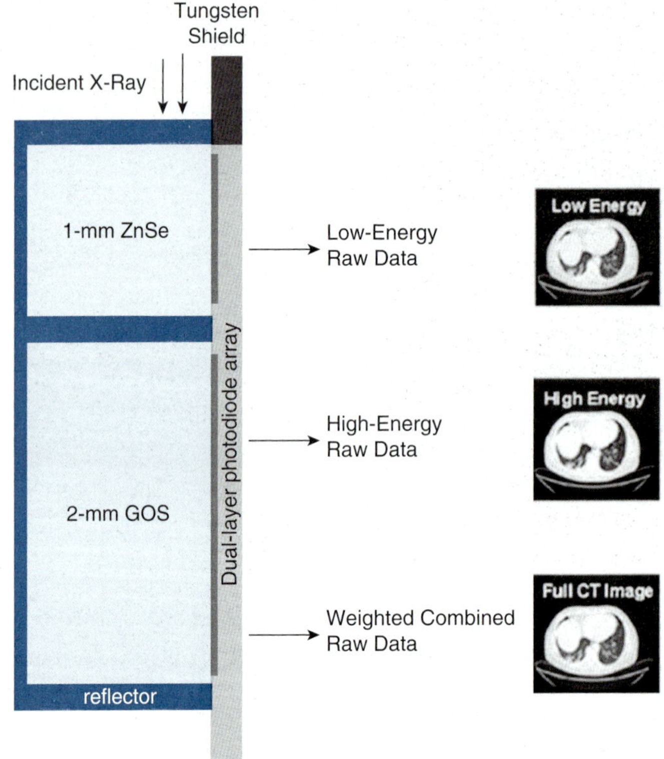


**FIGURE 4-37** Major components of the Philips Healthcare NanoPanel Prism Dual-Layer detector for detector-based spectral CT imaging. (See text for further explanation.) (From Shefer, E., Altman, A., Behling, R., et al. (2013). *Current Radiology Reports, 1*, 76-91. Reproduced by permission.)

In CT, essentially two *dual-energy methods* are used to extract spectral information from the x-rays transmitted through the patient during imaging. These include:

1. DSCT
2. Fast-kV switching CT

While Siemens Healthcare provides the DSCT system (Krauss et al., 2011), the fast-kV switching CT system is available from GE Healthcare (Chandra & Langan, 2011).

For a further description of dual-energy CT, the interested reader should refer to a recent paper by

Marin et al. (2014), which describes the basic principles of dual-energy CT including the physics of attenuation, different approaches to dual-energy CT (such as consecutive acquisition dual-energy CT, dual-energy CT, fast voltage switching dual-energy CT, and layer detector dual-energy CT), postprocessing tools (nonmaterial-specific display methods, material-specific methods, and energy-specific methods), and clinical applications.

DSCT is described further in Chapter 11.

## Multirow/Multislice Detectors

One major problem with single-slice, single-row detectors is related to the length of time needed to acquire data. The dual-slice, dual-row detector system was introduced to increase the volume coverage speed and thus decrease the time for data collection. CT scanners now use multirow detectors to image multislices during a 360-degree rotation. It is important to realize that other terms such as multidetector and multichannel have been used to describe the detectors for MSCT scanners (Douglas-Akinwande et al., 2006).

### Dual-Row/Dual-Slice Detectors

In 1992, Elscint introduced the first dual-slice volume CT scanner. The configuration of the dual-row detector system results in faster volume coverage compared with single-row CT systems (Fig. 4-38). This technology uses a dual-row, solid-state detector array coupled with a special x-ray tube based on a double-dynamic focus system. Figure 4-38 also shows the conventional beam geometry (single focal spot, single fan beam, and single detector arc array) and the beam geometry that arises as a result of the dynamic focal spot system. The dynamic focal spot is where the position of the focal spot is switched by a computer-controlled electron-optic system during each scan to double the sampling density and total number of measurements. Twin-beam technology results in the simultaneous scan of two contiguous slices with excellent resolution (Fig. 4-39) because the fan beam ray density and detector sampling are doubled twice, once for each of the two contiguous slices.

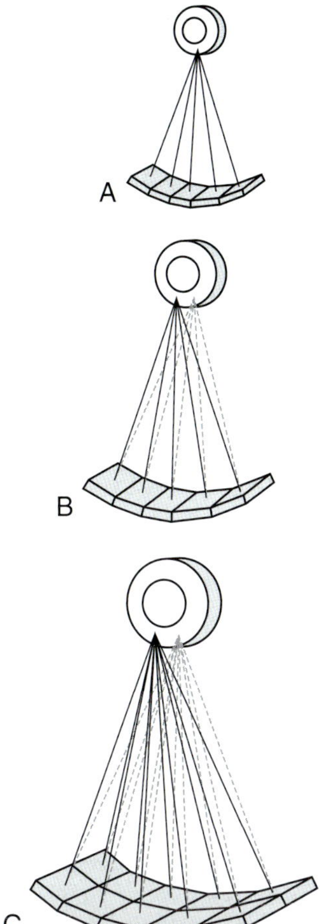


**FIGURE 4-38 A,** Conventional beam geometry with single focal spot, single fan beam, and single-detector arc array. **B,** Twin-beam geometry from Elscint's dynamic focal spot system. **C,** Dual-row, dual-detector system.

### Multirow/Multislice Detectors

The goal of multirow-multislice (MR-MS) detectors is to increase the volume coverage speed performance of both single-slice and dual-slice CT scanners. The MR-MS detector consists of one detector with rows of detector elements (Fig. 4-40). A detector with *n* rows will be *n* times faster than its single-row counterpart. MR-MS detectors are solid-state detectors that can acquire 4 to 64 to 320 slices per 360-degree rotation. In addition, the design of these detectors can influence the thickness of the slices.

An MR-MS detector is an array consisting of multiple separate detector rows. For example, these detector rows can range from 2 (Elscint dual-row detector) to 64 detector rows that can image simultaneously 2 to 64 slices, respectively, per 360-degree rotation. It is fairly obvious that the number of slices obtained per 360-degree rotation depends on the number of detector rows. For example, while a 16-detector row scanner can produce 16 images per 360-degree rotation, a 64-detector row scanner will produce 64 slices per 360-degree rotation.

Multirow CT detectors fall into two categories (Fig. 4-41): *matrix array detectors* and **adaptive array detectors** (Dalrymple et al., 2007; Flohr et al., 2005; Kalender, 2005). The matrix array detector

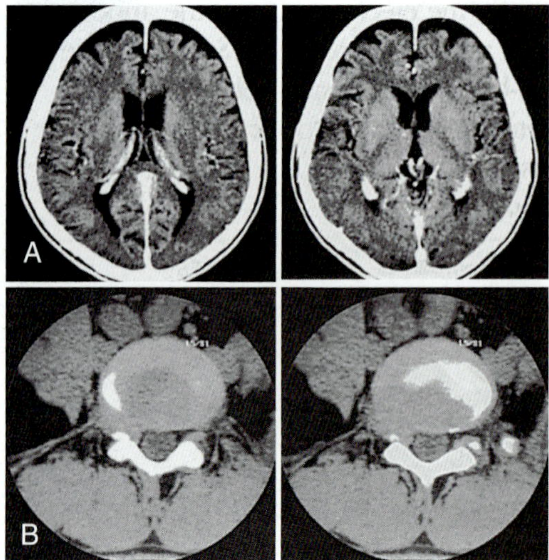


**FIGURE 4-39** Two contiguous slices acquired simultaneously for the brain **(A)** and spine **(B)**. The brain images are contiguous 10-mm slices and the spine images are contiguous 2.5-mm slices. (Courtesy Elscint, Hackensack, NJ.)

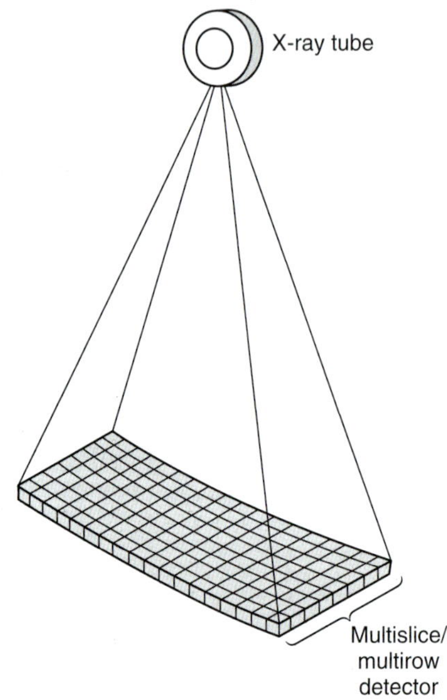


**FIGURE 4-40** The basic structure of a multislice/multirow detector used in multislice volume CT scanners.

(Fig. 4-41, *A*) is sometimes referred to as a **fixed array detector,** contains channels or cells, as they are often referred to, that are equal in all dimensions. Because of this, these detectors are sometimes referred to as *isotropic* in design, that is, all cells are perfect cubes. The adaptive array detector, on the other hand, is *anisotropic* in design (Kalender, 2005). This means that the cells are not equal; they

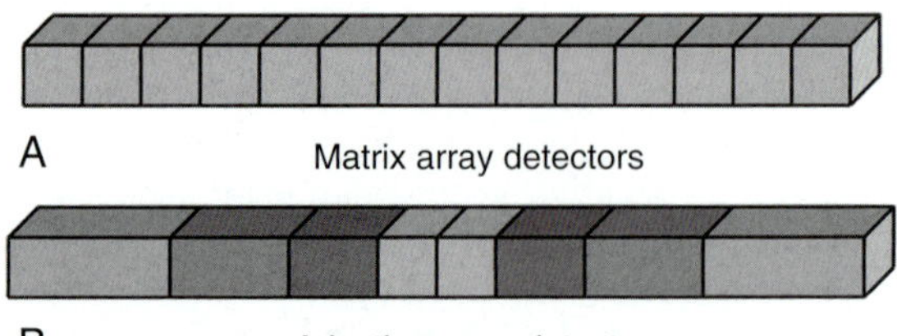


**FIGURE 4-41** Multirow CT detectors fall into two categories, namely, *matrix array detectors* **(A)** and *adaptive array detectors* **(B)**. (See text for further explanation.)

have different sizes (Fig. 4-41, *B*). The overall goal of isotropic imaging is to produce improved spatial resolution in both the longitudinal and transverse planes (Dalrymple et al., 2007).

During scanning, the number of slices and the thickness of each slice are determined by the detector configuration used. This configuration "describes the number of data collection channels and the effective section thickness determined by the data acquisition system settings" (Dalrymple et al., 2007). For the sake of simplicity, the detector configuration for a four-row matrix array detector is illustrated in Figure 4-42. In this example, each detector channel is 1.25 mm and four cells are activated or grouped together to produce four separate images of 1.25-mm thickness per 360-degree rotation. On the other hand, eight cells can be configured to produce four images of 2.5 mm thickness (1.25 mm + 1.25 mm = 2.5 mm) per 360-degree rotation, and so on. Multirow detectors are described further in Chapter 11.

Multirow detectors feature a number of imaging characteristics that are important to the technologist during scanning. These characteristics and specifications are shown in Table 4-3 from one CT vendor.

## Area Detectors

As discussed previously, several groups are investigating the use of area detectors for CT imaging and prototypes have been developed and are currently undergoing clinical testing. Two such CT scanners based on area detector technology are the 256-slice CT scanner prototype (Toshiba Aquilion, Toshiba Medical Systems, Japan) and the flat-panel CT scanner prototypes (one from Siemens Medical Solutions, and another from the Koning Corporation, United States).

### The 256-Slice CT Prototype Detector

An illustration of the gantry and detector for this scanner is shown in Chapter 1 (Fig 1-16). The detector is a wide area multirow array detector that has 912 channels × 256 segments and a beam width of 128 mm (four times larger than

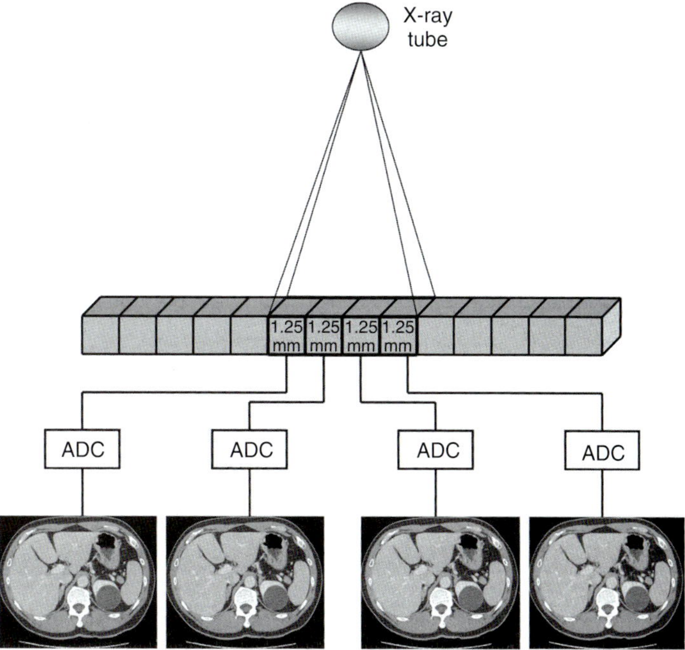


**FIGURE 4-42** The detector configuration for a four-row matrix array detector. In this example, each detector channel is 1.25 mm and four cells are activated or grouped together to produce four separate images of 1.25-mm thickness per 360-degree rotation.

the third-generation 16-slice Toshiba Aquilion CT scanner). This wide beam width makes it possible to scan larger volumes such as the entire heart in a single rotation (Mori et al., 2006; Mori, personal communications, 2006). This scanner is described further in Chapter 11.

### Flat-Panel Detectors

Flat-panel detectors similar to the ones used in digital radiography are being investigated for use in CT imaging. In this respect, several prototypes have been developed and are currently being evaluated for use in CT imaging. One such prototype is shown in Figure 4-10. Note that the detector is a flat-panel type and is based on the CsI indirect conversion digital radiography detector. More recently, flat-panel detectors are being investigated for use in breast CT, and several prototypes are now undergoing clinical testing (Glick et al., 2007; Kwan et al., 2007). Breast CT is described in Chapter 12.

**TABLE 4-3 Characteristics and Specifications of Multirow Detectors**

| Characteristics | Specifications |
|---|---|
| Material | Solid-state GOS |
| Number of elements | 43,008<br>86,016 effective with DFS |
| Dynamic range | 1,000,000 to 1 |
| Slip ring | Optical—up to 5.3 Gbps transfer rate |
| Data sampling rate | Up to 4640 views/revolution/element |
| Slice collimation | 2 × 0.5 mm, 16 × 2.5 mm, 32 × 1.25 mm, and 64 × 0.625 mm |
| Slice thickness | Spiral mode: 0.67 to 7.5 mm variable<br>Axial mode: 0.5 to 12 mm |
| Scan angles | 240, 360, and 420 degrees |
| Scan field of view | 250 and 500 mm |

Courtesy Philips Medical System.

## DETECTOR ELECTRONICS

### Function

The DAS refers to the detector electronics positioned between the detector array and the computer (Fig. 4-43). Because the DAS is located between the detectors and the computer, it performs three major functions: (1) measuring the transmitted radiation beam, (2) encoding these measurements into binary data, and (3) transmitting the binary data to the computer.

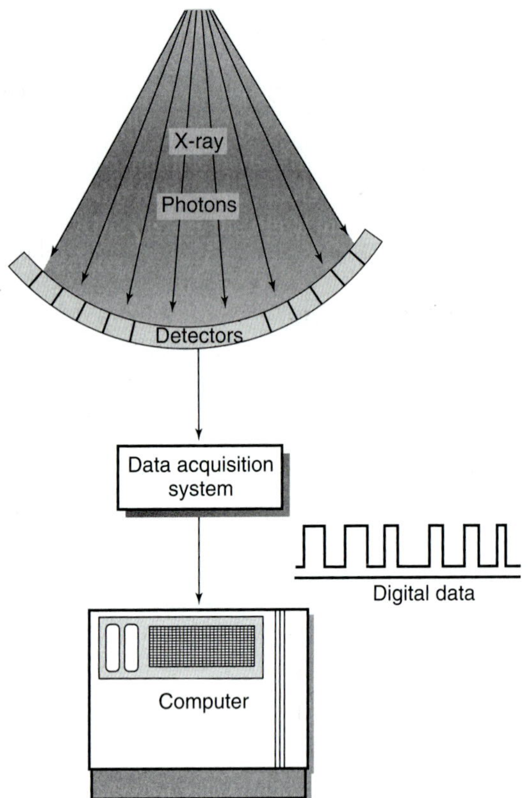


**FIGURE 4-43** Position of the data acquisition system in CT.

## Components

The detector measures the transmitted x rays from the patient and converts them into electrical energy. This electrical signal is so weak that it must be amplified by the preamplifier before it can be analyzed further (Fig. 4-44).

The transmission measurement data must be changed into attenuation and thickness data. This process (logarithmic conversion) can be expressed as follows:

$$\text{Attenuation} = \log \text{ of transmission} \cdot \text{thickness} \quad \textbf{(4-3)}$$

or

$$\mu_1 + \mu_2 + \mu_3 \ldots \mu_n = \ln I_0/I \cdot I/x$$

where μ is the linear attenuation coefficient, $I_0$ is the original intensity, $I$ is the transmitted intensity, and $x$ is the thickness of the object.

Logarithmic conversion is performed by the logarithmic amplifier, and these signals are subsequently directed to the ADC. The ADC divides the electrical signals into multiple parts—the more parts, the more accurate the ADC. These parts are measured in bits: a 1-bit ADC divides the signal into two digital values

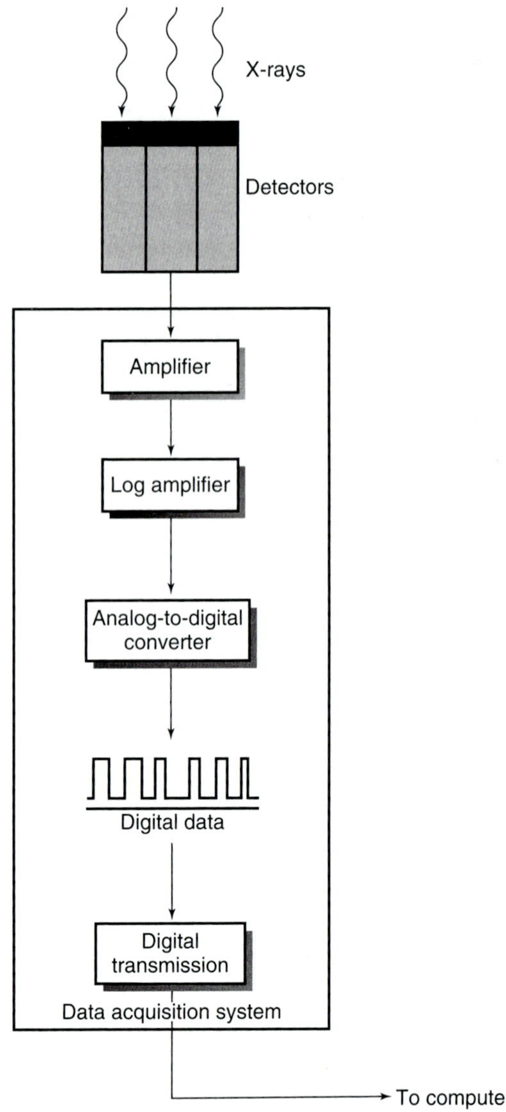


**FIGURE 4-44** Essential components of the data acquisition system in CT.

($2^1$), a 2-bit ADC generates four digital values ($2^2$), and a 12-bit ADC results in 4096 ($2^{12}$) digital values. These values help determine the grayscale resolution of the image. Modern CT scanners use 16-bit ADCs.

The final step performed by the DAS is data transmission to the computer. CT manufacturers have introduced optoelectronic data transmission schemes for this purpose because of the continuous rotation of the tube or detector arc and vast amount of data generated.

*Optoelectronics* refers to the use of lens and light diodes to facilitate data transmission (Fig. 4-45). Several optical transmitters send the data to the optical receiver array so that at least one transmitter and one receiver are always in optical contact. These receivers and transmitters are light-emitting diodes capable of

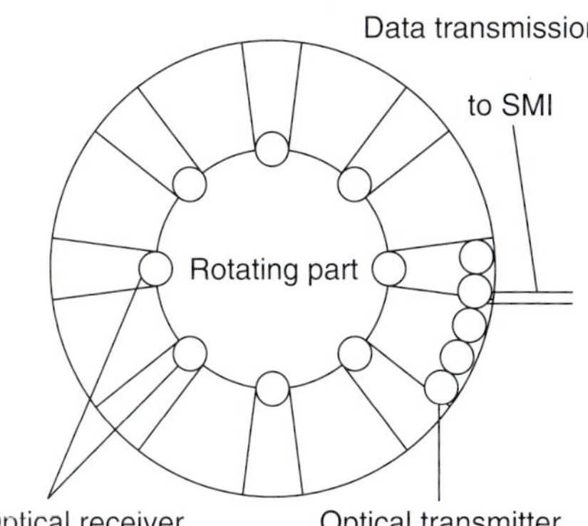


**FIGURE 4-45** Optoelectric data transmission. Optical transmitters on the gantry send data to the optical receiver array. At least one transmitter and one receiver are always in optical contact.

very high rates of data transmission; 50 million bits per second is common.

### Design Innovations

As described earlier in this chapter, the older conventional second-generation solid-state detectors employed separate electronics coupled to the ADC. A shortcoming of this design includes the use of several electrical components with long conducting wires, which not only increase electrical power consumption but more importantly produce electronic noise, thus compromising CT image quality. These problems are now overcome by another notable recent design innovation for CT detectors—miniaturized detector electronics through the use of *integrated microelectronic circuitry*. The purpose of such design elements is to reduce not only electronic noise but also to reduce power consumption. One such popular design is referred to as the *Application-Specific Integrated Circuit* (ASIC) for ADC.

The ASIC essentially contains the photodiodes and the ADCs, hence decreasing the distance through which electrical signals must travel. Furthermore, the ASIC design results in a much smaller and compact circuitry compared to second-generation conventional solid-state detectors. The results of the ASIC implementation are the reduction of electronic noise (thus improvement of image quality) and reduced electrical power consumption by the CT detectors.

Detectors such as Gemstone Clarity Detector (GE Healthcare), the Stellar Detector (Siemens Healthcare), PUREVision and the Quantum Vi Detectors (Toshiba Medical Systems), and the NanoPanel Prism Detector (Philips Healthcare) are all based on the integrated microelectronic circuitry design, sometimes also referred to as the integrated DAS circuitry. Figure 4-46 shows an example of the new detector miniaturized electronics design (Fig 4-46, *B*) compared with the conventional solid-state detector electronics, which includes the ADCs (Fig 4-46, *A*)

In summary, the ASIC component is an innovation in CT detector electronics design that ensures miniaturization of the electronic circuitry resulting in low power consumption and the use of shorter electrical wires that produce low electronic noise. The results of these innovations in CT detector technology are an improved signal-to-noise ratio and hence improved CT image quality, especially in low-dose CT imaging. In this regard, another CT **dose optimization** technique is the combined use of the new detector with iterative reconstruction algorithms. One such example is illustrated in Figure 4-47, which shows the visual image clarity of two images of a foot reconstructed with conventional CT technology (Fig 4-47, *A*) and the other reconstructed using the Stellar Detector (Fig 4-47, *B*) coupled with the use of an iterative reconstruction algorithm (Sinogram Affirmed Iterative Reconstruction-SAFIRE model-based reconstruction).

## DATA ACQUISITION AND SAMPLING

During data acquisition, the radiation beam transmitted through the patient falls on the detectors. Each detector then measures, or samples, the beam intensity incident on it. If enough samples are not obtained, artifacts, such as streaking (an aliasing artifact), appear on the reconstructed image. To solve this problem, the following methods have been devised to increase the number of samples available for image reconstruction and to thus improve the quality of the image:

- *Slice thickness*: The imaging of thin slices helps reduce streaking artifacts related to sampling.
- *Closely packed detectors*: When the detectors are closely packed, more detectors are available for data acquisition, which ensures more samples per view and an increase in the total measurements taken per scan. The innovations made to CT detectors recently allow for optimized sampling via improvements in detector characteristics such as fast decay time (primary speed) negligible afterglow. For example, the Gemstone Clarity Detector "has a primary decay time of only 30 microseconds, making it 100 times faster than GOS and .....it also has afterglow levels that reach only 25% of GOS levels making it ideal for fast sampling and high resolution" (Chandra, 2008). Figure 4-48 illustrates the effect of increased sampling on image resolution.

**Conventional Detector**

Conventional photodiode (PD)

Complex board w/ AD-converters

- Discrete PD and AD-converters → high number of electronic parts
- Long elec. connection distance
- Typical elec. noise contribution

**Stellar Detector**

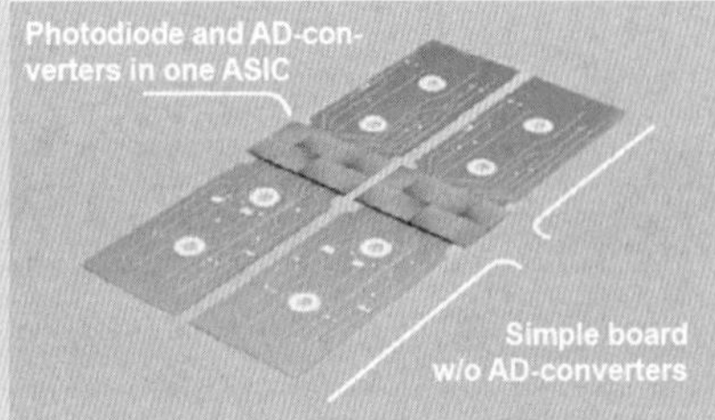


- Integrated PD and AD-converters in one ASIC
- Virtually no connection distance
- Significantly reduced elec. noise

**FIGURE 4-46** A comparison of the design of the electronic circuitry of the two generations of CT detectors. **A,** Conventional second-generation, solid-state electronic circuitry that includes the ADCs. **B,** The design difference characteristic of the Stellar Detector, in which the components are completely integrated with the photodiode, eliminating the need for these additional electronic components. (Courtesy Siemens Healthcare.)

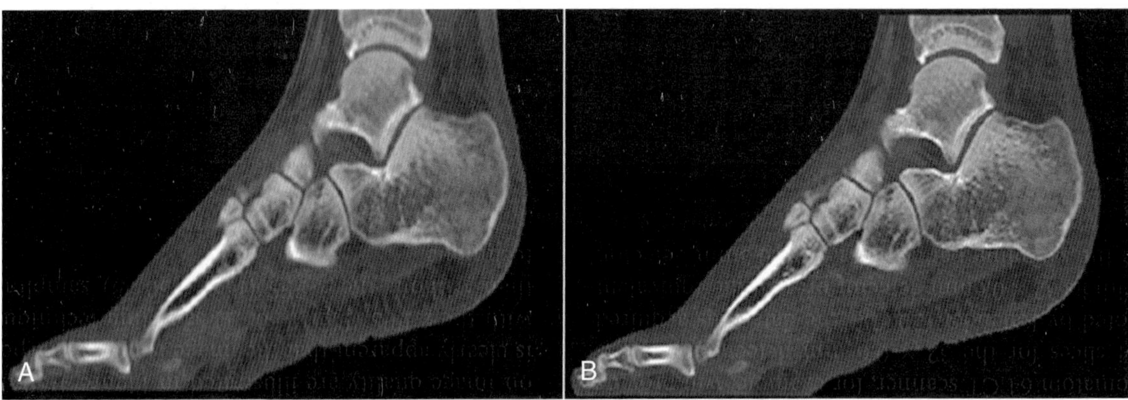


**FIGURE 4-47** A comparison of the visual image clarity of two images of a foot reconstructed with conventional CT technology **(A)** and the other reconstructed using the Stellar Detector **(B)** coupled with the use of an iterative reconstruction algorithm (Sinogram Affirmed Iterative Reconstruction-SAFIRE model-based reconstruction). (Courtesy Siemens Healthcare.)

- In the past, *the quarter-shifted detector arc* has been used: In conventional CT systems, the fan beam is composed of the same number of beams and detectors, and the spacing of the beams often causes sampling errors. These errors can be minimized if the detector arc is shifted by one-quarter detector space. The goal of detector shifting is to provide two sets of data that can be individually reconstructed or combined to provide a doubly fine sampling grid so more data are available for image reconstruction. In the Siemens Somatom Plus scanner, for example, this shifting is accomplished by the flying focal spot (dual focal spot x-ray tube). The same detector is used more than once to provide a large number of discrete measurements, which eliminates the aliasing artifact. This process is referred to as the *multifan measurement technique* (Siemens Medical Systems, 1999).
- The *double-dynamic focus* system used by Elscint in their CT twin scanner was yet another method of increasing detector sampling during data acquisition.

## New Sampling Technique: z-Sharp Technology

A more recent innovation is one that involves the use of the Straton x-ray tube described earlier in the

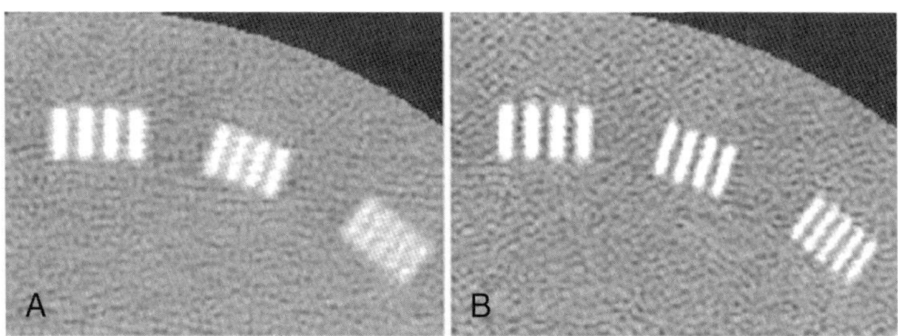


**FIGURE 4-48** The effect of increased sampling on the visual clarity (resolution) of the bar pattern. It is clear that compared to the standard sampling **(A)**, increased sampling results in a sharper image **(B)**. (Courtesy of GE Healthcare.)

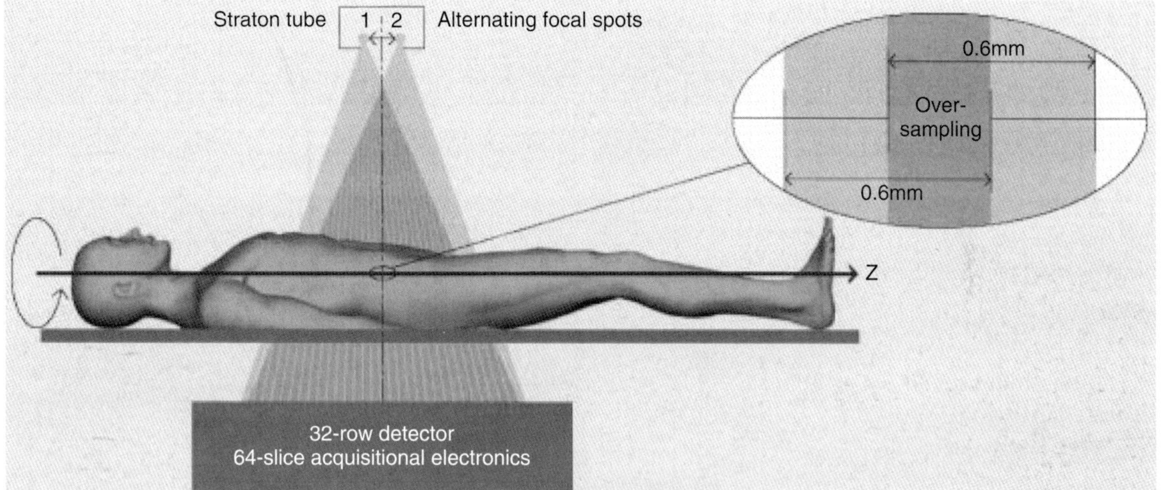


**FIGURE 4-49** The *z-flying focal spot technique* (referred to as the *z-Sharp technology*) provides doubling sampling, where two overlapping slices for each detector row are obtained at the same time per 360-degree rotation. (Courtesy Siemens Medical Solutions, Germany.)

chapter. As seen in Figure 4-49, the **z-flying focal spot technique** (referred to as the *z-Sharp technology*) provides doubling sampling, where two overlapping slices for each detector row are obtained at the same time per 360-degree rotation. The Siemens Somatom 64 CT scanner, for example, will provide 64 slices for the 32 × 0.6 mm detector array. As noted by Kalender (2005), "the data thus acquired with its 32 × 0.6mm detector present the equivalent to the sampling pattern of a 64 × 0.3mm detector. The data set results are representing 64 overlapping slices of 0.6mm width with a sampling distance of 0.3mm."

The results of double sampling in the *z*-direction by the *z-flying focal spot* (z-FFS) technique on image quality are illustrated in Figure 4-50. It is clearly apparent that the image is much sharper with the z-FFS (Fig. 4-50, *A*) sampling technique than without the z-FFS (Fig. 4-50, *B*) sampling technique.

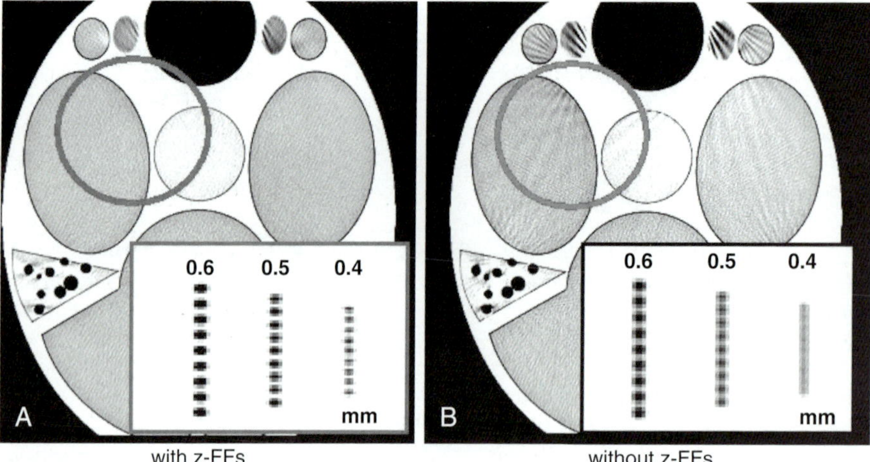


**FIGURE 4-50** The results of double sampling in the z-direction by the *z-flying focal spot* (z-FFS) technique on image quality. It is clearly apparent that the image is much sharper with the z-FFS **(A)** sampling technique than without the z-FFS **(B)** sampling technique. (Courtesy Siemens Medical Solutions, Germany.)

## REVIEW QUESTIONS

Answer the following questions to check your understanding of the materials studied.

1. Which of the following refers to the size, shape, motion, and path traced by the x-ray beam in CT scanning?
   A. Detector tracing
   B. Beam geometry
   C. Data acquisition
   D. Data projection
2. The data acquisition scheme using a fan beam of x rays and a 360° rotation of the x-ray tube and detectors is referred to as:
   A. first-generation scanning.
   B. second-generation scanning.
   C. third-generation scanning.
   D. fourth-generation scanning.
3. In which scanner is the apex of the fan beam at the detector?
   A. Fourth-generation scanner
   B. Third-generation scanner
   C. Fifth-generation scanner
   D. All of the above
4. The scanner based on slip-ring technology is:
   A. third-generation scanner.
   B. fourth-generation scanner.
   C. spiral/helical scanner.
   D. fifth-generation scanner.
5. Electromechanical devices made up of rings and brushes to transmit electricity across a rotating interface are called:
   A. target rings.
   B. helical rings.
   C. spiral rings.
   D. slip rings.
6. The x-ray generator used in modern CT scanners is the:
   A. singe-phase generator.
   B. constant potential generator.
   C. three-phase, six-pulse generator.
   D. high-frequency generator.
7. A filter is used in CT to:
   A. reduce the energy at the detector.
   B. protect the patient.
   C. decrease the intensity at the patient's skin.
   D. produce a more uniform beam at the detector.
8. The following crystals have been used in scintillation detectors in CT ***except***:
   A. gadolinium oxysulfide
   B. calcium tungstate
   C. ultrafast ceramic
   D. cadmium tungstate
9. A dual-layer detector such as the NanoPanel Prism Detector
   A. can be used for spectral CT imaging.
   B. is not used in current CT imaging.
   C. only provides information for high kVp techniques.
   D. can only be used for CT imaging at the molecular level.
10. The ratio of the largest signal to the smallest signal to be measured by a CT detector is referred to as the _______________ of the detector.
    A. stability
    B. response time
    C. efficiency
    D. dynamic range

## REFERENCES


Altman, A., et al. (2006). *Double decker detector for spectral CT*. US Patent US 7,968,853.

Arenson, J. (1995). Data collection strategies: gantries and detectors. In L. W. Goldman, & J. B. Fowlkes (Eds.), *Medical CT and ultrasound: current technology and applications* (pp. 329–347). College Park, MD: American Association of Physicists in Medicine.

Boyd, D. P., et al. (1979). A proposed dynamic cardiac 3-D densitometry for early detection and evaluation of heart disease. *IEEE Trans Nuclear Science, 26*, 2724–2727.

Boyd, D. P., & Lipton, M. J. (1983). Cardiac computed tomography. *Proceedings of the IEEE, 198*, 198–307.

Brooks, R. A., & Di Chiro, G. (1978). Split detector computed tomography: a preliminary report. *Radiology, 126*(1), 255–257.

Brunnett, C. J., et al. (1990). *CT design considerations and specifications*. Cleveland, OH: Picker International.

Carmi, R., et al., (2005). Material separation with dual layer CT. Presented at the *IEEE-MIC.Conference*. Puerto Rico, Wyndham El Conquistador, October 23–29.

Chandra, N. (2008). CT sampling technology, White Paper. *GE Healthcare*, 1–8.

Chandra, N., & Langan, D. A. (2011). Gemstone detector: dual energy imaging via fast kVp switching. In T. Johnson, C. Fink, S. O. Schonberg, & M. F. Reiser (Eds.), *Dual energy CT in clinical practice* (pp. 35–41). Berlin Heidelberg: Springer-Verlag.

Dalrymple, N. C., Prasad, S. R., El-Merhi, F. M., & Chintapalli, K. N. (2007). Price of isotropy in multidetector CT. *Radiographics, 27*, 49–62.

Deak, P. D., et al. (2009). Effects of adaptive section collimation on patient radiation dose in multisection spiral CT. *Radiology, 252*(1), 140–147.

Douglas-Akinwande, A. C., Buckwalter, K. A., Rydberg, J., Rankin, J. L., & Choplin, R. H. (2006). Multichannel CT: evaluating the spine in postoperative patients with orthopedic hardware. *Radiographics, 26*, S96–S110.

Flohr, T. G., Schaller, S., Stierstorfer, K., et al. (2005). Multi-detector row CT systems and image reconstruction techniques. *Radiology, 235*, 756–773.

Flohr, T. G., McCollough, C. H., Bruder, H., et al. (2006). First performance evaluation of a dual-source CT (DSCT) system. *European Radiology, 16*, 256–268.

Fox, S. H. (1995). CT tube technology. In L. W. Goldman, & J. B. Fowlkes (Eds.), *Medical CT and ultrasound: current technology and applications* (pp. 349–357). College Park, MD: American Association of Physicists in Medicine.

Gabbai, M., et al. (2014). The clinical impact of retrospective analysis in spectral detector dual energy body CT. *Radiological Society of North America 2013 Scientific Assembly and Annual Meeting*, December 1-6, 2013, Chicago IL. http://archive.rsna.org/2013/13018312.html Accessed March 19, 2014.

Glick, S. J., Thacker, S., Gong, X., & Liu, B. (2007). Evaluating the impact of x-ray spectral shape on image quality in flat-panel CT breast imaging. *Medical Physics, 34*, 5–20.

Goldman, L. W. (2000). Principles of CT and the evolution of CT technology. In L. W. Goldman, & J. B. Fowlkes (Eds.), *Categorical course in diagnostic radiology physics: CT and US cross sectional imaging*. Oak Brook, IL: Radiological Society of North America.

Goo, H. W. (2012). CT Radiation dose optimization and estimation: an update for radiologists. *Korean Journal of Radiology, 13*(1), 1–11.

Homberg, R., & Koppel, R. (1997). An x-ray tube assembly with rotating-anode spiral groove bearing of the second generation. *Electromedica, 66*, 65–66.

Hounsfield, G. N. (1973). Computerized transverse axial scanning (tomography). Part 1: Description of the system. *British Journal of Radiology, 46*, 1016–1022.

Kalender, W. A. (2005). *Computed tomography: fundamentals, system technology, image quality, applications* (2nd ed.). Erlangen, Germany: Publicis Corporate Publishing.

Kalender, W. A. (2014). Dose in x-ray computed tomography. *Physics in Medical Biology, 59*, R129–R150.

Krauss, B., et al. (2011). Dual source CT. In T. Johnson, C. Fink, S. O. Schonberg, & M. F. Reiser (Eds.), *Dual energy CT in clinical practice* (pp. 11–20). Berlin Heidelberg: Springer-Verlag.

Kwan, A. L. C., Boone, J. M., Yang, K., & Huang, S. Y. (2007). Evaluating the spatial resolution characteristics of a cone-beam breast CT scanner. *Medical Physics, 34*, 275–281.

Marin, D., Boll, D. T., Mileto, A., & Nelson, R. C. (2014). State of the art: dual-energy CT of the abdomen. *Radiology, 271*(2), 327–342.

McCollough, C. H. (1995). Principles and performance of electron beam CT. In L. W. Goldman, & J. B. Fowlkes (Eds.), *Medical CT and ultrasound, current technology and applications*. College Park, MD: American Association of Physicists in Medicine.

McCollough, C. H., Primak, A. N., Saba, O., et al. (2007). Dose performance of a 64-channel dual-source CT scanner. *Radiology, 243*, 775–784.

Mori, S., Endo, M., Nishizawa, K., et al. (2006). Comparison of patient doses in 256-slice CT and 16-slice CT scanners. *British Journal of Radiology, 79*, 56–61.

Parker, D. L., & Stanley, J. H. (1981). Glossary. In T. H. Newton, & D. G. Potts (Eds.), *Radiology of the skull and brain: technical aspects of computed tomography*. St. Louis, MO: Mosby.

Philips Healthcare (2005). MRC 800 X-ray tube technology *White Paper*. http://clinical.netforum.healthcare.philips.com/global/Explore/White-Papers/CT/MRC-800-X-ray-tube-technology. Accessed March 19, 2015.

Seeram, E. (2009). *Computed tomography technology*. Philadelphia: Elsevier.

Shefer, E., Altman, A., Behling, R., et al. (2013). State of the art of CT detectors and sources: a literature review. *Current Radiology Reports*, *1*, 76–91.

Siemens Medical Systems. (1999). *The technology and performance of the Somatom Plus*. Iselin, NJ: Siemens.

Ulzheimer, S., & Freund, J. (2012). The stellar detector. *White Paper*, 2–7 Siemens Healthcare.

Villafana, T. (1987). Physics and instrumentation: CT and MRI. In S. H. Lee, & K. C. V. G. Rao (Eds.), *Cranial computed tomography*. New York: McGraw-Hill.

Xu, C. (2012). *A segmented silicon strip detector for photon-counting spectral computed tomography (Doctoral Thesis)*. AlbaNova Universitetscentrum. Kungliga Tekniska Högskolan, Stockholm, Sweden.

Zhang, G., Marshall, N., Jacobs, R., Liu, Q., & Bosmas, H. (2013). Bowtie filtration for dedicated cone beam CT of the head and neck: a simulation study. *British Journal of Radiology*, *86*, 20130002.

5

# Image Reconstruction

## OUTLINE

**Basic Principles**
- Algorithms
- Fourier Transform
- Convolution
- Interpolation

**Image Reconstruction from Projections**
- Historical Perspective
- Problem in CT

**Reconstruction Algorithms**
- Back-Projection
- Iterative Algorithms
- Analytic Reconstruction Algorithms

**Types of Data**
- Measurement Data
- Raw Data
- Convolved Data
- Image Data

**Image Reconstruction in Single-Slice Spiral/Helical CT**

**Image Reconstruction in Multislice Spiral/Helical CT**

**Cone-Beam Algorithms for Multislice CT Scanners**
- Cone-Beam Geometry
- Cone-Beam Algorithms

**An Overview of Three-Dimensional Reconstruction Techniques**

## LEARNING OBJECTIVES

On completion of this chapter, you should be able to:

1. describe briefly what is meant by each of the following:
   - algorithms
   - fourier transform
   - convolution
   - interpolation.
2. explain briefly what is meant by the term "image reconstruction from projections."
3. trace the history of reconstruction techniques.
4. state the basic mathematical problem in CT.
5. identify three classes of reconstruction algorithms.
6. describe the back-projection reconstruction algorithm and state its fundamental limitation.
7. explain how the filtered back-projection algorithm works.
8. state the role of interpolation in image reconstruction in single- and multislice CT.
9. list four operations of a 3D surface display technique.

## KEY TERMS TO WATCH FOR AND REMEMBER

The following key terms/concepts are important to your understanding of this chapter.

**algorithm**
**analytic reconstruction algorithms**
**back projection**
**convolution**
**convolution method**
**filtered back-projection**
**Fourier coefficients**
**Fourier transform**
**frequency domain**
**interpolation**
**projection**
**ray sum**
**spatial domain surface shaded display**

## BASIC PRINCIPLES

For the computer to reconstruct an image of the patient by **computed tomography (CT),** the **x-ray tube** and detectors must rotate around the patient for at least 180 degrees plus the fan beam angle. Furthermore, Dual Source CT scanners are now available and in this case, the x-ray tubes and detectors need only rotate 90 degrees to get a full dataset. These scanners have **two** x-ray tubes (sources) and two detector arrays within the **gantry,** spaced at a 90-degree angle. The essential features of Dual Source CT scanners will be highlighted in Chapter 11.

In this way, sufficient x-ray transmission values or **attenuation** data are collected to satisfy the **image reconstruction** process that builds up an image of acceptable quality. The reconstruction process is based on the use of an algorithm that uses the attenuation data measured by the detectors to systematically build up the image for viewing and interpretation. The sequence of events after the data are collected from the detectors is shown in Figure 5-1. Although the older CT scanners collected data over 180 degrees, present-day CT scanners collect more attenuation data over 360 degrees to generate better quality images. The image reconstruction algorithms, as they are referred to, are numerous and have been developed and subsequently modified to meet the requirements of the new **generation** of CT scanners. Understanding these algorithms requires a basic introduction to several concepts, including the Fourier transform, convolution, and interpolation.

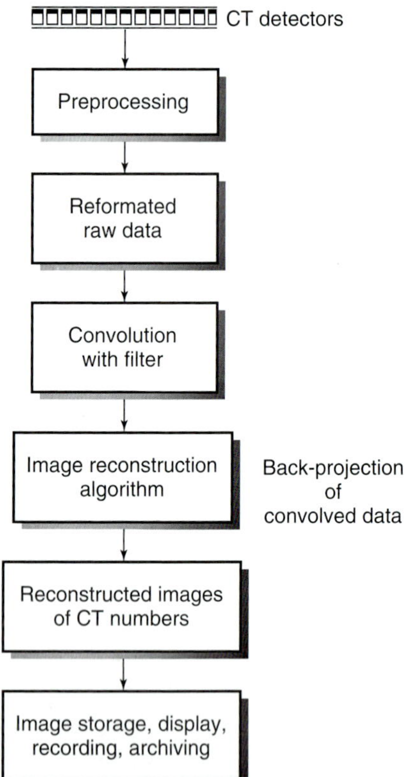


**FIGURE 5-1** Sequence of events after signals leave the detectors. The image reconstruction algorithms deal with the mathematics of the CT process.

The purpose of this chapter is to present a brief nonmathematical description of several image reconstruction algorithms to impress upon the technologist that the problem with CT is mathematical so mathematical solutions are needed to solve the problem. The description will begin with the algorithms used in the earlier conventional CT scanners, followed by a brief introduction to the algorithms used in both single-slice spiral/helical CT (SSCT) and multislice spiral/helical CT (MSCT) scanners. MSCT scanning principles are described in more detail in Chapter 11.

### Algorithms

The algorithm is now common in radiology because computers are used in many imaging and nonimaging applications. The word **algorithm** is derived from the name of the Persian scholar, Abu Ja'Far Mohammed ibn Mûsâ Alkowârîzmî, whose textbook on arithmetic (c. 825 CE) significantly influenced mathematics for many years (Knuth, 1977). According to Knuth, an algorithm is "a set of rules or directions for getting a specific **output** from a specific **input.** The distinguishing feature of an algorithm is that all vagueness must be eliminated; the rules must describe operations that are so simple and well defined, they can be executed by a machine. Furthermore, an algorithm must always terminate after a finite number of steps."

The solutions to mathematical problems in CT require image reconstruction algorithms, which are available as computer **software,** to reconstruct the image.

### Fourier Transform

The **Fourier transform,** which was developed by the mathematician Baron Jean-Baptiste-Joseph Fourier in 1807, is widely used in science and engineering. The Fourier transform is a useful analytical tool in mathematics, astronomy, chemistry, physics, medicine, and radiology. In radiology, the Fourier transform is used to reconstruct images of a patient's anatomy in CT and also in **magnetic resonance imaging (MRI).**

To understand the Fourier transform, Bracewell (1989) presented an analogy with the act of hearing. Incoming sound waves that enter the ear are separated into different signals and intensities. These signals arrive at the brain and are rearranged to produce a perception of the original sound. Bracewell (1989) defined the Fourier transform as "a function that describes the amplitude and phases of each sinusoid, which corresponds to a specific frequency. (Amplitude describes the height of the sinusoid; phase specifies the starting point in the sinusoid's cycle.)" In other words, the Fourier transform is a mathematical function that converts a signal in the **spatial domain** to a signal in the frequency domain.

The Fourier transform divides a waveform (sinusoid) into a series of sine and cosine functions of different frequencies and amplitudes. These components can then be separated. In imaging, when a beam of x rays passes through the patient, an image profile denoted by $f(x)$ is obtained. This can be expressed mathematically in the form of the Fourier series as follows:

$$\begin{aligned} f(x) = a_0/2 &+ (a_1 \cos x + b_1 \sin x) \\ &+ (a_2 \cos 2x + b_2 \sin 2x) \\ &+ (a_3 \cos 3x + b_3 \sin 3x) + \ldots \\ &+ (a_n \cos nx + b_n \sin nx) \end{aligned}$$

The constants—$a_0$, $a_1$, $b_1$, and so on—are called **Fourier coefficients** (Gibson, 1981) and can easily be calculated. Use of these Fourier coefficients makes it possible to reconstruct an image in CT.

## Convolution

**Convolution** is a digital **image-processing** technique used to modify images through a filter function (see Chapter 2). "The process involves multiplication of overlapping portions of the filter function and the detector response curve selectively to produce a third function which is used for image reconstruction" (Berland, 1987). (This will become clear during the discussion of the **filtered back-projection** algorithm.)

## Interpolation

Interpolation is used in CT in the image reconstruction process and the determination of slices in spiral/helical CT imaging. **Interpolation** is a mathematical technique used to estimate the value of a function from known values on either side of the function.

For example, if the speed of an engine controlled by a lever increases from 40 to 50 revolutions per second when the lever is pulled down by 4 cm, one can interpolate from this information and assume that moving it 2 cm gives 45 revolutions per second. This is *linear interpolation*, which is the simplest method of interpolation. If known values of one variable, $Y$, are plotted against the other variable, $X$, an estimate of an unknown value of $Y$ can be made by drawing a straight line between the two nearest known values.

The mathematical formula for linear interpolation is as follows:

$$Y_3 = Y_1 + (X_3 - X_1)(Y_2 - Y_1)/(X_2 - X_1)$$

where $Y_3$ is the unknown value of $Y$ (at $X_3$) and $Y_2$ and $Y_1$ (at $X_2$ and $X_1$) are the nearest known values between which the interpolation is made (Gibson, 1981).

# IMAGE RECONSTRUCTION FROM PROJECTIONS

## Historical Perspective

The history of reconstruction techniques dates back to 1917 when Radon developed mathematical solutions to the problem of image reconstruction from a set of its projections. He applied these techniques to gravitational problems. They were later used to solve problems in astronomy and optics, but they were not applied to medicine until 1961 (Fig. 5-2).

In his initial work, Hounsfield's images were noisy as a result of his chosen reconstruction technique. Special algorithms (convolution back-projection algorithms) were soon introduced. These algorithms were developed by Ramachandran and Lakshminarayanan (1971) and later used by Shepp and Logan (1974) to improve image quality and processing time.

## Problem in CT

Consider an object, $O$, represented by an $x$-$y$ coordinate system (Fig. 5-3). The spatial distribution of all attenuation coefficients, $\mu$, is given by $\mu(x,y)$, which varies between points in the object. Suppose a pencil

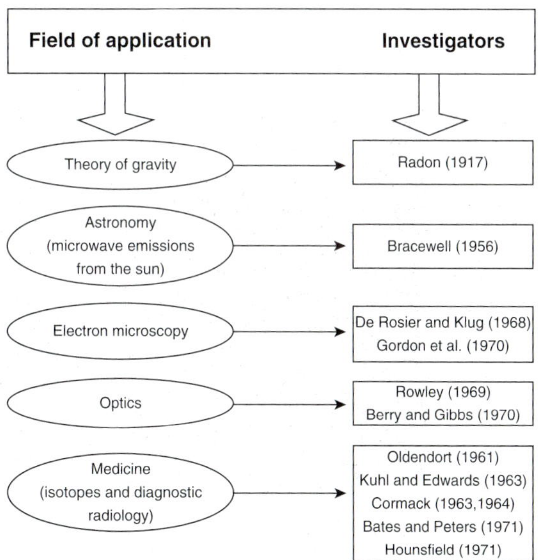


**FIGURE 5-2** Fields of application and principal investigators of image reconstruction techniques.

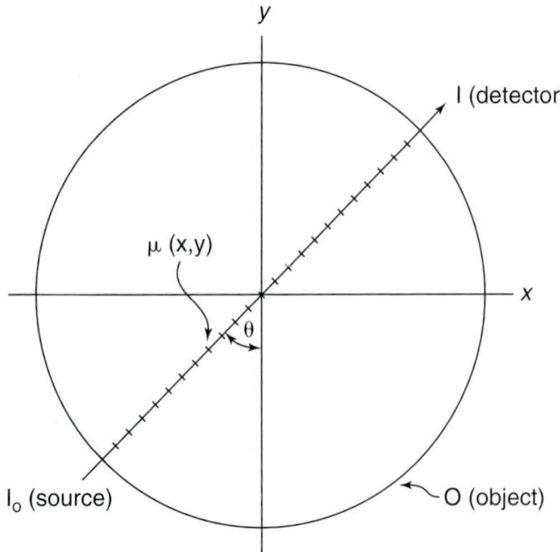


**FIGURE 5-3** The total distribution of attenuation coefficients in the object *O* is μ(*x,y*). The problem in CT is to calculate μ(*x,y*) from a set of projections specified by the angle θ. $I_0$ and *I* represent beam intensities from the source and at the detector, respectively. (From Seeram, E. (2001). *Computed tomography technology*. Philadelphia, PA: WB Saunders.)

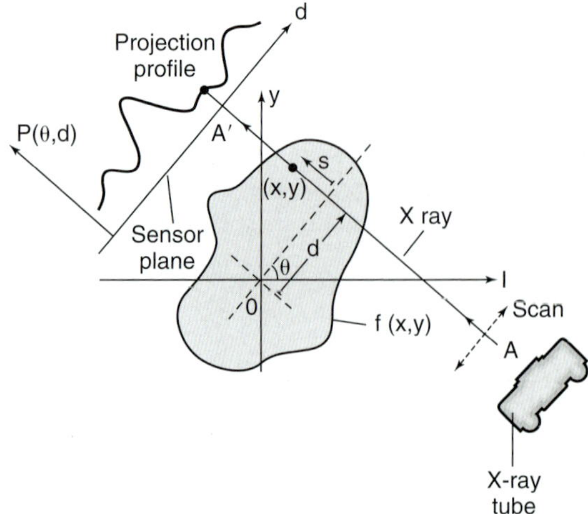


**FIGURE 5-4** Projection profile obtained when a parallel beam of x rays scans the object represented by *f*(*x,y*). (*d* is the distance of the ray *AA′* from the origin *0*.)

beam of x rays passes through the object along a straight path (arrow), and the intensity of the transmitted beam that falls on the CT detector is *I*. Then a projection is given by the line integral* of μ(*x,y*):

$$I = I_0 \exp\left[-\sum_{Source}^{Detector} \mu(x,y)\right] \quad (5\text{-}1)$$

By taking the negative logarithm, Equation 5-1 can be linearized to generate integral equations of the form

$$T_\theta(x) = \ln\frac{I}{I_0} \quad (5\text{-}2)$$

$$\ln\frac{I}{I_0} = -\sum_{Source}^{Detector} \mu(x,y) \quad (5\text{-}3)$$

where $T_0(x)$ is the x-ray transmission at angle θ, which is a measure of the total absorption along the straight line in Figure 5-3. $T_\theta(x)$ is referred to as the ***ray sum,*** which is the integral of μ(*x,y*) along the ray.

The computational problem in CT is to find μ(*x,y*) from the ray sums for a sufficiently large number of beams of known locations that pass through the object, *O*. The beam geometries discussed in Chapter 5 ensure that every point in the object is scanned successively by a large set of ray sums $T_\theta(x)$.

A set of ray sums is referred to as a **projection,** which can be generated as shown in Figure 5-4, as the x-ray tube and detector scan the object simultaneously. The ray *AA′* is equal to $x \cos\theta + y \sin\theta = d$. The projection is given by $P(\theta,d)$:

$$P(\theta,d) = \int_{AA'} f(x,y)\, ds \quad (5\text{-}4)$$

where *ds* is the differential along the path length *s*.

To understand the meaning of a projection, consider the following case in which a beam of intensity $I_{in}$ enters an object of thickness *x*:

$$I_{in} \rightarrow \boxed{\mu} \rightarrow I_{out}$$
$$\leftarrow x \rightarrow$$

The beam is attenuated according to the Lambert–Beer law, as follows:

$$I_{out} = I_{in} e^{-\mu x} \quad (5\text{-}5)$$

Because *x*, $I_{in}$, $I_{out}$, and *e* are known, μ can be calculated as follows:

$$\mu = \frac{1}{x} \cdot \log\frac{I_{in}}{I_{out}}$$

The following case represents the situation in the patient:

$$I_{in} \rightarrow \boxed{\mu_1|\mu_2|\mu_3|\ldots|\mu_n} \rightarrow I_{out}$$

From x–ray tube — $\leftarrow x_1 \rightarrow \leftarrow x_2 \rightarrow \leftarrow x_3 \ldots \leftarrow x_n \rightarrow$ — To the detector

$$I_{out} = I_{in} e^{-(\mu_1 x_1 + \mu_2 x_2 + \mu_3 x_3 + \ldots + \mu_n x_n)} \quad (5\text{-}6)$$

Because $x_1 = x_2 = x_3 \ldots = x_n$,

$$1/x \log I_{in}/I_{out} = \mu_1 + \mu_2 + \mu_3 \ldots + \mu_n \quad (5\text{-}7)$$

*A *line integral* is the integral (summation of values that are infinitesimally close to each other multiplied by the infinitesimal distance separating the values) of a 2D or 3D object along the point of a line (Parker & Stanley, 1981).

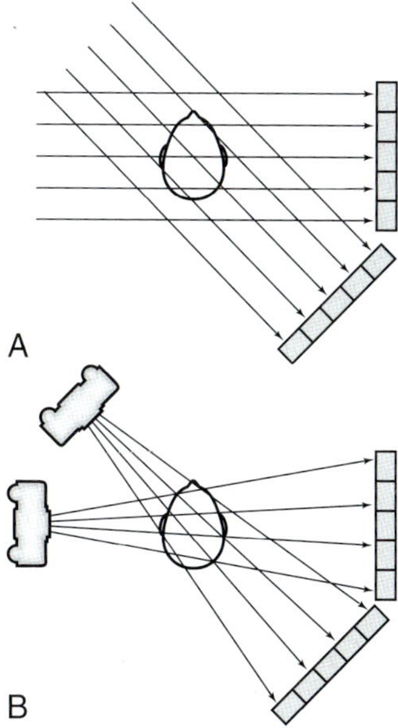


**FIGURE 5-5** Beam geometries used in CT to generate projection data. **A,** Parallel beam geometry used in the first CT scanners. **B,** Fan beam geometry was introduced to acquire the projection data faster than parallel beam geometries.

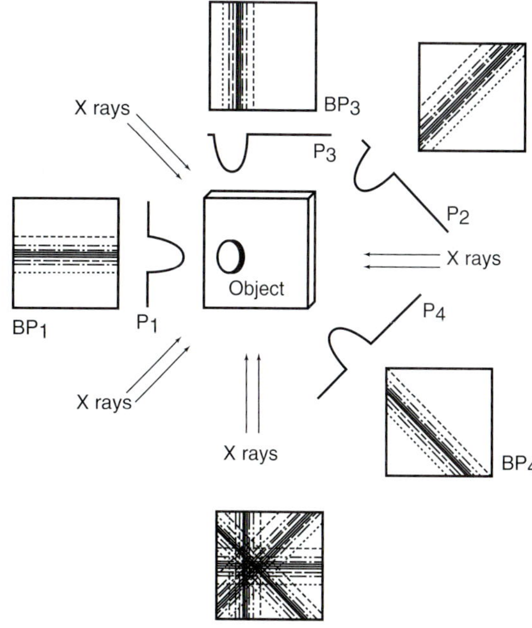


**FIGURE 5-6** Graphic representation of the back-projection reconstruction technique.

The problem in CT is to calculate all values for the μ terms for a large set of projections. Projections can be obtained through both parallel and fan beam geometries (Fig. 5-5). Hounsfield's original CT scanner used parallel beam projections acquired through a 180-degree rotation.

## RECONSTRUCTION ALGORITHMS

Image reconstruction from projections involves several algorithms to calculate all the μ terms in Equation 5-7 from a set of projection data. The algorithms applicable to CT include back-projection, iterative methods, and analytic methods.

### Back-Projection

**Back-projection** is a simple procedure that does not require much understanding of mathematics. Back-projection, also called the "summation method" or "linear superposition method," was first used by Oldendorf (1961) and Kühl and Edwards (1963). Back-projection can be best explained with a graphical or numerical approach.

Consider four beams of x rays that pass through an unknown object to produce four **projection profiles** $P_1$, $P_2$, $P_3$, and $P_4$ (Fig. 5-6). The problem involves the use of these profiles to reconstruct an image of the unknown object (black dot) in the box. The projected datasets are back-projected (i.e., linearly smeared) to form the corresponding images *BP1*, *BP2*, *BP3*, and *BP4*. The reconstruction involves summing these back-projected images to form an image of the object.

The problem with the back-projection technique is that it does not produce a sharp image of the object and therefore is not used in clinical CT. The most striking **artifact** of back-projection is the typical star pattern that occurs because points outside a high-density object receive some of the back-projected intensity of that object (Curry et al., 1990).

Back-projection can also be explained with the following 2 × 2 **matrix:**

$$\begin{array}{ccccc} I_0 \rightarrow & \mu_1 & \mu_2 & x \rightarrow I_1 \\ I_0 \rightarrow & \mu_3 & \mu_4 & x \rightarrow I_2 \\ & \leftarrow x \rightarrow & \leftarrow x \rightarrow & \\ & \downarrow & \downarrow & \\ & I_3 & I_4 & \end{array}$$

Four separate equations can be generated for the four unknowns, $\mu_1$, $\mu_2$, $\mu_3$, and $\mu_4$:

$$I_1 = I_0 e^{-(\mu_1 + \mu_2)x}$$
$$I_2 = I_0 e^{-(\mu_3 + \mu_4)x}$$
$$I_3 = I_0 e^{-(\mu_1 + \mu_3)x}$$
$$I_4 = I_0 e^{-(\mu_2 + \mu_4)x}$$

A computer can solve these equations very quickly.

A numerical example might help to give some insight into the calculations involved. Consider an object divided into four squares (2 × 2 matrix with four **pixels**), as shown on the following page.

Four projections are collected at four different known locations: 0, 45, 90, and 135 degrees.

To start, data are collected for four projections: 0, 45, 90, and 135 degrees.

1. The **ray** sum for the 0-degree projection on the left side is 1 (0 + 1).
2. The ray sum for the 0-degree projection on the right side is 5 (2 + 3).
3. The ray sums for the 45-degree projection are 0, 3 (2 + 1), and 3.
4. The ray sum for the 90-degree projection on the upper row is 2 (2 + 0).
5. The ray sum for the 90-degree projection on the lower row is 4 (3 + 1).
6. The ray sums for the 135-degree projection are 2, 3 (3 + 0), and 1.

These projection data—1, 5, 0, 3, 3, 2, 4, 2, 3, and 1—are then used systematically as defined by the algorithm to reconstruct the original image.

1. *First guess*: Place the data from the 0-degree projections into the matrix to obtain the first guess:

| | |
|---|---|
| 1 (0+1) | 5 (2+3) |
| 1 (0+1) | 5 (2+3) |

2. *Second guess*: Add the data from the 45-degree projections to the value of each square in the first guess:

| | |
|---|---|
| 1 (0+1) | 8 (5+3) |
| 4 (1+3) | 8 (5+3) |

3. *Third guess*: Add the data from the 90-degree projections to the value of each square in the second guess:

| | |
|---|---|
| 3 (1+2) | 10 (8+2) |
| 8 (4+4) | 12 (8+4) |

4. *Fourth guess*: Add the data from the 135-degree projections to the value of each square in the third guess:

| | |
|---|---|
| 6 (3+3) | 12 (10+2) |
| 9 (8+1) | 15 (12+3) |

The next step is to obtain the original matrix, as follows:

1. Subtract a constant value 6 (obtained by summing the values in the original matrix—0 + 1 + 2 + 3 = 6) from each square in the fourth guess:

| | |
|---|---|
| 0 (6–6) | 0 (12–6) |
| 3 (9–6) | 9 (15–6) |

2. Now reduce the preceding matrix to a simple ratio. By using the obvious common divisor, 3, the following is obtained:

| | |
|---|---|
| 0 (0/3) | 2 (6/3) |
| 1 (1/3) | 3 (9/3) |

This is the original 2 × 2 matrix.

## Iterative Algorithms

Another approach to image reconstruction is based on iterative techniques. "An iterative reconstruction starts with an assumption (for example, that all points in the matrix have the same value) and compares this assumption with measured values, makes corrections to bring the two into agreement, and then repeats this process over and over until the assumed and measured values are the same or within acceptable limits" (Curry et al., 1990).

Techniques include the simultaneous iterative reconstruction technique, the iterative least-squares technique, and the algebraic reconstruction technique (Brooks & Di Chiro, 1976; Gordon & Herman, 1974). These techniques differ in the application of corrections to subsequent **iterations.** The algebraic reconstruction technique was used by Hounsfield in the first EMI brain scanner (Hounsfield, 1972) and is detailed here.

Consider the following numeric illustration:

Original projection datasets (horizontal ray sums)

2 × 2 Matrix (4 elements)

| | | |
|---|---|---|
| 1 | 2 | → 3 |
| 3 | 4 | → 7 |
| ↓ 4 | ↓ 6 | |

1. Initial estimate: Compute the average of four elements and assign it to each pixel, that is, 1 + 2 + 3 + 4 = 10; 10/4 = 2.5

New projection datasets (horizontal ray sums)

| | | |
|---|---|---|
| 2.5 | 2.5 | → 5 |
| 2.5 | 2.5 | → 5 |

2. First correction for error (original horizontal ray sums minus the new horizontal ray sums divided by 2) = (3 – 5)/2 and (7 – 5)/2 = –2/2 and 2/2 = –1.0 and 1.0

| | |
|---|---|
| (2.5 − 1)<br>1.5 | (2.5 − 1)<br>1.5 |
| (2.5 − 1)<br>3.5 | (2.5 − 1)<br>3.5 |

3. Second estimate:

| | |
|---|---|
| 1.5 | 1.5 |
| 3.5 | 3.5 |
| ↓<br>5 | ↓<br>5 |

New projection datasets
(vertical ray sums)

4. Second correction for error (original vertical ray sums minus new vertical ray sums divided by 2) = (4 − 5)/2 and (6 − 5)/2 = −1.0/2 and +1.0/2 = −0.5 and +0.5:

| | |
|---|---|
| (1.5 − 0.5)<br>1 | (1.5 − 0.5)<br>2 |
| (3.5 − 0.5)<br>3 | (3.5 − 0.5)<br>4 |

The final matrix solution is thus

| | |
|---|---|
| 1 | 2 |
| 3 | 4 |

In the early years of CT use these iterative techniques were not used in commercial scanners because of the following limitations:

1. It is difficult to obtain accurate ray sums because of quantum **noise** and patient motion.
2. The procedure takes too long to generate the reconstructed image because the iteration can be done only after all projection datasets have been obtained, and because of the lack of computing power to solve these equations quickly.
3. To produce a "true" image, there should be more projection datasets than pixels. Therefore diagonal projection datasets are taken to eliminate ambiguity.

Today, iterative reconstruction algorithms have resurfaced because of the availability of high-speed computing (Beister et al., 2012). The primary advantages of iterative image reconstruction algorithms are to reduce image noise (Beister et al., 2012; Hsieh et al., 2013; Kaza et al., 2014) and minimize the higher radiation dose (Fleischmann & Boas, 2011; McCollough et al., 2012) inherent in the filtered back-projection algorithm.

All major CT manufacturers offer iterative reconstruction algorithms as of 2014. For example, while GE Healthcare and Philips Healthcare offer Adaptive Statistical Iterative Reconstruction (ASiR), Model-Based Iterative Reconstruction (MBIR), and Iterative Model Reconstruction, Siemens Healthcare offers Image Reconstruction in Image Space (IRIS) and Sinogram Affirmed Iterative Reconstruction (SAFIRE). Toshiba Medical Systems, on the other hand, offers the Adaptive Iterative Dose Reduction (AIDR) iterative algorithm.

Iterative reconstruction algorithms are described in more detail in Chapter 6.

## Analytic Reconstruction Algorithms

**Analytic reconstruction algorithms** were developed to overcome the limitations of back-projection and iterative algorithms and are used in modern CT scanners. Two analytic reconstruction algorithms are the Fourier reconstruction algorithm and filtered back-projection.

### Filtered Back-Projection

Filtered back-projection is also referred to as the **convolution method** (Fig. 5-7). The projection profile is filtered or convolved to remove the typical starlike blurring that is characteristic of the simple back-projection technique.

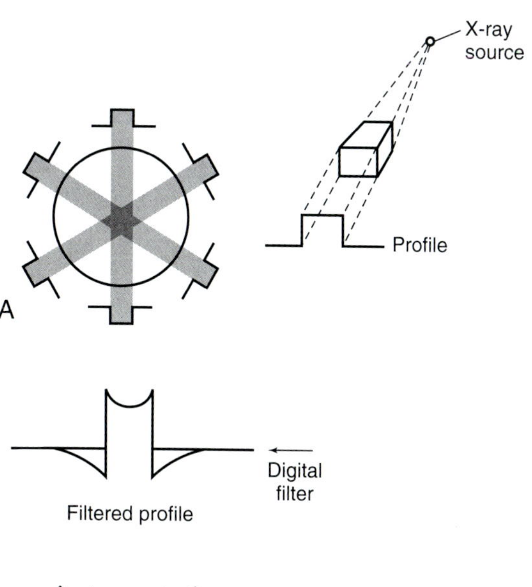


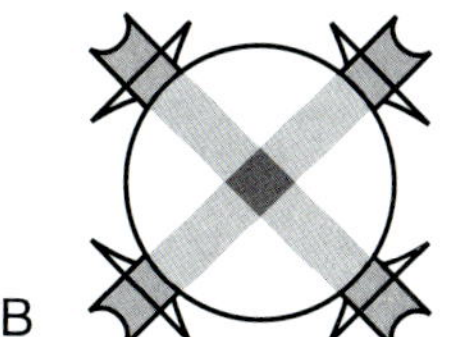


**FIGURE 5-7** Back-projection and filtered back-projection techniques used in CT. **A,** Back-projection results in an unsharp image. **B,** Filtered back-projection uses a digital filter (a convolution filter) to remove this blurring, which produces a sharp image.

The steps in the filtered back-projection method (Fig. 5-7, *B*) are as follows:

1. All projection profiles are obtained.
2. The logarithm of the data is obtained.
3. The logarithmic values are multiplied by a digital filter, or convolution filter, to generate a set of filtered profiles.
4. The filtered profiles are then back-projected.
5. The filtered projections are summed and the negative and positive components are therefore canceled, which produces an image free of blurring.

Major problems with the filtered back-projection algorithm include noise and streak artifact (Beister et al., 2012).

## Fourier Reconstruction

The Fourier reconstruction process is used in MRI but not in modern CT scanners because it requires more complicated mathematics than the filtered back-projection algorithm.

A radiograph can be considered an image in the **spatial domain;** that is, shades of gray represent various parts of the anatomy (e.g., bone is white and air is black) in space. With the Fourier transform, this spatial domain image—the radiograph represented by the function $f(x,y)$—can be transformed into a **frequency domain** image represented by the function $F(u,v)$. This frequency domain image consists of a range of high to low frequencies. In addition, this image can be retransformed into a spatial domain image with the inverse Fourier transform (Fig. 5-8).

There are several advantages to this transformation process. First, the image in the frequency domain can be manipulated (e.g., edge enhancement or smoothing) by changing the amplitudes of the frequency components. Second, a computer can perform those manipulations (digital image processing). Third, frequency information can be used to measure image quality through the point spread function, line spread function, and modulation transfer function (Huang, 1999).

The Fourier slice theorem states that the Fourier transform of the projection of an object at angle θ is equal to a slice of the Fourier transform of the object along angle θ (Fig. 5-9).

The Fourier reconstruction consists of the following steps (Fig. 5-10):

1. The object to be scanned is represented by the function $f(x,y)$.
2. Projection data are obtained from the object. A projection dataset for at least a 180-degree rotation is required for adequate reconstruction. These projections represent a spatial domain image.
3. Each projection is transformed into the frequency domain by the Fourier transform. This image must be converted into a clinically useful image.
4. Because CT scanners use a fast Fourier transform developed specifically for digital implementation, the frequency domain image must be placed on a rectangular grid (Fig. 5-10). This is accomplished by interpolation. The fast Fourier transform requires that the pixels in the grid array be 2, 4, 8, 16, 32, 64, 128, 256, 512, 1024, and so on.

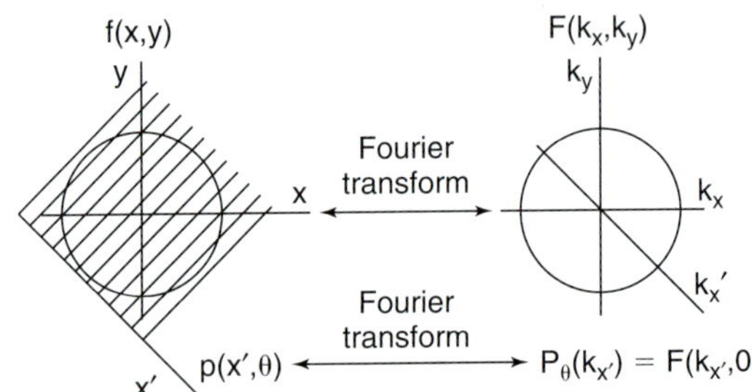


**FIGURE 5-9** The projection slice theorem forms the basis of Fourier reconstruction mathematics. The Fourier transform of the projection with respect to $x'$, $P_\theta(k_x)$ is equal to a slice of the Fourier transform $F(k_x, k_y)$ in the θ direction.

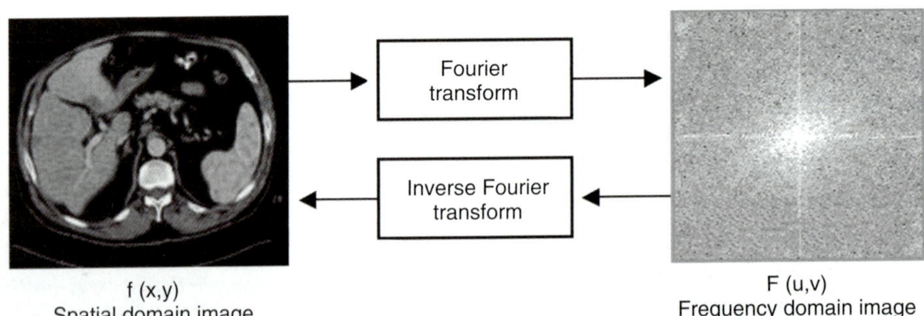


**FIGURE 5-8** Radiograph of an image represented in the spatial domain by the function $f(x,y)$. This can be transformed to an image in the frequency domain $F(u,v)$ with use of the Fourier transform. In addition, $F(u,v)$ can be retransformed into $f(x,y)$ with use of the inverse Fourier transform.

5. Finally, the interpolated image is transformed into a spatial domain image of the object through an inverse Fourier transform operation.

The Fourier reconstruction technique does not use any filtering because interpolation produces a similar result. Also, the 2D interpolation process may introduce artifacts if it is not conducted accurately; therefore it is not used in CT.

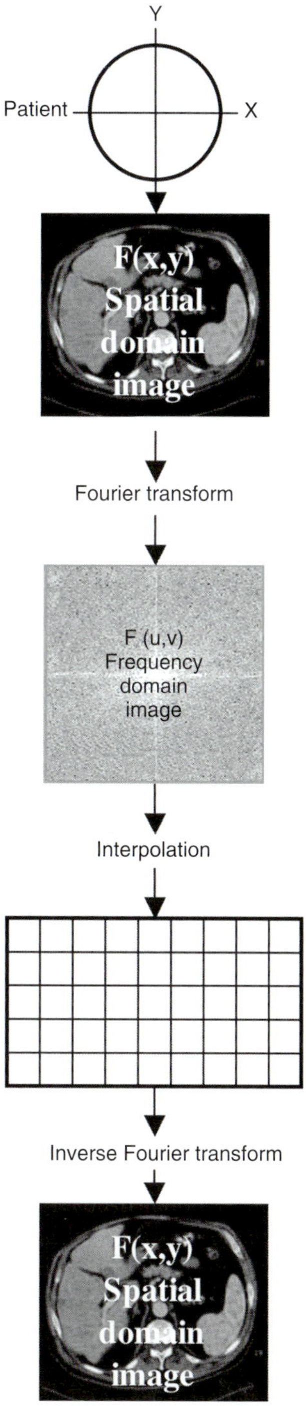

Y
Patient
X
F(x,y) Spatial domain image
Fourier transform
F (u,v) Frequency domain image
Interpolation
Inverse Fourier transform
F(x,y) Spatial domain image

**FIGURE 5-10** Steps involved in Fourier reconstruction.

## TYPES OF DATA

Figure 5-11 shows the data evolution from acquisition, reconstruction, and image display. Four data types are measurement data, **raw data,** filtered raw data or convolved data, and image data or reconstructed data.

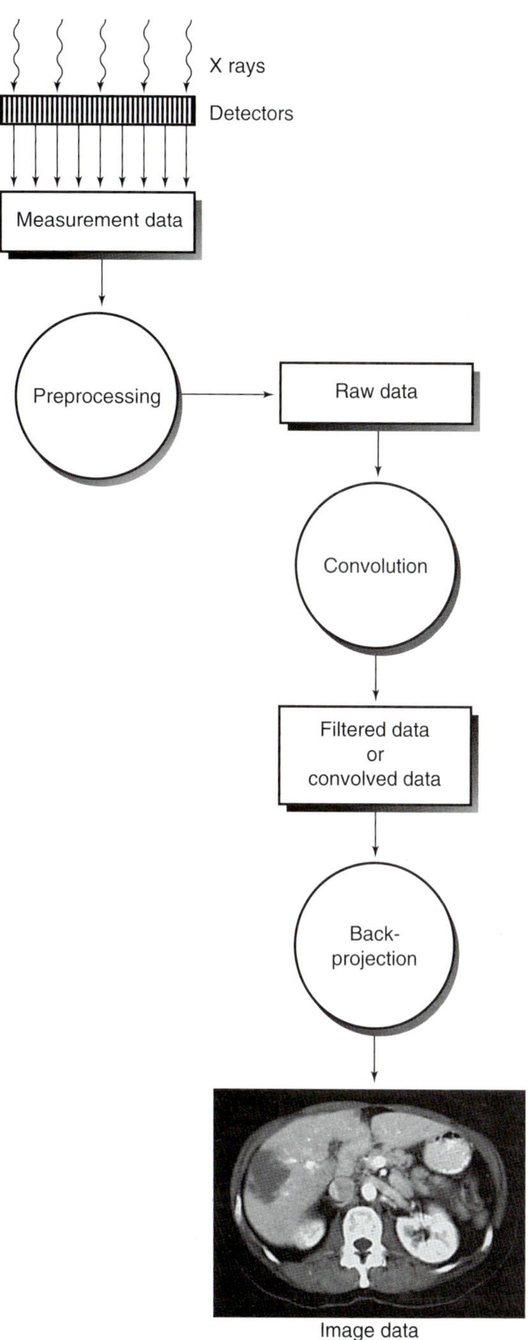


**FIGURE 5-11** The evolution of data in CT, from acquisition to image display on a monitor.

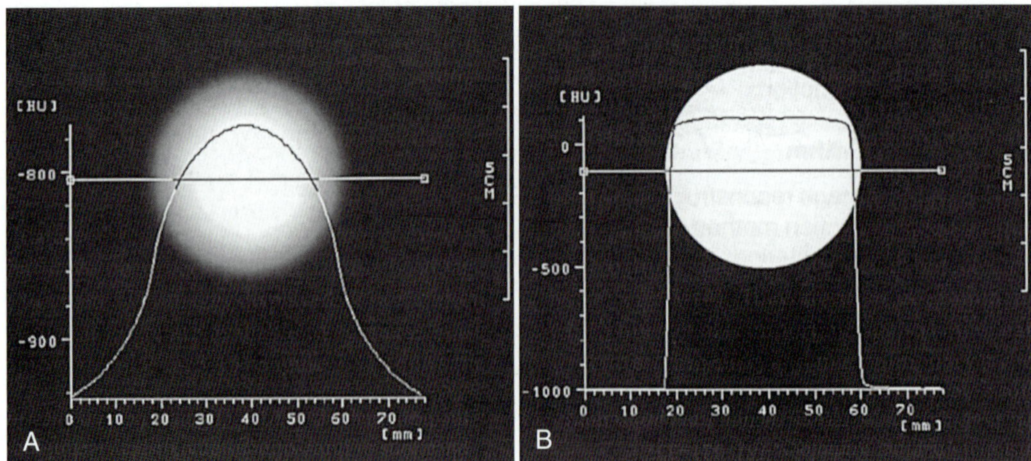


**FIGURE 5-12** The effect of convolution on image quality in CT. **A,** The image is back-projected without convolution. **B,** The dataset has been convolved before back-projection. (Courtesy Siemens Medical Systems, Iselin, NJ.)

## Measurement Data

Measurement data, or scan data, arise from the detectors. This dataset is subject to preprocessing to correct the measurement data before the image reconstruction algorithm is applied. Such corrections are necessary because of errors in the measurement data from **beam hardening,** adjustments for bad detector readings, or scattered radiation. If these errors are not corrected, they will cause poor image quality and generate image artifacts.

## Raw Data

Raw data are the result of preprocessed scan data and are subjected to the image reconstruction algorithm used by the scanner. These data can be stored and subsequently retrieved as needed.

## Convolved Data

The image reconstruction algorithm used by current CT scanners is the filtered back-projection algorithm, which includes both filtering and back-projection. Raw data must first be filtered with a mathematical filter, or kernel. This process is also referred to as the *convolution technique.* Convolution improves image quality through the removal of blur (Fig. 5-12). Figure 5-12, *A*, shows the degree of blurring present in an image before convolution. Figure 5-12, *B*, demonstrates image sharpening after convolution. **Convolution kernels** can only be applied to the raw data.

## Image Data

Image data, or reconstructed data, are convolved data that have been back-projected into the image matrix to create CT images displayed on a monitor. Various digital filters are available to suppress noise and improve detail (Fig. 5-13). Figure 5-13 shows the relationship between image noise and image detail of a standard algorithm, a smoothing algorithm, and an edge enhancement algorithm.

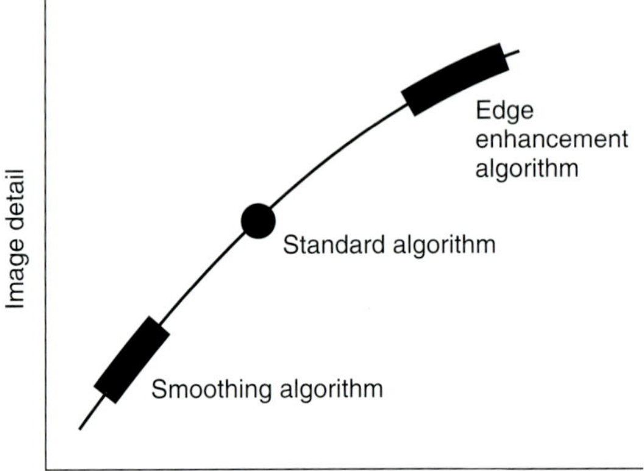


**FIGURE 5-13** The relationship between image detail and image noise for three digital filters in CT. Although edge enhancement algorithms provide good detail compared with smoothing algorithms, they also result in more noise. Smoothing algorithms reduce the image noise at the expense of detail but show good soft tissue structures.

The standard algorithm is usually used before the previous algorithms, especially when a balance between image noise and image detail is mandatory. Smoothing algorithms (Fig. 5-14) reduce image noise and show good soft tissue anatomy; they are used in examinations where soft tissue discrimination is important to visualize very low contrast structures. Edge enhancement algorithms emphasize the edges of structures and improve detail but create image noise (Fig. 5-14). They are used in examinations in which fine detail is important, such as inner ear, bone structures, thin slice, and fine pulmonary structures.

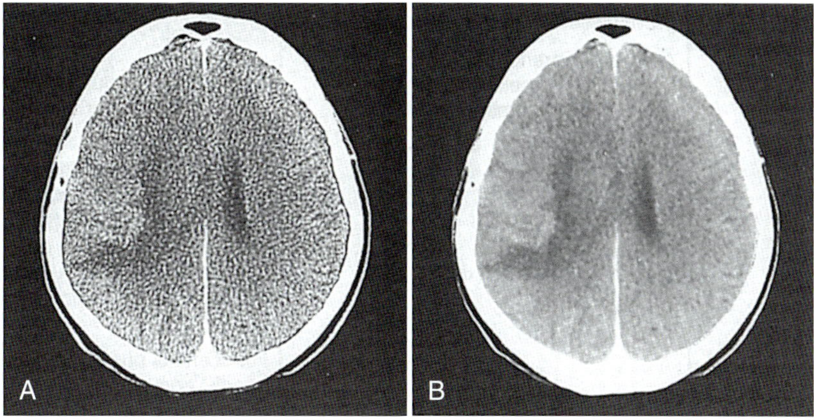


**FIGURE 5-14** The effect of two digital filters on the appearance of the CT image. **A,** An edge enhancement filter is used and more image noise is apparent. **B,** A smoothing digital filter is used and results in reduced image noise and good soft tissue discrimination. (Courtesy Siemens Medical Systems, Iselin, NJ.)

## IMAGE RECONSTRUCTION IN SINGLE-SLICE SPIRAL/HELICAL CT

The image reconstruction algorithms previously described apply to single-slice conventional CT. In SSCT, the same filtered back-projection algorithm is used with an additional consideration. Because the patient moves continuously through the gantry for a 360-degree rotation, the reconstructed image will be blurred so interpolation is necessary before the filtered back-projection is used. A planar section must first be computed from the volume dataset by using interpolation, after which images are generated with various interpolation algorithms. A more comprehensive description of these algorithms is presented in Chapter 11.

## IMAGE RECONSTRUCTION IN MULTISLICE SPIRAL/HELICAL CT

A notable difference between SSCT and MSCT is that the latter uses multiple detector rows that cover a larger volume at an increased speed and therefore require new algorithms. In general, for CT scanners with four detector rows, MSCT algorithms have been developed to allow for the reconstruction of variable **slice thicknesses** and address the problems of increased volume coverage and speed of the patient table. This is made possible by spiral/helical **scanning** with interlaced **sampling,** longitudinal interpolation, and fan beam reconstruction with the filtered back-projection algorithm. These three major steps are described further in Chapter 11.

The new generation of MSCT scanners (those with 16 and greater detector rows) requires modified image reconstruction algorithms. These algorithms are very complex and beyond the scope of this textbook; however, a few foundational concepts relating to these algorithms are introduced in the next section and further elaborated in Chapter 11, which deals specifically with MSCT principles and concepts.

## CONE-BEAM ALGORITHMS FOR MULTISLICE CT SCANNERS

A number of image reconstruction algorithms have been developed for conventional "stop-and-go" (or "step-and-shoot") CT scanners, SSCT scanners, and MSCT scanners with four detector rows.

There are several types of image reconstruction algorithms and specific beam geometries characteristic of the new CT scanners and these are described further in Chapter 11. Although conventional CT scanners use pencil beam and small fan beam geometries with the filtered back-projection image reconstruction algorithm, SSCT scanners use wide fan beam geometries. Here the image reconstruction algorithm is based on interpolation followed by filtered back-projection. MSCT scanners with four detector rows use a wider fan **beam geometry** (compared with SSCT scanners) and use a 2D reconstruction with interpolation and *z*-filtering, known as *z*-interpolation algorithms (Chen et al., 2003).

The algorithms for the SSCT and MSCT with four detector rows are referred to as spiral/helical fan beam approximation algorithms (Hu, 1999) simply because they are based on the fan beam geometry. According to Hein et al. (2003), the fan beam approximation algorithm "assumes that the source, detector, and slice of interest lie in the same plane, and that the projection of the slice of interest falls on a single detector row. This approximation is valid for small cone angles associated with one to four slice systems." The cone angle is associated with cone-beam geometry (Flohr et al., 2005).

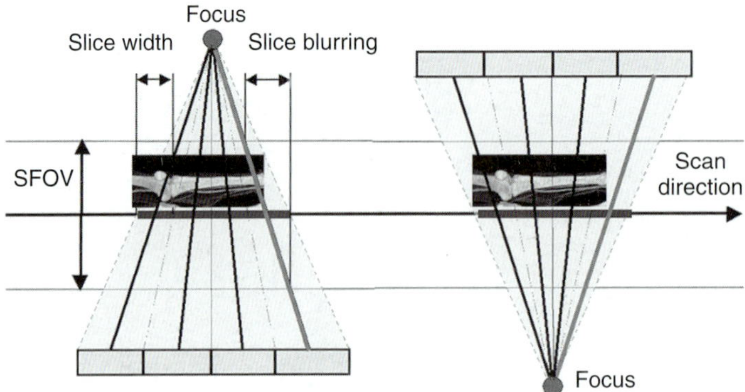


**FIGURE 5-15** Diagram shows geometry of four-section CT scanner demonstrating the cone-angle problem: measurement rays are tilted by the so-called cone angle with respect to the center plane. Left and right: Two view angles from sequential scan that are shifted by 180 degrees so that positions of x-ray tube and detector are interchanged. With single-section CT, identical measurement values would be acquired. With multidetector row CT, different measurement values are acquired. *SFOV*, Scan field of view. (From Flohr, T. G., Schaller, S., Stierstorfer, K., Bruder, H., Ohnesorge, B. M., & Schoepf, U. J. (2005). *Radiology, 235*, 756-773. Reproduced by permission of the Radiological Society of North America and the authors.)

### Cone-Beam Geometry

For a four-detector row MSCT scanner, the beam divergence from the x-ray tube to the outer edges of the detectors increases, as shown in Figure 5-15. Such a beam is called a cone beam. Within the cone beam, the rays that will be measured by the detectors are tilted at an angle relative to the central plane (plane perpendicular to the long axis of the patient, the **z-axis**). This angle is called the cone angle.

As the number of detector rows increases from 4 to 16 to 64 and 320, the cone angle becomes larger. The larger cone angles cause problems where the beam divergence along the *z*-axis becomes greater. This results in the plane of interest (planar section of slice of interest) being projected onto several detector rows (Hein et al., 2003). This situation generates inconsistent data that will lead to cone-beam artifacts, such as streaking and density changes, both of which will have a negative effect on image quality.

### Cone-Beam Algorithms

Fan beam approximation algorithms require that the data be consistent, that is, the x-ray beam from the tube to the detector and the section being imaged must be in the same plane. This is no longer the case for large cone angles characteristic of MSCT systems with larger than four detector rows. The fan beam approximation algorithms are not very accurate used with the new generation of MSCT scanners, so other image reconstruction algorithms are needed. These algorithms are called cone-beam algorithms, and they have been developed to eliminate the cone-beam artifacts previously mentioned. One such popular algorithm is the adaptive multiple plane reconstruction algorithm (Bruening & Flohr, 2003).

Essentially, several cone-beam algorithms have become available for use with the new generation of MSCT scanners, and they basically fall into two classes: exact cone-beam algorithms and approximate cone-beam algorithms (Kalender, 2005). These algorithms are described further in Chapter 11, because the terminology for these new MSCT scanners is an important requirement for understanding cone-beam algorithms.

## AN OVERVIEW OF THREE-DIMENSIONAL RECONSTRUCTION TECHNIQUES

The applications of 3D imaging are rapidly increasing (Calhoun et al., 1999; Cody, 2002; Dalrymple et al., 2005; Fishman et al., 2006; Logan, 2001; Udupa, 1999; Udupa & Herman, 2000). 3D imaging uses 3D surface and volumetric reconstruction. The algorithms for 3D imaging are based on those used in computer graphics and visual perception science. A 3D reconstruction technique for surface display (Fig. 5-16) is based on at least two processes, preprocessing and display, and consists of the following operations: interpolation, **segmentation,** surface formation, and projection (Cody, 2002; Philipp et al., 2003; Udupa & Herman, 2000; Zhang et al., 2011). 3D reconstruction techniques allow the user to "interactively visualize, manipulate, and measure large 3D objects on general purpose workstations" (Dalrymple et al., 2005; Fishman et al., 2006; Udupa & Herman, 2000).

3D reconstruction techniques are described in detail in Chapter 13.

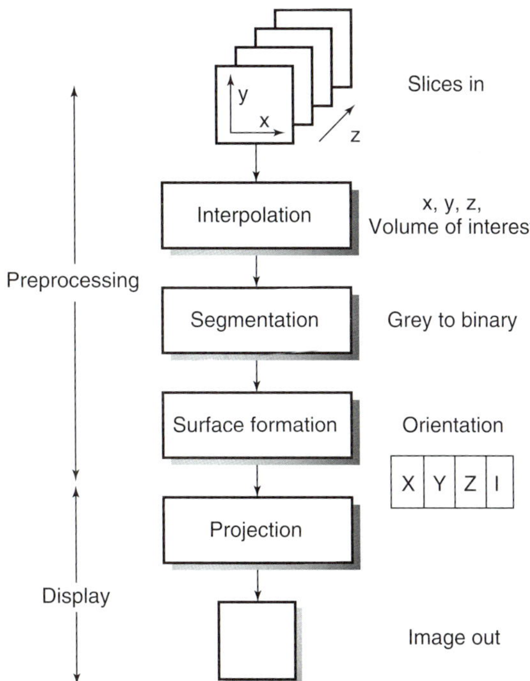


**FIGURE 5-16** A generalized algorithm for surface display of 3D images from a CT scanner.

## REVIEW QUESTIONS

Answer the following questions to check your understanding of the materials studied.

1. Which of the following changes a time domain signal into a frequency domain signal?
   A. Fourier transform
   B. Interpolation
   C. Convolution
   D. Algorithms
2. A measure of the total absorption of x rays along a straight line is referred to as:
   A. projection data.
   B. a projection profile.
   C. a ray sum.
   D. a view.
3. The basic problem in CT is to calculate:
   A. projection angles.
   B. the number of rays needed to image reconstruction.
   C. the number of rotations of the x-ray tube for one slice.
   D. μs for tissues from a large set of projection data.
4. The horizontal ray sums for the pixels shown below are:
   > 2 3 0 1 5 2 > ?
   A. 2.
   B. 152.
   C. 13.
   D. 12.
5. The back-projection technique results in:
   A. the classical star pattern in the image.
   B. image blur.
   C. poor image quality and, therefore, a diagnosis cannot be made.
   D. all are correct.
6. CT scanners now use the:
   A. back-projection algorithm.
   B. FT reconstruction.
   C. algebraic reconstruction method.
   D. filtered back-projection algorithm.
7. Image data are obtained:
   A. before back-projection.
   B. after back-projection.
   C. after preprocessing.
   D. after convolution.
8. The first operation to which raw data are subjected is referred to as:
   A. convolution.
   B. back-projection.
   C. 3D surface shading.
   D. preprocessing.

## REVIEW QUESTIONS—cont'd

9. Which of the following belongs to the class of analytic algorithms for CT?
   A. Back-projection
   B. Filtered back-projection
   C. Algebraic reconstruction technique
   D. All are correct

10. Which of the following uses a digital filter to modify an image matrix?
    A. Algorithm
    B. Interpolation
    C. FT
    D. Convolution

## REFERENCES


Beister, M., Kolditz, D., & Kalender, W. A. (2012). Iterative reconstruction methods in x ray CT. *Physica Medica, 28*(2), 94–108. http://dx.doi.org/10.1016/j.ejmp.2012.01.003.

Berland, L. L. (1987). *Practical CT: technology and techniques*. New York: Raven Press.

Bracewell, R. (1989). The Fourier transform. *Scientific American, 260*, 86–95.

Brooks, R. A., & Di Chiro, G. (1976). Principles of computer assisted tomography (CAT) in radiographic and radioisotopic imaging. *Physics in Medicine and Biology, 21*, 689–732.

Bruening, R., & Flohr, T. (2003). *Protocols for multislice CT—4 and 16 row applications*. New York: Springer Verlag.

Calhoun, P. S., Kuszyk, B. S., Heath, D. G., et al. (1999). Three-dimensional volume rendering of spiral CT data: theory and method. *Radiographics, 19*, 745–764.

Chen, L., Liang, Y., & Heuscher, D. J. (2003). General surface reconstruction for cone beam multislice spiral computed tomography. *Medica Physica, 30*, 2804–2812.

Cody, D. D. (2002). AAPM/RSNA physics tutorial for residents: topics in CT. Image processing in CT. *Radiographics, 22*, 1255–1268.

Curry, T. S., III, Dowdy, J. E., & Murry, R. C., Jr. (1990). *Christensen's physics of diagnostic radiology* (4th ed.). Philadelphia, PA: Lea & Febiger.

Dalrymple, N. C., Prasad, S. R., Freckleton, M. W., et al. (2005). Introduction to the language of three-dimensional imaging with multidetector CT. *Radiographics, 25*, 1409–1428.

Fishman, E. K., Ney, D. R., Health, D. G., Corl, F. M., Horton, K. M., & Johnson, P. T. (2006). Volume rendering versus maximum intensity projection in CT angiography: what works best, when, and why. *Radiographics, 26*, 905–922.

Fleischmann, D., & Boas, F. E. (2011). Computed tomography: old ideas and new technology. *European Radiology, 21*(3), 510–517. http://dx.doi.org/10.1007/s00330-011-2056-z.

Flohr, T. G., Schaller, S., Stierstorfer, K., Bruder, H., Ohnesorge, B. M., & Schoepf, U. J. (2005). Multi-detector row CT systems and image reconstruction techniques. *Radiology, 235*, 756–773.

Gibson, C. (Ed.). (1981). *The facts on file dictionary of mathematics*. New York: Facts on File.

Gordon, R., & Herman, G. T. (1974). Three-dimensional reconstruction from projections: a review of algorithms. *International Review of Cytology, 38*, 111–123.

Hein, I., Taguchi, K., Silver, M. D., Kazama, M., & Mori, I. (2003). Feldkamp-based cone beam reconstruction for gantry-tilted helical multislice CT. *Medica Physica, 30*, 3233–3242.

Hounsfield, G. H. (1972). *A method of and apparatus for examination of a body by radiation such as x or gamma radiation*. British Patent Office, Patent No. 1283915.

Hsieh, J., Nett, B., Zhou, Y., Sauer, K., Thibault, J.-B., & Bouman, C. A. (2013). Recent advances in CT image reconstruction. *Current Radiology Reports, 1*(1), 39–51. http://dx.doi.org/10.1007/s40134-012-0003-7.

Hu, H. (1999). Multislice helical CT: scan and reconstruction. *Medica Physica, 26*(5).

Huang, H. K. (1999). *PACS: basic principles and applications*. New York: Wiley-Liss.

Kalender, W. A. (2005). *Computed tomography: fundamentals, system technology, image quality, applications*. Erlangen, Germany: GWA.

Kaza, R. K., Platt, J. F., Goodsitt, M. M., et al. (2014). Emerging techniques for dose optimization in abdominal CT. *Radiographics, 34*(1), 4–17. http://dx.doi.org/10.1148/rg.341135038.

Knuth, D. E. (1977). Algorithms. *Scientific American, 236*, 63–80.

Kühl, D. E., & Edwards, R. Q. (1963). Image separation radioisotope scanning. *Radiology, 80*, 653–661.

Logan, L. (2001). Seeing the future in three dimensions. *Radiologic Technology, 15*, 483–487.

McCollough, C. H., Chen, G. H., Kalender, W., Leng, S., Samei, E., Taguchi, K., et al. (2012). Achieving routine submillisievert CT scanning: report from the summit on management of radiation dose in CT. *Radiology, 264*(2), 567–580.

Oldendorf, W. H. (1961). Isolated flying spot detection radio-density discontinuities displaying the internal structural pattern of a complex object. *IEEE Transactions on Biomedical Engineering, 8*, 68–72.

Parker, D. L., & Stanley, J. H. (1981). Glossary. In T. H. Newton, & D. G. Potts (Eds.), *Glossary radiology of the skull and brain: technical aspects of computed tomography*. St. Louis, MO: Mosby.

Philipp, M. O., Kubin, K., Mang, T., et al. (2003). Three-dimensional volume rendering of multidetector-row CT data: applicable for emergency radiology. *European Journal of Radiology, 48*, 33–38.

Ramachandran, G. N., & Lakshminarayanan, A. V. (1971). Three-dimensional reconstructions from radiographs and electron micrographs: application of convolution instead of Fourier transforms. *Proceedings of the National Academy of Science USA, 68*, 2236–2240.

Seeram, E. (2001). *Computed tomography technology*. Philadelphia, PA: WB Saunders.

Shepp, L. A., & Logan, B. F. (1974). The Fourier reconstruction of a head section. *IEEE Transactions on Nuclear Science, 21*, 21–43.

Udupa, J. K. (1999). Three-dimensional visualization and analysis methodologies: a current perspective. *Radiographics, 19*, 783–803.

Udupa, J. K., & Herman, G. T. (2000). *3D imaging in medicine*. Boca Raton, FL: CRC Press.

Zhang, Q., Eagleson, R., & Peters, T. M. (2011). Volume visualization: a technical overview with a focus on medical applications. *Journal of Digital Imaging, 24*(4), 640–664.

## BIBLIOGRAPHY

Cho, Z. H., & Ahn, I. S. (1975). Computer algorithms for the tomographic image reconstruction with x-ray transmission scans. *Computers and Biomedical Research, 8*, 8–25.

Fishman, E. K., Magid, D., Ney, D. R., et al. (1991). Three-dimensional imaging. *Radiology, 181*, 321–337.

Gabor, H. T. (1980). *Image reconstruction from projections*. New York: Academic Press.

Kalender, W. A., Seissler, W., Klotz, E., & Vock, P. (1989). Single-breath-hold spiral volumetric CT by continuous patient translation and scanner rotation. *Radiology, 173*, 414–419.

Strong, A. B., Lobregt, S., & Zonneveld, F. W. (1990). Applications of three-dimensional display techniques in medical imaging. *Journal of Biomedical Engineering, 12*, 233–238.

# 6

# Iterative Reconstruction Basics

## OUTLINE



## LEARNING OBJECTIVES

On completion of this chapter, you should be able to:

1. outline the assumptions made to derive the filtered back-projection (FBP) algorithm.
2. list 4 strategies to reduce noise in CT imaging.
3. state three categories of iterative reconstruction (IR) algorithms available from CT manufacturers.
4. describe three steps in a typical IR process without modeling.
5. state the meaning of the term "modeling" and list three models used in IR algorithms.
6. identify the points where these models are applied during the CT image reconstruction process.
7. state three goals of using IR algorithms in CT.
8. provide examples of various IR algorithms available from CT manufacturers.
9. list the characteristics on which the performance evaluation of IR algorithms compared with the FBP algorithm is based.

## KEY TERMS TO WATCH FOR AND REMEMBER

The following key terms/concepts are important to your understanding of this Chapter.

**forward projection**
**input**
**iterative reconstruction (IR)**
**IR Loop**
**IR process**
**iterations**
**measured projection data**
**modeling**
**noise statistics (noise model)**
**object and physics models**
**output**
**simulated projection data**
**system optics (optics model)**
**updated image**

In Chapter 5, **image reconstruction algorithms** for **computed tomography (CT)** were described in general, including a numerical illustration of the first **iterative reconstruction (IR)** algorithm used by Dr. Godfrey Hounsfield (1973), the inventor of CT. He shared the 1979 Nobel Prize in Medicine and Physiology with Professor Allan Cormack, a physics lecturer at the University of Cape Town, South Africa. The **filtered back-projection (FBP)** algorithm, an early analytical reconstruction algorithm, was also described in Chapter 5. It has been the major reconstruction algorithm used in CT since the 1970s. The basic framework of the FBP algorithm is shown in Figure 6-1. Essentially, the **measured projection data** (raw data) are subject to calibrations, corrections, and log conversion, and so on, followed by **convolution** filtering and back-projection (two key features of the FBP algorithm) to produce an image from which a diagnosis can be made.

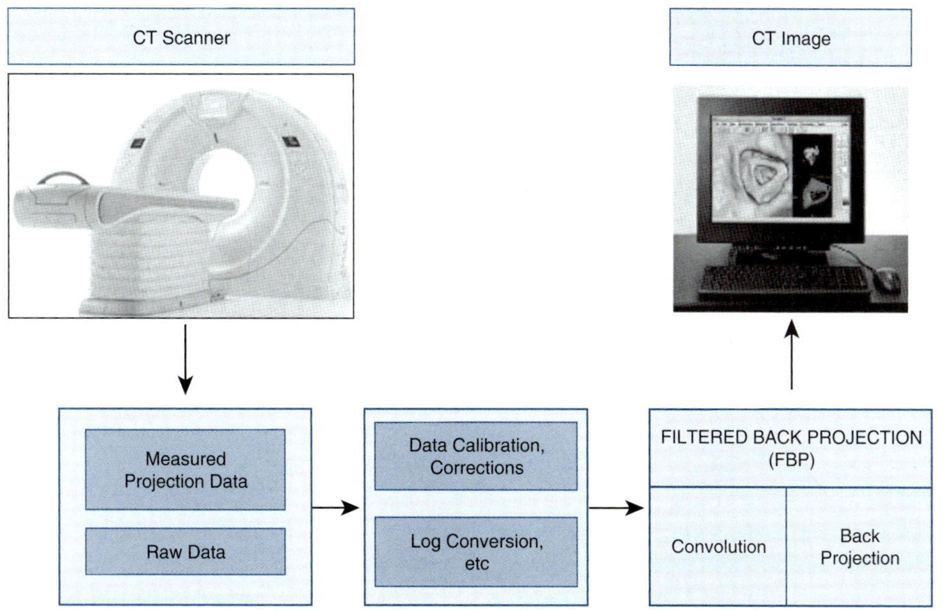


**FIGURE 6-1** The basic framework of the FBP CT reconstruction algorithm. (See text for further explanation).

The FBP algorithm is well recognized for its speed and "closed-form solution" (Hsieh, 2013), which is "available from a single pass over the acquired data" (Thibault, 2010). The FBP algorithm, however, has several limitations, including image **noise** and **artifact** creation (Hsieh et al., 2013; Thibault, 2010). While the noise problem can be overcome by increasing the milliamperes (mA) for the examination, radiation dose to the patient becomes a real challenge. This situation becomes more pronounced in low-dose CT examinations, in an effort to adhere to the as low as reasonably achievable (ALARA) philosophy of the International Commission on Radiological Protection. This philosophy tries to ensure that the lowest possible dose is used without compromising the diagnostic quality of the image.

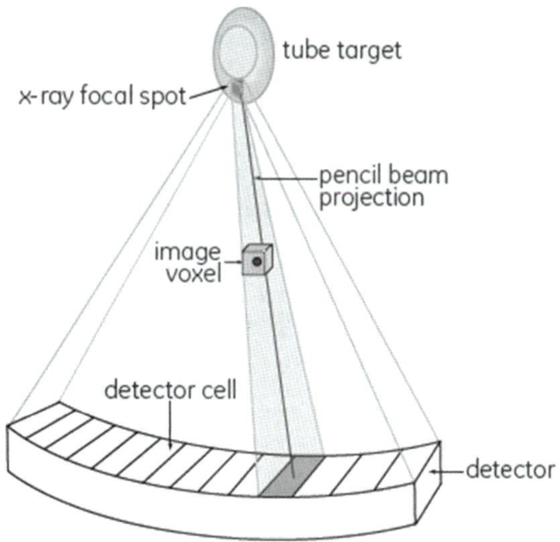


**FIGURE 6-2** Several components of the CT data acquisition process, including the sampling geometry, illustrating the nature of the assumptions made in deriving the FBP algorithm. (From Hsieh, J. (2008). Adaptive statistical iterative reconstruction. *GE Healthcare Whitepaper*. Courtesy GE Healthcare.)

## ASSUMPTIONS MADE TO DERIVE THE FBP ALGORITHM

The problems with the FBP algorithm are due to several "idealized" assumptions made when deriving the algorithm. Figure 6-2 has been used by Hsieh (2008) to illustrate the nature of these assumptions, which include:

1. The x-ray focal spot is a point source.
2. The size and shape of each detector cell is not taken into consideration.
3. "All x-ray photon interactions are assumed to take place at a point located in at the geometric center of the detector cell, not across the full area of the detector cell."
4. A pencil beam is used to "represent the line integral of the **attenuation** coefficient along the path" as shown in Figure 6-2.
5. The size and shape of the voxels are described as "infinitely small points located on a square grid."
6. The **projection** data are accurate and not affected by x-ray photon statistical changes and electronic noise.

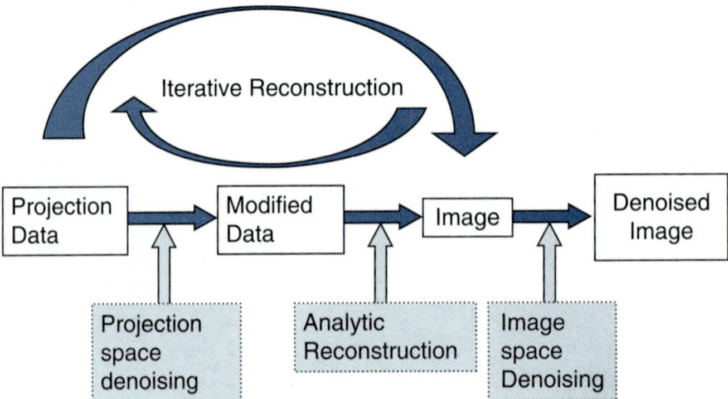


**FIGURE 6-3** Four denoising strategies and the exact points to which they are applied during CT image reconstruction. (From Ehman, E. C., Yu, L., Manduca, A., et al. (2013). *Radiographics, 34,* 849-862. Reproduced by permission of RSNA.)

The above assumptions of the CT system have been used successfully to derive the FBP algorithm. Such a CT system model "clearly does not represent physical reality" (Hsieh et al., 2013); therefore, other algorithms that model the CT system accurately are needed. These algorithms must consider accurate modeling of the CT system optics, the noise (noise model), and the image properties (image model). The highlights of modeling will be described later in the chapter. This is an important point to note, since accurate modeling results in improvements in image quality and noise reduction when compared with the FBP analytical algorithm.

## NOISE REDUCTION TECHNIQUES

The increasing use of CT has resulted in a corresponding increase in radiation dose to the patient and concerns about the potential biological effects of radiation **exposure** from CT examinations (Brenner & Hall, 2007; Pearce et al., 2012). Subsequently, these concerns have resulted in increasing awareness of various efforts to reduce the dose to the patient in CT **scanning** (Seeram, 2014).

It is well known that the use of low-dose techniques can produce noisy images; therefore, it is essential to consider various approaches to noise reduction, especially in low-dose CT imaging. Figure 6-3 shows four strategies to reduce the noise during CT image reconstruction. These include projection space denoising, analytical FBP denoising using standard reconstruction kernels (see Chapter 5), image space denoising, and the use of iterative image reconstruction (Ehman et al., 2014). While image space denoising and FBP-based analytic reconstruction use digital filters (e.g., smoothing filters, edge enhancement filters; see Chapter 2), projecting space denoising (filtering before image reconstruction) uses photon statistics to reduce noise through a statistical noise model or adaptive noise filtering (Ehman et al., 2014)

More recently, IR algorithms have been developed to reduce image noise when using lower exposure technique factors, and at the same time to preserve image quality (namely, **spatial resolution** and low-contrast detectability [LCD]) and reduce artifacts due to the presence of metal implants, **beam-hardening** effects, and photon starvation (Ehman et al., 2014). These artifacts (and more) are common when using the traditional FBP algorithm (Hsieh et al., 2013; Zeng & Zamyatin, 2013).

There are several IR algorithms commercially available from CT scanner manufacturers, based on different physical methods and concepts. These algorithms have been placed in the following three categories:

1. Iterative methods without modeling
2. Statistical methods with modeling of photon counting statistics
3. Model-based methods that exceed statistical modeling

## IR ALGORITHMS WITHOUT MODELING: FUNDAMENTAL CONCEPTS

A generalized or typical **IR process** consists of three steps as illustrated in Figure 6-4. These include **Input, IR Loop,** and **Output.**

### Input

In this step, the CT scanner produces **raw data** or measured projection data (projection data space). This raw dataset is then subjected to the standard

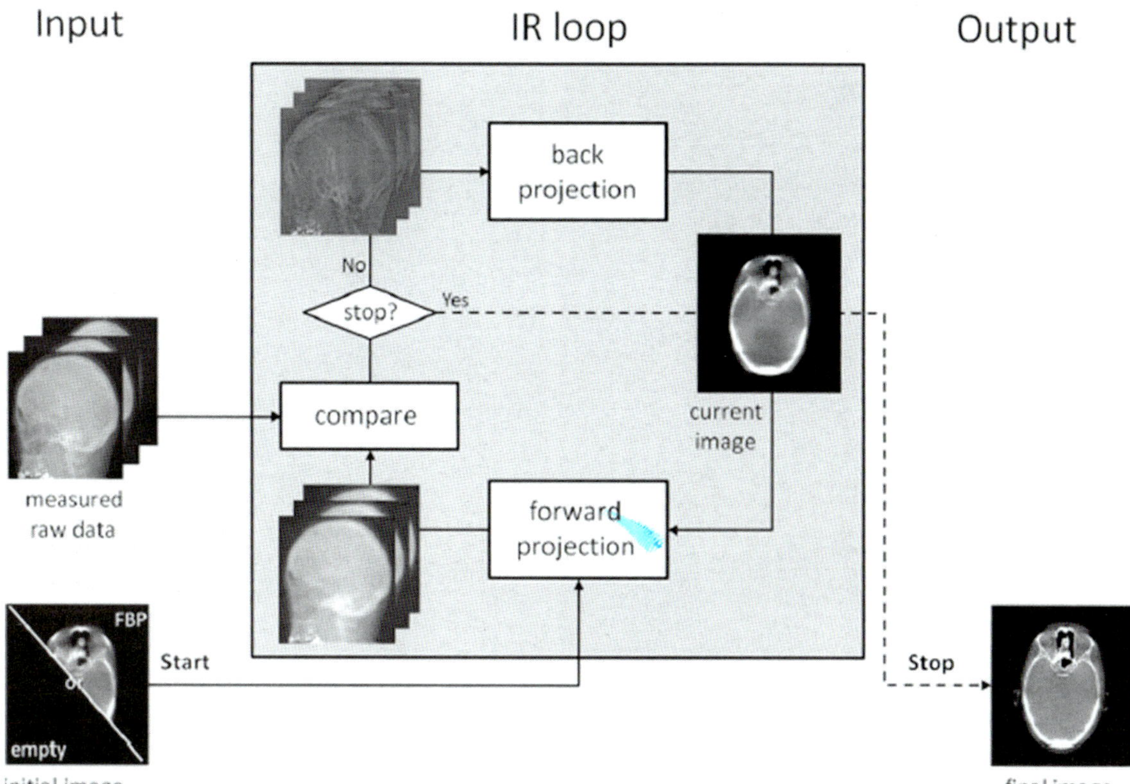


**FIGURE 6-4** A graphic illustration of the three steps involved in a generalized or typical IR process: Input, IR loop, and Output. (See text for further explanation). (From Beister, M., Kolditz, D., & Kalender, W. A. (2012). *Physica Medica*, *28*, 94 108. Reproduced by permission.)

FBP algorithm to generate the initial CT image (the current CT image).

## IR Loop

The IR loop forms the basis of the iterative reconstruction. There are three essential steps in this loop (Beister et al., 2012). First, a **forward projection** is applied to the initial CT image to create artificial raw data (also referred to as **simulated projection data**). Second, the simulated raw data are compared with the measured projection raw data (Fig. 6-4) and the difference is calculated to create an **updated image.** This difference is referred to as a "correction term," and, as noted by Biester et al. (2012), "the difference between the two shows the amount of adjustment or update needed for the current estimation of the object (image).One of the goals of image update (modification) is to minimize this difference." Third, the updated image is then back-projected (FBP algorithm) to the current CT image. "The iterative process is finished when either a fixed number of iterations is reached, or the update for the current image estimate is considered small enough, or when a predefined quality criterion in the image estimate is fulfilled" (Beister et al., 2012). In other words, IR algorithms focus on an optimization of the synthesized or artificial raw data (forward-projection data). Such optimization includes predetermined image quality criteria.

## Output

The output of the IR loop is a back-projection that results in the final volumetric image. A visual comparison of two sets of images reconstructed with the FBP algorithm and an IR algorithm is shown in Figure 6-5.

The accuracy of the estimate mentioned previously depends on what is referred to as modeling the CT system acquisition components and the object being imaged. These will be briefly described in the following section.

## MODELING APPROACHES IN IR ALGORITHMS: AN OVERVIEW

The term **modeling** is used to refer to the characteristics of the CT **imaging system** and the imaged object,

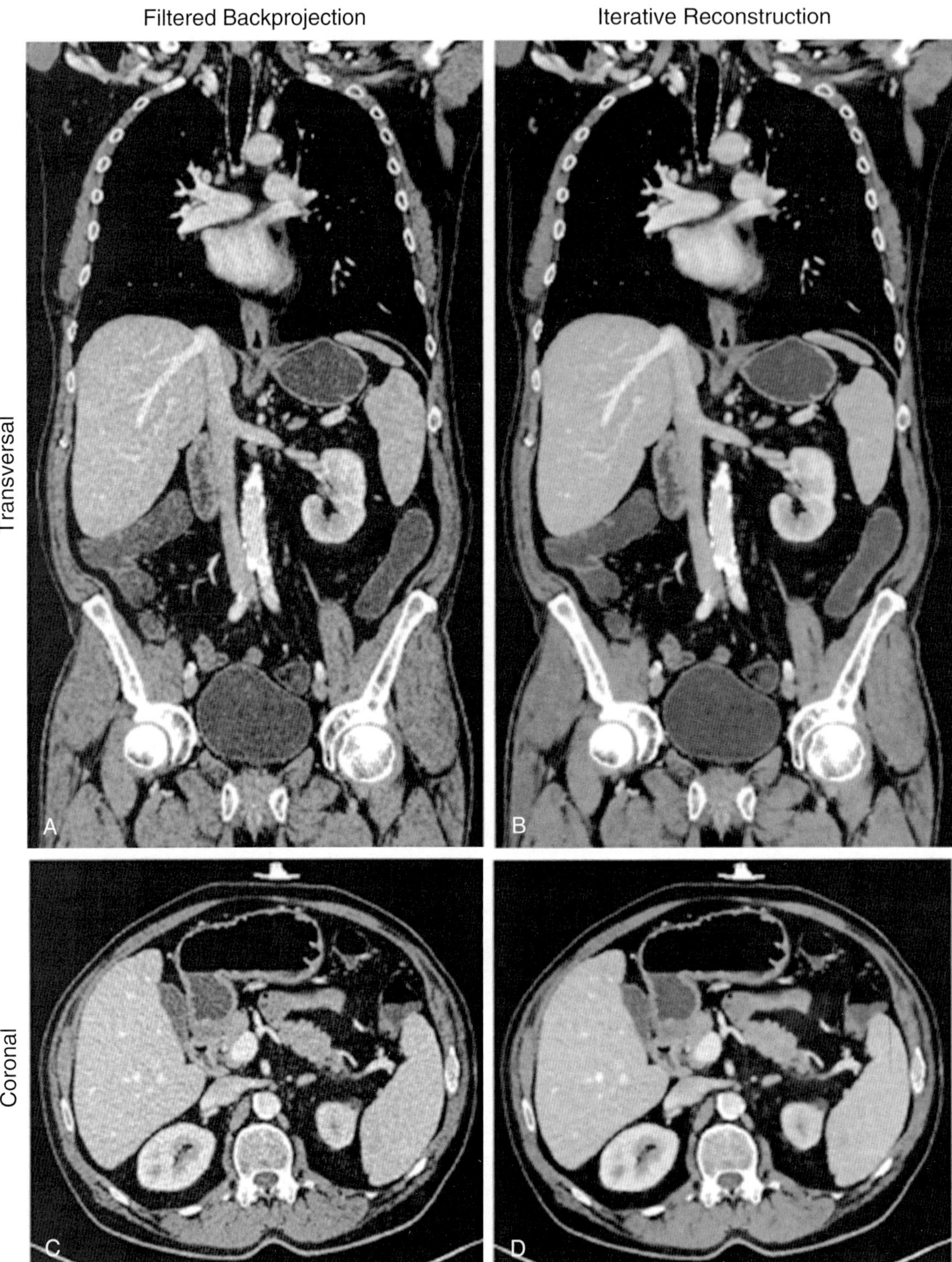


**FIGURE 6-5** A comparison of the image quality of two sets of images generated with the FBP algorithm and an IR algorithm. (From Beister, M., Kolditz, D., & Kalender, W. A. (2012). *Physica Medica, 28,* 94-108. Reproduced by permission.)

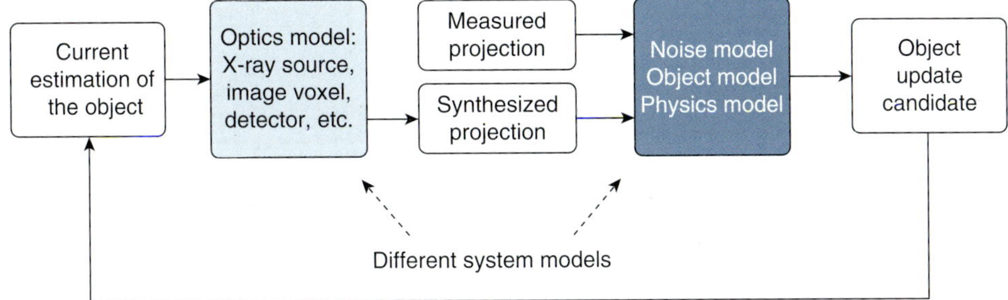


**FIGURE 6-6** Different system models and the points to which they are applied during the IR process. (From Fan, J. et al. (2014). Benefits of ASiR-V reconstruction for reduction of patient dose and preserving diagnostic quality in CT exams. *GE Healthcare Whitepaper*. Courtesy of GE Healthcare.)

and includes what has been popularly referred to as **system optics (optics model), noise statistics (noise model),** and **object and physics models.** These different system models are illustrated in Figure 6-6, where the points to which they are applied during the CT IR process are shown.

While the optics model or system optics addresses the x-ray source, image voxel, and detectors, and so on, the noise model takes into consideration the x-ray photon statistics (x-ray flux at the source and detector). The object model, on the other hand, deals with radiation attenuation through the patient, while the physics model examines the physics of CT **data acquisition.** The interested reader should refer to Beister et al. (2012) and Hsieh et al. (2013) for a more detailed account of these models.

While some IR algorithms model the system optics, others model the system noise statistics, physics, and objects. As noted by Hsieh et al. (2013), a "fully modeled IR is more computationally intensive than analytical reconstruction methods." Furthermore, Hsieh (2008) also points out that

> the computational intensity on the modeling of the noise portion of the system is not nearly as big as the modeling of the system optics. Therefore by focusing first on the modeling of the noise properties and the scanned object, we provide significant benefit for those examinations that may experience limitations due to noise in the reconstructed images, as a result of lower dose exams, large patients, thinner slices, etc. Phrased differently, we gain the dose benefit by lowering the noise in the reconstructed images, so that the scanning technique can be reduced with equivalent noise.

Iterative methods without modeling compute an initial estimate of the image from the projection data set (using the FBP image), subsequently improving the image (current estimate) using several **iterations** (a calculation process using a series of operations repeated several times). Statistical methods with modeling, on the other hand, use x-ray photons (photon counting statistics) during the IR process. Iterative statistical reconstruction algorithms can operate in the projection raw data domain (sonogram domain), in the image domain, and during the process of IR (Beister et al., 2012). Finally, as noted by Beister et al. (2012):

> ...model-based methods try to model the acquisition process as accurately as possible. The acquisition is a physical process in which photons with a spectrum of energies are emitted by the focus area of the anode of the **x-ray tube.** Subsequently, they travel through the object and are either registered within the area of the detector **pixel,** scattered outside of the detector, or are absorbed by the object. The better the forward projection is able to model this process, the better the artificial image can be matched to the acquired raw data. Better matching artificial raw data leads to better correction terms for the next image update step and, in consequence to an improved image quality in the reconstruction data.

Statistical and model-based methods are outside the scope of this book. The interested reader should refer to the paper by Beister et al. (2012) for a comprehensive description of these two methods. A graphic illustration of the statistical iterative reconstruction algorithm (ASiR) and a model-based IR algorithm (Veo; compared with the FBP analytical reconstruction algorithm) is shown in Figure 6-7.

Recall that the goals of IR algorithms compared with the FBP algorithm are to improve image quality (namely, spatial resolution or sharpness of the image), reduction of noise, better low-contrast detectability (LCD), and artifact reduction. Such image quality improvement is shown in Figure 6-8.

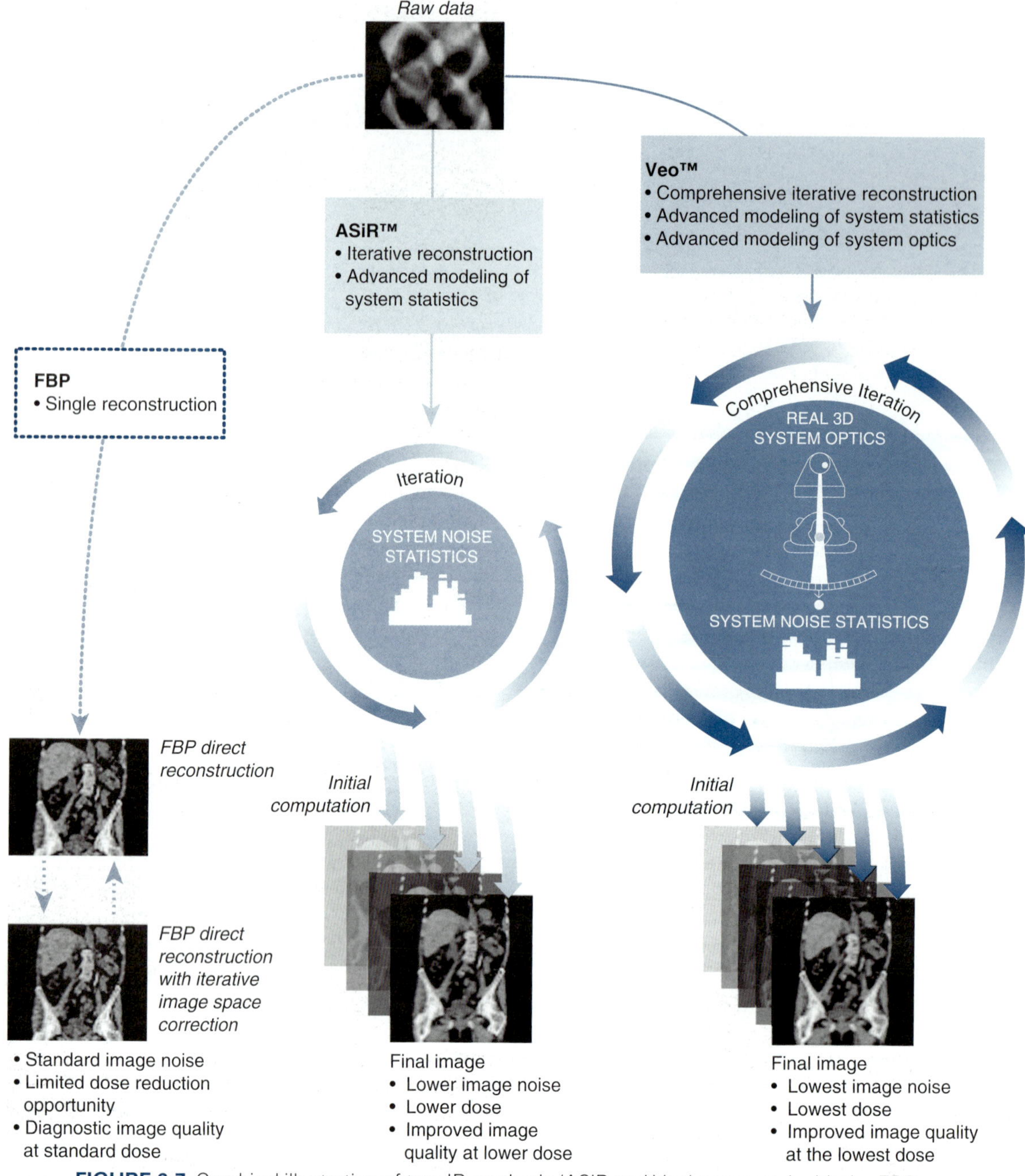


**FIGURE 6-7** Graphical illustration of two IR methods (ASiR and Veo) compared with the FBP analytical reconstruction. (From Thibault, J. B. (2010). Veo CT model-based iterative reconstruction. *GE Healthcare Whitepaper*. Courtesy of GE Healthcare.)

This image quality improvement and reduction of dose depend on accurate modeling. For the improvement of image quality, it is important that the system optics are modeled accurately in the reconstruction process. For reduced dose, better LCD, and artifact reduction, it is mandatory that the noise statistics, the physics, and the object are modeled accurately in the reconstruction process.

## EXAMPLES OF IR ALGORITHMS

There are several IR algorithms currently available from CT manufacturers GE Healthcare, Siemens Healthcare, Philips Healthcare, and Toshiba Medical Systems. Each vendor offers propriety algorithms that provide improved image quality and noise reduction in low-dose CT imaging (dose reduction) compared

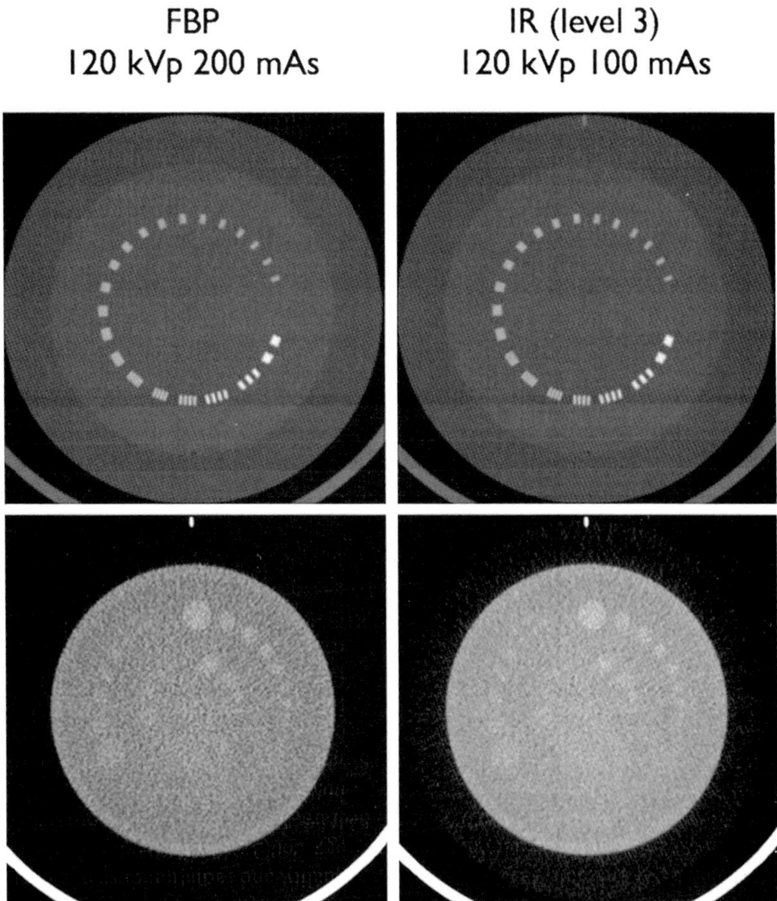


**FIGURE 6-8** Comparison of high-contrast spatial resolution (upper images; slice thickness, 0.615 mm; window setting, 450/1500) and low-contrast conspicuity objects (lower images; reformatted slice thickness, 5.0 mm; window setting, 60/360). FBP images (*left*) were acquired using 120 kV and 200 mA resulting in a $CTDI_{vol}$ of 13.5 mGy. IR images (*right*) were acquired using 120 kV and 100 mA resulting in a $CTDI_{vol}$ of 6.8 mGy. The reconstructions of both acquisitions result in comparable high-contrast spatial resolution and low-contrast conspicuity. (From Klink, T., Obmann, V., Heverhagen, J., Stork, A., Adam, G., & Begemann, P. (2014). *European Journal of Radiology, 83,* 1645-1654. Figure and legend reproduced by permission.)

with the FBP algorithm. Examples of these IR algorithms are listed in Table 6-1.

In 2008, the ASiR algorithm was the first IR algorithm commercially available (Beister et al., 2012; Fan et al., 2014). Subsequently other IR algorithms were developed. For example, in 2009, GE Healthcare introduced Veo model-based IR algorithm for their Discovery CT HD scanner. As noted earlier, this algorithm is based on the use of the statistical model as an optimization function. Other CT vendors such as Siemens Healthcare, Philips, and Toshiba Medical Systems introduced their propriety IR algorithms Image Reconstruction in Image Space (IRIS) in 2009 and Sinogram-Affirmed Image Reconstruction (SAFIRE) in 2010, iDose (iterative processing in projection [sinogram] and image domains) in 2009, and Adaptive Iterative Dose Reduction (AIDR) in 2010, respectively. It is not within the scope of this book to describe the details of these algorithms; however, two IR algorithms will be used to illustrate the steps involved in modeling and arriving at the final CT image. These two examples are from GE Healthcare and Toshiba Medical Systems. While GE Healthcare introduced ASIR-V as their next **generation** of ASiR (Fan et al., 2014), Toshiba now offers AIDR 3D as their most recent IR algorithm (Toshiba Medical Systems, 2015).

The ASIR-V algorithm is different from the earlier Veo CT model-based IR; it features more sophisticated noise modeling and object modeling, including a **bit** of physics modeling, and does not focus on the system optics modeling. This results in faster image

**TABLE 6-1 Examples of IR Algorithms Available from Four Major CT Vendors**

| CT Vendor | IR Algorithm | Acronym |
|---|---|---|
| GE Healthcare | Adaptive Statistical Iterative Reconstruction | ASiR |
| GE Healthcare | Veo Model-Based Iterative Reconstruction (with optimal use of statistical modeling) | Veo (MBIR) |
| GE Healthcare | ASIR-V (includes advanced noise and object models with some physics modeling) | ASIR-V |
| Siemens Healthcare | Image Reconstruction in Image Space | IRIS |
| Siemens Healthcare | Sinogram-Affirmed Image Reconstruction | SAFIRE |
| Siemens Healthcare | Advanced Modeled Iterative Reconstruction | ADMIRE |
| Philips | iDose (Iterative processing in projection [sinogram] and image domains) | iDose |
| Toshiba Medical Systems | Adaptive Iterative Dose Reduction | AIDR |
| Toshiba Medical Systems | Adaptive Iterative Dose Reduction 3D | AIDR 3D |

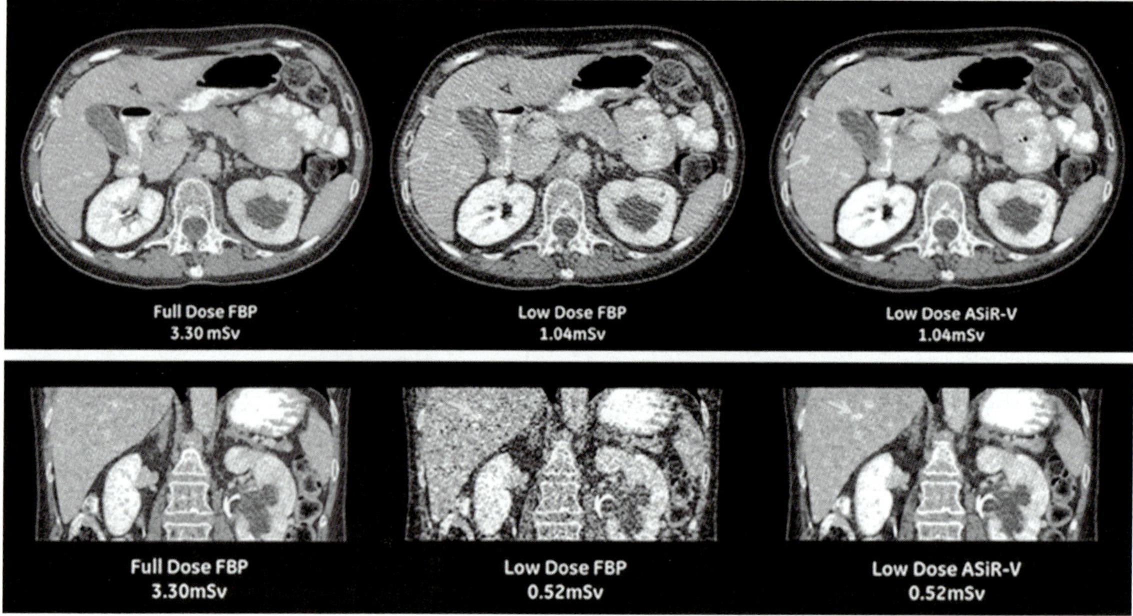


**FIGURE 6-9** Two clinical cases of dose reduction using the ASIR-V algorithm compared with the FPB algorithm with full-dose and low-dose implementation. While the images at the top show more than 3× dose reduction, the images at the bottom show more than 5× dose reduction. (Courtesy GE Healthcare.)

reconstruction similar to FBP. Another advantage of ASIR-V reconstruction is that it can be used with low-dose CT examinations and delivers a lower radiation dose to patients (Fig. 6-9), reduces streaks and noise (Fig. 6-10), and improves spatial resolution (Fig. 6-11) when compared with the FBP algorithm for equivalent image noise. The ASIR-V algorithm has been installed on several GE CT systems (Fan et al., 2014).

The AIDR 3D algorithm from Toshiba Medical Systems is illustrated in Figure 6-12. It is clear that this IR algorithm operates both in the raw data and reconstruction domains and is based on the scanner model that models the physical properties of the CT imaging system and a statistical noise model examining both quantum and electronic noise in the raw data. A further brief description is given by Toshiba (2015) as follows:

> The statistical and scanner models are used together with projection noise estimation for electronic noise reduction processing which takes place in the raw

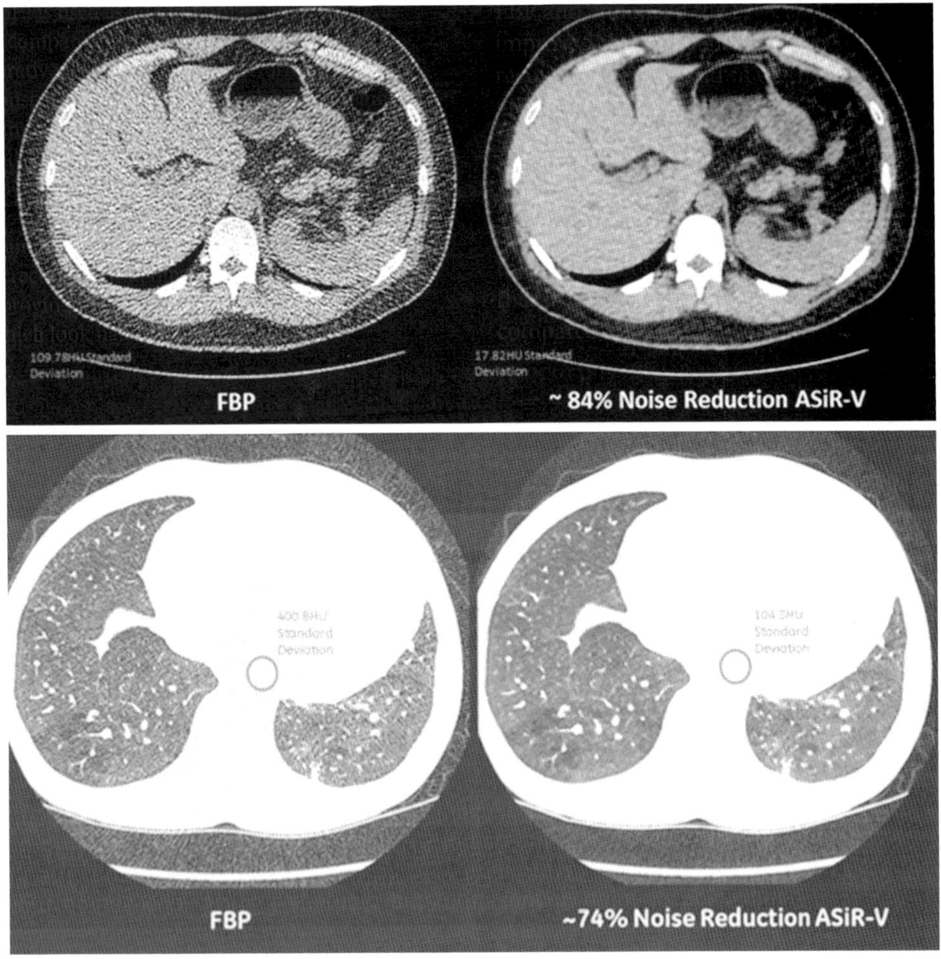


**FIGURE 6-10** ASIR-V reduces streaks and noise in clinical images. The top row shows an ultra-low-dose abdomen scan where ASIR-V significantly reduced low-signal streaks and image noise. The bottom row shows a pulmonary clinical case where ASIR-V reduced image noise to help visualize lung structure and low-density variations. (Courtesy GE Healthcare.)

data domain. The first model analyzes the physical properties of the CT system at the time of the acquisition, while the second model characterizes both electronic and quantum noise patterns in the raw data domain. The projection noise estimation takes care of noise and artifacts reduction. The initial image (FBP) is used as an input image in every iteration to be compared with the output image. A sophisticated iterative technique is then performed to optimize reconstructions for the particular body region being scanned by detecting and preserving sharp details and smoothing the image at the same time. Finally, a weighted blending is applied to the original reconstruction and the output of this iterative process to maintain the noise granularity. The complete AIDR 3D reconstruction therefore increases the SNR while improving the spatial resolution and produces images which look natural (Irwan et al., 2011).

A study by Kim et al. (2014) on "Adaptive Iterative Dose Reduction Algorithm in CT:

Effect on Image Quality Compared with Filtered Back Projection in Body Phantoms of Different Sizes" showed that "Adaptive iterative dose reduction 3D significantly reduced the image noise compared with FBP and enhanced the SNR and CNR ($p < 0.05$) with improved image quality ($p < 0.05$). When a stronger reconstruction algorithm was used, greater increase of SNR and CNR as well as noise reduction was achieved ($p < 0.05$). The noise reduction effect of AIDR 3D was significantly greater in the 40-cm phantom than in the 24-cm or 30-cm phantoms ($p < 0.05$)." These effects are visually demonstrated in **Figure 6-13** for three modes of operation of the AIDR 3D algorithm, that is mild (B), standard (C), and strong modes (D) compared with the FBP algorithm (A).

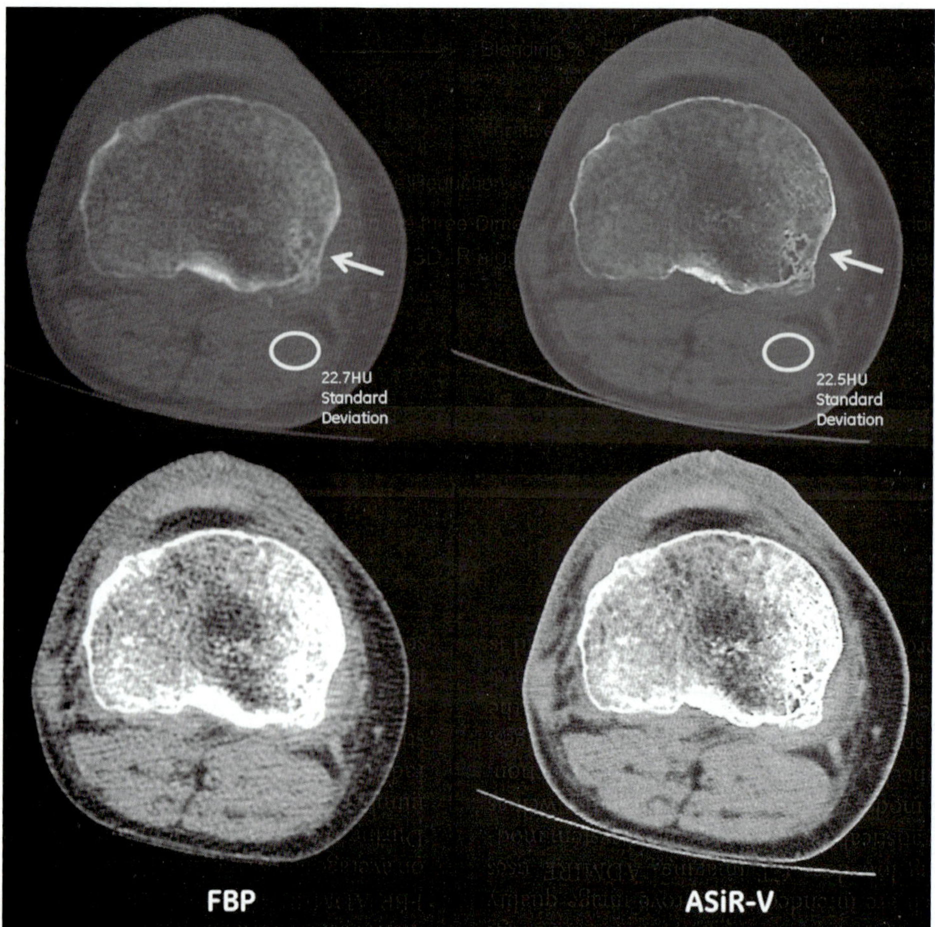


**FIGURE 6-11** A clinical ankle case. The FBP reconstruction clearly has lower resolution than the ASIR-V reconstruction, as pointed out by the arrows. The ASIR-V reconstruction displays a noise level similar to the FBP reconstruction, as shown by the ROI measurements. (Courtesy GE Healthcare.)

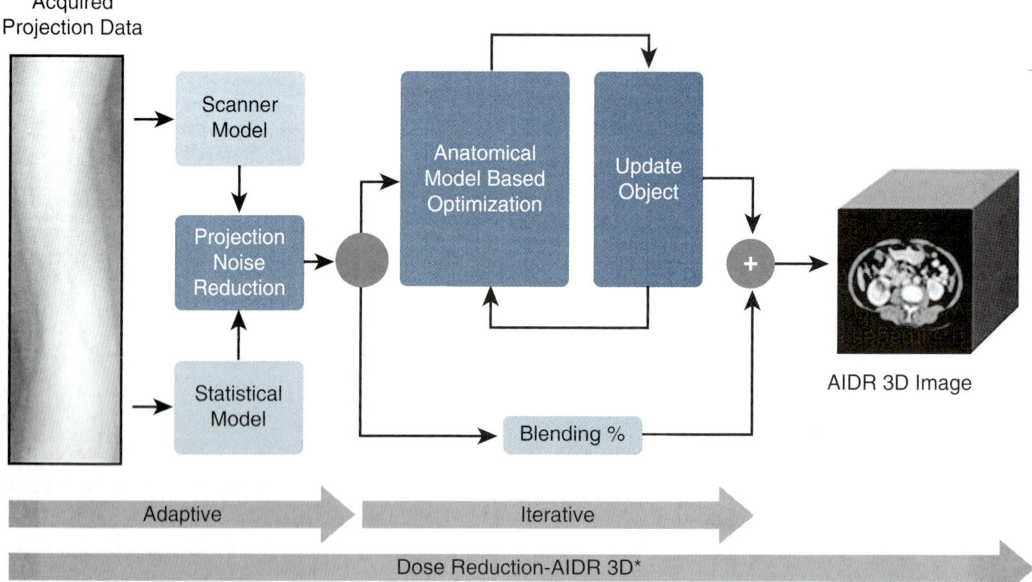


AIDR 3D* has been designed to work in both the three-Dimensional (3D) raw data and reconstruction domains.

**FIGURE 6-12** Graphic illustration of AIDR 3D IR algorithm. (Courtesy Toshiba Medical Systems.)

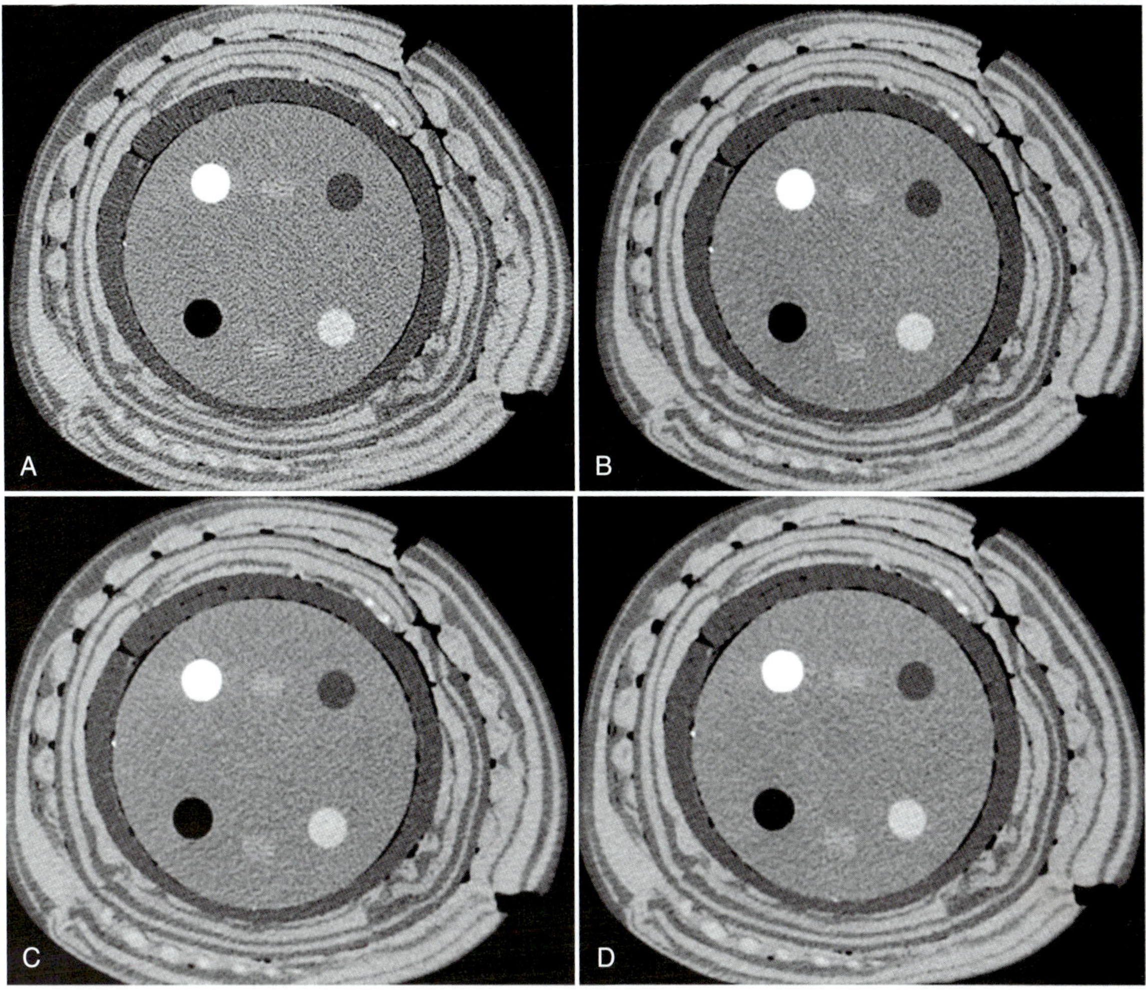


**FIGURE 6-13** A visual comparison between CT images obtained at 180 mAs reconstructed with filtered back-projection **(A),** adaptive iterative dose reduction three-dimensional mild **(B),** standard **(C),** and strong modes **(D)** (From Kim, M. et al. Adaptive iterative dose reduction algorithm in CT: effect on image quality compared with filtered back projection in body phantoms of different sizes, *Korean J Radiol, 15*(2):195-204, 2014. Reproduced by permission.)

A comparison between two images, one using AIDR 3D and one without AIDR 3D, is shown in Figure 6-13.

## PERFORMANCE EVALUATION STUDIES OF IR ALGORITHMS

An important step in the implementation of IR algorithms is the need for performance evaluation of these algorithms, particularly in CT clinical practice. The objectives of these algorithms are related to noise reduction, image quality improvement, and artifact reduction, which has resulted in a number of studies comparing IR algorithms with the FBP algorithm on noise reduction, dose reduction (e.g., performing CT examinations with lower milliamperes), and image quality improvements such as improved spatial resolution and improved LCD (Buxi et al., 2014; Chen et al., 2014; Kalender, 2014; Kordolaimi et al., 2013).

The literature is replete with studies based on both phantom and patient models (Beister et al., 2012; Buxi et al., 2014; Chen et al., 2014; Fan et al., 2014; Smith, 2013; Vardhanabhuti et al., 2013 a and b). It is not within the scope of this chapter to describe the details of these studies (such as methodologies and statistical analyses); however, the results of a few studies will be highlighted to illustrate the performance evaluation of IR algorithms. It is interesting to note that Beister et al. (2012), commenting on the earlier studies, stated that there have been "impressive improvements" in both noise reduction from −7% to −50%, and in image quality as well.

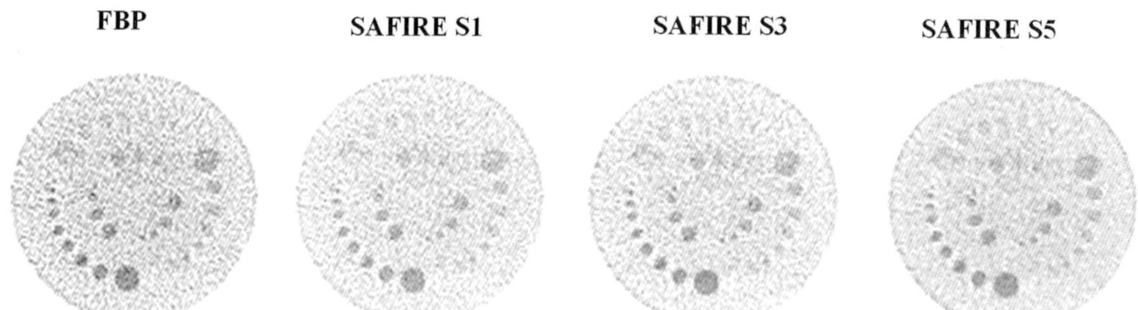


**FIGURE 6-14** A comparison of three levels of SAFIRE noise reduction strengths with the FBP algorithm. (From Ghetti, C., Palleri, F., Serreli, G., Ortenzi, O., Ruffini, L. (2013). *Journal of Applied Clinical Medical Physics, 14* (4). Reproduced by permission.)

As noted earlier in the chapter, the first IR algorithm (ASiR) was introduced by GE Healthcare in 2008. Subsequently, studies in performance evaluation published in 2010 (Leipsic et al., 2010; Prakash et al., 2010) and 2011 (Singh et al., 2011; Schindera et al., 2011) showed not only improved image quality, but also noise and dose reductions, when compared with the FBP algorithm. In a few of the studies cited next, short quotes will be used so as not to detract from the authors' original meaning.

## Examples of Studies in 2012

In 2012, other studies were published comparing the performance of the ASiR algorithm with the FBP algorithm (Protik et al., 2012; Singh et al., 2012). While Protik et al. (2012) found that there was a 26% to 30% reduction in image noise, and changes in noise texture associated with 50% ASiR, Singh et al. (2012) found that, compared with the FBP algorithm, the hybrid ASiR algorithm (used in the study) resulted in a dose reduction of 46.4% (3.7 mGy versus 6.9 mGy) for chest CT and 38.2% (5.0 mGy versus 8.1 mGy) for abdominal CT, and that at the low dose used in the study, the ASiR images "had substantially less objective noise that did FBP images."

## Examples in 2013

Studies of IR algorithm performance compared with the FBP algorithm were performed by Vardhanabhuti et al. (2013a,b), Ghetti et al. (2013), Metha et al. (2013), and Choi et al. (2013). Vardhanabhuti et al. (2013a) compared the FBP algorithm with the ASiR and the MBIR algorithms using standard and low-dose techniques for chest CT examinations. Their results showed that the MBIR algorithm produced "significant noise reduction" in low-dose CT scans.

The purpose of the study by Ghetti et al. (2013) was to assess the performance of the IR algorithm, SAFIRE, on image-quality parameters, such as **low-contrast resolution** and spatial resolution, compared with the FBP algorithm. Figure 6-14 shows a comparison of three levels of SAFIRE noise reduction strengths (using the low-contrast module of the Catphan 600) with the FBP algorithm. The authors reported that the images of the low-contrast resolution phantom are "sharper with less background noise" compared with the FBP image, and as the SAFIRE strength increased, image texture changes increased, resulting in an improvement in image quality. They also reported that the spatial resolution (detail visualization) with the FBP algorithm is about the same when using the SAFIRE algorithm at strength 5, as is illustrated in Figure 6-15. Finally Ghetti et al. (2013) found that "... at different dose levels SAFIRE preserves the CT number accuracy, **linearity,** and spatial resolution, both in the transverse and coronal planes. These results confirm that SAFIRE allows for image noise reduction with preserved image quality."

Vardhanabhuti et al. (2013b) compared the effects of different kilovolts (kV) and automatic tube current modulation of MBIR and ASiR with the FBP algorithm in abdominopelvic CT. It was found that the MBIR algorithm resulted in significant noise reduction compared with ASiR and the FBP algorithms at 17 levels of Noise Index (NI) used at 120 kV. They also reported that "when lowering the kV, the subjective image quality was improved, but when this is performed in conjunction with increasing NI, image quality was maintained only at moderately high NI of 50, but was degraded at higher NIs despite improving contrast-to-noise ratio."

Metha et al. (2013) explored the performance of the Philips Healthcare Iterative Model Reconstruction (IMR), referred to as iDose, using a phantom model. The results showed that the iDose algorithm may "simultaneously enable 60%-80% lower radiation dose, 43%-80% low contrast detectability

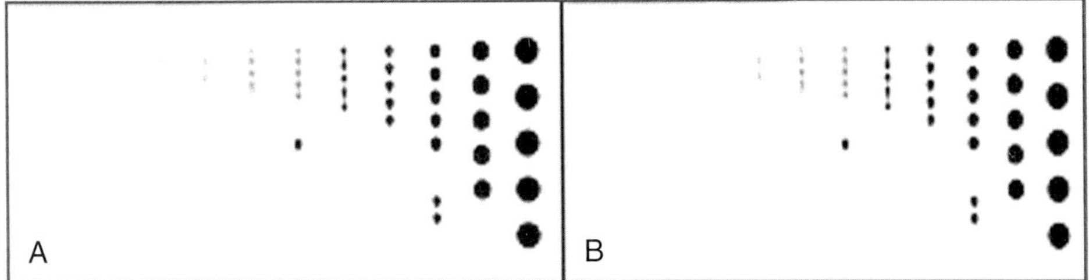


**FIGURE 6-15** The spatial resolution (detail visualization) with the FBP algorithm is about the same when using the SAFIRE algorithm at strength 5. (From Ghetti C., Palleri, F., Serreli, G., Ortenzi, O., Ruffini, L. (2013). *Journal of Applied Clinical Medical Physics, 14* (4). Reproduced by permission.)

improvement, and 70%-83% less image noise relative to the FBP algorithm." They also reported that iDose "may enable 1.2x-1.7x high-contrast spatial resolution improvement; or 2.5x-3.6x low-contrast detectability improvement; or 73%-90% image noise reduction, relative to filtered **back projection**."

Choi et al. (2013) used a phantom model of a pancreas embedded with 16 small lesions and scanned using four different CT scanners and the IR-specific algorithms from GE Healthcare, Philips Healthcare, Siemens Healthcare, and Toshiba Medical Systems (using 70 mA to 250 mA) to assess the image quality, dose reduction, and figure of merit (FOM) compared with the FBP images (labeled reference images) taken at 250 mA. The results showed that "image noise was markedly improved with the IR; therefore, a 36 to 60% dose reduction was possible. As a result, the final CT dose index volume ($CTDI_{vol}$) can be diminished to 7.05 to 11.40 mGy with the IR algorithms. The IR demonstrated 1.52 to 7.84 times higher FOM than that of FBP. Particularly, an advanced fully IR showed outstanding results of FOM (6.06-7.84 times)."

## Examples in 2014

The performance evaluation of IR algorithms such as MBIR (Smith et al., 2014) and SAFIRE (Goenka et al., 2014) continued in 2014. For example, Kim et al. (2014) compared the performance of the AIDR 3D algorithm with the FBP algorithm on noise reduction and image quality improvements. The conclusions drawn from this study showed that the AIDR 3D is effective in both noise reduction and image quality improvements compared with the FBP algorithm. Furthermore the AIDR 3D algorithm's "effectiveness may increase as the phantom size increases."

Yet another study in 2014 by Klink et al. (2014) compared the performance of iDose IR algorithm with the FBP algorithm on the influence of scan and reconstruction parameters on image quality and $CTDI_{vol}$ described in Chapter 10. The results of this study showed that

> ...noise reduction was significantly improved using IR with increasing iterations, independent of tissue, scan-mode, tube voltage, current, and kernel. IR did not affect high-contrast resolution. Low-contrast resolution was also not negatively affected, but improved in scans with doses <5 mGy, although object detectability generally decreased with lowering of the exposure. At comparable image quality levels, the $CTDI_{vol}$ was reduced 26%-50% using IR. In patients, applying IR vs FBP resulted in good to excellent image quality while tube voltage and current settings could be significantly decreased.

Another interesting study is by Samei et al. (2014) who compared the performance of the IRIS algorithm with the FBP algorithm on image quality and dose using different kilovolt settings with a phantom model. Imaging was done at a 0.5 seconds rotation time; 80 kV, 100 kV, 120 kV, and 140 kV; 64 mA to 640 mA; and 220-mm to 250-mm field of **view**. The results of this study demonstrated the following:

1. Compared with the FBP, IRIS resulted in greater reduction of the dose, even with thinner slices, and an improvement in image quality at constant dose.
2. While 80 kV to 100 kV proved optimum for the small phantom, it was 100 kV to 120 kV for the large phantom.
3. "...that noise cannot be a sole predictor of image quality across reconstruction algorithms...the performance of FBP and IRIS does not overlap even though the spatial resolution, pixel noise, kVp, and object contrast are exactly the same in both sets of images."

## Examples in 2015

Another IR algorithm study comparing its performance with the FBP algorithm was done by Khawaja et al. (2015). In this study, the researchers compared the performance of a knowledge-based IMR (Philips

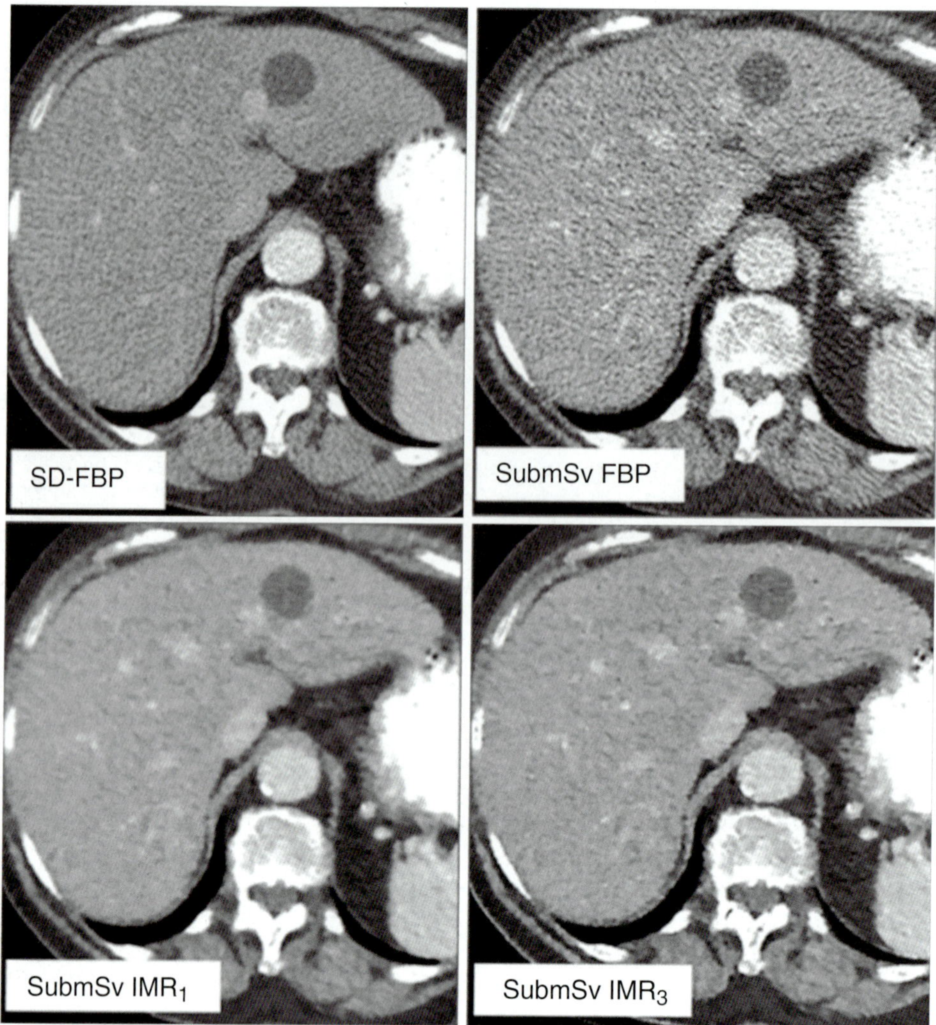


**FIGURE 6-16** Transverse abdominal CT ($CTDI_{vol}$, 6 mGy; SubmSv scan, 1.2 mGy) images of a 64-year-old woman (BMI, 29 kg/m$^2$) with known Hodgkin disease show a low attenuation liver lesion. Both liver parenchyma and lesion were acceptable for SubmSv $IMR_{1-2}$ images and unacceptable with SubmSv-FBP (too noisy) and SubmSv-$IMR_3$ images. (From Khawaja, R. D. A., Singh, S. L., Blake, M., Harisinghani, M., Choy, G., et al. (2015). *European Journal of Radiology, 84*, 2-10. Images and legend reproduced by permission.)

Healthcare) algorithm with that of the FBP algorithm at standard dose (SD) on lesion detection at reduced dose (RD = submillisievert) in abdominal CT scans and performance on image quality. The results showed that "all true lesions (ranging from 32 to 55) on SD FBP images were detected on RD IMR images across all patients. RD FBP images were unacceptable for subjective image quality. Subjective ratings showed acceptable image quality for IMR for organ margins, soft-tissue structures, and retroperitoneal **lymphadenopathy,** compared with RD FBP in patients with a BMI ≤ 25 kg/m$^2$ (median-range, 2-3). Irrespective of patient BMI, subjective ratings for hepatic/renal cysts, stones and colonic diverticula were significantly better with RD IMR images (P < 0.01). Objective image noise for RD FBP was 57-66% higher, and for RD IMR was 8-56% lower than that for SD-FBP (P < 0.01). Noise spectral density (NSD) showed significantly lower noise in the **frequency domain** with IMR in all patients compared to FBP.

Figure 6-16 shows that for visualization of liver margins and parenchyma, RD $IMR_1$ images were significantly better ($p < 0.01$) compared with the images obtained with RD $IMR_3$ images. Furthermore, Figure 6-17 illustrates that RD $IMR_1$ images showed liver lesions significantly better ($p < 0.01$) than the RD FBP images; however, RD $IMR_3$ images appear the same as RD FBP images ($P > 0.05$"); (Khawaja et al., 2015).

A more recent study on the performance evaluation of the Advanced Modeled Iterative Reconstruction (ADMIRE) algorithm is one by Solomon et al.

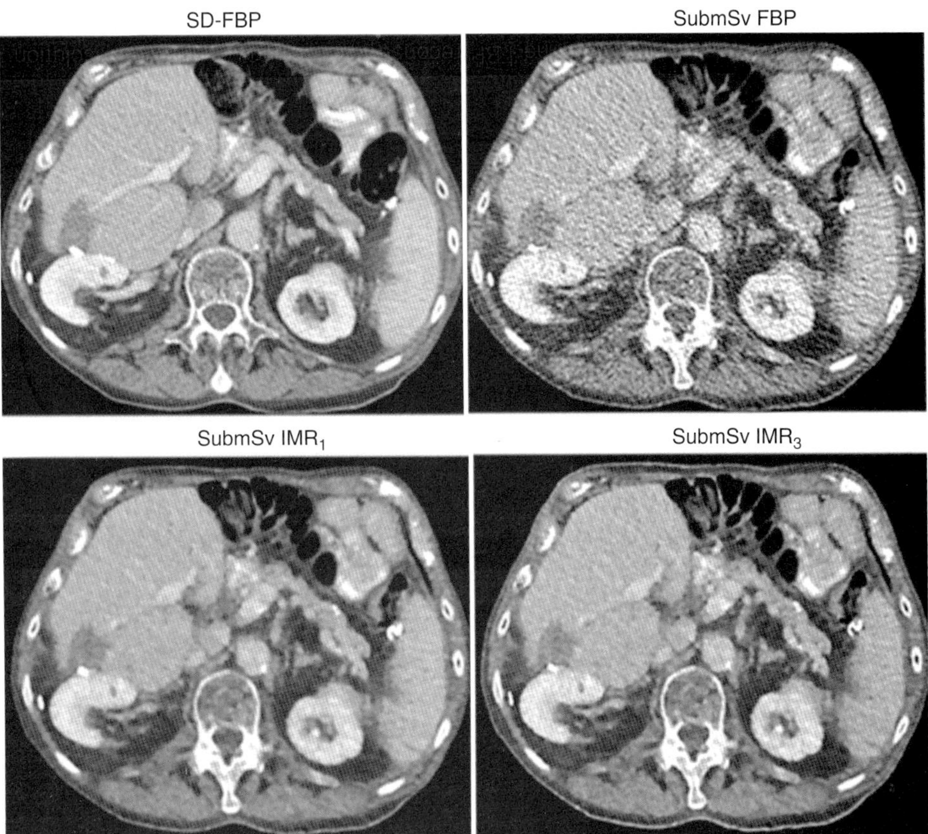


**FIGURE 6-17** Transverse abdominal CT ($CTDI_{vol}$, 6 mGy; SubmSv scan,1.2 mGy) images of a 78-year-old man (BMI, 21 kg/m$^2$) with known primary hepatocellular carcinoma show a low-attenuation renal lesion in right kidney. Both renal margins and lesion were acceptable for all SubmSv $IMR_{1-2}$ images and unacceptable with SubmSv-FBP (too noisy) and SubmSv-$IMR_3$ images. (From Khawaja, R. D. A., Singh, S. L., Blake, M., Harisinghani, M., Choy, G., et al. (2015). *European Journal of Radiology, 84,* 2-10. Reproduced by permission.)

(2015). Before looking at the results of this study, a brief description of the ADMIRE IR algorithm from Siemens Healthcare is in order.

The Food and Drug Administration (FDA) has recently provided 510(k) clearance to this third-generation IR algorithm (Godt, 2014). The overall operating technical principles of ADMIRE are illustrated in **Figure 6-18.** This algorithm provides an extension of the previously cleared Sinogram Affirmed Iterative Reconstruction (SAFIRE) reconstruction algorithm. Essentially, it involves the integration of a number of additional steps in reconstruction, of the final image all of which are intended to improve image quality while using low-dose CT imaging. ADMIRE uses raw data statistical modeling, advanced system modeling, and model-based noise cancellation as well as artifact cancellation. The result is noise reduction, improved spatial resolution at high-contrast edges, and images free from artifacts. Furthermore, the ADMIRE algorithm also provides a noise texture, which approaches that of the FBP algorithm, and is implemented on the Somatom Force, Siemens' dual-source CT system.

A comparison of images acquired with the ADMIRE IR algorithm compared with the FBP algorithm is shown in **Figure 6-19**.

The study by Solomon et al. (2015) assessed the ADMIRE algorithm on low-contrast detectability in a contrast-detail phantom, against the FBP algorithm. The results showed that "during the first session, detection accuracy increased with increasing contrast, size, and dose index (diagnostic accuracy range, 50%-87%; interobserver variability, ±7%). When compared with FBP, ADMIRE improved detection accuracy by 5.2% on average across the investigated variables ($P < .001$). During the second session, a significantly increased number of visible objects was noted with increasing radiation dose index, section thickness, and ADMIRE strength over FBP (up to 80% more visible objects, $P < .001$). Radiation dose reduction potential ranged from 56% to 60% and from 4% to 80% during the two sessions, respectively."

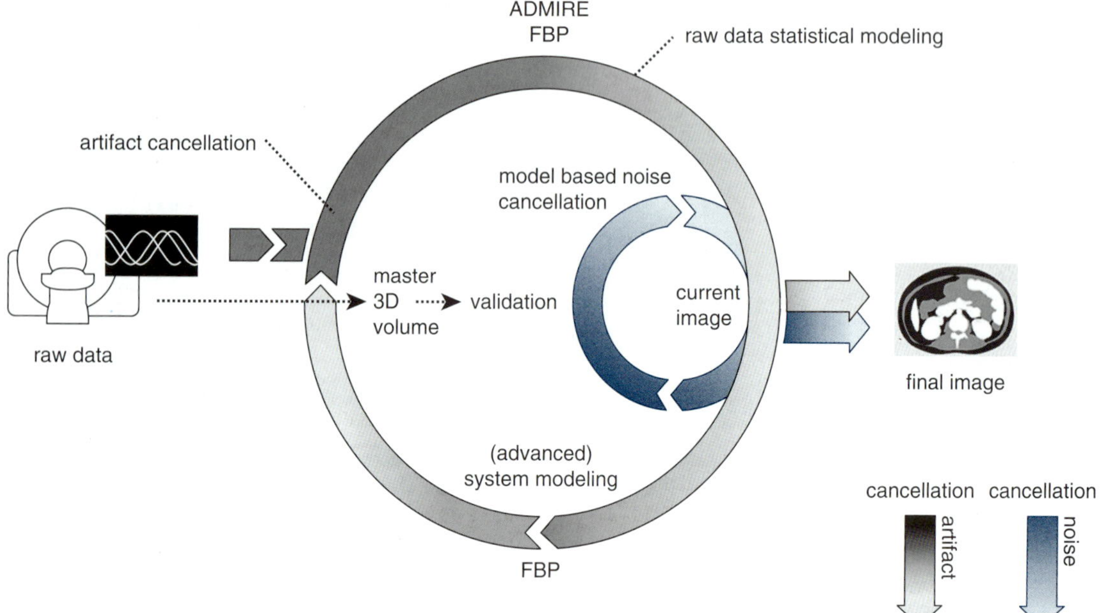


**FIGURE 6-18** The overall technical principles of the ADMIRE IR algorithm involve the integration of a number of additional steps in reconstruction of the final image all of which are intended to improve image quality while using low-dose CT imaging. ADMIRE uses raw data statistical modeling, advanced system modeling, and model-based noise cancellation as well as artifact cancellation. (Courtesy of Siemens Healthcare.)

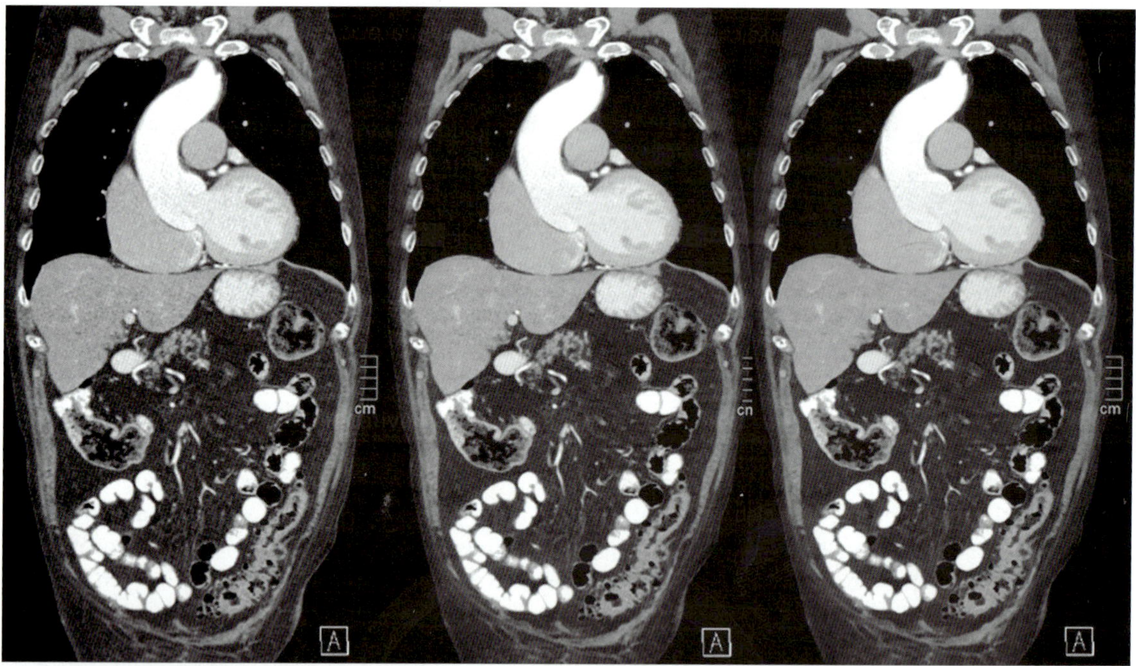


**FIGURE 6-19** A comparison of three images from the Siemens FORCE (dual-source mode, p=1.55; scan time <2s; 100kV; DLP 707mGycm) with FBP, ADMIRE 3 and 5 recon. The FBP image is shown on the left, images with the use of ADMIR 3 in the middle, and ADMIRE 5 on the right side. (Courtesy of Prof. Dr. med. Michael Lell, Professor of Radiology, Department of Radiology, University Erlangen.)

## CONCLUSION: A NOTEWORTHY PERSPECTIVE

Several studies from 2012 to 2015 comparing the performance of IR algorithms with the FBP algorithm have been cited above with definitive conclusions that IR algorithms provide noise and dose reduction, improve image quality (namely, spatial and low-contrast resolution), and reduce artifacts compared with the FBP algorithm. It is important, however, to understand what Beister et al. (2012) stated so authoritatively:

> The image quality performance of different products is hard to compare in general since they are scanner-specific and many other system parameters can also have a noteworthy influence on the reconstruction performance. At best, a comparison of complete systems may be possible. There appears to be a consensus, however, that MBIR approaches including geometric modeling reliably reduce noise and improve image sharpness at the same time.

## REVIEW QUESTIONS

Answer the following questions to check your understanding of the materials studied.

1. Which of the following is not a key feature of the FBP algorithm-measured projection data (raw data)?
   A. Calibrations and correction
   B. Log conversion
   C. Adaptive section collimation
   D. Convolution and back-projection
2. Which of the following occurs as the last step before the image is created using the FBP algorithm?
   A. Back-projection
   B. Convolution
   C. Beam-hardening correction
   D. Log conversion
3. The following are assumptions of the FBP algorithm ***except***:
   A. projection data is shaped by a special filter
   B. the x-ray focal spot is a point source
   C. the detector cell size and shape are not considered
   D. the projection data is accurate and not influenced by electronic noise
4. The most recent method to reduce noise in low-dose CT imaging is to:
   A. use the FBP algorithm denoising with a standard reconstruction kernel.
   B. use high mAs techniques.
   C. use a smoothing digital filter.
   D. use an iterative reconstruction (IR) algorithm.
5. The following refers to IR algorithms currently available from CT manufacturers:
   A. statistical methods with modeling photon statistics
   B. iterative methods without modeling
   C. model-based methods
   D. all are correct
6. With IR algorithms without modeling:
   A. low mAs techniques are used to reduce noise.
   B. the FBP algorithm is applied to the raw data to produce an initial CT image.
   C. high kVp techniques are essential to reduce dose.
   D. the final CT image is not as accurate when using IR algorithms with modeling.
7. Which of the following is not as essential step in an IR algorithm without modeling?
   A. Simulated projection data are created from the forward projection dataset
   B. Simulated raw data are compared with the measured projection data
   C. Optimization of the forward projection data
   D. Predetermined image quality criteria are not necessary
8. A IR algorithm that models the x-ray tube, image voxels and detectors, etc. is referred to as the:
   A. object model.
   B. physics model.
   C. optics or system model.
   D. noise model.
9. Compared to the FBP algorithm, IR algorithms result in all of the following ***except***:
   A. reduction in image noise
   B. improvement in image quality such as spatial resolution
   C. faster production of the final CT image
   D. reduction of image artifacts
10. Performance evaluation studies have compared IR algorithms with the FBP algorithm on all of the following characteristics ***except***:
    A. the speed of obtaining the final image
    B. image quality improvement
    C. noise reduction
    D. dose reduction

## REFERENCES


Beister, D., Kolditz, D., & Kalender, W. A. (2012). Iterative reconstruction methods in x-ray CT. *Physica Medica, 28*, 94–108.

Brenner, D. J., & Hall, E. J. (2007). Computed tomography: an increasing source of radiation exposure. *New England Journal of Medicine, 357*, 2277–2284.

Buxi, T. B. S., Yadav, A., Singh Rawat, K., & Singh Ghuman, S. (2014). Effect of iterative reconstructions in low dose computed tomography. *Journal of Biomedical Graphics and Computing, 4*(3), 1–9.

Chen, B., Ramizrez Giraldo, J. C., Solomon, J., & Samei, E. (2014). Evaluating iterative reconstruction performance in computed tomography. *Medical Physics, 41*(12), 121913.

Choi, J. W., Lee, J. M., Yoon, J. H., Baek, J. H., Han, J. K., & Choi, B. I. (2013). Iterative reconstruction algorithms of computed tomography for the assessment of small pancreatic lesions: phantom study. *Journal of Computer Assisted Tomography, 37*(6), 911–923.

Ehman, E. C., Yu, L., Manduca, A., et al. (2014). Methods for clinical evaluation of noise reduction techniques in abdominopelvic CT. *Radiographics, 34*, 849–862.

Fan, J., et al. (2014). Benefits of ASiR-V reconstruction for reducing patient radiation dose and preserving diagnostic quality in CT exams. *Whitepaper, GE Healthcare.*

Ghetti, C., Palleri, F., Serreli, G., Ortenzi, O., & Ruffini, L. (2013). Physical characterization of a new CT iterative reconstruction algorithm method operating in sonogram space. *Journal of Applied Clinical Medical Physics, 14*(4), 263–271.

Godt, E. *FDA clears latest CT reconstruction algorithm from Siemens.* http://www.healthimaging.com/topics/advanced-visualization/fda-clears-latest-ct-reconstruction-algorithm-siemens, August 18, 2014.

Goenka, A. H., Herts, B. R., Obuchowski, N. A., et al. (2014). Effect of reduced radiation exposure and iterative reconstruction on detection of low-contrast low-attenuation lesions in an anthropomorphic liver phantom: an 18 reader study. *Radiology, 272*(1), 154–163.

Gordic, S., et al. (2014). Advanced modelled iterative reconstruction for abdominal CT: qualitative and quantitative evaluation. *Clinical Radiology, 69*(12), e497–504.

Hounsfield, G. N. (1973). Computerized transverse axial scanning (tomography), Part 1: description of the system. *British Journal of Radiology, 46*, 1016–1022.

Hsieh, J. (2008). Adaptive statistical iterative reconstruction. *Whitepaper, GE Healthcare.*

Hsieh, J., Nett, B., Yu, Z., Sauer, K., & Thibault, J.-B. (2013). Recent advances in CT image reconstruction. *Current Radiology Reports.* http://dx.doi.org/10.1007/s40134-012-0003-7. Published Online January 16.

Irwan, R., et al. (2011). AIDR 3D—reduces dose and simultaneously improves image quality. *Whitepaper, Toshiba Medical Systems* Europe BV.

Kalender, W. (2014). Dose in x-ray computed tomography. *Physics in Medicine and Biology, 59*, R129–R150.

Khawaja, R. D. A., Singh, S., Blake, M., Harisinghani, M., Choy, G., et al. (2015). Ultra-low dose abdominal MDCT: Using a knowledge-based Iterative Model Reconstruction technique for substantial dose reduction in a prospective clinical study. *European Journal of Radiology, 84*, 2–10.

Kim, M., et al. (2014). Adaptive iterative dose reduction algorithm in CT: effect on image quality compared with filtered back projection in body phantoms of different sizes. *Korean Journal of Radiology, 15*(2), 195–204.

Klink, T., Obmann, V., Heverhagen, J., Stork, A., Adam, G., & Begemann, P. (2014). Reducing CT radiation dose with iterative reconstruction algorithms: the influence of scan and reconstruction parameters on image quality and $CTDI_{vol}$. *European Journal of Radiology, 83*, 1645–1654.

Kordolaimi, S. D., Argentos, S., Pantos, I., Kelekis, N. L., & Efstathopoulos, E. P. (2013). A new era in computed tomography dose optimization: The impact of iterative reconstruction on image quality and radiation dose. *Journal of Computer Assisted Tomography, 37*, 924–931.

Leipsic, J., et al. (2010). Estimated radiation dose using adaptive statistical iterative reconstruction in coronary CT angiography: The ERASIR study, *Am J Roentgenol, 195*, 655–660.

Metha, D., et al. (2013). Iterative model reconstruction: simultaneously lowered radiation dose and improve image quality. *Medical Physics International Journal, 1*(2), 147–155.

Pearce, M. S., Salotti, J. A., Little, M. P., et al. (2012). Radiation exposure from CT scans in childhood and subsequent risk of leukemia and brain tumors: a retrospective cohort study. *Lancet, 380*(9840), 499–505.

Prakash, P., et al. (2010). Radiation dose reduction with chest computed tomography using adaptive statistical reconstruction technique: initial experience. *Journal of Computer Assisted Tomography, 34*(1), 40–45.

Protik, A., Thomas, K., Babyn, P., & Ford, N. L. (2012). Phantom study of the impact of adaptive statistical iterative reconstruction (ASiR) on image quality for pediatric computed tomography. *Journal of Biomedical Science and Engineering, 5*, 793–803.

Samei, E., Richard, S., & Lurwitz, L. (2014). Model-based CT performance assessment and optimization of iodinated and non-iodinated imaging tasks as a function of kVp and body size. *Medical Physics, 41*(8), 081910.

Schindera, S. T., et al. (2011). Iterative reconstruction algorithm for abdominal multidetector CT at different tube voltages: assessment of diagnostic accuracy, image quality, and radiation dose in a phantom study. *Radiology, 260*(2), 454–462.

Seeram, E. (2014). CT dose optimization. *Radiologic Technology, 85*(6), 655–675.

Singh, S., et al. (2011). Adaptive statistical iterative reconstruction technique for radiation dose reduction in chest CT: a pilot study. *Radiology, 259*(2), 565–573.

Singh, S., Kalra, M. K., Shenoy-Bhangle, A. S., et al. (2012). Radiation dose reduction with hybrid iterative reconstruction for pediatric CT. *Radiology, 263*(2), 537–546.

Smith, E. A., Dillman, J. R., Goodsitt, M. M., et al. (2014). Model-based iterative reconstruction: effect of patient dose and image quality in pediatric body CT. *Radiology, 270*, 526–534.

Smith, K. (2013). Iterative reconstruction in computed tomography. *Imaging and Therapy Practice*, January, 15–17.

Solomon J et al.: Diagnostic performance of an advanced modeled iterative reconstruction algorithm for low-contrast detectability with a third-generation dual-source multidetector CT scanner: potential for radiation dose reduction in a multireader study, *Radiology*, Mar 4:142005, 2015. [Epub ahead of print]

Thibault, J. B. (2010). Veo CT model-based iterative reconstruction. *GE Healthcare Whitepaper*.

Toshiba Medical Systems. AIDR 3D (2015). <http://www.toshiba-medical.co.jp/tmd/english/products/dose/aidr3d/index.html > Accessed March 2015.

Vardhanabhuti, V., Loader, R., & Roobottom, C. A. (2013a). Assessment of image quality on effects of varying tube voltage and automatic tube current modulation with hybrid and pure iterative reconstruction techniques in abdominal and pelvic CT. *Investigative Radiology, 48*(3), 167–174.

Vardhanabhuti, V., et al. (2013b). Image quality assessment of standard and low-dose chest CT using filtered back projection (FBP), adaptive statistical iterative reconstruction (ASIR) and novel model-based iterative reconstruction (MBIR) algorithms. *American Journal of Roentgenology, 200*, 545–552.

Zeng, G. L., & Zamyatin, A. (2013). A filtered back projection algorithm with ray-by-ray noise weighting. *Medical Physics, 40*(13), 031113.

# 7

# Basic Instrumentation

## OUTLINE

**Computer Systems**
- Definition
- Hardware Organization

**Software Concepts**

**Computer Architectures and Processing Operations**
- Types
- Terminology

**CT Scanner—Basic Equipment Configuration**

**Imaging System**
- Gantry
- Patient Table

**CT Computer and Image-Processing System**
- Processing Architectures and Hardware
- The Graphics Processing Unit
- Scanner Control and Image Reconstruction
- Image Display and Manipulation
- Operating Systems
- CT Software

**Image Display, Storage, Recording, and Communications**
- Image Display
- Image Storage
- Laser Recording System
- Communications

**CT and Picture Archiving and Communications Systems**
- Picture Archiving and Communications Systems: A Definition
- PACS: Major Components
- PACS and CT Interfacing
- PACS and Information Systems Integration

**CT Control Console**

**Options and Accessories for CT Systems**
- Options
- Accessories

**Other Considerations**
- Modular Design Concept
- Operating Modes of the Scanner
- Room Layout for CT Equipment
- Equipment Specifications

## LEARNING OBJECTIVES

On completion of this chapter, you should be able to:

1. describe the fundamental differences between computer hardware and computer software.
2. identify the different types of computer architectures and processing operations.
3. describe the components of three major subsystems of a CT scanner.
4. describe the characteristics of the CT gantry and the patient couch.
5. describe each of the following elements of a CT computer and image-processing system:
   - processing architecture
   - hardware
   - software.
6. state what is meant by the graphics processing unit (GPU) and identify its role in CT imaging
7. outline the characteristic features of CT image display, recording, and storage.
8. describe the major components of a picture archiving and communications system (PACS) and how it interfaces with a CT scanner.
9. outline the main features of a CT control console.
10. describe several hardware and software options for CT scanners.
11. identify various accessories for use in CT.
12. describe what is meant by the modular design concept and operating modes of a scanner.
13. describe a typical room layout for a CT scanner.
14. identify the major technical specifications for a CT scanner.

## KEY TERMS TO WATCH FOR AND REMEMBER

The following key terms/concepts are important to your understanding of this chapter.

**accessories**
**applications software**
**communications**
**computer architecture**
**computer system**
**connectivity**
**graphics pipeline**
**hardware**
**imaging system**
**integrated control console**
**input hardware**
**modular design concept**
**operating mode**
**parallel processing**
**picture archiving and communication systems (PACS)**
**pipeline processing**
**processing hardware**
**processing operations**
**software**
**systems software**

In Chapter 1, an overview of **computed tomography (CT)** was presented and a brief history reviewed, followed by an outline of the growth of CT technology from the time it was invented to its current clinical applications and uses in nonclinical areas, such as **scanning** baggage at airports. An important point made in Chapter 1 emphasized that computers play an important role in the production of a CT image, and that they are a major component of the CT **imaging system.** Because of this, it is mandatory for technologists to have a general understanding of what a computer is and how it works.

This chapter reviews a few important basic technical elements of computers and outlines the major equipment components of the CT scanner, including the imaging system, the CT computer and processing system, image display, storage, recording, and communications, CT and **picture archiving and communication systems (PACS),** and CT control console and options and accessories for CT systems. A number of other considerations, such as the modular design concept, **operating modes** of the scanner, room layout for CT equipment, and equipment specifications, will be highlighted.

## COMPUTER SYSTEMS

### Definition

A computer is a machine for solving problems. Specifically, the modern computer is a high-speed electronic computational machine that accepts information in the form of data and instructions through an **input** device and processes this information with arithmetic and logic operations from a program stored in its memory. The results of the processing can be displayed, stored, or recorded by suitable **output** devices or transmitted to another location.

Essentially, people can perform these same tasks; the word computer historically referred to a person. A **computer system,** on the other hand, consists of at least three elements: hardware, software, and computer users (Fig. 7-1). **Hardware** refers to the physical components of the machine, and **software** refers to the instructions that make the hardware work to solve problems. People are essential to computer systems because they design, develop, and operate hardware and software.

These elements result in three core characteristics that reflect the usefulness of computers: speed (solve problems very quickly), reliability (not prone to errors—computers are only as good as the people who program them), and storage capability (storage of a vast amount of data and information (Capron, 2005).

### Hardware Organization

A computer processes the data or information it receives from people or other computers and outputs the results in a form suitable to the needs of the user. This is a three-step process (Fig. 7-2).

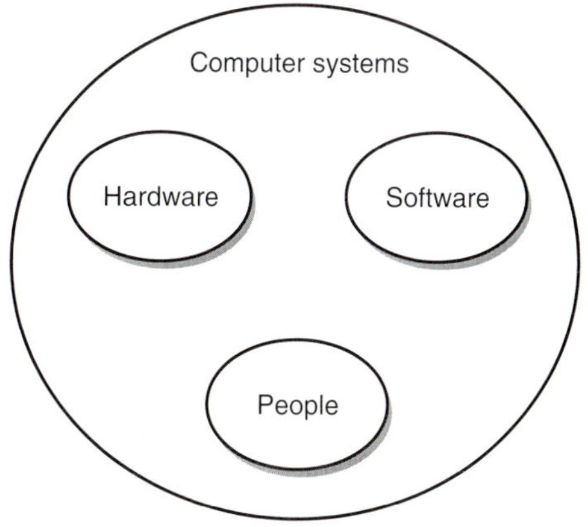


**FIGURE 7-1** The three essential elements of a computer system.

The organization of a computer includes at least five hardware components: an input device, a central processing unit (CPU), internal memory, an output device, and external memory or storage (Fig. 7-3). **Input hardware** refers to input devices such as a keyboard from which information can be sent to the processor. **Processing hardware** includes the CPU and internal memory. The CPU is the brain of the computer; it consists of a control unit that directs the activities of the machine and an arithmetic-logic unit to perform mathematical calculations and data comparisons. In addition, the CPU includes an internal memory, or main memory, for the permanent storage of software instructions and data.

After data are processed, results are sent to an output device in the form of a hard or soft copy. One popular hard-copy output device is a printer. If the results are displayed on a monitor for direct viewing, then the term *soft copy* is used. Finally, processing results can be stored on external storage devices. These include magnetic storage devices, such as disks and tapes, and optical storage devices.

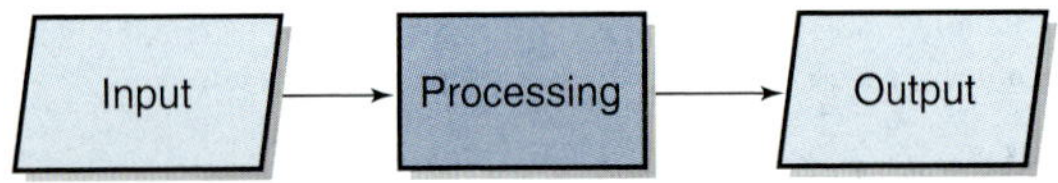


**FIGURE 7-2** Computer processing involves input, processing, and output.

## SOFTWARE CONCEPTS

The hardware receives its instructions from the software. The instructions are written in steps that specify ways to solve problems. These sets of instructions are called *programs.*

The three categories of software are (1) **systems software,** (2) applications software, and (3) software development tools. *Systems software* refers to programs that start up the computer and coordinate the activities of all hardware components and applications software. **Applications software** refers to programs developed by computer systems users to solve specific problems. Software development tools include computer or programming languages such as BASIC, FORTRAN, COBOL, Pascal, DELPHI, C, and C++. Other tools are now available to simplify and expedite the software development process.

## COMPUTER ARCHITECTURES AND PROCESSING OPERATIONS

**Computer architecture** refers to the general structure of a computer and includes both the elements of hardware and software. Specifically, it refers to computer systems, computer chips, circuitry, and systems software.

### Types

Essentially, the two types of CPU architectures are complex instruction set computing (CISC)

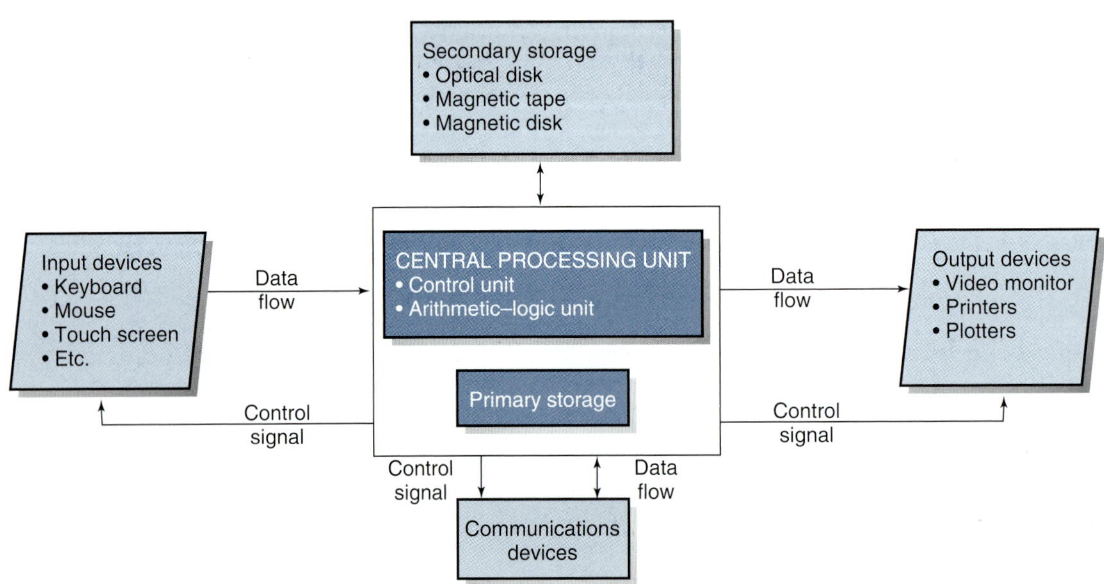


**FIGURE 7-3** Organization of the hardware components of a computer.

architecture and reduced instruction set computing (RISC) architecture. The CISC microprocessor design has more built-in operations compared with the RISC microprocessor design. Computers with CISC architecture include the IBM 3090 mainframe computer and nearly all microcomputers. Computers with RISC architecture are the IBM 6000, Sun Microsystems SPARC, and Motorola 88000. According to Covington (1991), "RISC is faster if memory is relatively fast so that no time is wasted fetching instructions. CISC is faster if memory is relatively slow because the same work can be done without fetching as many instruction codes."

These architectures are capable of **processing operations** such as serial or sequential processing, distributed processing, multiprocessing, multitasking, **parallel processing,** and pipelining. CT technologists should understand the meaning of these terms because they are used in the CT literature and manufacturers' brochures.

### Terminology

The following definitions are taken from the most recent edition of the *Microsoft Computer Dictionary*, published by Microsoft Press.

- *Serial or sequential processing*: Information (data and instructions) is processed in the order in which items are entered and stored in the computer. It is a simple form of processing data, one instruction at a time.
- *Distributed processing*: The information is processed by several computers connected by a network. True distributed processing "has separate computers that perform different tasks in such a way that their combined work can contribute to a larger goal .... It requires a highly structured environment that allows hardware and software to communicate, share resources, and exchange information freely."
- *Multitasking*: The computer works on more than one task at a time.
- *Multiprocessing*: Multiprocessing uses two or more connected processing units. "In multiprocessing, each processing unit works on a different set of instructions (or on different parts of the same process). The objective is increased speed or computing power, the same as in parallel processing, and the use of special units called *co-processors*."
- *Parallel processing*: This is a "method of processing that can run only on a type of computer containing two or more processors running simultaneously. Parallel processing differs from multiprocessing in the way a task is distributed over the available processors; in multiprocessing, a process might be divided up into sequential blocks, with one processor managing access to a database, another analyzing the data, and a third handling graphical output to the screen." A number of processes can be carried out at the same time.
- *Pipelining*: A "method of fetching and decoding instructions in which, at any given time, several program instructions are in various stages of being fetched or decoded. Ideally, pipelining speeds execution time by ensuring that the microprocessor does not have to wait for instructions; when it completes execution of one instruction, the next is ready and waiting .... In parallel processing, *pipelining* can also refer to a method in which instructions are passed from one processing unit to another, as on an assembly line, and each unit is specialized for performing a particular type of operation."

## CT SCANNER—BASIC EQUIPMENT CONFIGURATION

The basic equipment configuration for CT is illustrated in Figure 7-4. Three major systems are the imaging system, the computer system, and the image display, recording, storage, and communication system. Figure 7-5 shows an earlier unit with the associated major system components.

The three major systems are housed in separate rooms, as follows:

1. The imaging system is located in the scanner room.
2. The computer system is located in the computer room.
3. The display, recording, and storage system is located in the operator's room.

Today, CT scanners are typically housed in similar physical spaces that contain the three system components identified in Figure 7-5.

The purpose of the imaging system is to produce x rays, shape and filter the x-ray beam to pass through only a defined cross section of the patient, detect and measure the radiation passing through the cross section, and convert the transmitted photons into digital information. The major components of the imaging system are the **x-ray tube** and generator, collimators, filter, detectors, and detector electronics. The x-ray tube and generator are responsible for x-ray production. The radiation beam that emanates from the tube is filtered through a specially designed filter that protects the patient from low-energy rays and ensures beam uniformity at the detectors. The collimators

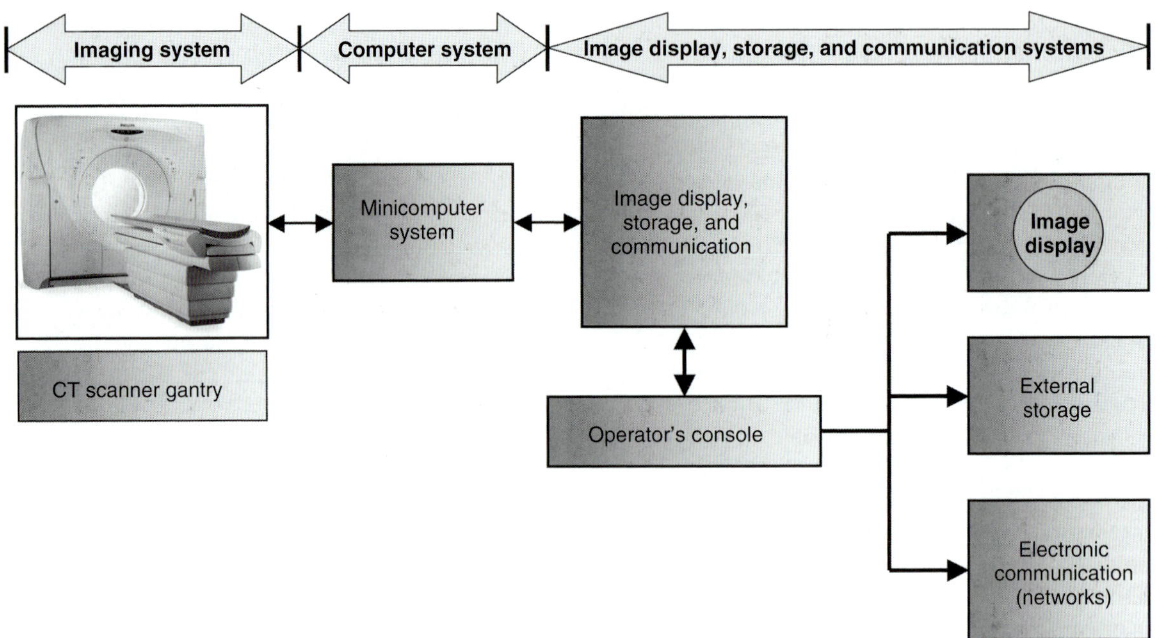


**FIGURE 7-4** Basic equipment configuration for CT, showing the major technical components.

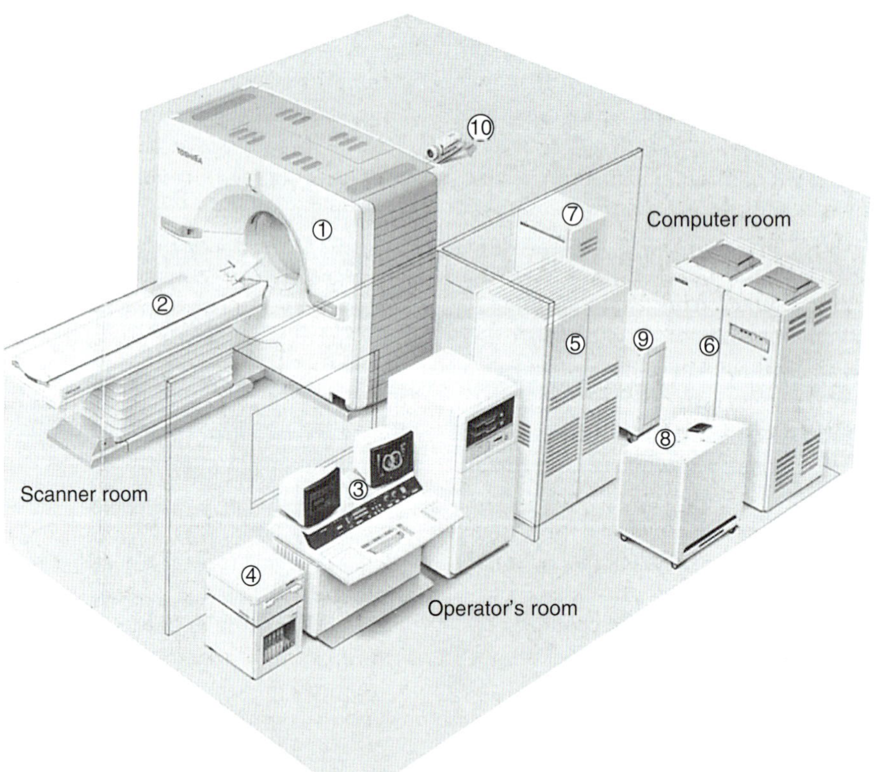


**FIGURE 7-5** Components of a CT imaging system. *1,* Gantry; *2,* patient couch; *3,* integrated console; *4,* optical disk system including cassette storage; *5,* high-speed processor system; *6,* x-ray high-voltage generator; *7,* couch control unit; *8,* system transformer I; *9,* system transformer II; *10,* patient observation system. (Courtesy Toshiba America Medical Systems, Tustin, Calif.)

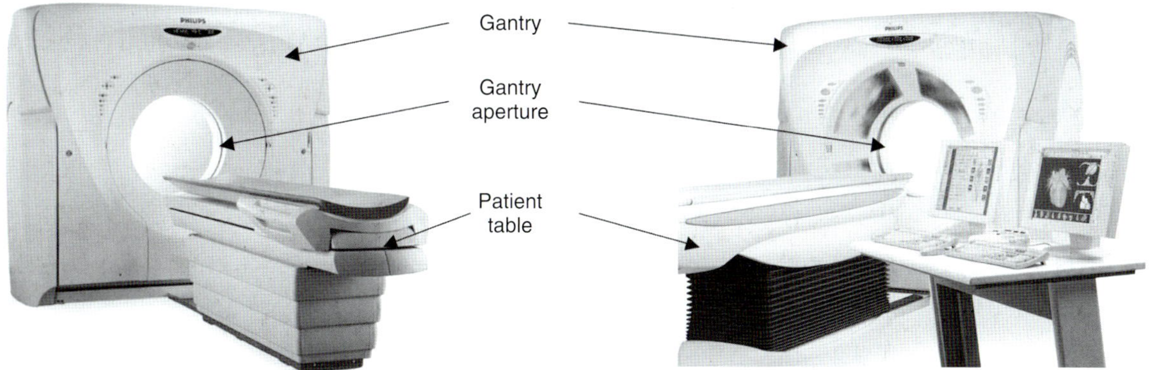


**FIGURE 7-6** The external appearance of a CT scanner, showing the gantry, the gantry aperture, and the patient table. (Courtesy Philips Medical Systems.)

help define the **slice thickness** and restrict the x-ray beam to the cross section of interest. The detectors capture the x-ray photons and convert them into electrical signals (analog information); the detector electronics, or **data acquisition system (DAS),** converts this information into digital data.

The computer system receives the digital data from the DAS and processes it to reconstruct an image of the cross-sectional anatomy. In addition, the computer system performs image manipulation and various **image-processing** operations such as **windowing,** image enhancement, image enlargement and measurements, multiplanar reconstruction, 3D imaging, and quantitative measurements.

The computer system generally includes input–output devices, CPUs, array processors, interface devices, back-projector processors, storage devices, and communications hardware. The computer system also includes software that allows each hardware component to perform specific tasks. The software enables scanning procedures to be created and activated from an input device and extensive image display and analysis functions, such as image pan and zoom, image annotation, multiple image display, windowing, reverse video, image rotation, and collage and sagittal-coronal display.

The purpose of the image display, recording, storage, and communication system is to

1. Display the output digital image from the computer in a form meaningful to the observer or diagnostician. CT images are now displayed on flat panel monitors or on cathode ray tube (CRT) monitors. These are highlighted subsequently.
2. Provide a hard copy of the image on a recording medium that provides a permanent copy of the reconstructed image and accommodates the preference of the radiologist during diagnostic interpretation. Today, film images are no longer available and radiologists now have to make the primary diagnosis from a display monitor in the total digital imaging department.
3. Facilitate the storage and retrieval of digital data to address the problems of film storage and archiving and the environmental concerns of film manufacturing, consumption, and disposal. The filmless imaging department now stores images in the PACS.
4. Communicate images, diagnostic reports, and patient demographic data in an electronic communications network environment such as PACS and radiology information systems.

## IMAGING SYSTEM

The imaging system comprises several components housed in the **gantry** that work together to acquire an image from the patient. The gantry and patient table (couch) are often referred to as the *scanner* (Fig. 7-6).

### Gantry

The **gantry** is a mounted framework that surrounds the patient in a vertical plane. It contains a rotating scan frame onto which the x-ray generator, x-ray tube, and other components are mounted. It houses imaging components (Fig. 7-7) such as the slip rings, x-ray tube, high-voltage generator, collimators, detectors, and the DAS.

The x-ray tubes of slip-ring scanners require high instantaneous power and have larger anodes with a typical diameter of 5 inches or more. Some CT scanners may incorporate an on-board oil-to-air heat exchanger to assist in cooling the x-ray tube during operation.

The generator in the gantry is usually a small, solid-state **high-frequency generator** mounted on the rotating scan frames. Because it is located close to the x-ray tube, only a short high-tension cable is required to couple the x-ray tube and generator. This design eliminates external x-ray control cabinets and long high-tension cables like the older CT imaging systems.

The power ratings of generators typically range from 30 kW to 60 kW, depending on the scanner. These ratings enable a large selection of **exposure** techniques (values such as 80 kV, 100 kV, 120 kV, 130 kV, and 140 kV and about 20 mA to 500 mA, in 1-mA increments, are not uncommon).

Gantry cooling is a prime consideration because the ambient air temperature affects several components. In the past, air conditioners were placed in the gantry. Modern cooling systems circulate ambient air from the scanner room throughout the gantry.

Two important features of the gantry are the gantry aperture and gantry tilting range. The gantry aperture is the opening in which the patient is positioned during the scanning procedure (Fig. 7-8). The technologist can approach the patient from both the front and back of the gantry. Most scanners have a 70-cm aperture that facilitates patient positioning and helps provide access to patients in emergency situations.

The CT gantry must be capable of tilting (Fig. 7-9) to accommodate all patients and clinical examinations. The degree of tilt varies between systems, but ±12 to ±30 degrees in 0.5-degree increments is somewhat standard. The gantry also includes a set of laser beams to aid patient positioning. Other gantry characteristics include scan control panels (controls gantry tilt and patient table elevation), scan control box (controls emergency stop, intercom, and scan enable and pause functions), slice **position** indicator, radiation indicator, and intercom systems with multilingual autovoice to facilitate communication with the patient in one of several languages.

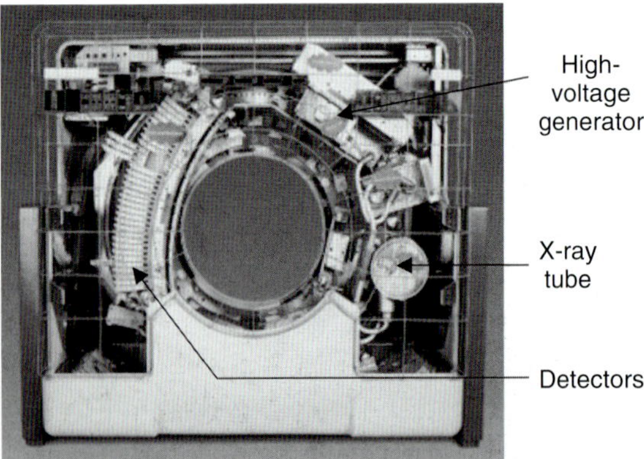


**FIGURE 7-7** The gantry houses imaging components such as the x-ray tube and generator, slip rings, collimators, detectors, and detector electronics. (Courtesy Philips Medical Systems.)

## Patient Table

The patient couch, or patient table, provides a platform on which the patient lies during the examination (Fig. 7-6). The couch should be strong and rigid to support the weight of the patient. Additionally, it should provide for safety and comfort of the patient during the examination.

The couch consists of a support referred to as the *table top*, which floats and rests on a pedestal. The couch top is usually made of carbon fiber composites because they have low absorption and provide

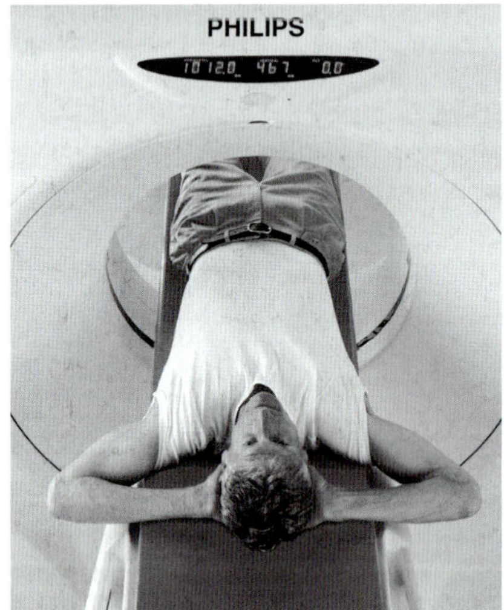


**FIGURE 7-8** The gantry aperture is the opening in the gantry in which the patient is positioned for the examination. The diameter of the aperture shown is 700 mm. (Courtesy Philips Medical Systems.)

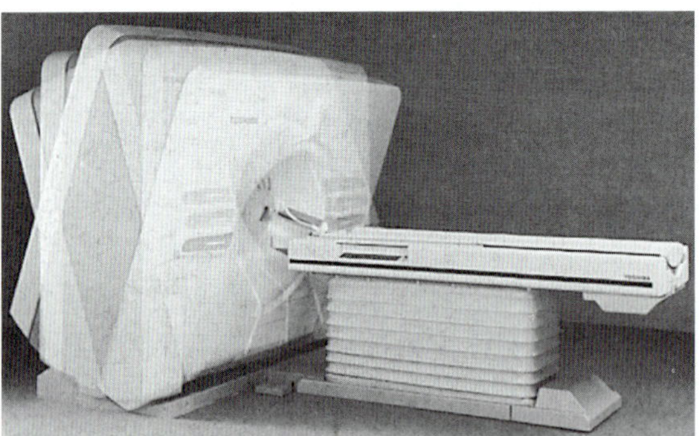

**FIGURE 7-9** The tilting range of the gantry. (Courtesy Toshiba America Medical Systems, Tustin, Calif.)

excellent vibration-damping features and meet the strength requirements necessary to take images of heavy patients. The technologist has ample room between the gantry and table for patient access and positioning (Fig. 7-10). The pedestal houses the mechanical and electrical components that facilitate vertical and horizontal couch movements. The vertical movement should provide a range of heights to make it easy for patients to mount and dismount the table (Fig. 7-11). This feature is especially useful in the examination of geriatric, trauma, and **pediatric patients.** Horizontal or longitudinal couch movements should enable the patient to be scanned from head to thighs without repositioning (Fig. 7-12).

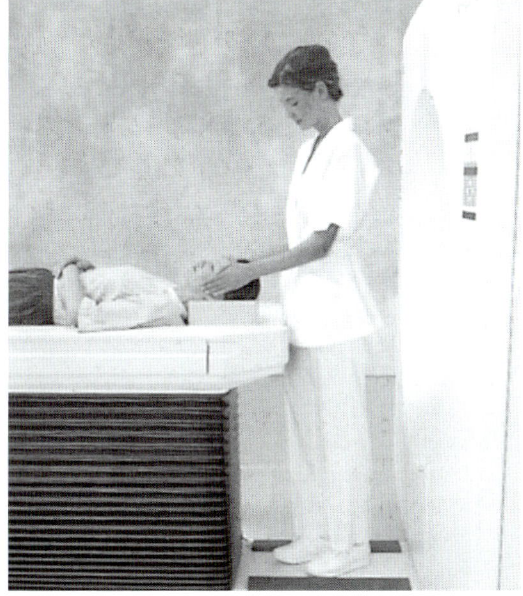

**FIGURE 7-10** A design feature of the gantry and table of a CT scanner that facilitates both access to and positioning of the patient. (Courtesy Siemens Medical Solutions USA, Inc.)

Box 7-1 lists the table characteristics for one CT system.

## CT COMPUTER AND IMAGE-PROCESSING SYSTEM

Computers are classified according to their processing capabilities, storage capacity, size, and cost. At present, computers are grouped in four main classes: supercomputers, mainframe computers, minicomputers, and microcomputers.

Midrange computers were once referred to as minicomputers, an old term that has been defined as "a mid-level computer built to perform complex computations while dealing efficiently with a high level of input and output from users connected via terminals (Microsoft, 2002). Midrange computers are also frequently connected to other midrange computers on a network and distribute processing among other computers such as personal computers (PCs). Midrange computers are used in CT and MRI.

Microcomputers are small digital computers available in a variety of sizes such as laptops or tablets. One category of microcomputers is the workstation, an upper-end PC. Workstations are now commonplace in radiology and are used in several digital imaging modalities including CT and MRI.

### Processing Architectures and Hardware

Various computer architectures for CT have been developed to accommodate fast **image reconstruction** and other image-processing functions such as image manipulation and visualization software. For example, the evolution of computer architectures for CT scanners first used **pipeline processing**

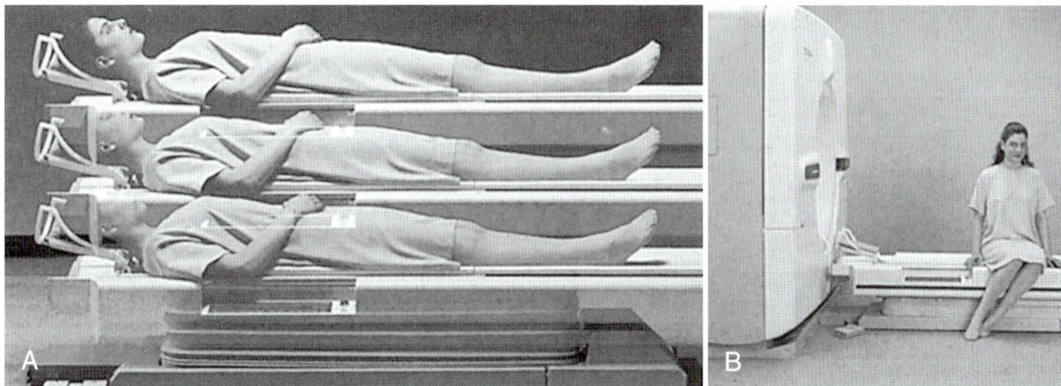


**FIGURE 7-11** The vertical movement of the couch can provide a range of heights **(A)** and allow the patient to mount and dismount the table with little effort **(B)**. (Courtesy Toshiba America Medical Systems, Tustin, Calif.)

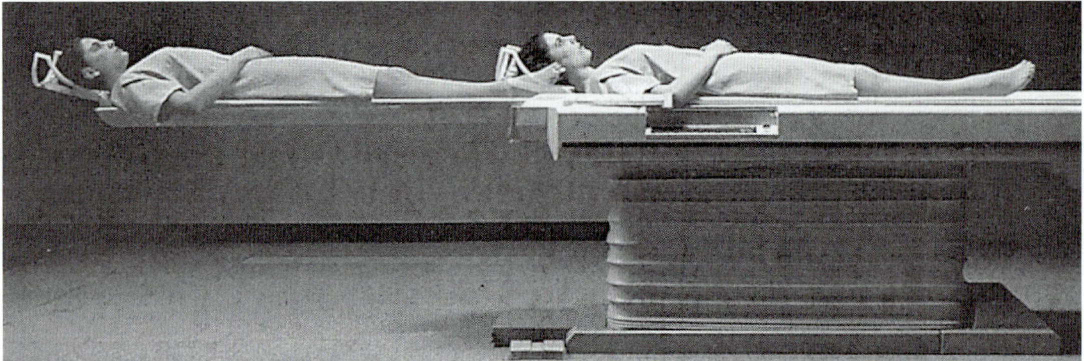

**FIGURE 7-12** Longitudinal or horizontal movement of the CT couch (*top*) should allow the patient to be scanned from head to thigh without repositioning. (Courtesy Toshiba America Medical Systems, Tustin, Calif.)

**BOX 7-1 Characteristics of the Brilliance Computed Tomography Scanner Table**

**Longitudinal Motion**
Stroke: 1900 mm
Scannable range: 1620 mm
Speed: 0.5-143 mm/s
Position accuracy: ±0.25 mm

**Vertical Motion**
Range: 526 mm to 1040 mm, 1.0 inch
Speed: 2.5-50 mm/s

**Table Load Capacity**
204 kg (450 pounds) with full accuracy

**Floating Table Top**
Carbon-fiber table top with foot pedal and hand control for easy positioning and quick release

Courtesy Philips Medical Systems.

architectures (Fig. 7-13), followed by the use of parallel and distributed processing architectures, as the processing and clinical application tasks became more sophisticated. An earlier example of the latter is illustrated in Figure 7-14. The basis for these architectures depends on the way that the computer assigns various tasks (e.g., preprocessing **raw data, convolution, back-projection,** and visualization tasks such as 3D imaging, **CT angiography,** and virtual reality imaging) to the numerous processors in its electronic circuits.

An important component of computer-processing architectures for CT and magnetic resonance imaging is the **array processor,** which is a dedicated electronic circuit capable of the high-speed calculations needed in CT. Array processors feature key elements such as speed, power, flexibility, and expandability. To accommodate these elements, the array processor architecture may consist of the following:

- Multiple dedicated processors (voxel processor) and storage to accommodate high-speed data acquisition such as spiral/helical imaging and 2D, 3D, and 4D image reconstruction, storage, display, and recording.
- Dedicated image storage and independent manipulation of data that includes raw spiral/helical data.
- The Digital Imaging and Communications in Medicine (DICOM) network is the standard for connectivity in radiology. It allows multimodality and multivendor equipment to connect electronically to facilitate data and image communications. DICOM functionality includes Service Class User and Service Class Provider, DICOM Print, Query/Retrieve, Storage Commitment, and Modality Worklist, to mention only a few.

## The Graphics Processing Unit

Medical imaging and radiation therapy involve technologies that generate large amounts of datasets that "comprise a large number of similar elements, such as voxels in tomographic imaging, beamlets in intensity-modulated radiation therapy (IMRT) optimization, k-space samples in **Magnetic Resonance Imaging (MRI),** projective measurements in x-ray CT, and coincidence events in PET" (Pratx & Xing, 2011). Fast processing of such vast datasets becomes a challenge for the CPUs of present computers used in imaging and therapy.

It is now recognized that CT produces massive acquisition datasets during an examination. These datasets are used to reconstruct images using sophisticated reconstruction algorithms such as the **filtered back-projection (FBP),** the Feldkamp-Davis-Kress (FDK) **algorithm,** and **iterative reconstruction (IR)**

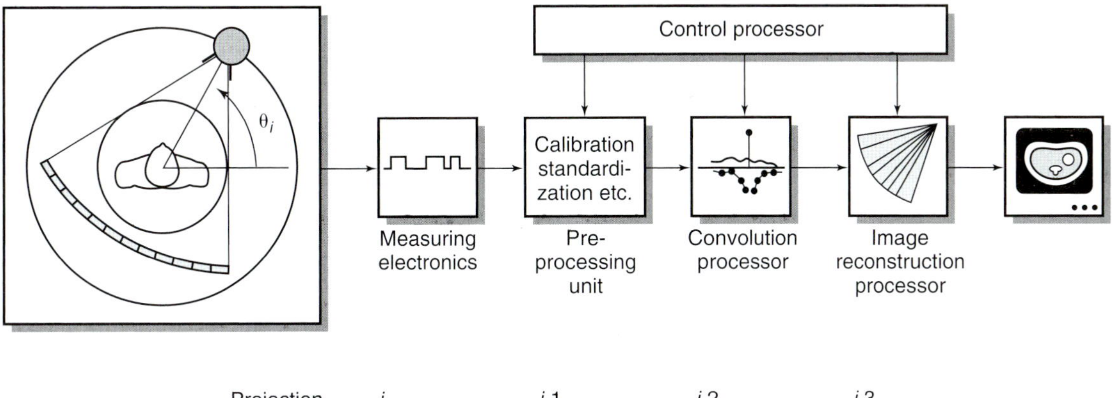


**FIGURE 7-13** An historical illustration of a computer configuration of the Siemens Somatom whole-body CT scanner with pipeline processing. The reconstruction steps of preprocessing, convolution, and basic projection are assigned to separate processors.

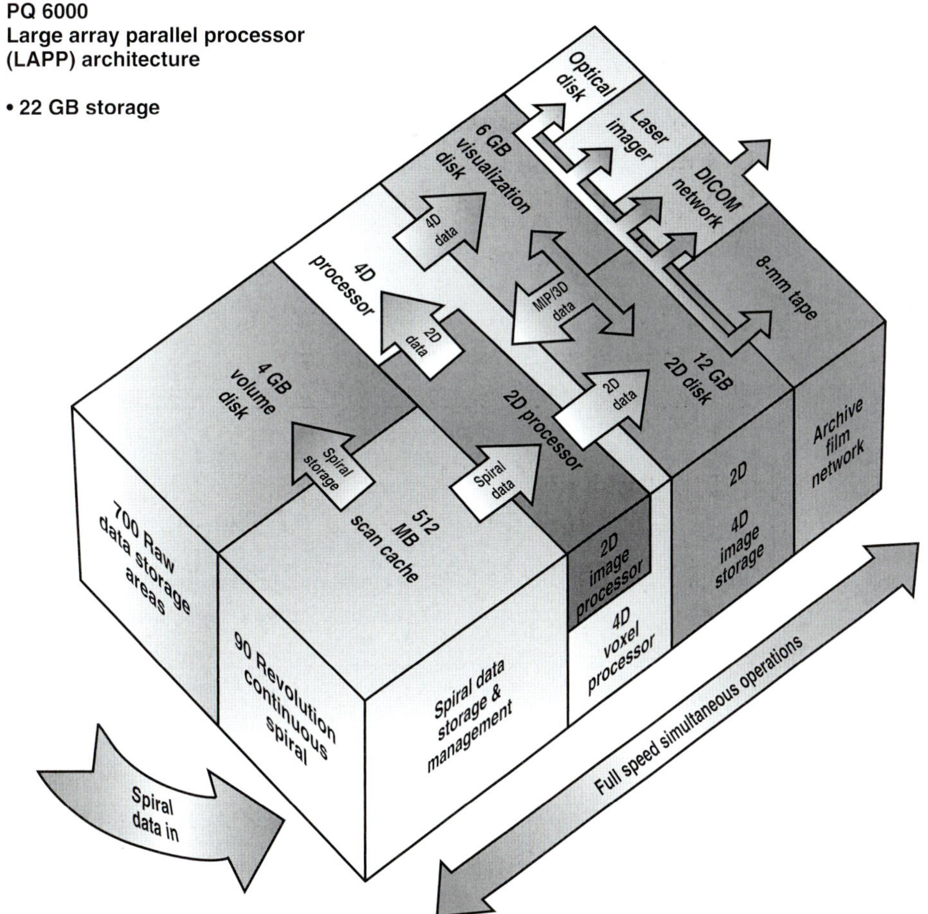


**FIGURE 7-14** The Picker PQ 6000 CT Imaging System is based on a largearray parallel processor architecture. (Courtesy Picker International, Cleveland, Ohio.)

algorithms, which are now present on all modern CT scanners (see Chapter 6). One of the major limitations of IR algorithms, compared with the FBP algorithm, relates to the large amount of **iterations** needed to complete the computationally intensive reconstruction operations to provide the observer with the final image. Such iterations require increased computational power, which is now possible with the use of the *graphic processing unit* (GPU), and can be used to reduce the processing requirements of the CPU.

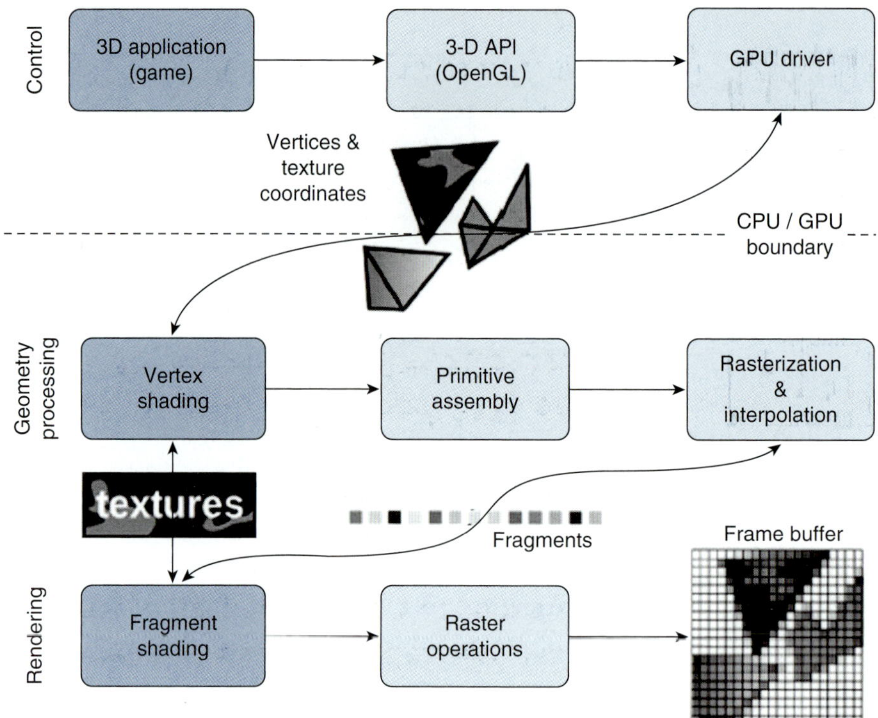


**FIGURE 7-15** The graphics pipeline used by GPU computing. See text for further explanation (From Pratx, G., & Xing L. (2011). *Medical Physics, 38* (5). Reproduced by permission of the AAPM and the authors.)

A characteristic feature of "normal" CPUs is that they use serial processing compared with the parallel processing of the GPU, and thus are capable of fast mathematical processing (Owens, 2005).

GPUs have been used in the computer graphics in the video gaming industry. The GPU is fast and can "render complex 3-D scenes in tens of milliseconds" (Pratx & Xing, 2011).

## GPU Architecture

The GPU architecture is beyond the scope of this book; however, one of the main features of the architecture is the **graphics pipeline,** which includes several graphics processors (parallel processors) that can perform mathematically intensive operations (Xu & Mueller, 2003).

Briefly, Lefohn et al. (2006) indicated that

> GPUs incorporate multi-pipelined stream processors and high bandwidth memory access, and include their own DRAM (device memory) optimized to process 2D and 3D geometries in parallel. Data are transferred between the CPU main memory and the GPU graphics memory via a dedicated Accelerated Graphics Port or a Peripheral Component Interconnect Express (PCI-Express) bus. Modern GPUs are programmable and employ a SWAR (SIMD, i.e., Single Instruction Stream Multiple Data Stream).

The graphics pipeline "decomposes graphics computation into a sequence of stages that exposes both task parallelism and data parallelism (Fig 7-15). Task parallelism is achieved when different tasks are performed simultaneously at different stages of the pipeline. Data parallelism is achieved when the same task is performed simultaneously on different data. The computational **efficiency** is further improved by implementing each stage of the graphics pipeline using custom rather than general-purpose hardware" (Pratx & Xing, 2011). For a more detailed description of the graphics pipeline, the GPU computing model, and performance optimization, the reader is referred to an excellent review article by Pratx & Xing (2011).

## Imaging and Radiation Therapy Applications

In 2004, Xu and Mueller (2004) published an article titled "Ultra-Fast 3D Filtered Backprojection on Commodity Graphics Hardware," which described using the GPU to process the FDK algorithm in CT. Using a number of techniques, the researchers showed that the GPU ran the algorithm about 7.5 times faster compared with a CPU, without compromising the image quality.

As reviewed by Pratx & Xing (2011), the GPU is now used in the following areas:

1. Image reconstruction
2. Image processing
3. Dose calculation and treatment plan optimization
4. Other applications

In image reconstruction, for example, IR algorithms on CT scanners "can profit greatly from the highly parallel architecture of GPUs" (Beister et al., 2012). In addition, the back-projection technique "fits the GPU pipeline formidably well" (Pratx & Xing, 2011).

In image processing, operations such as image registration and image **segmentation,** which are "computationally demanding" operations, fit the GPU pipeline processing very well. The GPU has been used in other areas, such as "cardiac CT scans, coregistered multimodal cardiac studies, CT-based virtual colonoscopy, and sinus virtual endoscopy. GPU computing techniques have also been developed to aid surgical planning, for instance, through illustrative visualization or biomechanical simulation" (Pratx & Xing, 2011).

For a more comprehensive discussion of the applications of the GPU in medical physics and medical imaging, the interested reader is referred to the paper by Pratx and Xing (2011).

### Scanner Control and Image Reconstruction

The operator must be able to communicate with the system to enable scanning, which may be activated through keyboard commands or a touch screen. With the touch screen, the operator can select prestored protocols; modify protocol parameters; or select the sharp, smooth, or standard algorithm, depending on the CT examination. PC interfaces that use a mouse and drop-down Windows-based menus are becoming commonplace.

### Image Display and Manipulation

A wide range of image display and manipulation techniques is afforded by the CT software. Software is highlighted in a later subsection.

### Operating Systems

Operating systems are programs that control the hardware components and the overall operation of the computer; they also enable the computer to run other programs. The operating system consists of a major program called the *supervisor*, which resides in primary memory and controls all other portions of the operating system. CT computers often use interleaved processing techniques such as multitasking, multiprocessing, and multiprogramming, which allow computers to process several programs simultaneously, thus increasing the number of jobs the computer can handle at any given time. The system also runs rapidly and efficiently. The operating system used in some CT systems is UNIX compatible and facilitates multiuser and multitasking capabilities. Microsoft Windows NT and XP operating systems are commonplace in CT scanning.

### CT Software

CT software is a special topic that is beyond the scope of this book. It should be noted, however, that the software for CT has been evolving rapidly as more and more clinical applications are made possible by multislice CT scanners, which provide 16 to 64 or more slices per revolution of the tube and detectors.

CT software can be placed in one of three categories: reconstruction software, preprocessing software, and **image postprocessing** software. Reconstruction software, which builds up the image from the raw data collected from the detectors, consists of very sophisticated algorithms with thousands of lines of coding. Preprocessing software, on the other hand, performs corrections on the data collected from the detectors before the data are sent to the reconstruction computer. **Beam-hardening** corrections and corrections for bad detector readings are examples of these corrections. Finally, image postprocessing software operates on reconstructed images displayed for viewing to facilitate diagnostic interpretation. A list of what has been popularly referred to as visualization and analysis software is shown in Box 7-2. This software can be placed into two categories: basic and advanced image visualization and analysis tools.

Box 7-3 provides a brief description of several image visualization and analysis software tools. These include tools such as the CT viewer, multiplanar reformation (MPR), maximum or minimum intensity **projection** (MIP), 3D surface-shaded display reconstruction, RelateSlice, MasterCut, and custom image filters.

Box 7-4 briefly describes several other tools, such as 3D small volume analysis, quantitative CT angiography (Q-CTA), combine images, and CT time lapse. Advanced clinical applications tools such as CT/MR Fusion, functional CT, brain perfusion, and virtual colonoscopy are also included.

## IMAGE DISPLAY, STORAGE, RECORDING, AND COMMUNICATIONS

### Image Display

A display device for CT is generally a black-and-white or color monitor (Fig. 7-16). These can be CRT flat display or liquid crystal display flat-panel display devices, with the latter replacing the former.

**BOX 7-2 Examples of Visualization and Image Analysis Software Tools from One Computed Tomography Vendor**

Volume rendering
Brain perfusion
ViewForum
Cardiac review
Cardiac CT angio
Cardiac CT Left Ventricle (LV)/ Right Ventricle (RV) function
Calcium scoring
CT endoscopy
Real-time MPR
Dental planning
DICOM remote viewer
Image fusion
Advanced vessel analysis
General reporting
Application reporting
Lung nodule assessment (LNA)
MasterCut
Stent planning
RelateSlice
Bone removal
Slab viewer
Combine images
CT perfusion
3D shaded surface display
Custom image filters
MIP
Multiplanar reconstruction
Q-BMAP II bone mineral analysis
Q-CTA
CT viewer
Rapid view remote reconstruction
3-D small volume analysis
CT time lapse
LNA reporting
Stereotaxis
Stenosis analysis
Bone mineral analysis
CT/MR Fusion
Endo 3D

Courtesy Philips Medical Systems.

Although images are usually displayed in grayscale, nonimage data such as text fields, patient data, and option selections can be displayed in color.

The image display system includes features such as the display **matrix, pixel size, bit** depth, CT value scale, grayscale, image monitor and the number of lines, selectable window width and window center, single and double windows, and highlighting. CT manufacturers provide detailed specifications for each of these features.

## Image Storage

Data are stored in digital form to preserve the wide **dynamic range** of images, including the capability for image processing and intensity transformations, and to decrease the possibility of lost records and reduce the space needed for archiving.

Digital images are stored in 2D pixel arrays; each pixel point is represented by a number of bits that determine how many gray levels can be represented by a particular pixel. CT image size varies according to the anatomy being examined. A typical CT image has a matrix size of 512 × 512 × 8 bytes (12 bits). In this case, each has a gray-level range of 512 ($2^8$) to 4096 ($2^{12}$).

A CT image of 512 × 512 × 2 bytes (16 bits) would require 0.5 megabytes (MB) of storage. If the CT examination contains about 50 images, then 25 MB of storage is needed. If 50 examinations are performed in one day, then 1.25 gigabytes (GB) of storage is needed.

Storage devices for CT include magnetic tape and disks, digital videotape, optical disks, and optical tape. It is interesting to note that the capacity of an optical disk simply is so much more than that of magnetic tapes. This is clearly illustrated in Figure 7-17 from the early days of image storage discussions. Today, CD writers can be used for archiving CT images as well.

The type of storage devices used, their respective storage capacities, and the typical number of images that can be stored on each device will be different, depending on the manufacturer.

## Laser Recording System

In the past, the requirements for hard-copy recording of CT images were a major consideration during CT imaging because the images were used for diagnostic interpretation. The requirements were broad grayscale contrast resolution to enable the perception of subtle differences in tissue contrast and high **spatial resolution** to detect boundaries of different tissues.

Laser image recording systems were used to meet these requirements. Although multiformat video cameras were popular in the past, laser cameras, or laser imagers, replaced the video camera technology. Two types of lasers were used for film recording in CT: solid-state laser diodes and gas lasers, such as helium-neon (He-Ne), helium, cadmium, argon, carbon dioxide, and nitrogen. The He-Ne laser is the simplest and most reliable gas laser. The solid-state laser, typical of the 3M laser imaging systems, has a wavelength of 820 nanometers (nm), but the He-Ne laser has a wavelength of 633 nm. Both systems use

**BOX 7-3 Brief Description of Several Image Visualization and Analysis Software Tools from One CT Vendor**

Features

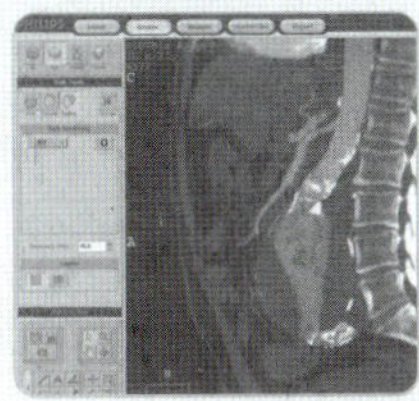

**CT Viewer**

A powerful and easy to use general viewing environment with Slab, Planar, Endoscopy and Volume review modes that utilize any rendering technique (Volume Rendering, Minimum & Maximum MIP; Volume Intensity Projection (VIP); and Average modes) for rapid inspection of large volume CT datasets.

- Slab inspection mode allows user to rotate around any structure such as an aneurysm, while keeping area of interest in view

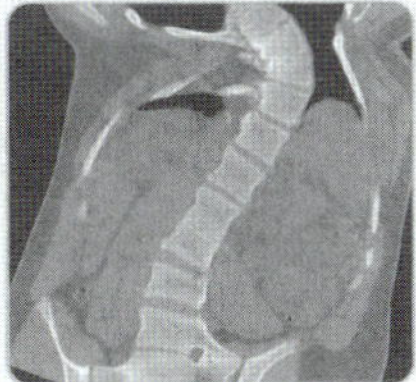

**MPR- Multiplanar Reformation**

Real-time reformation of axial images into any user-defined plane - coronal, sagittal or general oblique – or curved plane. Interactive and friendly user interface is provided. The user defines the number of planes, their position, orientation, thickness and spacing and the reformatted image is displayed in real-time. Zoom, pan, leaf and window are available.

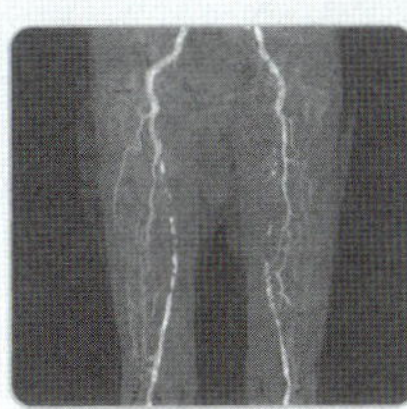

**Maximum or Minimum Intensity Projection (MIP)**

CT and MR Angiography Maximum Intensity Projection (MIP) images, from a volumetric set of images, can be quickly reconstructed to demonstrate enhanced vascular structures. The projection images can be interactively generated in any arbitrary viewing angle, and can be windowed, zoomed and panned.

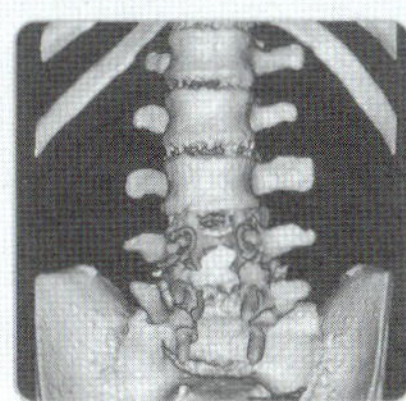

**3-D SSD Reconstruction**

Provides fast reconstruction of three-dimensional images of up to 15 different tissues or organs and easy to understand presentation of complex anatomy. Real-time manipulation of 3-D images includes zoom, pan, rotation around any axis, and cutting of the organs with a user-defined viewing aperture to expose underlying tissues. Making a tissue transparent enables viewing of underlying organs.

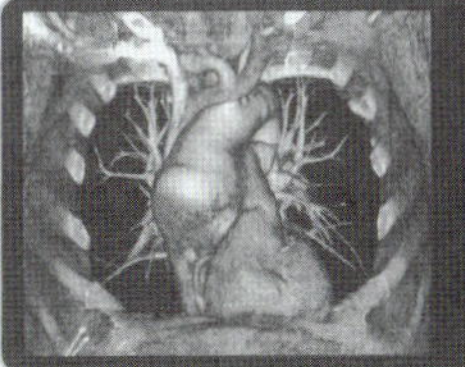

**RelateSlice™**

Displays corresponding 2-D axial information of areas identified on volume-rendered, MIP or virtual endoscopy images.

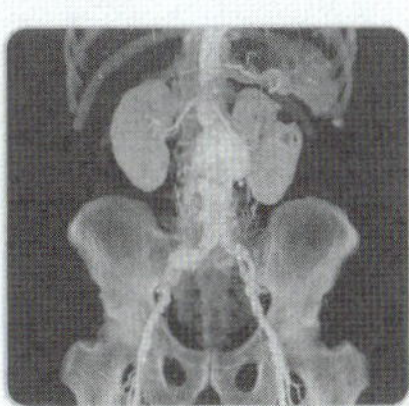

**MasterCut™**

Defines MPR curved cuts along vascular structures on MIP or volume-rendered images for panoramic and cross-sectional views.

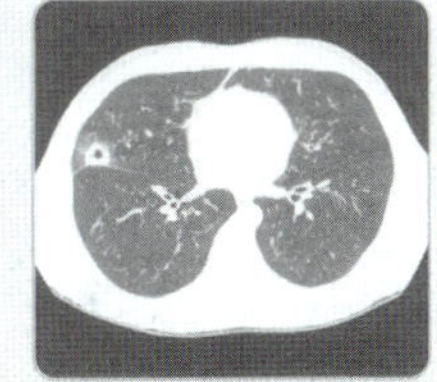

**Custom Image Filters**

Automated real-time image enhancement or smoothing, defined for up to three independent density ranges such as lung, soft tissue and bone.

Courtesy Philips Medical Systems.

infrared-sensitive films (820 nm) and He-Ne laser films sensitive to the 633-nm wavelength beam. Today laser printing on film is obsolete and is not described further in this book.

## Communications

**Communications** refers to electronic networking or connectivity by using a local-area or wide-area network (LAN or WAN). **Connectivity** ensures the transfer of data and images from multivendor and multimodality equipment according to the DICOM standard.

CT scanners must support various network speeds such as 10/100/1000 megabits per second and Ethernet switching for very fast image transfer. CT scanners now feature full implementation of the DICOM

**BOX 7-4 Several Other Image Visualization and Analysis Software Tools from One CT Vendor, Including Tools for Advanced Clinical Applications**

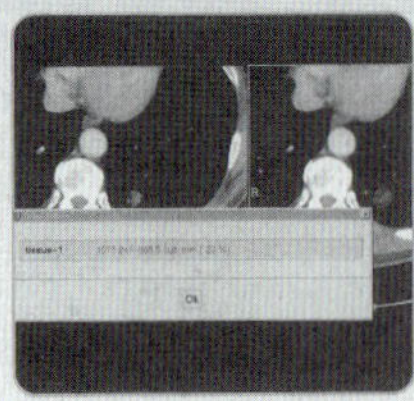

**3-D Small Volume Analysis**

Enables tumor or nodule characterization with respect to growth rates within the 3-D application. This tool uses automatic segmentation to help in identifying a solitary nodule or tumor (early staging of lung cancer) and measures volumetric parameters such as nodule volume, long axis, and short axis for follow-up purposes.

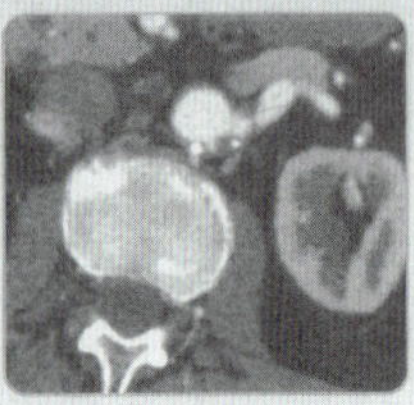

**Quantitative CTA (Q-CTA)**

Q-CTA is a tool kit for taking quantitative measurements of anatomic structures, including vasculature from the 2-D, 3-D or 4-D Angio volume-rendered image. This is accomplished by semi-automatically defining the dimensions of the vessel.

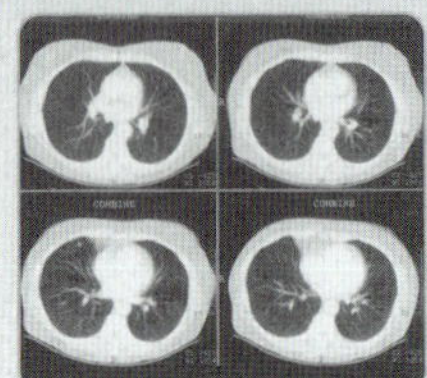

**Combine Images**

Post processing function enabling linear combination of axial images. Used for filming and reviewing thick slices from thin slice acquisitions, helping to manage large datasets. Does not require raw data or office processing.

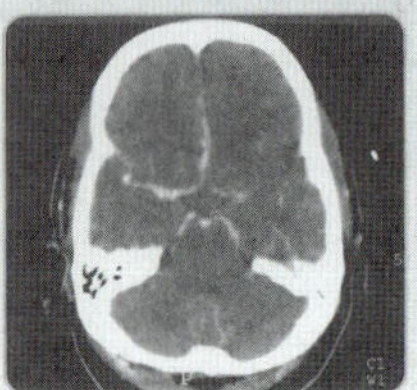

**CT Time Lapse**

Graphic display of CT pixel values vs. time is available for analysis of uptake and perfusion of contrast media with time.

Advanced Clinical Applications

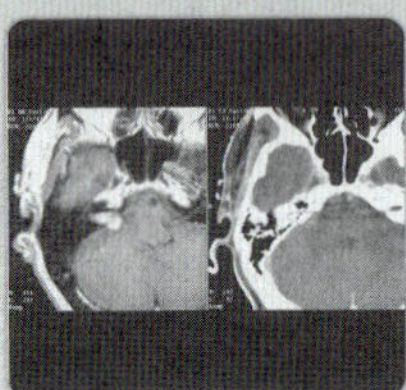

**CT/MR Fusion™***

Allows for the three-dimensional coregistration of studies acquired in different modalities (CT and MR) or in the same modality at different times or with different scan conditions.

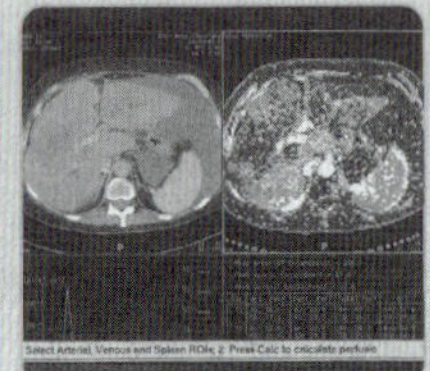

**Functional CT***

Delivers whole organ liver perfusion. Capable of evaluating tumor perfusion to improve your ability to characterize known lesions. Provides both arterial and portal perfusion measurements for whole liver or single location liver studies.

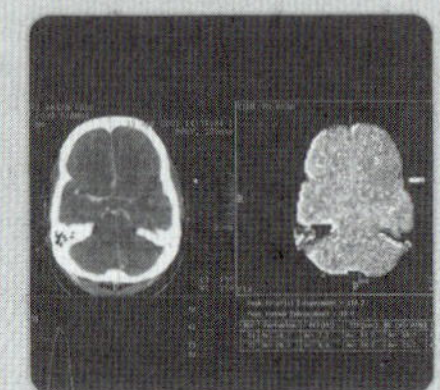

**Brain Perfusion***

Brain Perfusion delivers quantifiable brain perfusion results to evaluate the acute or chronic stroke patient. This technique is further enhanced by extended coverage of 40mm and new acquisition techniques. With its powerful clinical tools, including large coverage and low dose imaging, the brain perfusion application allows users to evaluate tissue perfusion for improved characterization of known or suspected lesions.

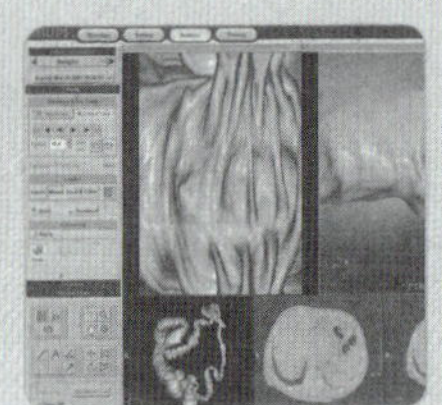

**Virtual Colonoscopy***

Provides many exclusive features to improve time-to-diagnosis and significantly increase clinical confidence such as real-time Filet View mode to view 100% of colon surface and MIP colonoscopy view display for identifying contrast-enhanced lesions such as polyps, tumors, or even inflammatory disease.

Courtesy Philips Medical Systems.

communication protocol, which allows connectivity to various scanners and workstations in the digital radiology department. CT communication systems are described in the next section.

## CT AND PICTURE ARCHIVING AND COMMUNICATIONS SYSTEMS

The CT scanner is now connected to the PACS, so a brief overview of PACS is included here.

### Picture Archiving and Communications Systems: A Definition

What is PACS exactly? Some researchers believe that it should be called IMACS (image management and communication systems); however, the more popular acronym is PACS.

There are several comprehensive definitions of PACS. As early as 2002, Siegel and Reiner (2002) offered one such definition "... PACS refer to a

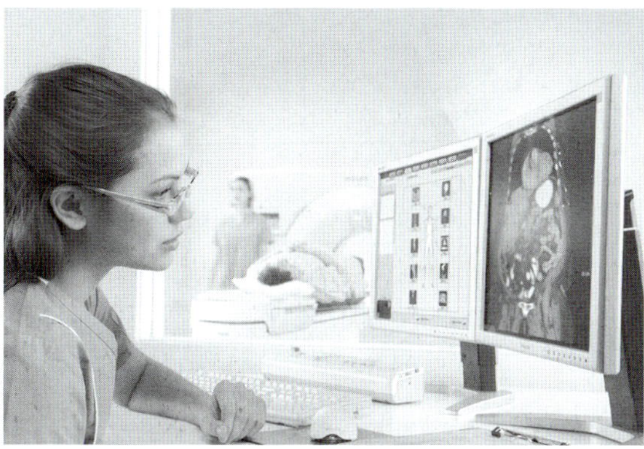

**FIGURE 7-16** A display device for CT is generally a black-and-white or color monitor. These can be CRT flat display (as shown) or liquid crystal display flat-panel display devices, with the latter replacing the former.

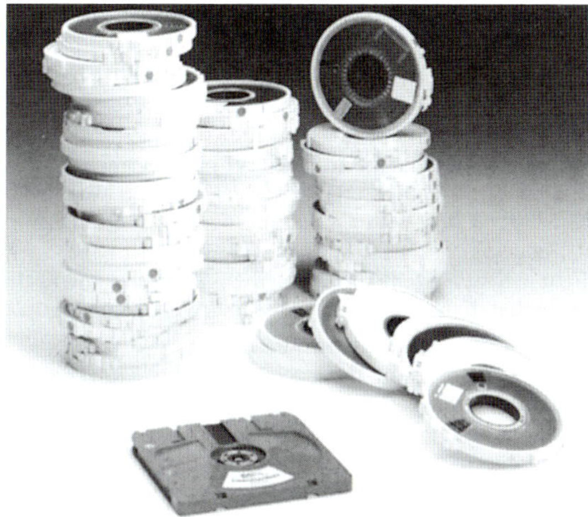

**FIGURE 7-17** Optical disk for CT image storage. A single disk can hold the equivalent of 70 magnetic tapes.

computer system that is used to capture, store, distribute, and then display medical images. For diagnostic imaging applications, PACS technology can be utilized to achieve near filmless operation."

A more detailed definition as provided by Arenson et al. (2000) is that PACS

> ... are a collection of technologies used to carry out digital medical imaging. PACS are used to digitally acquire medical images from various modalities such as CT, MRI, Ultrasound (US), Nuclear Medicine (NM), and digital projection radiography. The image data and pertinent information are transmitted to other and possibly remote locations over network, where they can be displayed on computer workstations for soft-copy viewing in multiple locations simultaneously. Data are secured and archived on digital media such as optical disks or tape and can be automatically retrieved as necessary.

Basically, the two definitions convey the same idea and meaning of PACS, except that the second one offers a more detailed picture of PACS.

## PACS: Major Components

The major components of a CT PACS and their functional relationships are shown in Figure 7-18. The essential elements include the CT scanner, various interfaces, and a PACS controller (as it is often referred to), which includes a database/image server, archive server, short- and long-term archives, RIS/HIS system, web server, and image display, all connected by computer networks. To extend its functionality and usefulness, the PACS is integrated with the RIS and HIS again through computer communication networks. Note that the devices within the PACS communicate with each other, whereas the PACS is integrated with the Radiology Information System (RIS) as well as the Hospital Information System (HIS). This communication and integration requires the use of communication protocol standards. In this regard, two *communication protocol standards* are now commonplace in the digital radiology environment, including the CT scanner.

### Communication Protocol Standards

Connectivity refers to a measure of the effectiveness and efficiency of computers and computer-based devices to communicate and share information and messages without human intervention (Capron, 2005; Laudon, 1994).

The use of communication protocol standards is integral to achieving connectivity. Although a *protocol* deals with the specifics of how a certain task will be done, a *standard* is an "approved reference model and protocol determined by standard-setting groups for building or developing products and services" (Laudon, 1994).

In health care, HIS, RIS, and PACS integration is based on different communication protocol standards. Two such popular standards are health level 7 (HL-7) and DICOM. HL-7 is the standard application protocol for use in most HIS and RIS systems; DICOM is the imaging communication protocol for PACS (Creighton, 1999). DICOM was developed by the American College of Radiology and the National Electrical Manufacturers Association. In a PACS environment DICOM conformance is mandatory. In a CT-PACS environment, certain DICOM standards are applicable to CT. Some examples of these include storage service class, query and retrieve, print, HIS/RIS, and worklist.

Essential features of an image management and archiving system that is compliant with DICOM and compatible with HIS and RIS include examination

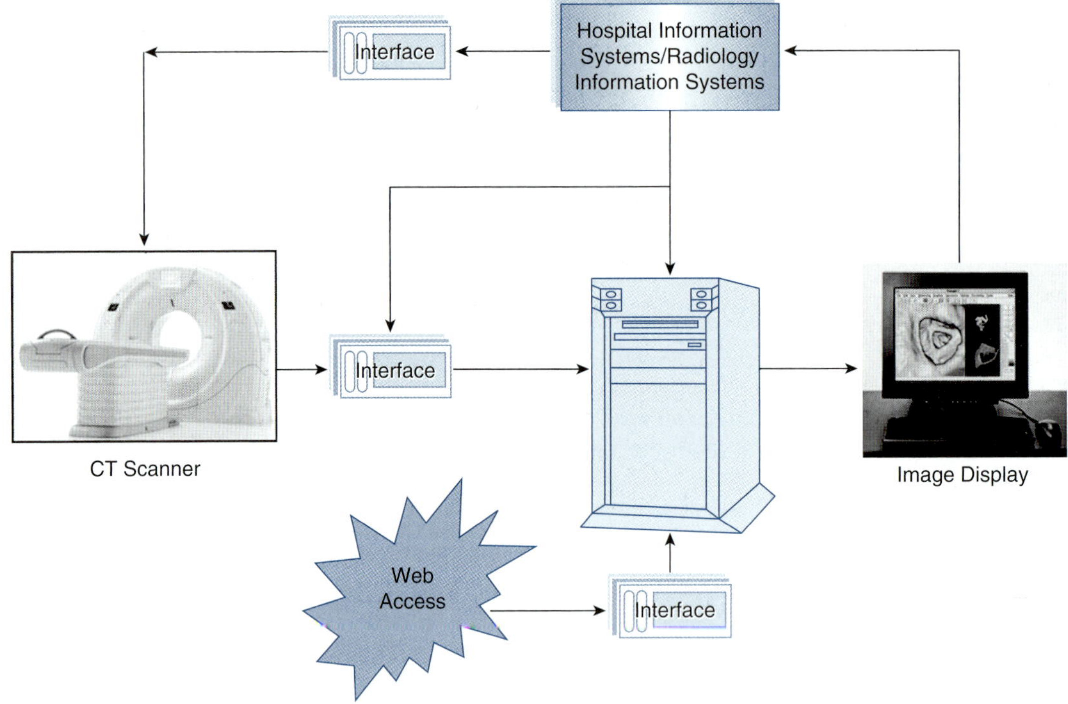


**FIGURE 7-18** The major components of a CT PACS and their functional relationships.

acquisition (acquisition of patient demographics) and image acquisition; workflow management; diagnostic, clinical, and enterprise display; and hard-copy output. The enterprise display component allows users to view, retrieve, and distribute image data and radiology reports online by using the DICOM web server. The nature of possible network systems in radiology is complex.

PACS can be classified according to its size and scope. If a PACS is dedicated to a single digital imaging modality such as a CT or MRI scanner, it is usually called a mini-PACS, in which case a single LAN is a central feature.

Networking consists of both hardware components and the necessary software to enable the hardware to function. Networks can be discussed in terms of LANs or WANs. The basis for this classification is the **distance** covered by the network. A LAN connects computers separated by short distances, such as in a radiology department or in a building or two or more buildings. A WAN, on the other hand, connects computers separated by large distances, such as in another province or country. The Internet is a perfect example of a WAN.

## Image Compression

Once images are acquired and sent through the computer network, they are generally displayed for viewing and stored temporarily or permanently for retrospective viewing and analysis.

The digital images acquired in a total digital radiology department are large files with varying matrix sizes. For example, a CT image can be a 512 × 512 matrix by 2 bytes per pixel (bit depth). These two characteristics alone (matrix size and bit depth) place huge demands on storage requirements and the speed of transmission over the network.

One effective way to manage the size of image files for transmission and storage is that of image compression. Image compression is a complex topic that is beyond the scope of this chapter; however, it is described in more detail in Chapter 2. In this chapter, the following basic facts are noteworthy for CT technologists:

- The purpose of compression is to speed up transmission of information (textual data and images) and to reduce storage requirements.
- Several image compression methods are available, each providing advantages and disadvantages. Compression can be either:
    1. *Lossless or reversible,* where no information is lost in the process
    2. *Lossy or irreversible,* where some information is lost in the process (Seeram, 2011; Seeram & Seeram, 2008)

### PACS and CT Interfacing

There are several issues related to interfacing a CT scanner to the PACS. These are related to the CT workstation, worklists, image distribution, information systems (RIS/HIS), RIS/HIS/PACS integration, and DICOM specifications. Each of these will be reviewed briefly.

Workstations will be used for primary diagnosis and other viewing tasks; therefore, an immediate concern is to orient radiologists, physicians, and technologists to the nature of the workstation for soft-copy display of images. General hardware and software concerns must be addressed, especially software that allows sophisticated image processing such as 3D imaging and virtual reality imaging.

Worklists are used to match cases from the CT scanner to various workstations; therefore, a PACS must be capable of creating and using worklists effectively (the worklist assignment algorithm is critical).

Image distribution is an important issue for CT PACS. The system must have the ability to send images to a referring physician and the radiation treatment planning department, for example. In this case, DICOM conformance is critical. PACS also should be capable of teleradiology applications; for example, images from a CT scanner could be sent to a radiologist's home where he can download them for interpretation. This would certainly save the radiologist travel time late at night.

### PACS and Information Systems Integration

The integration of a CT scanner and PACS is critical. Equally important is the PACS integration with the HIS/RIS. Therefore connectivity is important. Bushberg et al. (2012) and Dreyer et al. (2006) have discussed the role of information systems integration in radiology. They identified at least five separate information systems for digital radiography (DR), including PACS, RIS, HIS, a voice-recognition direction system, and the electronic teaching/research file system.

Integration of these systems is essential because it is intended to solve many problems with DR. This is not within the scope of this chapter; however, it is important to delineate between an HIS and an RIS. According to the experts (Van Musen and Bemmel, 2002, HIS is "an information system used to collect, store, process, retrieve, and communicate patient care and administrative information for all hospital-affiliated activities and to satisfy the functional requirements of all authorized users."

An RIS could be a stand-alone system or it may be integrated into an HIS. Some of the functions performed by the RIS are patient registration, examination scheduling, patient tracking, film archiving, report **generation,** administration and billing, and documentation.

## CT CONTROL CONSOLE

CT control consoles have evolved into what is commonly referred to as the integrated console. This multimedia concept allows the operator full control of the physical system (e.g., gantry control) and allows for real-time processing such as multiplanar reformatting, 3D manipulation, zoom, and pan. The **integrated console controls** the entire system and enables the operation of various functions.

Typically, an integrated console consists of the following components:

- *Floating keyboard*: Important components include alphanumerical and special function keys, the trackball or mouse, and window controls.
- *Touch panel*: Allows system parameters such as scan setup and control parameters to be actuated without typed keyboard commands.
- *Window controls*: Include the window width and window level controls, which alter picture contrast. *Window width* refers to the range of **CT numbers.** *Window level* is the center of the range.
- *Image display*: CT images are displayed on monitors for viewing and manipulation by the operator before the final image is communicated to the PACS.
- *High-capacity optical disk drive and CD writer*: A 9.1-GB erasable optical disk drive is not uncommon.
- *Control functions*: Various automated functions such as autoarchive, autowindow, and autovoice are featured on CT control consoles. These allow the technologist to devote more time to the scanning procedure and the needs of the patient.

## OPTIONS AND ACCESSORIES FOR CT SYSTEMS

### Options

A number of options, both hardware and software, are currently available for CT scanners. The hardware options may include optical disks, optical cartridge tape, remote diagnostic stations, independent workstations, and so forth.

Software options (Box 7-4) include packages for bone mineral analysis, dynamic scan, 3D image reconstruction, volumetric MPR, evaluation of regional cerebral blood flow (xenon CT), perfusion CT, dental CT, and networking.

### Accessories

**Accessories** support and provide excellent **immobilization** of the patient to enhance the overall efficiency of the CT examination. These accessories include pediatric cradles, arm and leg supports, elevated and flat head holders, table mattresses, side rails, table extenders, knee supports, head pillows with hand rests, axial and coronal head holders, and radiation therapy table tops.

## OTHER CONSIDERATIONS

### Modular Design Concept

The **modular design concept** is intended to simplify the upgrading of scanners. The hardware modular design concept features detector modules, analog-to-digital conversion cards, tubes, generators and subassemblies, memory boards, array processors, back-projectors, display camera interfaces, and network interface boards. Software modules allow for the easy modification, updating, and revision of software packages to meet the demands of the clinical environment.

### Operating Modes of the Scanner

A modern CT scanner can operate in a variety of modes to meet the requirements of various clinical examinations. Typical operating modes include routine scan mode and rapid or dynamic scan mode. Various spiral/helical scan modes such as overlap scan, skip scan, and tilt scan are available to suit the needs of the examination (Fig. 7-19).

### Room Layout for CT Equipment

The room layout for CT scanners varies among institutions and depends on the particular type of scanner. A typical room layout (Fig. 7-20) includes at least three sections or rooms to house different components of the scanner:

1. The scanning room houses the gantry and patient couch. This room should be large enough to accommodate gurneys and emergency equipment.
2. The computer room generally houses the **host computer** and other peripheral computing equipment.
3. The control room houses the control console and film recording equipment.

### Equipment Specifications

The acquisition of a CT scanner is an interesting experience, and the CT technologist should take advantage of the opportunity to participate in such an activity. The CT department or purchasing committee generally informs the vendor of the necessary equipment specifications. In addition, vendors will have equipment specifications available for review.

In general, several major technical specifications and features of a CT scanner to be considered are as follows:

1. *X-ray generator*: Both physical and operating parameters
2. *X-ray tube and detectors*: Heat storage capacity and cooling rates of the tube and the type, quantum detection, and conversion efficiencies of detectors
3. *Scanning gantry*: Aperture size, tilting range, and laser positioning aids and controls
4. *Patient couch*: Movement characteristics and strength of the couch top
5. *Operator's console*: Characteristics of the display monitor, keyboard, and touch panel control and general ergonomics and storage considerations
6. *Physician's console*: Hardware and software
7. *Computer hardware*: The main central processing unit, operating system, and storage device type and capacity
8. *Computer software*: Image reconstruction, display, visualization, and analysis packages
9. *Workstations*: both hardware and software
10. *Accessories*
11. *Quality control equipment*: Includes phantoms for quality control and radiation dose measurements

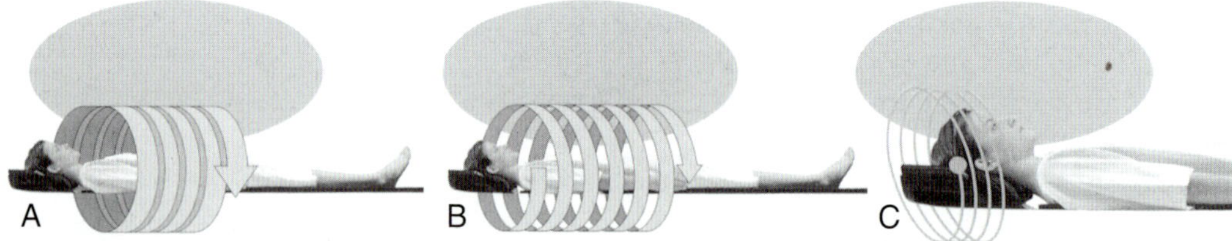


**FIGURE 7-19** Three scan modes for spiral/helical CT scanning. Each scan mode includes overlap scan, which is useful to make high-quality 3D images. Skip scan can be used to scan a wide area in a short amount of time. Tilt scan is used with various gantry tilts. **A,** High-quality 3D images: overlap scan. **B,** Short time/wide range scan: skip scan. **C,** According to head OM line: tilt scan. (Courtesy Shimadzu Medical Systems, Seattle, Wash.)

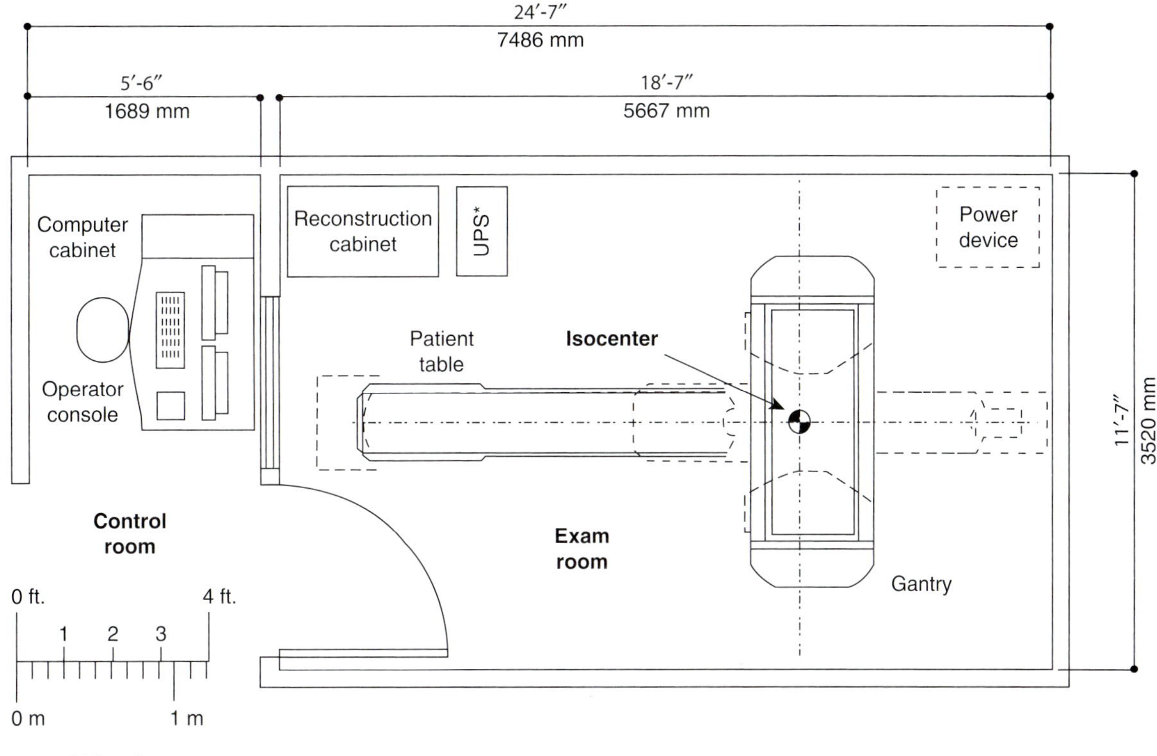


**FIGURE 7-20** Typical room layout for CT scanning equipment. (Courtesy Philips Medical Systems.)

## REVIEW QUESTIONS

Answer the following questions to check your understanding of the materials studied.

1. The purpose of the CT imaging system is to
   1. convert x-rays to digital data.
   2. detect and measure the radiation transmitted through the patient.
   3. produce, shape, and filter the x-ray beam.

   A. 1 only
   B. 1 and 2
   C. 2 and 3
   D. 1, 2, and 3
2. Which of the following houses the x-ray tube and detectors?
   A. the gantry
   B. the housing of the x-ray tube
   C. the generator
   D. the detector box
3. Which is not a component of the imaging system?
   A. laser printer
   B. x-ray tube
   C. collimator
   D. detectors
4. Which of the following generators is used in a modern CT scanner?
   A. single-phase
   B. constant potential
   C. three-phase
   D. high-frequency
5. The computer and image-processing systems of a CT scanner system consist of all of the following ***except***:
   A. software
   B. data acquisition system
   C. hardware
   D. processing architecture
6. A hard copy (film image) is produced by a:
   A. television monitor.
   B. laser optical disk.
   C. laser imager (printer).
   D. magnetic disk.
7. Which of the following (on the control console) controls picture contrast?
   A. touch panel
   B. floppy disk drive
   C. keyboard
   D. window controls (WW)

8. CT software refers to all of the following ***except***:
   A. UNIX
   B. operating systems
   C. applications software
   D. magneto-optical disks
9. Modular design concept is intended to:
   A. simplify technologist operation.
   B. simplify upgrading of scanners.
   C. simplify radiologist performance.
   D. make the patient more comfortable.
10. A hardware option for CT scanners is:
   A. xenon CT.
   B. bone mineral analysis package.
   C. 3D imaging package.
   D. independent workstation.

## REFERENCES


Alexander, J., & Krumme, H. J. (1988). *Electromedica, 56*, 50–56.

Arenson, R. L., et al. (2000). Computers in imaging and healthcare: Now and in the future. *Journal of Digital Imaging, 13*(4), 145–156.

Beister., et al. (2012). Iterative reconstruction methods in x-ray CT. *Physica Medica, 28*, 94–108.

Bushberg, J. T., et al. (2012). *The Essential Physics of Medical Imaging*. Philadelphia: Wolters Kluwer/Lippincott Williams & Wilkins.

Capron, H. L. (2005). *Computers: tools for an information age*. Upper Saddle River, NJ: Prentice Hall.

Covington, M. A. (1991). *Computer Science-Outline notes*. New York: Barron's.

Creighton, C. (1999). A literature review on communications between picture archiving and communication systems and radiology information systems and/or hospital information systems. *Journal of Digital Imaging, 12*, 138–143.

Dreyer, K. J., et al. (2006). *PACS: A guide to the digital revolution* (ed 2). New York: Springer Science + Business Media.

Dümmling, K. (1984). *Electromedica, 52*, 13–28.

Laudon, K. C. (1994). *Management information systems: organization and technology*. Englewood Cliffs, NJ: Macmillan.

Lefohn, A. E., Kniss, J., Strzodka, R., Shubhabrata, S., & Owens, J. D. (2006). Glift: generic, efficient, random-access GPU data structures. *ACM Transactions on Graphics, 25*(1), 60–99.

Microsoft. (2002). *Microsoft Press-Computer Dictionary*. Redmond, CA: Microsoft Press.

Musen, M. A., & Bemmel, J. van (2002). *Handbook of Medical Informatics*. Heidelberg, Germany: Springer-Verlag.

Owens, J. (2005). Streaming architectures and technology trends. In M. Pharr (Ed.), *GPU gems 2*. Upper Saddle River, NJ: Addison-Wesley.

Pratx, G., & Xing, L. (2011). GPU computing in medical physics: a review. *Medical Physics, 38*(5), 2685–2687.

Seeram, E., & Seeram, D. (2008). Image postprocessing in digital radiology: a primer for technologists. *Journal of Medical Imaging and Radiation Sciences, 39*, 23–41.

Seeram, E. (2011). *Digital Radiography-An Introduction*. Clifton Park, NY: Delmar, Cengage Learning.

Siegel, E., & Reiner, B. (2002). *Image Workflow*. In K. J. Dreyer, et al. (Ed.), *PACS: A Guide to the digital revolution*. New York: Springer-Verlag: New York Inc.

Xu, F., & Mueller, K. (2003). Towards a unified framework for rapid 3D computed tomography on commodity GPUs. Portland, OR: *IEEE medical imaging conference*.

Xu, F., & Mueller, K. (2004). *Ultra-fast 3D filtered backprojection on commodity graphics hardware*. Washington D.C.: IEEE international symposium on biomedical imaging.


## BIBLIOGRAPHY


Alexander, J., & Krumme, H. J. (1998). Somatom Plus: new perspectives in computerized tomography. *Electromedica, 56*, 50–56.

Fugita, K., et al. (1992). Advanced computer architecture for CT. *Radiology*, S63.

Philips Medical Systems. (2007). *Brilliance™ CT-64 channel configuration*. The Netherlands: Global Information Center.

Siemens Medical Solutions. (2007). *CT SOMATOM Sensation, SOMATOM Emotion, and SOMATOM Spirit—product data*. Malvern, PA: Siemens Medical Solutions USA.

Toshiba America (2007). Medical Systems. *Aquilion 64 CT scanner*. Tustin, CA: Toshiba America Medical Systems.

8

# Image Postprocessing and Visualization Tools

## OUTLINE



## LEARNING OBJECTIVES

On completion of this chapter, you should be able to:

1. list two major classes of image manipulation techniques and provide examples of each.
2. explain the concept of windowing in CT.
3. define window width (WW) and window level (WL).
4. evaluate the effect of WW and WL on image contrast and image brightness respectively.
5. describe briefly specialized computer programs for image manipulation:
6. explain briefly how CT is used in radiation treatment planning.
7. identify basic and advanced visualization tools for use in CT.
8. identify the hardware components of advanced visualization and analysis CT workstations.

## KEY TERMS TO WATCH FOR AND REMEMBER

The following key terms/concepts are important to your understanding of this Chapter.

**advanced quantitative measurement tools**
**advanced visualization tools**
**basic visualization tools**
**cine visualization tools**
**image postprocessing**
**interactive visualization tools**
**multimodality image fusion tools**
**multiplanar reconstruction (MPR)**
**reference point**
**region of interest (ROI)**
**virtual reality visualization tools**
**visualization tools**

---

Image postprocessing and visualization techniques belong to the domain of digital **image processing** (see Chapter 2). Image postprocessing has become an integral part of the operation of the **computed tomography (CT)** department. Today, more and more techniques are available for modifying the original reconstructed image displayed for viewing by the technologist and interpretation by the radiologist.

This chapter elaborates on several image postprocessing techniques used routinely in CT that allow the observer to manipulate or change the image quality characteristics such as brightness and contrast, to enhance diagnostic interpretation of images. In this respect, the operations are essentially postprocessing digital operations intended to display the acquired axial images in other 2D formats, such as sagittal, coronal, and oblique images, and 3D image displays, such as surface-shaded displays (SSD), **projection** displays (maximum and minimum intensity projections), and volume-rendered (VR) images. Additionally, 3D-rendered images can be used to generate another technical application referred to as virtual reality imaging (Kalender, 2005). This chapter also includes an overview of basic and advanced visualization tools integrated into the CT **imaging system**.

## IMAGE POSTPROCESSING

### Definition

Image postprocessing refers to the use of various techniques (image processing **software** or algorithms) that modify the reconstructed images displayed for viewing and interpretation. These operations or techniques are used to change the overall appearance of the displayed image to enhance the visualization of structures in the image. For example, image characteristics such as brightness and contrast can be changed to suit viewing needs. It is very important to note that these **postprocessing operations** do not produce more information content. As a result, "the information content in the processed image is always less than or equal to that in the original image" (Glen et al., 1981).

### Techniques

Image-processing operations such as point, local, and global processing operations or techniques are described in Chapter 2. Essentially, these operations fall into two categories: linear and nonlinear. Linear techniques include image smoothing and image enhancement, and nonlinear techniques are concerned with grayscale manipulation with which the grayscale of the image can be modified with different **algorithms**. This chapter discusses nonlinear techniques.

A common algorithm used routinely in CT by technologists and radiologists is based on a point processing technique (see Chapter 2) referred to as **gray-level mapping**, which is also popularly referred to as "contrast enhancement," "contrast stretching," "histogram modification," "**histogram** stretching," or "**windowing**." Because windowing is the most common image-processing technique used in CT, it is described in detail in the next section. Furthermore, image postprocessing uses the axial image dataset stored in the computer to produce new 2D and 3D images. As mentioned earlier, although the 2D images are reformatted images such as coronal, sagittal, and oblique views, 3D images are displayed as maximum and minimum intensity, SSD, and VR images. 3D imaging will be described in detail in Chapter 13.

## WINDOWING

The CT image is reconstructed from projection data collected from the patient. The result of **image reconstruction** is a numerical image. This image must be changed into a grayscale image to be viewed by technologists and radiologists. The process is outlined graphically in Figure 8-1. The numerical image consists of a range of **CT numbers** (gray levels), and these numbers are converted into grayscale, with the lower numbers assigned black and the higher numbers assigned white (see Chapter 3).

Windowing refers to a method by which the CT image grayscale can be manipulated with the CT numbers of the image (Kalender, 2005; Seeram, 2005 2010; Seeram & Seeram, 2008; Xue et al., 2012). The operator (or observer) can alter these numbers to optimize the demonstration of the different structures as shown in Figure 8-2. By manipulating CT numbers of various tissues, the picture can be changed to show soft tissues and dense structures such as bone.

The picture contrast and brightness are easily changed with two control mechanisms: the **window width (WW)** and the **window level (WL)**, respectively.

### Window Width and Window Level

#### Definitions

By definition, the range of the CT numbers in the image is referred to as the *window width*. It determines the maximum number of shades of gray that can be displayed on the CT monitor. The *window level* is defined as the center or midpoint of the range of CT numbers (Fig. 8-3). In Figure 8-3 the WW is 2000 (1000 + 1000), the WL is 0, and the number of shades of gray assigned is 256.

When the WW and WL are changed, the image contrast and brightness can be optimized to suit the viewing needs of the observer. "Specifically, a large window width indicates that there is a relatively long grayscale or a large block of CT numbers that will be assigned some value of gray. Thus, the transition zone between the lower CT numbers portrayed as black and the higher CT numbers portrayed as white will be large. A narrow window width implies that the transition from black to white will take place over a relatively few CT numbers" (Moran, 1983). Figure 8-4 illustrates the effect of

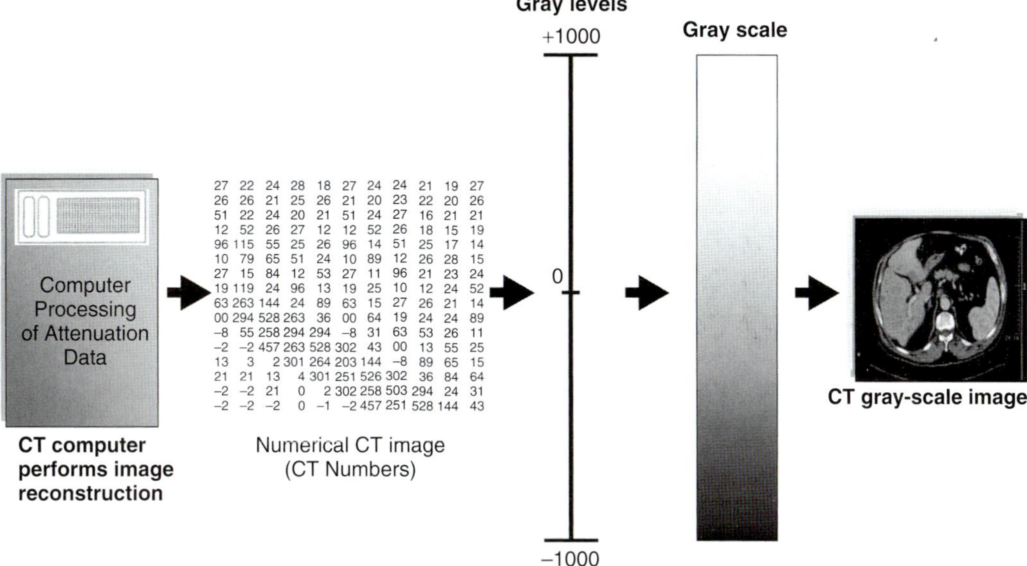


**FIGURE 8-1** The computer processes attenuation data collected from the patient to generate CT numbers. These numbers represent a numerical image (digital image) that is subsequently converted into a grayscale image displayed for viewing by an observer. This image is now subject to digital image postprocessing, such as windowing.

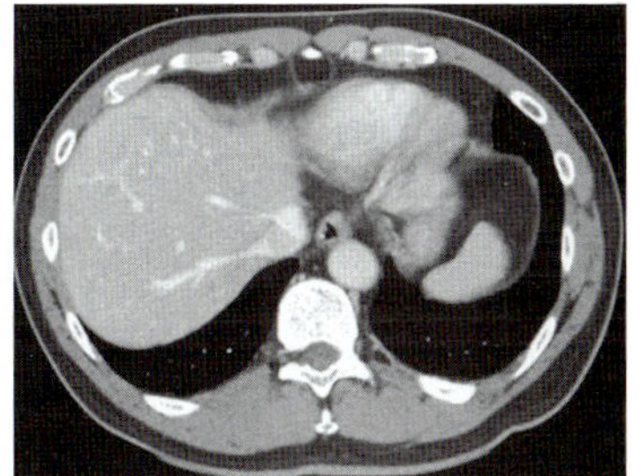
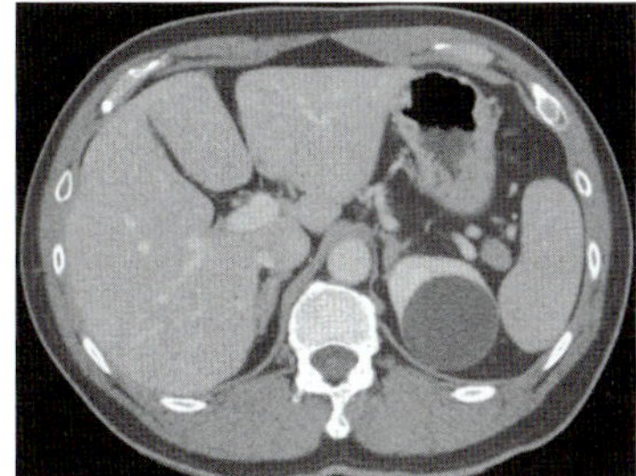
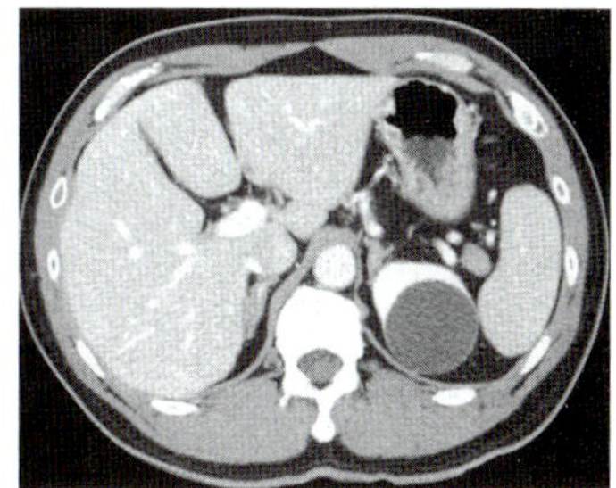

**FIGURE 8-2** Different structures of the abdomen can be optimized for viewing through windowing, a digital image postprocessing technique used to manipulate the grayscale image by using the CT numbers that comprise the image.

a wide WW (WW = 2000) on the image grayscale, and Figure 8-5 shows the effect of using a narrow WW (WW = 1000) on image grayscale to optimize image contrast. As shown in Figure 8-5, *A*, the upper and lower limits of the gray levels can be calculated by using the values of the WW and WL through the following relationships:

- The upper gray level value = WL + WW ÷ 2
- The lower gray level = WL − WW ÷ 2

## Manipulating Window Width and Window Level

A graphic illustration of the effect of different WW and WL settings is shown in Figure 8-6. For ease of explanation and simplicity, a WW of 2000 and a WL of 0 will be used here. In Figure 8-6, *A*, the CT numbers range from +1000 for bone to −1000 for air. In this case, the WW is 2000; that is, there are 1000 CT numbers above 0 and another 1000 numbers below 0. The midpoint of the range (WL) is 0; this is referred to as a **reference point,** which in this case represents water. Air, which is assigned a CT number of −1000, is also considered a reference point.

In Figure 8-6, *B*, the WW is 200 and the WL is 40. At this setting, all CT numbers greater than +100 appear white and those less than −100 appear black, whereas those between +100 and −100 appear as shades of gray.

In Figure 8-6, *C*, the WW is 200 and the WL is +40. CT numbers less than −60 appear black, those greater than +140 appear white, and those between +140 and −60 appear as shades of gray.

In Figure 8-6, *D*, the WW is 400 and the WL is 0. All CT numbers greater than +200 appear white, those less than −200 appear black, and those between +200 and −200 appear as shades of gray. If the entire

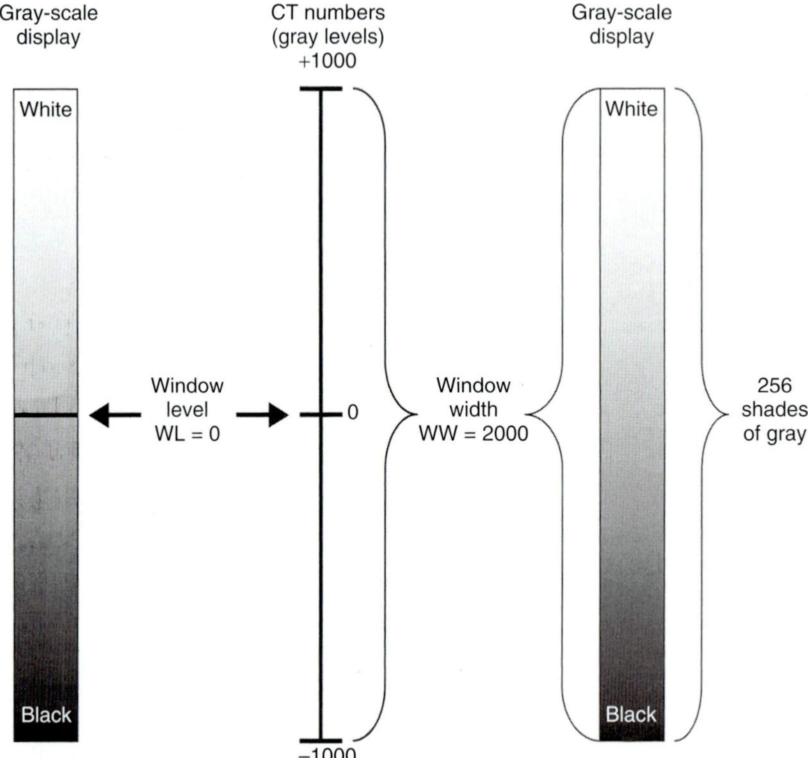


**FIGURE 8-3** The concepts of WW and WL and corresponding gray levels and grayscale. While the WW is the range of the CT numbers that make up an image, the WL is defined as the center of the range of numbers.

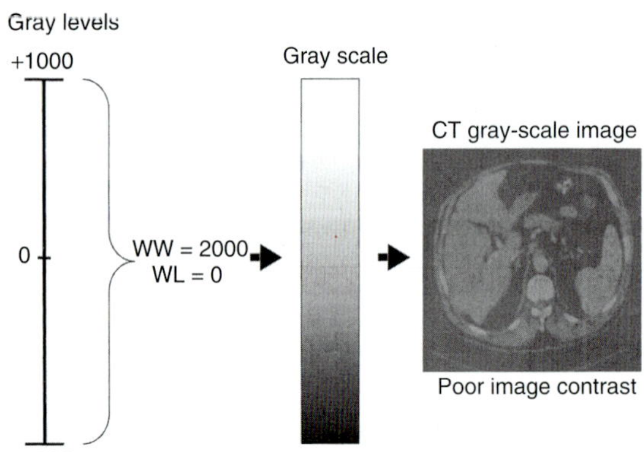


**FIGURE 8-4** The effect of a wide WW on the image grayscale. In this case wide WW of 2000 produces an image with poor contrast. The WL is set at 0.

range of CT numbers (the entire WW) is displayed, rather than a portion of the range, "small differences in **attenuation** between soft tissues will be obscured" (Zatz, 1984).

It is important to note that the CT number range varies among scanners. Although the range for some CT scanners varies from −1000 to +3095 Hounsfield units (HU; 4095 CT numbers), the range for other scanners may be −2048 to +6143 HU (8191 CT numbers). The tissue grayscale is stretched out with white at one end, black at the other, and shades of gray in between. The grayscale changes as the WW is expanded or narrowed. For bone structures, the WW must include the higher CT numbers on the scale. For structures that contain air, the WW moves toward the lower CT numbers on the scale. Similarly, the WL can fall anywhere on the scale, depending on the structures of interest (Fig. 8-7). An example of the effect of WW and WL adjustment on the appearance of the CT image is shown for the thorax in Figure 8-8.

In his discussion of the proper use of WW and WL in clinical CT, Berland (1987) noted the following:

1. Wide windows (400 HU to 2000 HU) should be used to encompass tissues of greatly differing attenuation within the image. For example, body scans are usually filmed at 350 HU to 600 HU to encompass the attenuation numbers of fat, fluid, and muscle. Lung and bone are filmed at 1000 HU to 2000 HU to include air spaces and vessels for lungs and cortex and marrow for bone.
2. Narrow windows (50 HU to 350 HU) should be used to display soft tissues within structures that contain different tissues of similar densities. For example, brain may be displayed at 80 HU to 150 HU to show differences between gray and

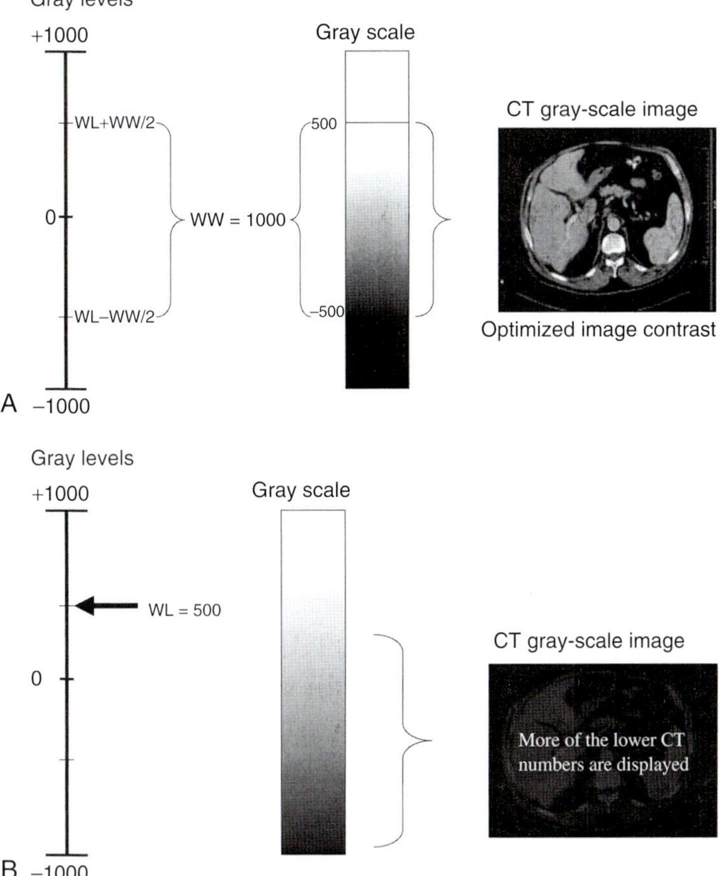


**FIGURE 8-5** The effect of a narrow WW on image grayscale. In this case the WW of 1000 produces an image with optimized image contrast compared with a WW of 2000, as shown in Figure 8-4. The WL is set at 0. Although the upper limit of the grayscale is calculated by the relationship WL + WW/2 (0 + 1000/2 = 500), the lower limit of the scale is equal to WL – WW/2 (0 – 1000/2 = –500).

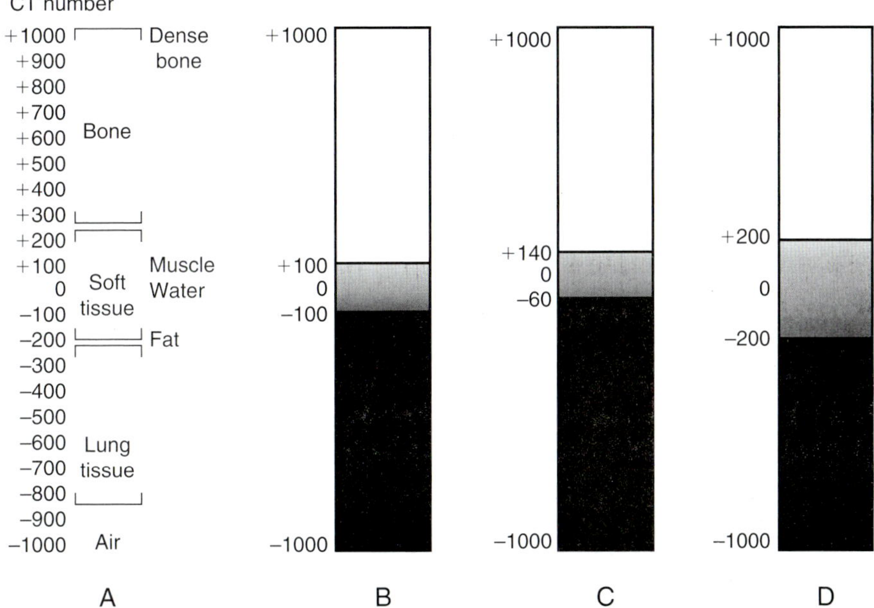


**FIGURE 8-6** Graphic illustration of the effect of different WW and WL settings on the appearance of the CT image. (See text for further explanation.)

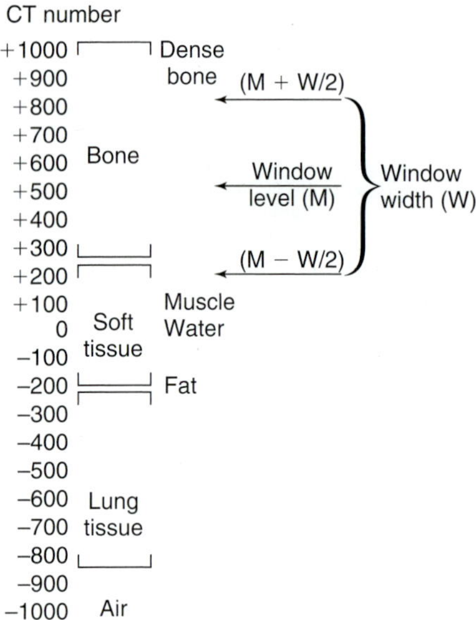


FIGURE 8-7 The relationship between WL and WW. These windows can be moved along the scale to optimize images of particular structures.

white matter. Liver may be viewed at 100 HU to 250 HU to highlight liver metastases. The effects of both wide and narrow window widths on image appearance are shown in Figure 8-9.

3. Levels should be centered near the average attenuation of the tissues of interest. For example, attenuation body scans may be viewed at a level of 0 HU to 60 HU because fat has attenuation numbers from −60 HU to −100 HU, whereas the attenuation numbers of muscle and organs may range from 60 HU to 150 HU with intravenous contrast. Lung is viewed at a level of −600 HU to −750 HU.

## Effect of Window Width on Image Contrast

In general, the viewer can alter the contrast of the CT image by changing the WW (Figure 8-10). When the WW is large (wide WW), the three different structures—the lung, liver (soft tissues), and pelvis (bone)—have the same gray tone (bottom of diagram). With a narrow WW, there is very sharp contrast to the point where the lungs appear black, bone appears white, and the liver is shown as gray tones.

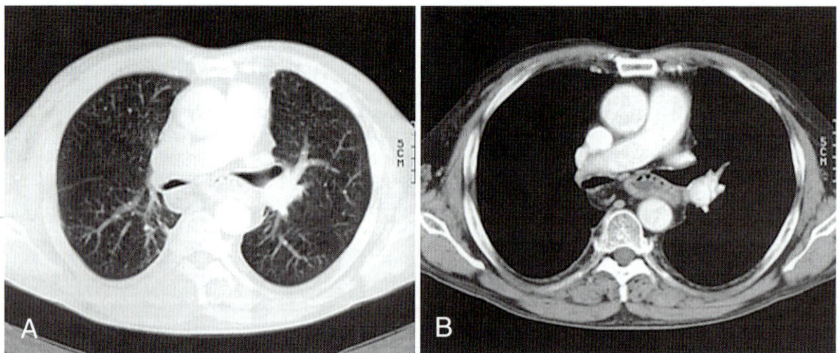


FIGURE 8-8 The effect of WW and WL adjustments on image appearance. **A,** A lung WW of 1500 HU and a WL of −530 HU are used. **B,** Soft tissue WW of 500 HU and a WL of +40 HU are used. (Courtesy Siemens Medical Systems.)

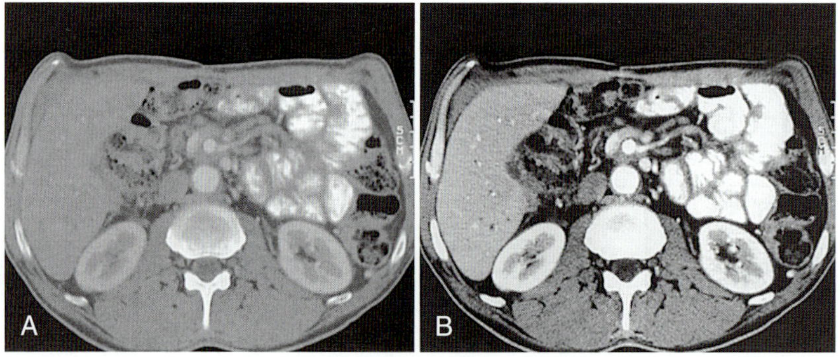


FIGURE 8-9 The effect of a wide WW **(A)** and a narrow WW **(B)** on the appearance of the CT image. (Courtesy Siemens Medical Systems.)

Finally, image contrast is optimized with the use of a medium WW (middle of diagram).

The effect of different WW settings (603, 499, 249, and 95) on an abdominal CT image with a fixed WL (+40) is clearly shown in Figure 8-11. The following conclusions may be drawn:

1. As the WW increases, the contrast decreases (Fig. 8-11, *A*).
2. As the WW decreases, the contrast becomes greater. The image appears totally black and white with a WW of 95 (Fig. 8-11, *D*).
3. Contrast is optimized with medium WW settings and is probably best (depending on the observer's subjective impression) when the image is recorded with a WW of 499 for the optimization of certain abdominal structures (Fig. 8-11, *B*).

## Effect of Window Level on Image Brightness

Figure 8-3 shows the WL as the CT number in the middle of the WW and represents the medium gray-scale. As graphically illustrated in Figure 8-12, when the WL is centered on the lungs (lower CT numbers), the image display is optimized for that structure, and the liver (soft tissue) and pelvis (bone) are displayed as white. On the other hand, when the WL is centered on the pelvis (higher CT numbers), the image display is optimized for the pelvis, and the lungs and

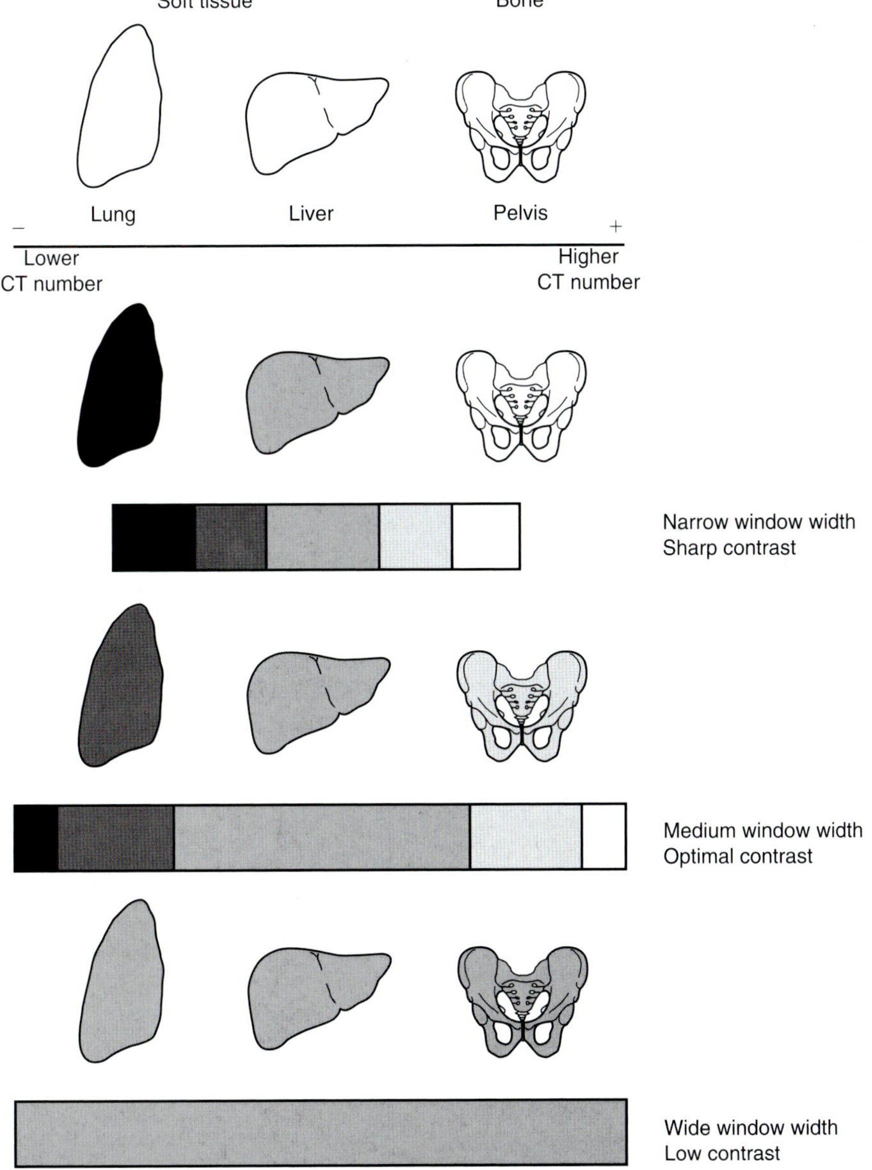


**FIGURE 8-10** The effect of WW on the appearance of different organs with widely varying CT numbers.

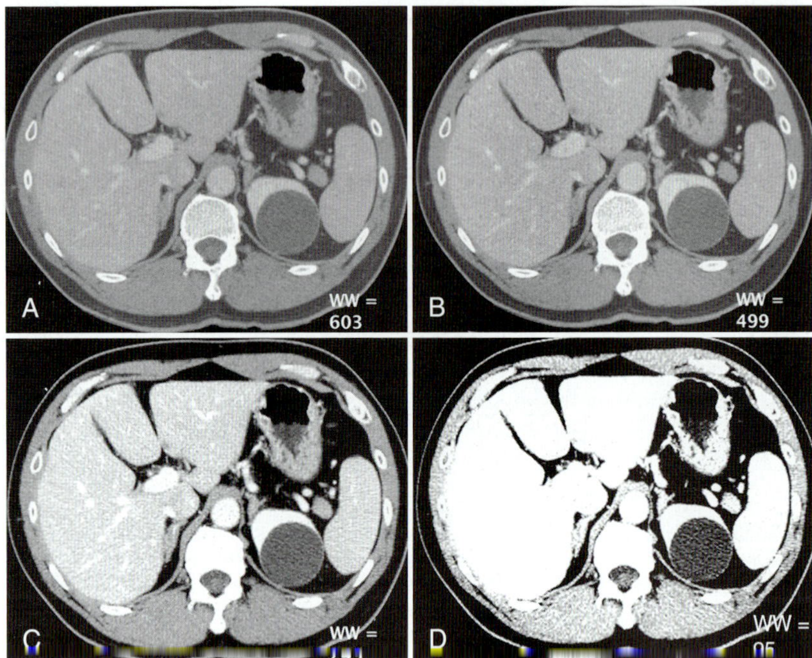


**FIGURE 8-11** Effect of different WW settings (with a fixed WL = +40) on image contrast with a fixed WL setting. As WW decreases from 603 **(A)**, 499 **(B)**, 249 **(C)**, to 95 **(D)**, contrast improves.

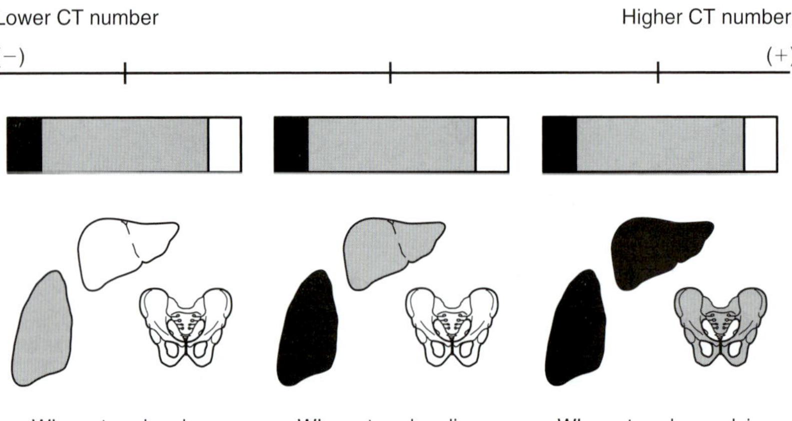


**FIGURE 8-12** Graphic illustration of the effect of WL on gray-tone appearance of different organs.

liver appear black. Finally, with the WL centered on the liver (middle CT numbers), the pelvis appears white, and the liver is optimized for viewing.

The effects of different WL settings (with fixed WW) on the display of images of the abdomen are shown in Figure 8-13. As the WL decreases from +248 to −106, the picture changes from black (Fig. 8-13, *A*) to white (Fig. 8-13, *D*). A graphic illustration of this effect is clearly apparent in Figure 8-14. As the WL moves toward the higher CT numbers (generally white), more CT numbers with lower values (generally black) are displayed. In addition, as the WL moves toward the lower CT numbers, more CT numbers with higher values are displayed, and the image looks white.

## Preset Windows

Preset windows are available on scanners to optimize windowing. For example, a double (dual) window display will facilitate the simultaneous display of two different density ranges. Both windows have different window widths and window levels (Fig. 8-15). Although a single window setting displays one anatomic region, a double (or dual) window display provides well-defined contours to separate two different anatomic areas (Fig. 8-16).

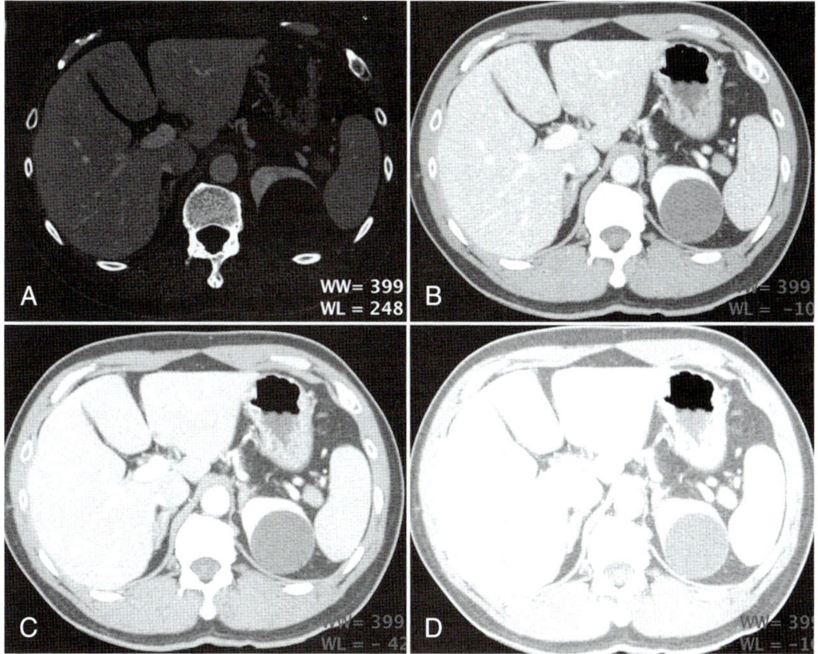


**FIGURE 8-13** Effect of different WL settings on image display with a fixed WW. As the WL decreases from +248 to −106, the picture changes from black **(A)** to white **(D)**.

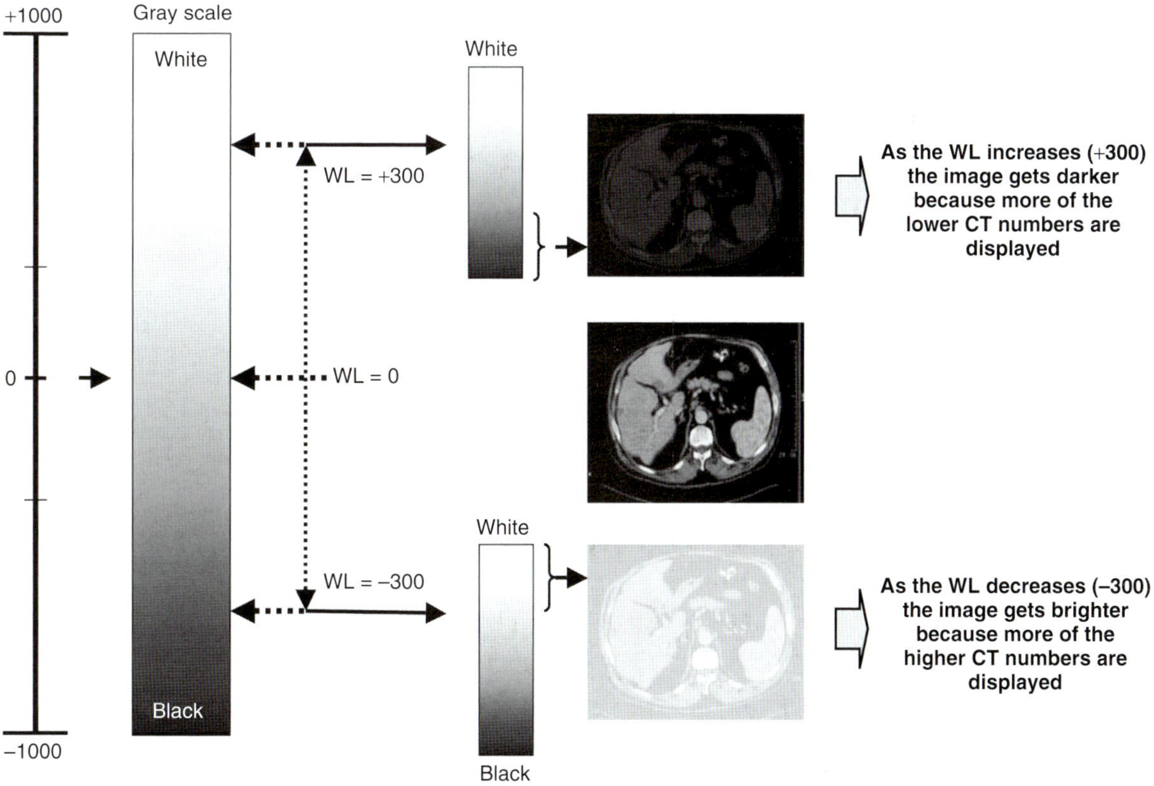

+1000
Gray scale
White
White
WL = +300
**As the WL increases (+300) the image gets darker because more of the lower CT numbers are displayed**
0
WL = 0
White
WL = −300
**As the WL decreases (−300) the image gets brighter because more of the higher CT numbers are displayed**
Black
−1000
Black

**FIGURE 8-14** Graphic illustration of this effect (Fig. 8-13). As the WL moves toward the higher CT numbers (generally white), more CT numbers with lower values (generally black) are displayed. As the WL moves toward the lower CT numbers, more CT numbers with higher values are displayed, and the image looks white.

# TWO-DIMENSIONAL IMAGE PROCESSING: CT IMAGE REFORMATTING TECHNIQUES

## Multiplanar Reconstruction

**Multiplanar reconstruction (MPR),** sometimes referred to as *image reformatting* or *image reformation* (not to be confused with image reconstruction), is a computer program that can create coronal, sagittal, and paraxial images from a stack of contiguous transverse axial scans (Fig. 8-17).

The sagittal image defines a plane that passes through an anatomic region from anterior to posterior and divides the body into right and left sections; the coronal image defines a plane that passes through the body region from right to left (or left to right), dividing the region into anterior and posterior sections. The paraxial image, on the other hand, defines a plane that cuts through the coronal and sagittal planes in the longitudinal direction of an anatomica region.

Irregular, oblique, and other views can also be generated. The irregular **view** (e.g., linear or curved)

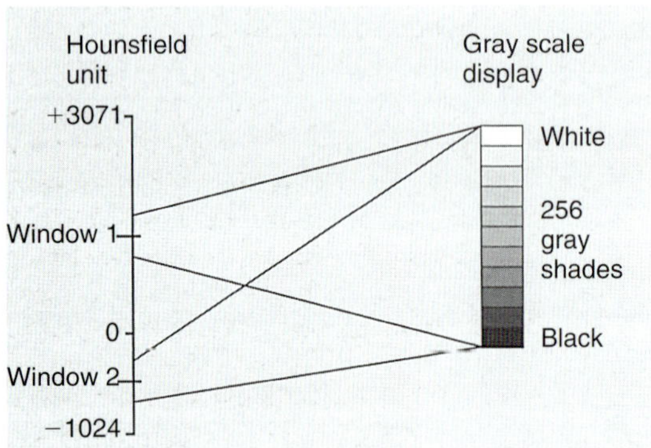


**FIGURE 8-15** The fundamental principles of the double (dual) window setting. (Courtesy Siemens Medical Systems, Iselin, NJ.)

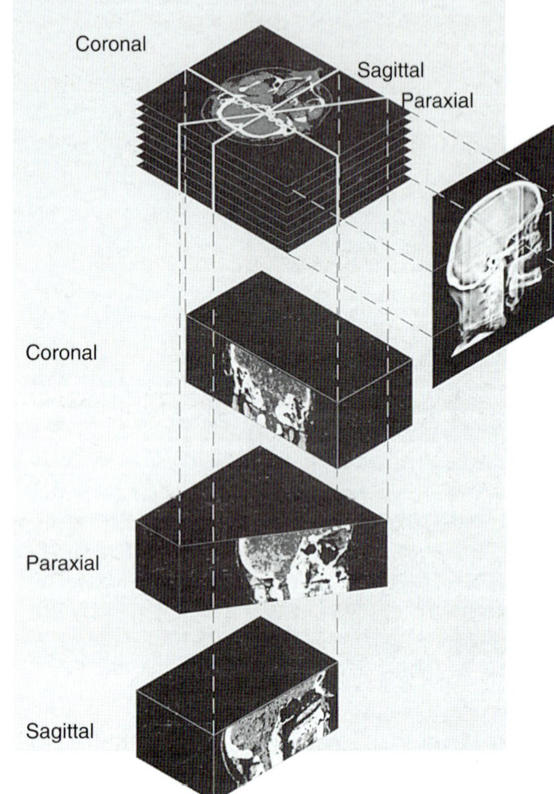


**FIGURE 8-17** Multiplanar reconstruction involves the use of a computer program to reformat sagittal, paraxial, and coronal views from a stack of contiguous transverse axial images. (Courtesy Siemens Medical Systems, Iselin, NJ.)

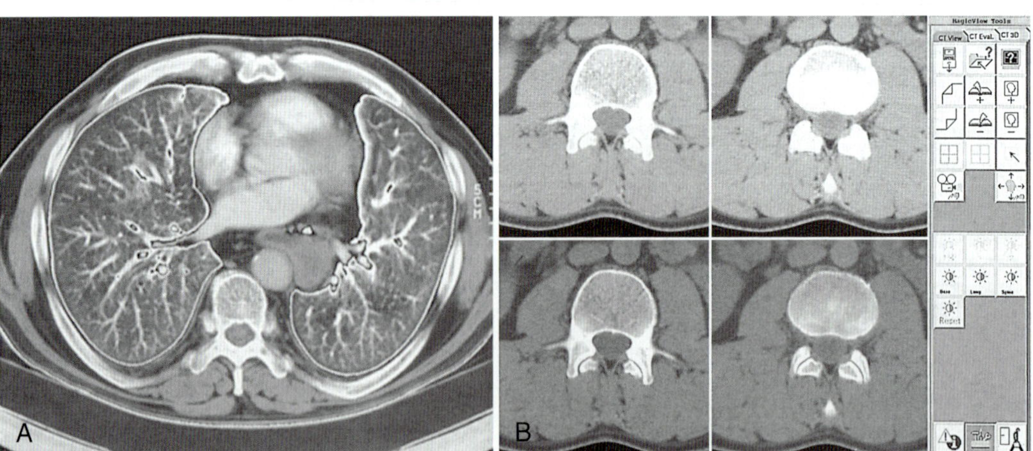


**FIGURE 8-16** **A,** A double (dual) window display with a WW and WL of 750 HU and −730 HU, respectively, with a WW and a WL of 500 HU and 35 HU, respectively. **B,** Dual windows allow the observer to view bone and soft tissue windows of the same images simultaneously. (Courtesy Siemens Medical Systems, Iselin, NJ.)

can be reconstructed from a stack of contiguous transverse images (Fig. 8-18). The oblique view can be reconstructed with at least three arbitrarily definable points in different transverse images (Fig. 8-19).

In the conceptual framework to generate these images (Fig. 8-20), the voxel on the left represents the information contained and stored in a specific volume of tissue. In reformatting, the computer program uses any set of points to build an image of the selected plane. Mackay (1984) noted the following:

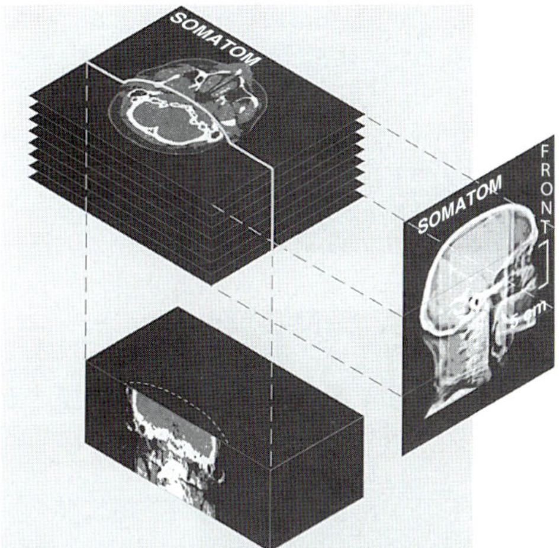


**FIGURE 8-18** Irregular views can be created through multiplanar reconstruction techniques using the images from a stack of contiguous transaxial slices. (Courtesy Siemens Medical Systems, Iselin, NJ.)

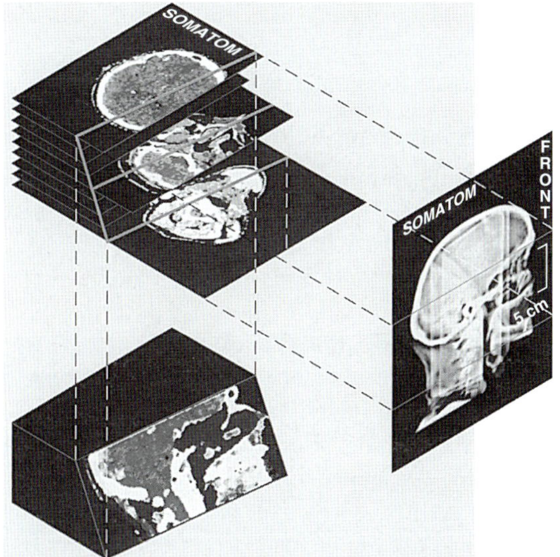


**FIGURE 8-19** Oblique views can be reconstructed by multiplanar reconstruction techniques using definable points in different transaxial slices. (Courtesy Siemens Medical Systems, Iselin, NJ.)

> Suppose in the figure that the first image computed and stored was the left-hand face of the cube, followed by the plane parallel to it with the number 2, after which the third set of projections would be collected to form the parallel plane containing the number 3, and so on. All the points in the cube would gradually be accumulated and stored in the computer, and it is convenient to think of the **position** of the storage of a number as corresponding to the position of a point in the cube. Any of the original planes could be displayed by "calling up" the number representing the points in that plane and producing a proportional brightness on the oscilloscope screen at the corresponding position. On the screen instead could be displayed the dots shown at the center section [of Fig. 8-20]. On the lower left of the screen would be displayed the point designated (1, B, a), which came from the first section, for example. Next to it would be displayed a point from the bottom of the second section and in one increment from the right side, and so on. By sequentially calling up all the points located inward one increment from the right face of the cube one can display a section through the subject perpendicular to all the planes that were originally scanned. In the display one can instead move to the left one increment from each successive step inward to a new line on the television screen; this results in the display of a plane at an angle through the body as shown in the right-hand part of the figure. It should be clear that from this array of computed data one can display any section through the volume. Often the sections across a subject are more widely spaced than are the lines across the section in making the original projections, in which case the resolution in a tilted display will not be the same up and down as across the image.

There are both advantages and disadvantages to reformatted images (see Box 8-1). Major advantages include the following:

1. To enable the visualization of specific structures such as the optic nerves and lesions in relation to surrounding structures
2. To determine the true extent of lesions or fractures and to help localize lesions and intra-articular bone fragments or foreign bodies

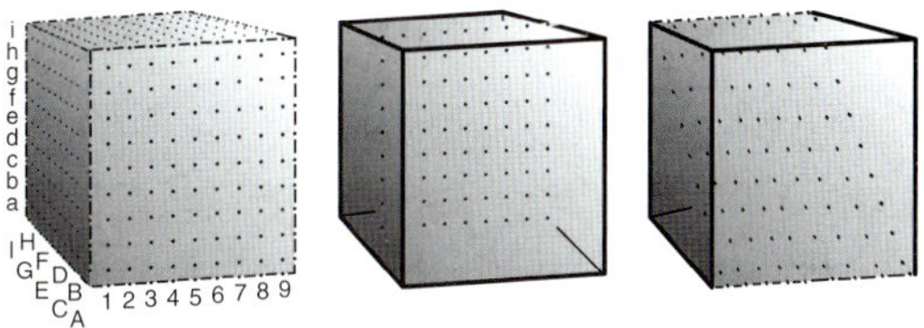


**FIGURE 8-20** A conceptual framework for generating reformatted images in CT.

**BOX 8-1 Reformatted Images**

**Advantages**
- Enables visualization of specific structures in relation to surrounding structures
- Determines extent of lesions or fractures
- Helps to localize lesions, bone fragments, or foreign bodies

**Disadvantage**
- Loss of image detail

One major disadvantage of MPR is image quality. Image detail is not as good as that obtained in transaxial images. The reformatted image quality depends on the quality of the axial images, and it is therefore important that the patient does not move or breathe during the **scanning** procedure (Box 8-1). In addition, the plane thickness affects image detail; thus thick planes result in blurring and loss of structural detail. Today, multislice CT scanners capable of **isotropic** imaging (see Chapter 11) solve these problems, because all dimensions of the voxel are equal—the voxel is a perfect cube.

# THREE-DIMENSIONAL IMAGE PROCESSING

## Three-Dimensional Imaging: An Overview

3D imaging in CT belongs to a class of digital image processing referred to as image synthesis (see Chapter 2). Image synthesis operations "create images from other images or non-image data. These operations are used when a desired image is either physically impossible or impractical to acquire, or does not exist in a physical form at all" (Baxes, 1994). Synthesis operations include image reconstruction techniques (see Chapters 5 and 6) that are the basis for CT and magnetic resonance (MR) images and 3D visualization techniques that are based on computer graphics technology. Special software gathers information from the transaxial scan data to display 3D images on a 2D television screen.

A thorough description of 3D CT imaging is not within the scope of this chapter, but it is elaborated in Chapter 13. It is important, however, to introduce some of the language of 3D imaging here.

3D imaging is gaining widespread attention in radiology (Bolan, 2013; Calhoun et al., 1999; Choplin et al., 2004; Cody, 2002; Dalrymple et al., 2005; Fatterpekar et al., 2006; Fishman et al., 2006; Kalender, 2005; Lell et al., 2006; Philipp et al., 2003; Seeram, 2001; 2005; Seeram & Seeram, 2008; Udupa, 1999; Zhang et al., 2011). Already it is used in CT, MR imaging, and other imaging modalities to provide both qualitative and **quantitative information** from images to facilitate and enhance diagnosis.

The general framework of 3D imaging (Fig. 8-21) includes four major steps: **data acquisition,** creation of 3D space (all voxel information is stored in the computer), processing for 3D image display, and, finally, 3D image display. Images can be displayed as projection images, such as **maximum intensity projection (MIP)** and minimum intensity projection images (MinIP), SSD images, VR images, and virtual reality images. The principles of the **generation** of each of these are elaborated in Chapter 13.

Digital image postprocessing allows the observer to view all aspects of 3D space, a technique referred to as 3D visualization. The application of 3D visualization techniques in radiology is referred to as 3D medical imaging. Basic and advanced visualization tools in 3D medical imaging are highlighted later.

Dr. Jayaram Udupa (1999), an expert in 3D imaging from the Department of Radiology at the University of Pennsylvania, noted that there are four classes of 3D imaging operations: preprocessing, visualization, manipulation, and analysis. For example, as noted by Dr. Udupa, visualization operations are intended "to create renditions from a given set of scenes or objects that facilitate the visual perception of object information." These four classes of operations are described further in Chapter 13.

# VISUALIZATION TOOLS

**Visualization tools** such as windowing are computer programs that provide the observer-diagnostician with additional information to facilitate diagnosis. Visualization tools range from basic to advanced.

## Basic Tools

**Basic visualization tools** are basic computer programs integrated into the CT system with the following capabilities (Fig. 8-22):

1. Multiple imaging and multiple windows (Fig. 8-22, *A*)
2. Image magnification (Fig. 8-22, *B*)
3. Evaluation of geometric characteristics such as distances and angles (Fig. 8-22, *C*)
4. Superimposition of coordinates on the image to provide a reference for biopsies (Fig. 8-22, *D*)
5. Highlighting, in which the pixels in certain regions of the image can be made to appear brighter (Fig. 8-22, *E*)
6. CT histogram, which is a plot of the pixel values, as a function of the frequency with which each value occurs; this can be done for the entire image

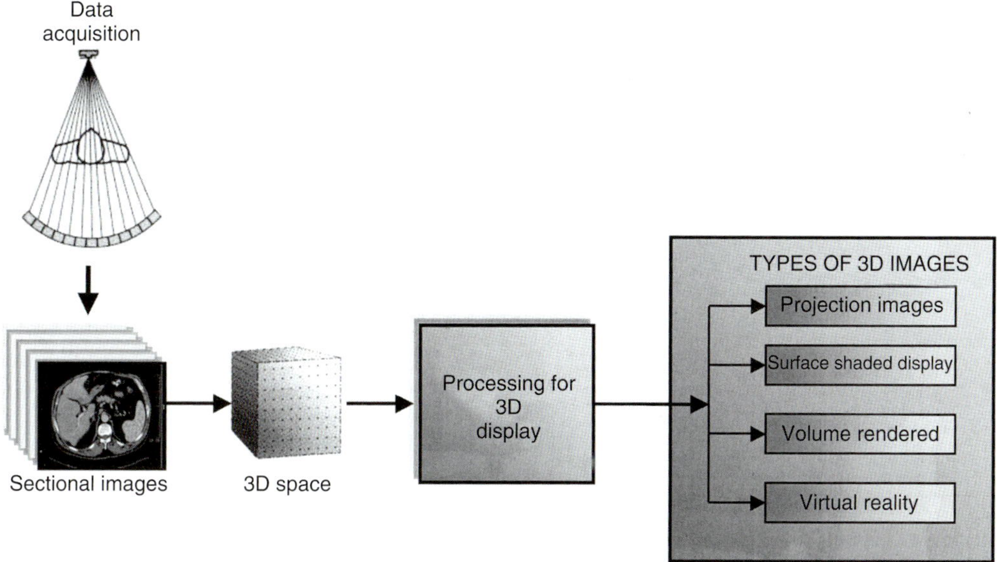


**FIGURE 8-21** The general framework of 3D imaging includes four major steps: data acquisition, creation of what is referred to as 3D space, digital image processing for 3D image display, and finally, 3D image display. As noted, several different types of 3D images can be displayed to suit the needs of the observer.

or a portion of the image, as defined by the **region of interest** (**ROI;** Fig. 8-22, *F*)

7. ROI statistics, which allow for statistical calculations such as the mean and standard deviation within the ROI
8. ROI transfer, whereby the ROI can be transferred from slice to slice
9. Split imaging, in which an image can be split into two detailed thin slices, and fused imaging, in which two contiguous thin slices can be fused into a single thick slice

Optional software packages are also available for dental CT applications, dynamic CT, networking, workstations, and 3D imaging.

## Advanced Tools

**Advanced visualization tools** require powerful computer workstations with advanced image-processing capabilities and increased memory to handle the vast amount of data used in various visualization techniques. An example of this type of workstation is shown in Figure 8-23. Currently, a wide variety of advanced visualization tools are commercially available:

- 3D visualization tools allow the user to render various 3D images from the axial dataset. 3D **rendering** falls into three categories: SSD (surface rendering), VR, and MIP and MinIP. As noted by Zhang et al. (2011), "more recently, further efficiencies have been attained by designing and implementing **volume rendering** algorithms on graphic processing units (GPUs)." Basic highlights of the GPU are presented in Chapter 7.
- Computed tomography angiography (CTA) is a relatively new technique based on **volume scanning** principles. It is an application of 3D imaging and is becoming more popular in the examination of the circulatory system. Examples of CTA visualization tools include 4D angio, vessel tracking, skull removal, and multiple target volume.
- In 4D angio, the fourth dimension is opacity instead of time and is based on VR technology. Changes in the opacity values of various tissues enable the observer to simultaneously visualize bone, soft tissues, and vascular structures; therefore both foreground and background structures are visible. 4D angio is preferred over conventional MIP techniques for the visualization of aortic aneurysms, renal arteries, stents, and carotid bifurcation. Target volume MIP allows the user to render only a selected volume of data and does not require **segmentation** techniques.
- The vessel-tracking tool allows the user to produce a set of MPR images (batches), including curved MPR images, for the entire vessel. The skull removal tool facilitates the subtraction of bones of the skull from the CTA image and allows the observer to visualize very detailed images of the vessels and soft tissues.
- MPR tools display all types of MPR images from the axial dataset in the axial, coronal, sagittal, and oblique planes, as described earlier in this chapter.

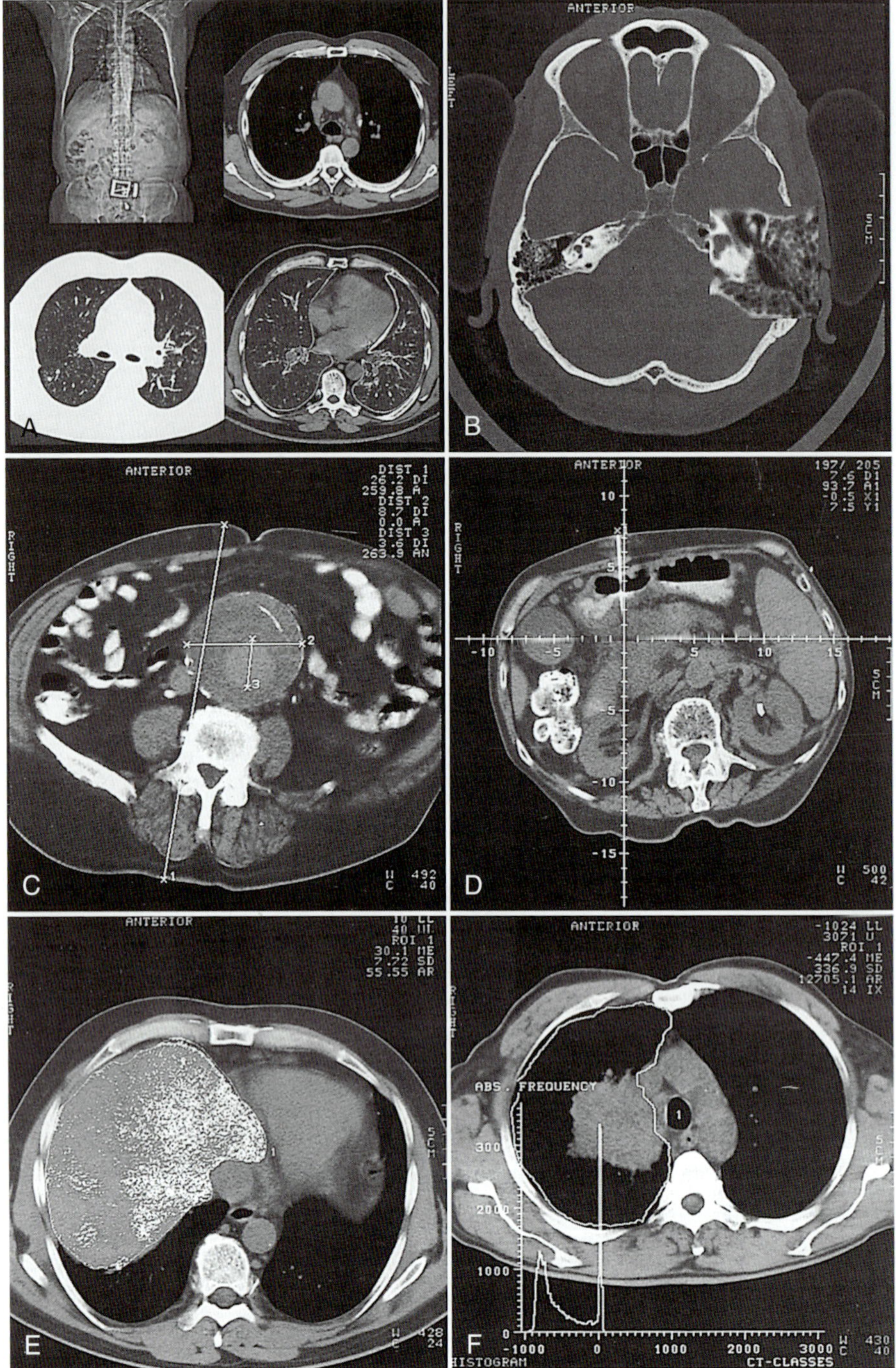


**FIGURE 8-22** Other computer programs for CT are capable of the following: **A,** multiple imaging and windows; **B,** image magnification; **C,** measurement of distances; **D,** superimposition of coordinates on the image; **E,** highlights; and **F,** histogram. (Courtesy Siemens Medical Systems, Iselin, NJ.)

- **Interactive visualization tools** offer the following features in any 3D-rendering mode: window/level adjustment, volume of interest adjustment, scan information display, movie creation and playback, split screen presentation, zoom, and measurements.
- **Cine visualization tools** allow the user to view a large set of images very quickly.
- **Advanced quantitative measurement tools** facilitate measurements such as distances, angles, areas, mean, standard deviation, minimum and maximum voxel values, density value in HU,

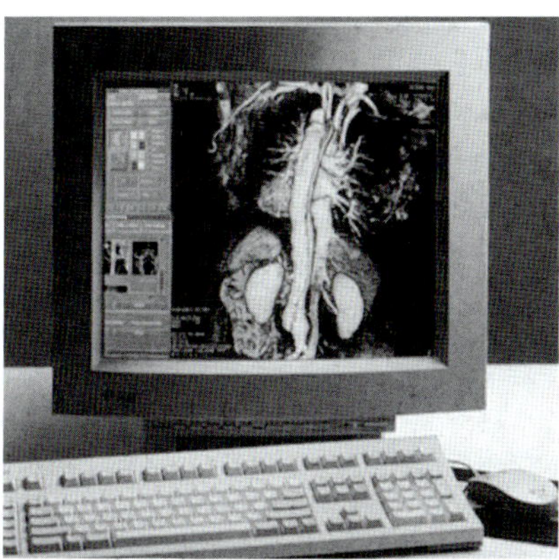

**FIGURE 8-23** Example of a workstation for advanced image processing. (Courtesy Philips Medical Systems.)

density histogram for a particular ROI, and volume of 3D objects.

- **Multimodality image fusion tools** allow the user to combine images from a wide variety of imaging modalities such as CT, MR imaging, positron emission tomography, and single-photon **emission CT** to facilitate diagnosis of tumor localization and quantification, surgical planning, and oncology planning.
- **Virtual reality visualization tools** include Voyager and 3D Navigator. These tools create 3D and 4D images of tubular structures such as the colon and bronchi and allow the user to "fly through" the images of hollow organs in a technique referred to as *CT virtual endoscopy*, which is gaining widespread attention in radiologic imaging.

## ADVANCED VISUALIZATION AND ANALYSIS WORKSTATIONS

### Hardware Components

**Hardware** components include the central processing unit, various processors, and data and image storage devices. The **host computer** of an advanced visualization and analysis workstation can be a Sun SPARC (Sun Microsystems) or a Silicon Graphics platform with varying amounts of random access memory, depending on the cost of the system. The operating system of both platforms is the UNIX multitasking system, which provides optimum speed and system response. In addition, these workstations feature various microprocessors to improve **data processing**.

The monitor of the workstation must provide good image quality and offer a maximum luminance of at least 50 foot-lamberts (American College of Radiology, 2006). These monitors are usually cathode **ray** tubes or flat-panel displays with at least 2.5 K × 2 K pixel resolution and should be capable of a wide range of display formats. The keyboard is a full alphanumerical keyboard with function, archiving, and display keys. Additionally, a mouse can be used to communicate with the computer.

Data and image storage devices include hard disks and magnetic tape. The storage capacity of these media varies depending on the system.

### Connectivity

**Connectivity,** or networking, is an important feature of current workstations because of the trend toward filmless radiology departments through the implementation of picture archiving and communication systems, radiology information systems, and hospital information systems (see Chapter 7).

The transfer of data and images to and from the CT scanner and workstations is an essential component of connectivity. Such transfer must comply with industry standards for electronic **communications** between different imaging modalities and devices from multiple vendors. One such standard is the Digital Imaging and Communications in Medicine (DICOM), and workstations for CT, MR imaging, and other imaging modalities must be DICOM compliant.

## REVIEW QUESTIONS

Answer the following questions to check your understanding of the materials studied.

1. Gray-level mapping is also referred to as all of the following ***except***:
   A. contrast stretching
   B. windowing
   C. image enhancement
   D. histogram modification
2. In CT, windowing is an example of:
   A. local processing of raw data.
   B. convolution.
   C. gray-level mapping.
   D. image smoothing.
3. In CT, the window width is the:
   A. region of interest.
   B. pixel depth.
   C. range of CT numbers.
   D. center of the range of CT numbers.
4. The window level in CT is defined as the:
   A. middle of the range of CT numbers.
   B. CT number in the middle of the image.
   C. range of CT numbers in the image.
   D. dimension of the matrix.

## REVIEW QUESTIONS—cont'd

5. The contrast of the CT image is controlled by the:
   A. kVp.
   B. WW.
   C. WL.
   D. mA.
6. The brightness of the image can be altered by the:
   A. kVp.
   B. mA.
   C. WW.
   D. WL.
7. When the WL changes from −100 to +400, the picture changes from:
   A. white to black.
   B. black to white.
   C. gray to white.
   D. gray to dark green.
8. The software program that generates sagittal and coronal images from the transaxial dataset is referred to as:
   A. multislice CT.
   B. multiplanar reformatting.
   C. multidectector CT.
   D. multireconstruction of CT slices.
9. Which of the following is ***not*** an example of a basic visualization tool?
   A. image magnification
   B. statistics
   C. CT histogram
   D. 3D imaging
10. The following are examples of advanced visualization software tools ***except***:
    A. 3D imaging.
    B. CTA
    C. split imaging
    D. virtual reality imaging

## REFERENCES


American College of Radiology. (2006). *ACR technical standard for digital image data management*. Reston, VA: American College of Radiology.

Baxes, G. A. (1994). *Digital image processing: principles and applications*. New York: John Wiley.

Berland, L. L. (1987). *Practical CT: technology and techniques*. New York: Raven Press.

Bolan, C. (2013). Routine 3D imaging becomes a reality. *Applied Radiology*, July 27–31.

Choplin, R. H., et al. (2004). CT with 3D rendering of the tendons of the foot and ankle: technique, normal anatomy, and disease. *RadioGraphics, 24*, 343–356.

Cody, D. (2002). Image processing in CT. *Radiographics, 22*, 1255–1268.

Dalrymple, N. C., Prasad, S. R., Freckleton, M. W., & Chintapalli, K. N. (2005). Informatics in radiology (infoRAD): introduction to the language of three-dimensional imaging with multidetector CT. *Radiographics, 25*, 1409–1428.

Fatterpekar, G. M., Doshi, A. H., Dugar, M., Delman, B. N., Naidich, T. P., & Som, P. M. (2006). Role of 3D CT in the evaluation of the temporal bone. *Radiographics, 26*, S117–S132.

Fishman, E. K., Ney, D. R., Heath, D. G., Corl, F. M., Horton, K. M., & Johnson, P. T. (2006). Volume rendering versus maximum intensity projection in CT angiography: what works best, when and why? *Radiographics, 26*, 905–921.

Girish et al.: Role of 3D CT in the evaluation of the temporal bone, *Radiographics, 26*: S117–S132, 2006.

Glen, W., et al. (1981). Image manipulation and pattern recognition. In T. H. Newton, & D. G. Potts (Eds.), *Radiology of the skull and brain: technical aspects of computed tomography*. St. Louis, MO: Mosby.

Kalender, W. (2005). *Computed tomography: fundamentals, system technology, image quality, applications*. Erlangen, Germany: Publicis Corporate Publishing.

Lell, M. M., Anders, K., Uder, M., Klotz, E., et al. (2006). New techniques in CT angiography. *Radiographics, 26*, S45–S62.

Mackay, R. S. (1984). *Medical images and displays*. New York: John Wiley.

Morgan, C. L. (1983). *Basic principles of computed tomography*. Baltimore, MD: University Park Press.

Philipp, M. O., Kubin, K., Mang, T., Hormann, M., & Metz, V. M. (2003). Three-dimensional volume rendering of multidetector-row CT data: applicable for emergency radiology. *European Journal of Radiology, 48*, 33–38.

Seeram, E. (2001). *Computed tomography technology*. Philadelphia, PA: WB Saunders.

Seeram, E. (2005). Digital image processing. *Radiologic Technology, 76*, 435–452.

Seeram, E. (2010). Computed tomography: physical principles and recent technical advances. *Journal of Medical Imaging Radiation Sciences, 41*, 87–109.

Seeram, E., & Seeram, D. (2008). Image postprocessing in digital radiology: a primer for technologists. *Journal of Medical Imaging Radiation Sciences, 39*, 23–43.

Udupa, J. K. (1999). Three-dimensional visualization and analysis methodologies: A current perspective. *Radiographics, 19*, 783–806.

Xue, Z., Antani, S., Long, L. R., Demner-Fushman, D., & Thoma, G. R. (2012). window classification of brain CT images in biomedical articles. *AMIA Annual Symposium Proceedings, 2012*, 1023–1029.

Zatz, L. M. (1984). Basic principles of computed tomography scanning. In T. H. Newton, & D. G. Potts (Eds.), *Radiology of the skull and brain: technical aspects of computed tomography*. St. Louis, MO: Mosby.

Zhang, Q., Eagleson, R., & Peters, T. M. (2011). Volume visualization: a technical overview with a focus on medical applications. *Journal of Digital Imaging, 24*(4), 640–664.

Zhiyun X et al.: Window Classification of Brain CT Images in Biomedical Articles, *AMIA Annu Symp Proc.* 2012, 1023–1029, 2012.

9

# Image Quality

*Jiang Hsieh*

## OUTLINE



## LEARNING OBJECTIVES

On completion of this chapter, you should be able to:

1. identify several types of phantoms for measuring image quality in CT.
2. define each of the following:
   - spatial resolution
   - low-contrast resolution
   - temporal resolution
   - noise
   - CT number accuracy and linearity
   - uniformity.
3. discuss the factors affecting spatial and contrast resolution in CT.
4. discuss the factors affecting noise in CT.
5. define the term "artifact."
6. discuss the types, causes, and reduction of artifacts in CT.

## KEY TERMS TO WATCH FOR AND REMEMBER

The following key terms/concepts are important to your understanding of this Chapter.

**artifact**
**beam hardening**
**full-width at half-maximum (FWHM)**
**full-width at tenth-maximum (FWTM)**
**linearity**
**low-contrast resolution**
**modulation transfer function (MTF)**
**noise**
**partial volume averaging**
**slice sensitivity profile (SSP)**
**spatial resolution**
**temporal resolution**

In general, the image quality of a **computed tomography (CT)** scanner can be described by several key performance parameters: high-contrast spatial resolution, low-contrast resolution, temporal resolution, CT number uniformity and accuracy, **noise,** and artifacts. These parameters are influenced not only by the CT system performance but also by the operator's selection of protocols such as **x-ray tube** voltage (in kilovolts [kV]), tube current (in milliamperes [mA]), **slice thickness,** helical **pitch,** reconstruction parameters, and scan speed. The introduction of new technologies, such as **iterative reconstruction (IR)** and dual-energy, has made the determination of these parameters even more complex. Like real-life problems, trade-offs have to be made between image quality, dose to the patient, system limitations, patient conditions, and clinical indications. Many studies have been conducted to understand such trade-offs (Barnes & Lakshminarayan, 1981; Blumenfeld & Glover, 1981; Hanson, 1981; Hsieh, 2009; Kalender & Polacin, 1995; McCollough & Zink, 2000; Morgan, 1983; Pfeiler et al., 1976; Robb & Mortin, 1991). Clearly, trade-off decisions between various performance parameters are not as straightforward as would be hoped. Although the design of CT scanners has evolved significantly to minimize the complexity of parameter selection, even state-of-the-art scanners still depend, in various degrees, on the experience of the operator to produce optimal image quality.

Given the limited scope of this chapter, it is impossible to discuss all factors that affect the image quality of a CT scanner, let alone the trade-offs among these factors. Instead, only the most important performance parameters are the focus and, whenever possible, some of the common factors that influence the CT performance and phantoms used to perform quantitative measurements are briefly discussed. Because of the wide availability of the helical/spiral and multislice/volumetric CT scanners, their specific characteristics and requirements are incorporated into the discussion of each topic, rather than isolated in a separate section.

# SPATIAL RESOLUTION

**Spatial resolution** of a CT scanner describes the scanner's ability to resolve closely placed objects that are significantly different from their background. That is, the contrast of these objects to their background is high. This is different from the low-contrast resolution that will be discussed in a later section where the CT number difference between the objects and background is small. Historically, spatial resolution was defined and measured predominately within the **scanning** plane. With the popularity of the multislice/volumetric helical CT, however, the cross-plane resolution becomes just as important.

## In-Plane Spatial Resolution

### Definition and Measurements

The term "in-plane" refers to the fact that the spatial resolution is measured in the axial plane (*x-y* plane) of the CT. The in-plane resolution is specified in terms of line pairs per centimeter (lp/cm) or line pairs per millimeter (lp/mm). A line pair is a pair of equal-sized black–white bars. Therefore, a bar pattern representing 10 lp/cm is a set of uniformly spaced combshaped bars with 0.5-mm wide teeth. Because the CT acquisition and reconstruction process is band-limited (high-frequency contents are suppressed or eliminated), the reconstructed image of a bar pattern is a blurred version of the original object, as illustrated in Figure 9-1. The edges of the bars are softened, and the magnitude of the bar pattern is reduced. If the peak-to-valley magnitude of the original object is normalized as unity, the reconstructed peak to valley is smaller. For example, in Figure 9-1, at 1 lp/cm spatial frequency, the reconstructed peak-to-valley magnitude is 0.88; at 2 lp/cm, the magnitude is 0.59, and so on. In general, the magnitude reduces as the frequency (lp/cm) of the bar pattern increases. If the spatial frequency is plotted as a function of the image fidelity, a smooth curve is obtained (Fig. 9-2). This is often referred to as the **modulation transfer function (MTF)** of the

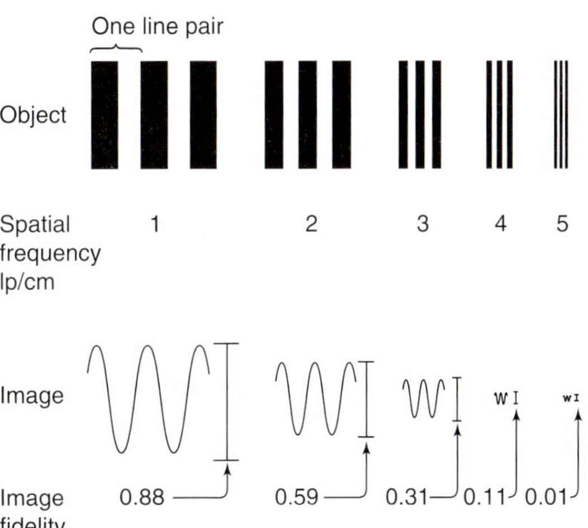


**FIGURE 9-1** A bar pattern (object) consists of line pairs (one line pair equals one bar plus one space). The number of line pairs per unit length is called the spatial frequency. Large objects have a low spatial frequency, whereas small objects have a high spatial frequency. *lp*, line pair.

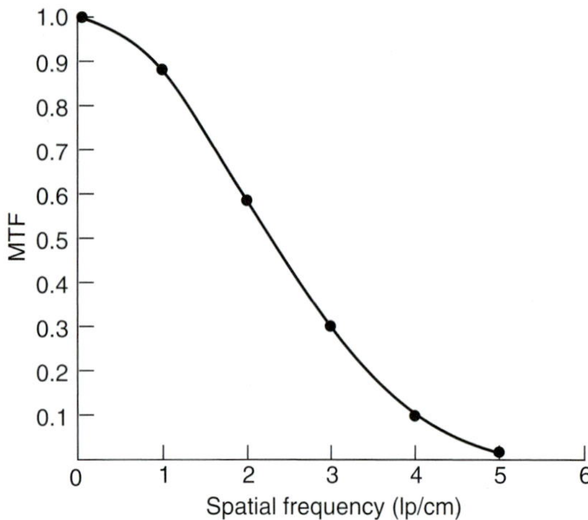


**FIGURE 9-2** A modulation transfer function (*MTF*) curve obtained from the data given in Figure 9-1.

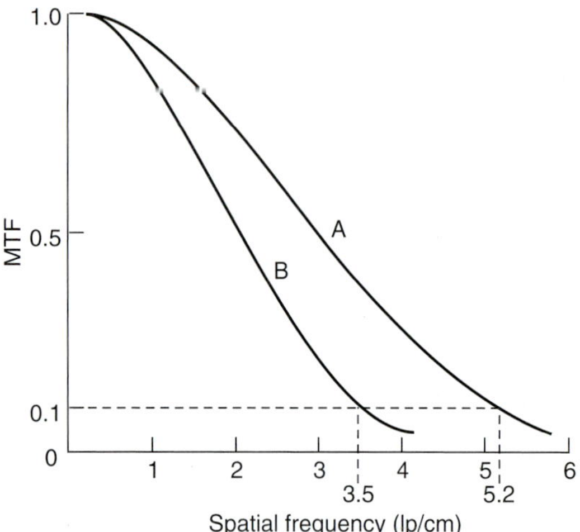


**FIGURE 9-3** MTF curves for two CT scanners.

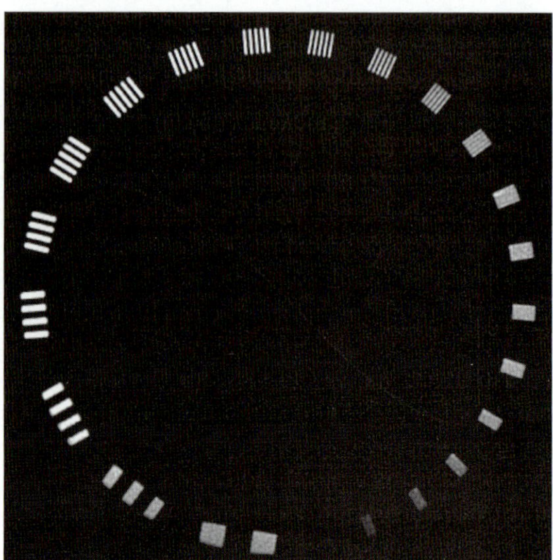

**FIGURE 9-4** Image of a Catphan high-resolution insert. Bar patterns range from 1 lp/cm to 21 lp/cm.

system. MTF can be used as part of the quality assurance to determine a scanner's resolution capability or used to compare the performance of different CT systems. For example, scanner A can image 5.2 lp/cm at 10% MTF compared with scanner B, which can only image 3.5 lp/cm at 10% MTF (Fig. 9-3). This simply means that scanner A has a better spatial resolution capability than scanner B.

An ideal system would have a flat MTF curve, a unity response independent of frequency. Such a system ensures that the object can be reproduced exactly. For practical systems, however, the frequency response falls off quickly as the frequency increases. Three points on the MTF curve are of particular interest: 50%, 10%, and 0%. The 50% MTF refers to the frequency at which the magnitude of the MTF curve drops to 50% of its peak value. Similarly, the 10% and 0% MTF refer to the frequencies at which the MTF drops to 10% and 0% of the peak value. Although the value of 50% MTF and 10% MTF are measured experimentally, the 0% MTF is sometimes calculated theoretically based on the **sampling** theory. Various phantoms have been designed specifically to measure the MTF of the system. For example, the Catphan High Resolution Insert contains high-density metal bar patterns ranging from 1 lp/cm to 21 lp/cm, as shown in Figure 9-4.

Alternatively, the MTF of a system can be derived from the point spread function (PSF) of the system (Hsieh, 2009). PSF is defined as the system response to a Dirac delta function. If the scanned object is a high-density thin wire placed perpendicular to the scanning plane, and as long as the diameter of the wire is significantly smaller than the spatial resolution of the system, the wire can be considered as a Dirac delta function. The reconstructed image of such wire is then simply the PSF of the system. By definition, MTF is related to PSF by the magnitude of the **Fourier transform.** Figure 9-5 depicts a GE Performance Phantom with a 0.08-mm diameter tungsten wire submerged in water. If we isolate the wire portion of the image, remove its background (Fig. 9-6, *A*), and take the Fourier transform of this image (Fig. 9-6, *B*), the MTF of the CT system can be obtained by averaging the **frequency domain** image over 360 degrees, as shown by the curve in Figure 9-6.

## Factors Affecting Resolution

Many factors affect the in-plane spatial resolution. The most dominating factors are the x-ray focal

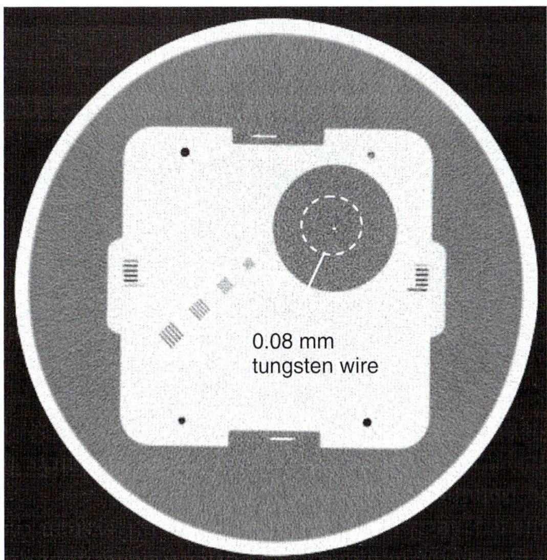


**FIGURE 9-5** Image of a GE Performance Phantom. A thin tungsten wire is submerged in water for MTF measurement.

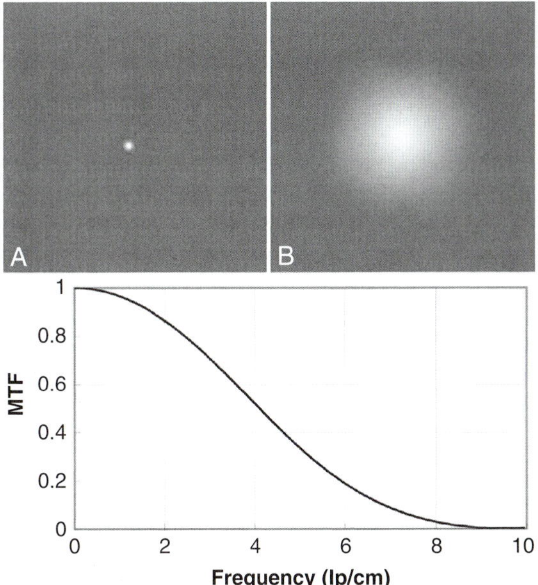


**FIGURE 9-6** MTF measurement with a thin wire. **A,** A tungsten wire reconstructed with standard algorithm to approximate PSF. **B,** Magnitude of the Fourier transform of the PSF image. The MTF curve is averaged over 360 degrees.

spot size and shape, detector cell size, scanner geometry, and sampling frequency. Although these factors are largely determined by CT manufacturers, operators do have limited control. For example, most CT scanners have more than one x-ray focal spot to account for an increased tube loading. By properly selecting the x-ray tube current, an operator has the option to use either the small spot (lower tube current, higher spatial resolution) or the large spot (higher tube current, lower spatial resolution).

The in-plane resolution is also strongly influenced by the reconstruction **algorithm.** Chapter 5 indicates that **image reconstruction** involves two mathematical procedures: **convolution** and **back-projection.** Essentially, if the **projection profiles** are back-projected without correction, blurring results (Fig. 9-7, *A*). To sharpen the image, a convolution process (a ramp filter) is applied to modify the frequency contents of the **projection** before back-projection (Fig. 9-7, *B*). The convolution algorithm, or kernel, affects the appearance of image structures. Convolution algorithms have been developed for each anatomic-specific application. In general, these algorithms are applied to emphasize soft tissue (standard algorithm) and bone (bone algorithm). The former is applied to the mid brain, pancreas, adrenal, or any soft tissue region, and the latter is applied to bony structures such as the inner ear and extremities. As an illustration, two images in Figure 9-8 are reconstructed from the same scan data with two different reconstruction kernels. Figure 9-8, *A*, was reconstructed with a standard kernel and Figure 9-8, *B*, with a bone kernel. It is clear that the bone kernel produces a much sharper image (higher spatial resolution) as demonstrated by a better visualization of the bar patterns. It is also worth pointing out that increased noise often accompanies the spatial resolution improvement. Similar clinical examples are given in Figure 9-9, where a lung scan was reconstructed with a standard (*A*) and a lung kernel (*B*).

Another parameter that affects the spatial resolution is the reconstruction **field of view (FOV).** On the basis of the Nyquist sampling theory (to fully reproduce the original signal, the sampling frequency needs to be at least twice the highest frequency present in the signal), the sampling interval **(pixel size)** has to be sufficiently small to support the reconstruction and visualization of small objects. The **pixel** size is related to the reconstruction FOV by the following equation:

$$\text{Pixel size} = \frac{\text{FOV}}{\text{Matrix size}} \quad \textbf{(9-1)}$$

The reconstruction FOV, sometimes called the display FOV or DFOV, refers to the diameter of the reconstructed area in millimeters or centimeters covered by the image. This is different from the scan FOV, which refers the *maximum* size that a scanner

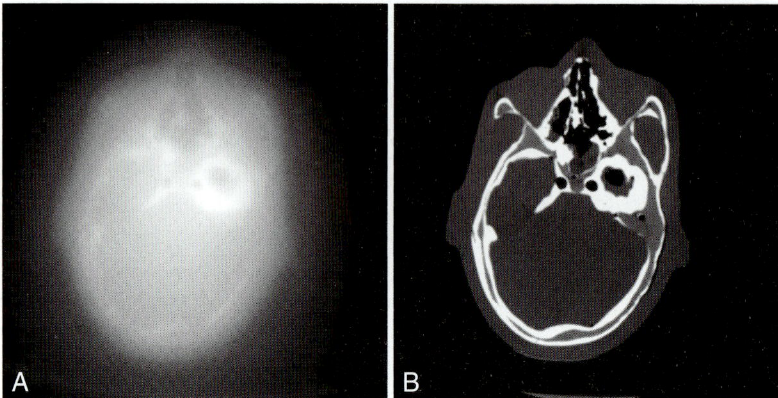


**FIGURE 9-7** Images of a head phantom to illustrate the impact of the convolution process. **A,** Reconstructed with back-projection only. **B,** Reconstructed with filtered back-projection.

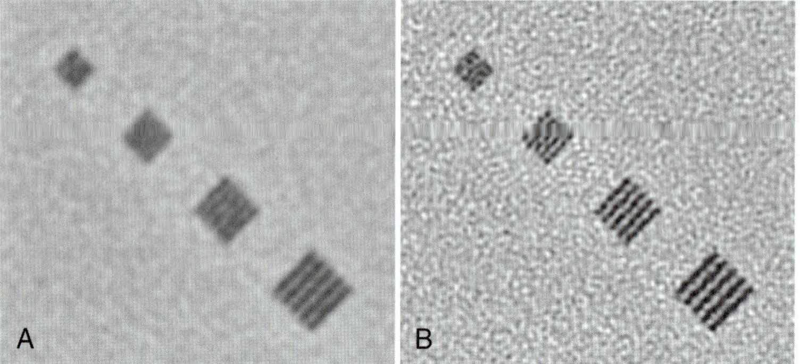


**FIGURE 9-8** Impact of the selection of reconstruction kernel on spatial resolution. **A,** Reconstructed with a standard kernel. **B,** Reconstructed with a bone kernel.

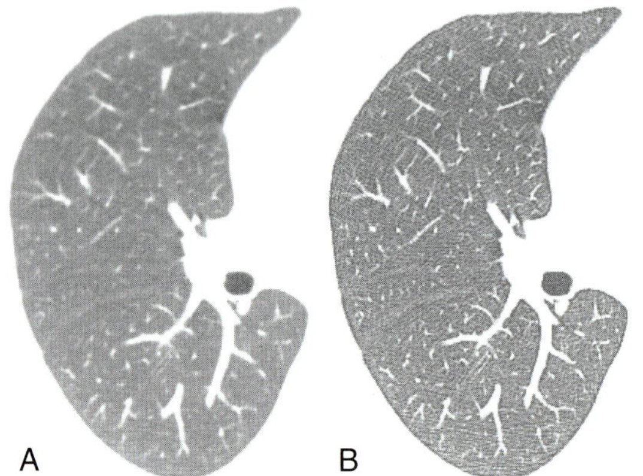


**FIGURE 9-9** A patient chest scan reconstructed with different kernels. **A,** Standard algorithm. **B,** Lung algorithm.

is *capable* of covering. For a 50-cm reconstruction FOV at a **matrix** size of 512 × 512, the pixel size is 0.98 mm (500 mm/512), and if the FOV is reduced to 10 cm, the pixel size is 0.20 mm. (This is often referred to as targeting.) To illustrate the impact of pixel size, Figure 9-10 depicts images reconstructed with the same projection dataset at two different FOVs. Figure 9-10, *A* and *B*, was reconstructed with a 50-cm FOV. The reconstructed image was then interpolated in image space to a 10-cm FOV to produce Figure 9-10, *B*. Figure 9-10, *C*, was reconstructed directly to 10-cm FOV. Note that for the 10-cm target-reconstructed image, all bar patterns are clearly visible, whereas even the fourth largest bar pattern is barely visible for the reconstructed images with 50-cm FOV.

## Cross-Plane Spatial Resolution

The introduction of helical/spiral and multislice/volumetric CT has fundamentally changed the way many radiologists **view** CT images. Historically, CT images were always viewed one slice at a time. New technologies have enabled radiologists to view images in three dimensions by using multiplanar reformat (MPR), **maximum intensity projection (MIP),** or **volume rendering** (VR). An example is shown in Figure 9-11, where a coronal view of a patient study is displayed. It is difficult to tell from the image alone whether the data were acquired

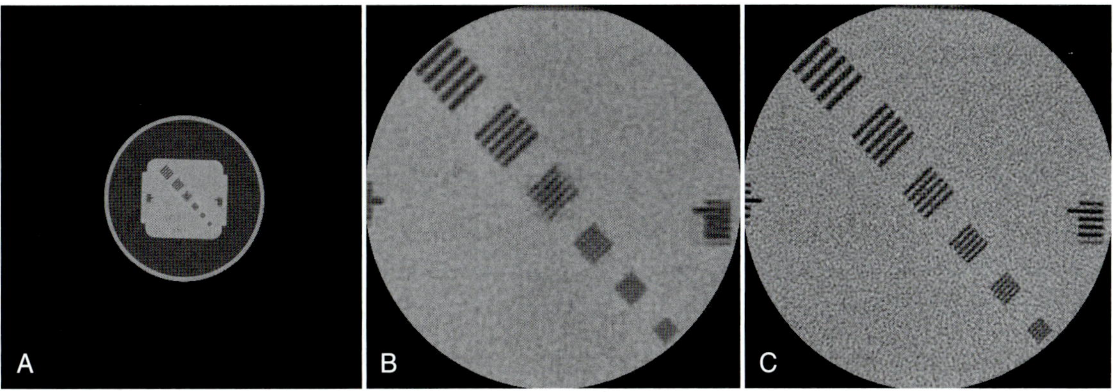


**FIGURE 9-10** Images reconstructed with different FOVs. **A,** Reconstructed with 50-cm FOV. **B,** Reconstructed with 50-cm FOV and interpolated to 10-cm FOV. **C,** Targeted reconstruction to 10-cm FOV.

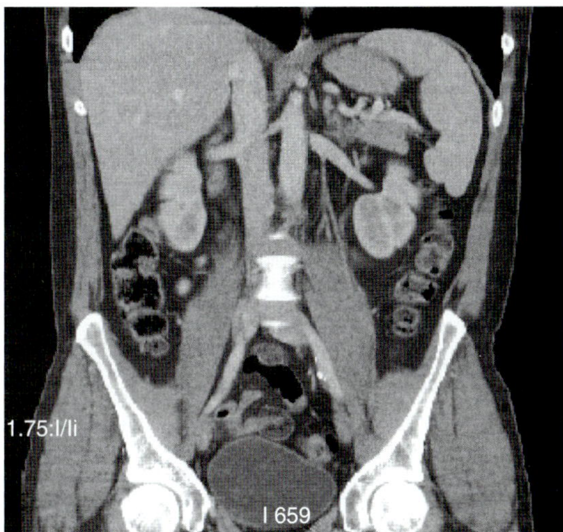


**FIGURE 9-11** Coronal view of a patient study scanned on a LightSpeed scanner.

slice by slice or directly in the coronal plane. This demonstrates that the spatial resolution of the state-of-the-art scanner is nearly **isotropic.** That is, the spatial resolution is roughly the same in all directions.

Improved cross-plane spatial resolution also reduces artifacts caused by partial volume averaging (detailed discussions will be provided in the Image Artifact section). Figure 9-12 presents a comparison of the spatial resolution afforded by two slices of different thicknesses. Thin-slice imaging of lung "is currently the most accurate noninvasive tool for evaluation of lung structure" (Mayo, 1991).

Cross-plane spatial resolution is traditionally described by the **slice sensitivity profile (SSP).** Similar to the in-plane resolution, SSP represents the system response to a Dirac delta function and is typically graphed as intensity vs. location (in $z$). The full-width at half-maximum (FWHM) of SSP is often referred to as the slice thickness. In practice, the Dirac delta function is often approximated by an object whose thickness is significantly smaller than the slice thickness of the system. For example, researchers use a small bead or a thin disk to perform SSP measurement. The disk is placed perpendicular to the **z-axis** and a series of scans are collected to construct the SSP. In many cases, the SSP curve itself is replaced by two numbers: the **full-width at half-maximum (FWHM)** and the **full-width at tenth-maximum (FWTM).** Definitions of FWHM and FWTM are illustrated in Figure 9-13, where FWHM represents the **distance** between two points on the SSP curve whose intensity is 50% of the peak and FWTM represents the distance between two points on the SSP whose intensity is 10% of the peak.

A more convenient method of measuring SSP is to use a shallow-angled slice ramp (Goodenough et al., 1977; Hsieh, 2001). A wire or thin strip is placed at a shallow angle with respect to the $x$-$y$ plane. During the scan, the line or thin strip is projected onto the $x$-$y$ plane, as shown in Figure 9-14. On the basis of simple trigonometry, the SSP in $z$ is magnified by a factor, $1/\tan(\theta)$, where $\theta$ is the angle of the strip formed with the $x$-$y$ plane. When $\theta$ is small, the magnification factor is large. For example, Catphan phantom uses a 23-degree ramp to produce a 2.4-fold enlargement in the measured SSP. Therefore, the FWHM of the system, $Z_{FWHM}$, can be calculated from the FWHM measurement of the wire in the reconstructed image, $W_{FWHM}$, by the following:

$$Z_{FWHM} = \frac{W_{FWHM}}{2.4} \tag{9-2}$$

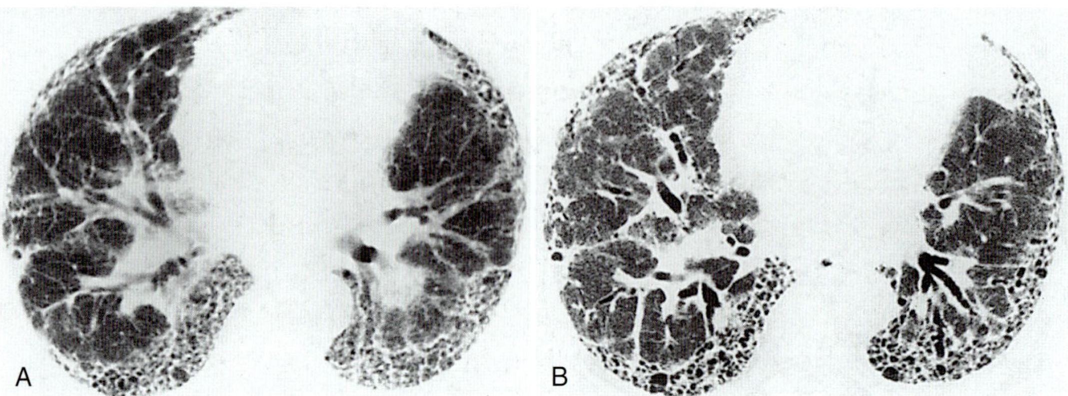


**FIGURE 9-12** Comparison of the degree of spatial resolution of slices with two different thicknesses. The spatial resolution of the thinner slice **(B)** taken with 1.5-mm collimation is apparent when compared with the image of the slice taken with 10-mm collimation **(A)**. (From Mayo, J. R., (1991). *Radiology Clinics of North America, 29,* 1043-1048.)

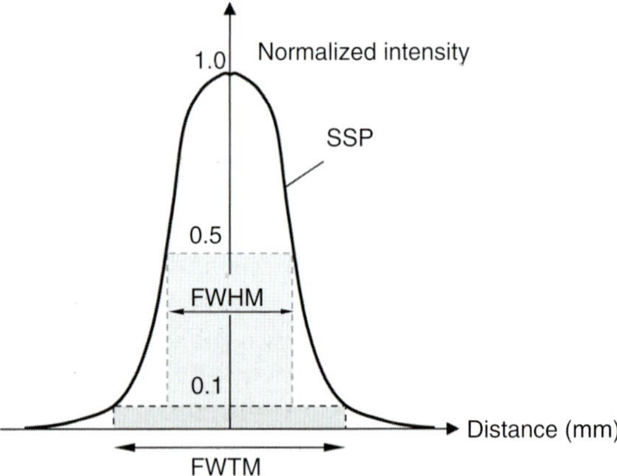


**FIGURE 9-13** Illustration of FWHM and FWTM. FWHM represents the distance between two points on the SSP curve whose intensity is 50% of the peak. FWTM represents the distance between two points on the SSP whose intensity is 10% of the peak.

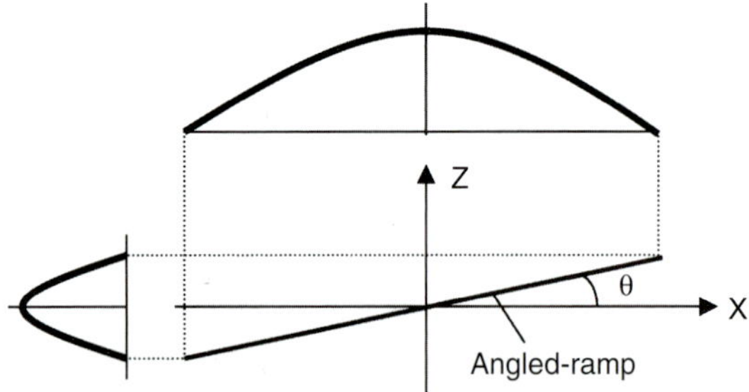


**FIGURE 9-14** Illustration of measurement of slice-sensitivity profile by a shallow-angled slice ramp. The slice ramp is projected onto the *x-y* plane during reconstruction. A magnified version of the SSP is produced.

Figure 9-15 shows a GE Performance Phantom scanned with a 5-mm and a 10-mm detector aperture in step-and-shoot mode. It is clear from the figure that the image of the slice ramp is twice as wide at 10 mm, indicating a linear relationship between the width of the reconstructed wire and the thickness of the slice. It is also clear that a significant reduction in contrast is observed at 10 mm as a result of the partial volume effect.

It should be noted that once the SSP is obtained, MTF can be calculated straightforwardly by taking the Fourier transform of the SSP. As the spatial resolutions in all orientations become isotropic, it is more convenient and reasonable to specify both the in-plane and cross-plane resolution in a similar fashion, such as MTF.

## LOW-CONTRAST RESOLUTION

### Definition and Measurements

One of the key advantages of CT over conventional radiography is its ability to observe low-contrast objects whose density is slightly different from the background. In CT, this is sometimes referred to as the **sensitivity** *of the system* (Hounsfield, 1978). To understand **low-contrast resolution,** consider three tissues of different densities and atomic number (*Z*), as shown in Figure 9-16. If these tissues were imaged by conventional radiography, the obtained image would have shown good contrast between bone and soft tissue (muscle and fat) only. The values of the density and *Z* for muscle and fat are too close to be clearly distinguished by radiography, and they appear as "soft tissue shadows." The contrast between bone with a *Z* of 13.8 and soft tissue with a *Z* of 7.4 is apparent because of

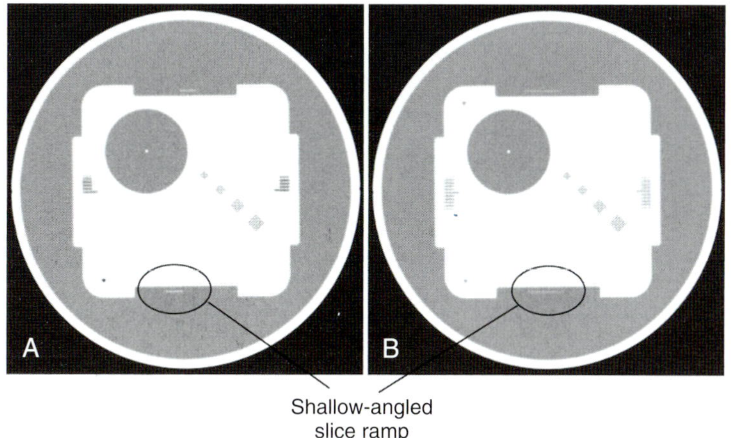


**FIGURE 9-15** Illustration of the use of slice ramp to measure SSP. **A,** Acquired with 5-mm slice thickness in step-and-shoot mode. **B,** Acquired with 10-mm slice thickness in step-and-shoot mode.

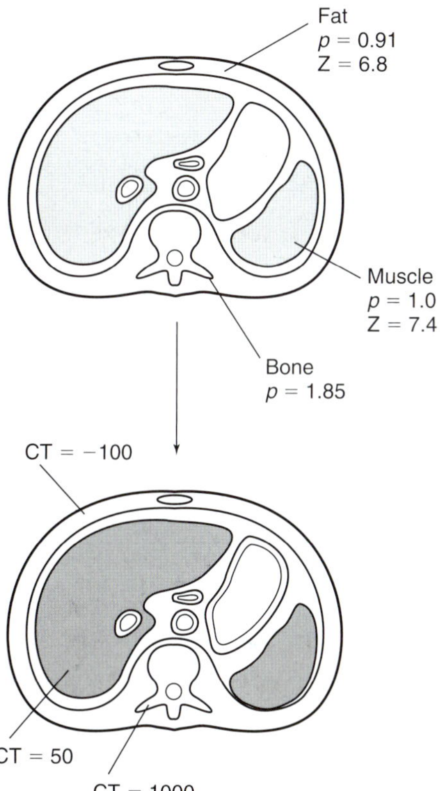


**FIGURE 9-16** Densities (*p*) and atomic numbers (*Z*) for three types of tissue. When they are imaged by CT, excellent low-contrast resolution is obtained. (From Bushong, S. (2009). *Radiologic science for technologists* (9th ed.). St. Louis, MO: Mosby.)

the significant difference between the densities and *Z* of these two tissues. CT, on the other hand, can image tissues that vary only slightly in density and atomic number. Although radiography can discriminate a density difference of approximately 10% (Curry et al., 1990), CT can detect density differences from 0.25% to 0.5%, depending on the scanner (Hsieh, 2009).

Low-contrast resolution can be measured with phantoms that contain low-contrast objects of different sizes. The low-contrast performance or low-contrast detectability (LCD) of the scanner is typically defined as the smallest object that can be visualized at a given contrast level and dose. Figure 9-17 shows the low-contrast portion of a Catphan (The Phantom Laboratory, Salem, New York, USA). This phantom has been used extensively by the physicist community to perform quality assurance tests of CT scanners. There are three sets of disks with contrasts of 0.3%, 0.5%, and 1.0%, and the sizes of the disks are 2 mm, 3 mm, 4 mm, 5 mm, 6 mm, 7 mm, 8 mm, 9 mm, and 15 mm. In CT, the contrast level is specified in terms of the percentage CT number difference between the object and the background relative to the CT number difference between the background and air. A 1% contrast means that the mean CT number of the object differs from its background by 10 Hounsfield units (HU).

## Factors That Affect Low-Contrast Detectability

From the definition of LCD, it can easily be concluded that the visibility of an object depends on its size and on its contrast (intensity difference) to the background. This is easily demonstrated with the Catphan. Note that the three sets of objects are of matching sizes. The disks located from the 10 o'clock to 2 o'clock **positions** are more easily visualized than those located from the 2 o'clock to 6 o'clock positions. The difference in contrast between these two sets is 7 HU. Figure 9-17 also illustrates the impact of the object size on the LCD. As the object size decreases,

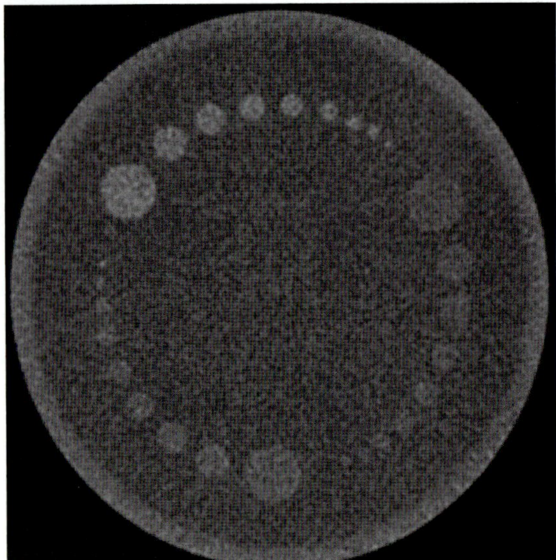

**FIGURE 9-17** Image of a low-contrast portion of the Catphan phantom.

the confidence level of identifying a 0.3% contrast disk decreases.

The LCD definition also implies that an object's visibility is highly influenced by the presence of noise. To demonstrate this effect, the low-contrast portion of a GE Performance Phantom was scanned with two different tube currents, 200 mA and 50 mA, while all other acquisition parameters were kept the same; the reconstructed images are shown in Figure 9-18. The noise for the 50-mA scan is a factor of two higher compared with the 200-mA case (one fourth of the dose). For the 200-mA scan, all four low-density holes are clearly identifiable, whereas the smallest hole is obscured by the noise for the 50-mA scan.

Many factors affect the noise level in the reconstructed images. Some of them can be controlled by the operator, and others are outside the operator's reach. The parameters under operator control include x-ray tube voltage (in kV), tube current (in mA), scan speed (in seconds), helical pitch, slice thickness, and, more recently, the use of IR algorithms. The selection of the parameters, however, is not straightforward. For example, by increasing the tube current, a noise reduction and better LCD can be achieved. However, increased tube current translates to a higher dose to the patient (linear relationship) and, potentially, runs the risk of a tube cooling (forced delay during scans to prevent the tube from overheating). Similarly, although the use of a higher tube voltage (kV) results in improved x-ray photon statistics (therefore lower noise in the image), the quality of the x-ray beam is somewhat compromised because the visibility of low-contrast objects depends on the presence of low-energy photons, which are disproportionally less for the higher tube voltage. Consequently, LCD may be degraded with an increased kV. The same applies to the selection of slice thickness. Although an image with a thicker slice generally contains more x-ray photons (less noise), the partial volume effect can reduce the visibility of smaller objects. This is illustrated in Figure 9-19, where the low-contrast portion of the GE Performance Phantom was reconstructed with 3.75-mm and 7.5-mm slice thickness. Because the phantom is made of a thin plate (less than 1 mm in thickness), a thicker slice produces a larger partial volume effect and reduces the contrast of the object. As a result, although the noise is reduced with the 7.5-mm thickness, the LCD of the low-density objects is actually reduced.

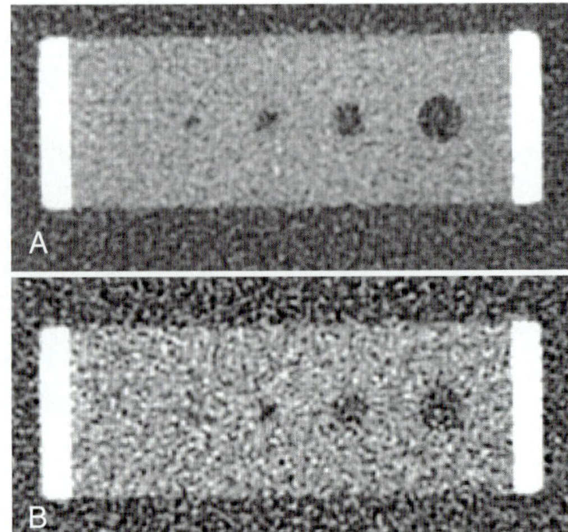


**FIGURE 9-18** Illustration of the impact of noise to low-contrast detectability. **A,** Acquired with 200 mA and standard algorithm. **B,** Acquired with 50 mA and standard algorithm.

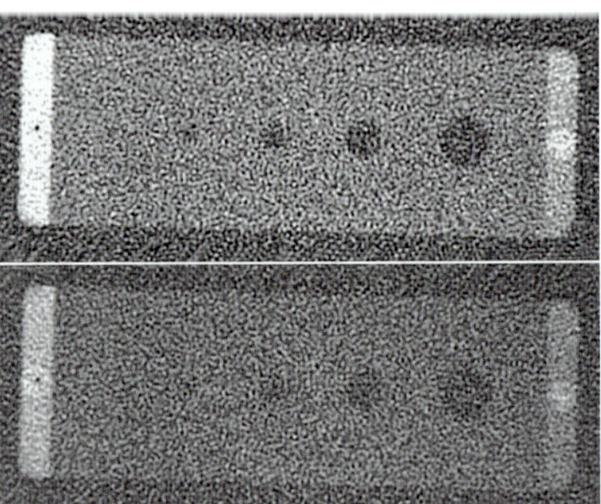

**FIGURE 9-19** Illustration of the impact of slice thickness, at 3.75 mm (*top*) and 7.5 mm (*bottom*).

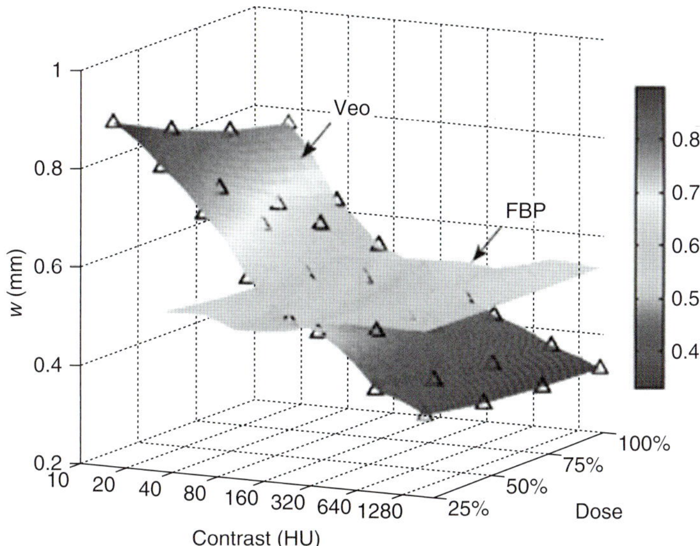


**FIGURE 9-20** Illustration of the contrast, dose-dependence of the figure-of-merit spatial resolution (*w*). (Figure courtesy GuangHong Chen, printed with permission.)

In recent years, a variety of IR algorithms was introduced to commercial CT products. Given the large amount of literature on the subject, a review article is provided for reference (Hsieh et al., 2013). The goal of the IR algorithms, in general, is to reduce the noise in the reconstructed images while maintaining the CT number accuracies and the contrast of the reconstructed objects. The reduced noise can translate to a reduction in radiation dose while maintaining the same image quality. What makes the situation more complex is the nonlinear behavior of IR algorithms relative to the dose and noise. Unlike the linear relationship between dose and variance (noise) in the **filtered back-projection (FBP)** reconstructed images when noise is dominated by the x-ray photon statistics, such a relationship often does not exist for IR algorithms. The behavioral difference between FBP and IR is not limited to dose versus variance (noise). For example, a recent study showed that the spatial resolution of the IR reconstructed image can be contrast- and dose-dependent, while the spatial resolution of FBP is contrast- and dose-independent, as shown in Figure 9-20 (Li, 2014).

## TEMPORAL RESOLUTION

**Temporal resolution** is an indication of a CT system's ability to freeze motion of the scanned object. An oversimplified analogy is the "shutter" speed of a camera. When a photo is taken at a sports event, a higher shutter speed should be used to reduce the blurring effects caused by the moving athletes. The awareness and importance of the temporal resolution for CT scanners has increased significantly in recent years thanks to an increased clinical utility of cardiac imaging. Because the heart motion is continuous and often irregular, cardiac imaging is one of the most challenging clinical applications for CT.

### Factors That Affect Temporal Resolution

There are several methods that improve a CT scanner's ability to freeze cardiac motion. The most straightforward way to reduce or eliminate the motion impact is to increase the scan speed. The state-of-the-art third-generation multislice scanners are capable of rotating at speeds of less than 0.3 seconds per **gantry** rotation. Considering the size of a typical CT gantry (1 m), and the weight of the components on the rotating side (hundreds of pounds), the centrifugal force is huge. One attempt to overcome the mechanical difficulty is to use an electron-beam scanner in which high-speed electrons are deflected by the specially designed magnetic field so that x-ray photons are generated along an arc surrounding the patient. Because there is no moving part for this scanner, scan speeds as high as 33 ms can be achieved.

Even at the speed of 33 ms, it is insufficient to completely freeze the cardiac motion. Therefore all third-generation CT scanners also rely on reconstruction algorithms that use less than a full rotation of projection data for reconstruction. The most commonly used algorithm is the so-called half-scan algorithm in which the projection dataset in the view range of 180 degrees plus fan angle are used (Parker, 1982). For typical CT scanner geometries, this represents a 220-degree, or approximately 40%, improvement in terms of temporal resolution. To further improve the temporal resolution of the scanner, multisector reconstruction is also used in which the 220 degrees of projection data are acquired over multiple cardiac cycles (Hsieh, 2009). Typically, the dataset is uniformly divided over the heart cycles to optimize the performance. For a two-sector reconstruction, for example, only slightly over 110 degrees of projections are collected over a single cardiac cycle. This type of approach relies on the repeatability of heart motion from cycle to cycle. To overcome this constraint, dual-source CT scanners was introduced in recent years where two sets of tube-detector pair, offset roughly by 90-degrees, are mounted on a single gantry (Petersilka, 2008). When the gantry rotates slightly over a quarter of a rotation, the combined data cover the required half-scan range and enable image reconstruction over a single cardiac cycle. Because of the limited scope of this chapter, the details are not discussed.

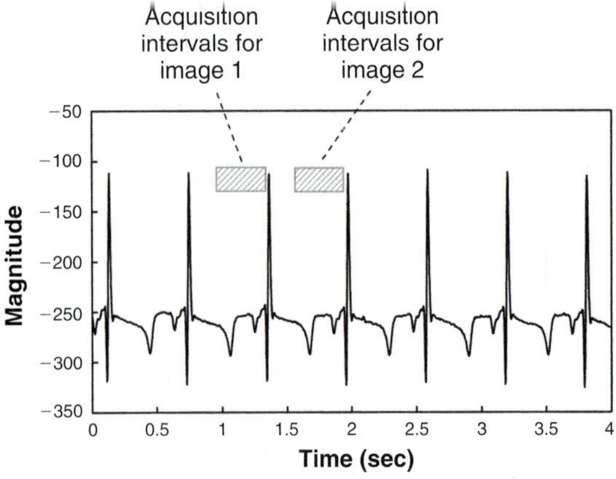


**FIGURE 9-21** Illustration of ECG-gated acquisition.

## Techniques to Reduce Motion Impact

A technique used by all CT vendors incorporates a physiological gating device for cardiac imaging (Hsieh et al., 1999; Kachelriess et al., 2000). Although this approach does not improve the temporal resolution of the scanner, it helps to minimize the heart motion. In a typical cardiac cycle, there are quiescent time periods in which the heart is in a relatively motionless state. These correspond to the diastole and systole phases of the heart. If the **data acquisition** takes place during these time periods, fewer motion artifacts can be expected. This is often accomplished by synchronizing the data acquisition and reconstruction with an electrocardiographic (ECG) signal, either retrospectively or prospectively, as shown in Figure 9-21. The advantage of a prospective gating is the reduction in x-ray dose to the patient, since the x-ray tube can be shut off during the non–data-acquisition periods to minimize the x-ray **exposure.** The disadvantage of the prospective gating is its reliance on the regularity of the heart motion because the data acquisition timing for the current cardiac cycle has to be predicted on the basis of previous heart cycles. For compromise, automatic exposure control is often used in practice in which the x-ray tube current is reduced to a fraction of the peak current during the nonquiescent time periods to provide a balance between patient dose and robustness. To illustrate the impact of ECG gating, Figure 9-22 depicts two reconstructed cardiac images, with

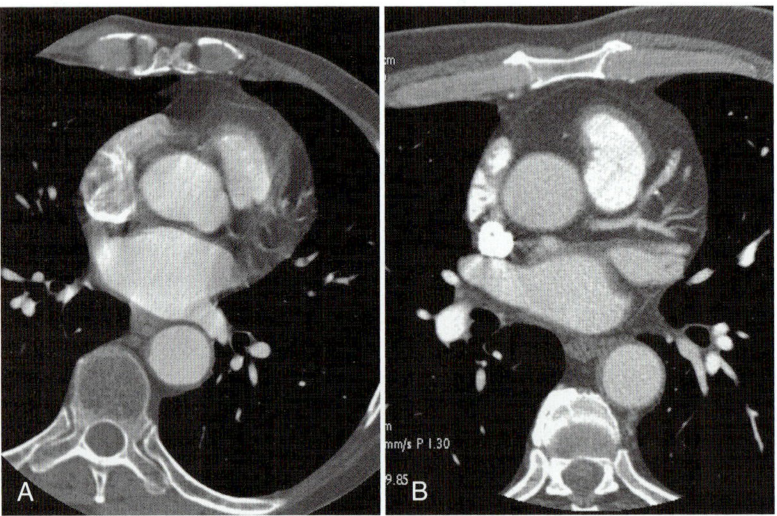


**FIGURE 9-22** Impact of ECG gating in cardiac imaging. **A,** Nongated cardiac acquisition. **B,** ECG-gated acquisition.

and without the proper ECG gating. Motion artifact reduction with ECG gating is obvious.

For cardiac imaging, there is another important factor that affects the image quality: coverage. Note that not all commercially available CT scanners can cover the entire heart (12 cm to 16 cm) in a single rotation. Consequently, the heart volume is often scanned over multiple heart cycles, with each cycle covering a subsection of the heart. Superb temporal resolution only ensures that within each subsection the motion-induced image degradation is kept to a minimum. It does not guarantee, however, that the heart is in exactly the same state from one subsection to the next and the contrast enhancement level is consistent among all subsections. Studies have shown that the probability of a stable heart rate decreases quickly as the total data acquisition time increases. The total data acquisition time is determined by the gantry speed, helical pitch, and detector coverage. For the same gantry speed and helical pitch, a larger detector coverage translates to a faster study time and, in turn, an improved probability of a consistent cardiac volume. Figure 9-23, *A*, shows a reformatted image of a heart vessel with phase misregistration. The vessel looks discontinuous and can lead to misdiagnosis. When a heart is scanned on a state-of-the-art CT system with 16 cm *z*-coverage, misregistration is completely eliminated, since the entire heart is imaged in a single cardiac cycle, as shown in Figure 9-23, *B*.

Recently, advanced reconstruction algorithms have been utilized to combat motion artifact in cardiac imaging (Bhagalia et al., 2012; Isola et al., 2010; Taguchi et al., 2007). Some of the algorithms rely on segmenting the coronary arteries in the initial seed images reconstructed with the conventional methods, estimating the motion based on the arteries, and compensating for the motion in either projection space or image space. Projection-space algorithms work exclusively on the measured projections prior to the image reconstruction, while image-space algorithms work only on the reconstructed images. When combined with the advanced CT **hardware** design this algorithm can produce reliable results, even under unstable heart rate conditions (Fig. 9-24).

## CT NUMBER ACCURACY AND UNIFORMITY

### Accuracy and Linearity

The CT number is related to the **attenuation** coefficient of the object, $\mu$, by the following equation:

$$\text{CT number} = \frac{\mu - \mu_w}{\mu_w} \times 1000 \qquad \textbf{(9-3)}$$

where $\mu_w$ is the attenuation coefficient of water. On the basis of this definition, two points are defined precisely on the CT number scale. The first is water with a CT number of 0 and the second is air with a CT number of −1000. Because water is similar to the soft tissue in terms of attenuation characteristics, it is important to establish its accuracy for CT scanners.

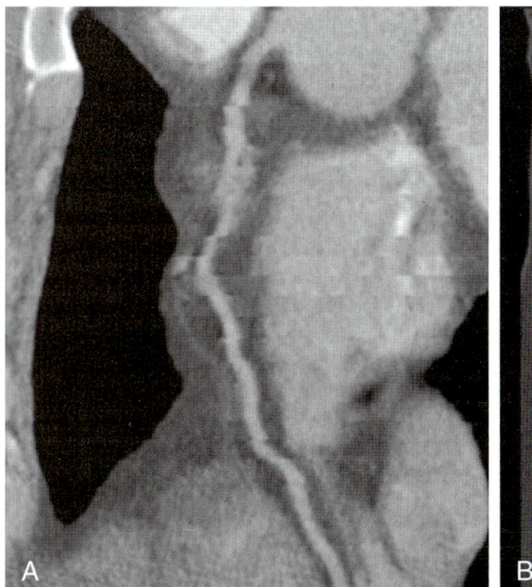


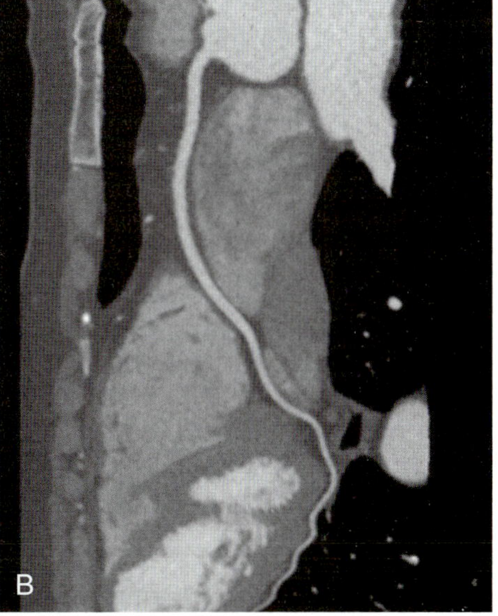


**FIGURE 9-23** **A,** Illustration of phase misregistration in cardiac imaging. **B,** Illustration of a cardiac scan performed on a 16cm detector system where misregistration is completely eliminated.

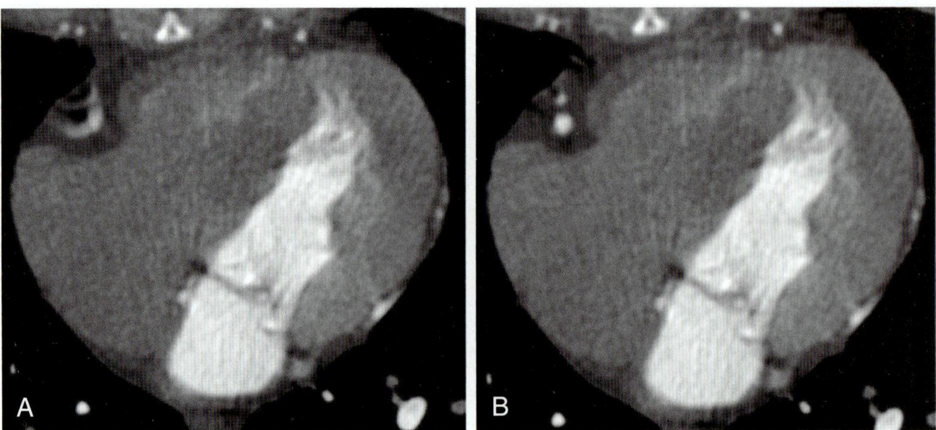


**FIGURE 9-24** Clinical images of a cardiac study. **A,** Original image. **B,** With a motion-correction algorithm.

**TABLE 9-1 Characteristics of the American Association of Physicists in Medicine Computed Tomography Phantom**

| Material | Density (g/ml) | Linear Attenuation Coefficient ($cm^{-1}$) at 60 keV | Approximate CT Number |
|---|---|---|---|
| Polyethylene, $C_2H_4$ | 0.94 | 0.185 | −85 |
| Polystyrene, $C_8H_8$ | 1.05 | 0.196 | −10 |
| Nylon, $C_6H_{11}NO$ | 1.15 | 0.222 | 100 |
| Lexan, $C_{16}H_{14}O$ | 1.20 | 0.223 | 115 |
| Plexiglas, $C_5H_8O_2$ | 1.19 | 0.229 | 130 |
| Water, $H_2O$ | 1.00 | 0.206 | 0 |

Modified from Bushong, S. (2009). *Radiologic science for technologists* (9th ed.). St. Louis, MO: Mosby.

Nearly all CT manufacturers provide phantoms filled with water for this type of testing. When the phantom is scanned, the average CT number in the water portion should be fairly close to 0.

Linearity is another important parameter in CT image quality. **Linearity** refers to the linear relationship of **CT numbers** to the **linear attenuation coefficients** of the object to be imaged. This can be checked by a daily calibration test, during which an appropriate phantom is scanned to ensure that the CT numbers for water and other known materials are correct. These phantom characteristics are listed in Table 9-1. Figure 9-25 depicts a linearity section of the Catphan with the large cylinders filled with Teflon, Delrin, acrylic, polystyrene, air, polymethylpentene, and low-density polyethylene. The CT numbers of the reconstructed cylinders are used to determine the acceptance of the CT system. The average CT numbers can also be plotted as a function of the attenuation coefficients of the phantom materials. The relationship should be a straight line (Fig. 9-26) if the scanner is in good working order (Bushong, 1997).

CT number accuracy, or more precisely the accuracy of the reconstructed image values, has an increased level of importance with the introduction of dual-energy (DE) imaging. Although the concept of DECT was introduced soon after the installation of the very first CT scanner (Hounsfield, 1973), its clinical utility is available only recently thanks to significant advancements in CT hardware. One of the key advantages of DECT is its ability to perform material decomposition (Chandra et al., 2011; McCollough et al., 2011; Thorsten et al., 2011). In DECT, each object is scanned with two different x-ray tube potentials (e.g., 80 kVp and 140 kVp). When ignoring the k-edge effect, the attenuation coefficient of any material can be expressed as the linear combination of the attenuation coefficients of the "basis-material" pairs, such as water and iodine. The process to map from the projection data collected under different kVps to the projection data representing the equivalent densities of the basis-material is often called material decomposition (Hsieh 2009). The reconstruction of the basis-material density images allows CT

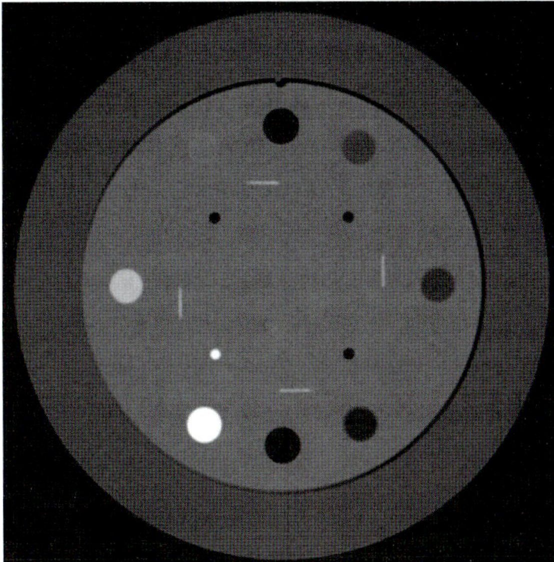

**FIGURE 9-25** Linearity insert of the Catphan. The eight larger cylinders are filled with Teflon, Delrin, acrylic, polystyrene, air, PMP, and LDPE.

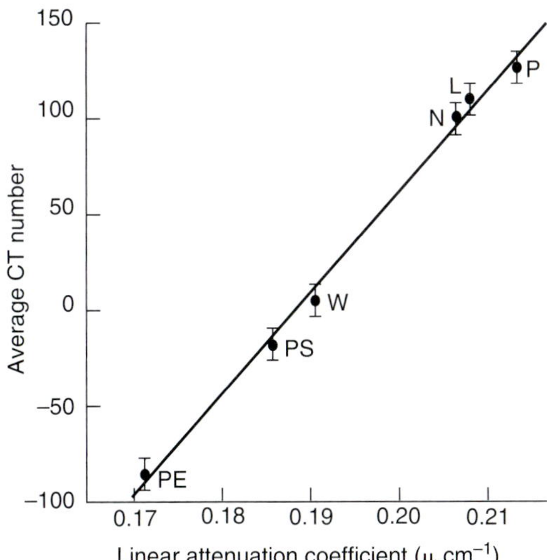


**FIGURE 9-26** Plot of average CT numbers as a function of linear attenuation coefficients. This indicates acceptable CT linearity if the relationship is a straight line. (From Bushong, S. (2009). *Radiologic science for technologists* (9th ed.). St. Louis, MO: Mosby.)

to differentiate materials that may appear to be the same under conventional CT imaging, such as different types of kidney stones. The accuracy of the material differentiation, of course, depends on the accuracy of the reconstructed basis-material densities. This accuracy can be significantly impacted by many factors, such as beam hardening and scatter. Therefore, proper compensation of nonideal conditions of CT scans is crucial. DECT application to identify different types of tumors based on their contrast uptake characteristics is seen in Figure 9-27.

### Uniformity

CT number uniformity dictates that for a uniform phantom, the CT number measurement should not change with the location of the selected regions of interest (ROIs) or with the phantom position relative to the isocenter of the scanner. A reconstructed 20-cm water phantom is seen in Figure 9-28. Theoretically, the average CT numbers in two ROI locations should be identical. Because of the effect of beam hardening, scatter, **stability** of the CT system, and many other factors, the CT number uniformity can only be maintained within a reasonable range (typically a few HUs). As long as the operator understands the system limitations (based on system specifications or phantom testing results) and the factors that influence the performance, he or she can avoid the potential pitfalls of using absolute CT numbers for diagnosis.

## NOISE

### Measurements

On the basis of the discussion on LCD, the importance of image noise is obvious. **Image noise** is measured typically on uniform phantoms. To perform noise measurement, the standard deviation, σ, within

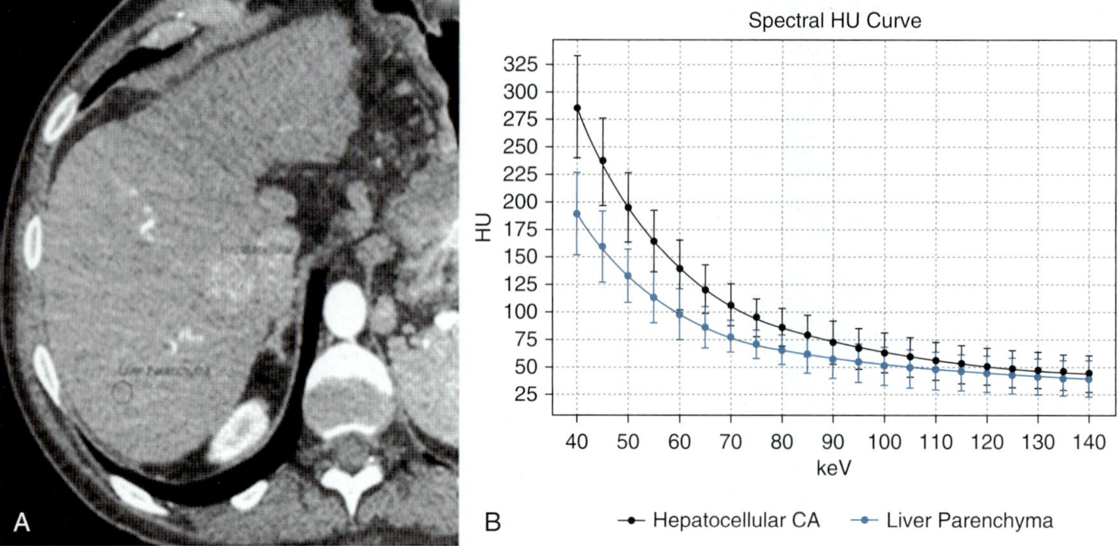


**FIGURE 9-27** Clinical example of a liver tumor **(A)** monochromatic image at 65keV **(B)** spectral curves of two ROIs. Blue, background tissue curve; Black, tumor tissue curve.

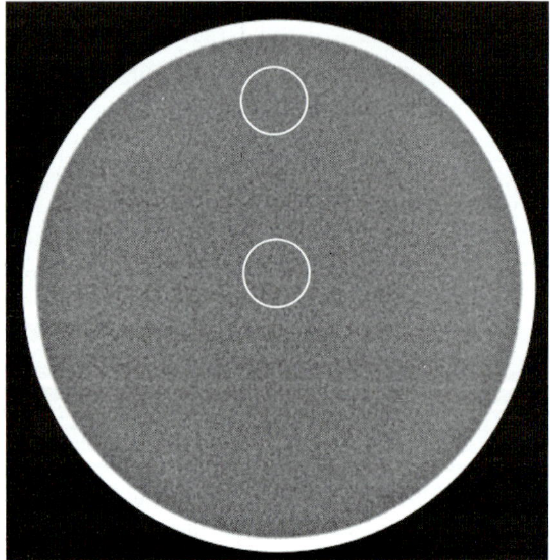

**FIGURE 9-28** Water phantom for CT number uniformity measurement.

an ROI of the reconstructed image, $f(i, j)$, is calculated as follows:

$$\delta = \sqrt{\frac{\sum_{i,j \in \text{ROI}} \left[ f(i,j) - \bar{f} \right]^2}{N-1}} \tag{9-4}$$

where $i$ and $j$ are indices of the 2D image, $N$ is the total number of pixels inside the ROI, and $\bar{f}$ is the average pixel intensity and is calculated by the following equation:

$$\bar{f} = \frac{1}{N} \sum_{i,j \in \text{ROI}} f(i,j) \tag{9-5}$$

In both equations, the summation is 2D over the ROI. Note that most CT scanners provide tools to calculate the standard deviation over the ROI defined by the operator, and rarely require the operator to perform calculations based on the above equations. For robustness, several ROIs are often used and the average value of the measured standard deviations is reported.

## Noise Sources

Three major sources contribute to the noise in the image. The first source is the quantum noise determined by the x-ray flux or the number of detected x-ray photons. It is influenced by the scanning techniques (e.g., x-ray tube voltage, tube current, slice thickness, scan speed, helical pitch), the scanner **efficiency** (e.g., detector quantum efficiency, detector geometrical efficiency, amber-penumbra ratio), and patient (e.g., patient size, amount of bones and soft tissues in the scanning plane). The scanning technique dictates the number of x-ray photons that reach the patient, and the scanner efficiency determines the percentage of the x-ray photons exiting the patient that are converted to useful signals. The LCD section briefly discusses

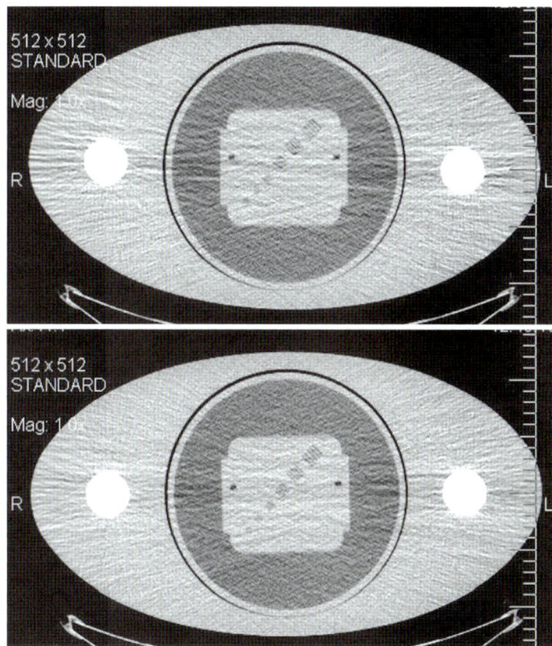


**FIGURE 9-29** Illustration of DAS noise impact. *Top*, Old vintage DAS; *bottom*, new low-noise DAS.

the trade-offs of different acquisition parameters. As long as the trade-offs are well understood, these options can be used effectively to combat noise. More advanced scanners offer features that allow the operator to select a noise level, and the CT system will determine the x-ray tube current required to achieve a specified noise level. Because the patient anatomy changes with location, the x-ray tube current typically changes as a function of tube angle as well as the location along the patient long axis.

The second source that influences the noise performance is the inherent physical limitations of the system. These include the electronic noise in the detector photodiode, the electronic noise in the **data acquisition system (DAS),** scattered radiation, and many other factors. Figure 9-29 shows an oval phantom scanned with two different DASs while all other acquisition parameters were kept constant. Significant reduction in image noise can be observed with the lower noise DAS.

The third noise-influencing factor is the reconstruction parameters. In general, a high-resolution reconstruction kernel produces an increased noise level, since this kernel preserves or enhances high-frequency contents in the projection. Unfortunately, most noise presents itself as high-frequency signals and is enhanced at the same time. An example of the noise impact of filter kernel selection for an FBP algorithm is shown in Figure 9-8. Note that the noise level of Figure 9-8, *B*, is significantly higher than that of Figure 9-8, *A*.

### Noise Power Spectrum

It should be pointed out that standard deviation alone is insufficient to fully characterize the noise in the image, since noise in the reconstructed images is no longer white. This characteristic can be described by the noise power spectrum (NPS), or Wiener spectrum (Riederer et al., 1978). The NPS is obtained with the Fourier transform to break down the image noise into its frequency components as illustrated in Figure. 9-30. To demonstrate the impact of noise spectrum on the image, Figure 9-31 shows a low-contrast phantom scanned with different tube currents and reconstructed with different kernels, one with the standard kernel and the other with the bone kernel. The tube currents were selected so that both images have the same standard deviation. However, the visibility of the low-contrast objects is clearly different. This example demonstrates nicely that to fully characterize the noise in the image standard deviation alone is insufficient.

## IMAGE ARTIFACT

### Definition and General Discussion

Artifacts can degrade image quality, affect the perceptibility of detail, or even lead to misdiagnosis. They can cause serious problems for the radiologist who has to provide a diagnosis from images obtained by the CT scanner. Therefore it is mandatory that the technologist understand the nature of artifacts in CT.

In general, an **artifact** is "a distortion or error in an image that is unrelated to the subject being studied" (Morgan, 1983). Specifically, a *CT image artifact* is defined as "any discrepancy between the reconstructed CT numbers in the image and the true attenuation coefficients of the object" (Hsieh, 1995). This definition is comprehensive and implies that anything that causes an incorrect measurement of transmission readings by the detectors or an inconsistency between the measurement and reconstruction will result in an image artifact. Because CT numbers represent gray shades in the image, incorrect measurements will produce incorrect CT numbers that do not represent the attenuation coefficients of the object. These errors result in various artifacts that affect the appearance of the CT image.

In CT, artifacts arise from a number of sources, including the patient, inappropriate selection of protocols, reconstruction process, problems relating to the equipment such as malfunctions or imperfections,

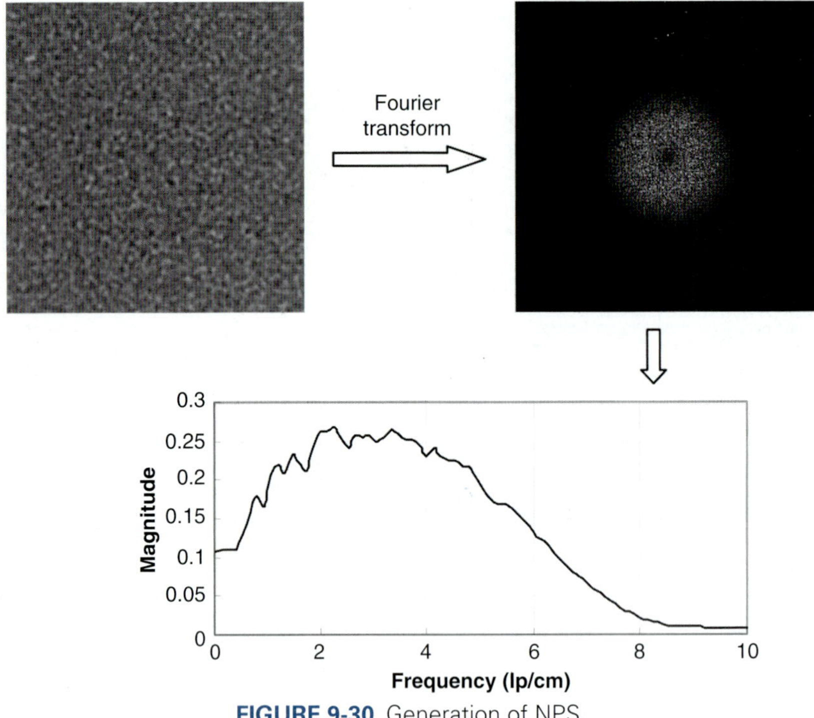

**FIGURE 9-30** Generation of NPS.

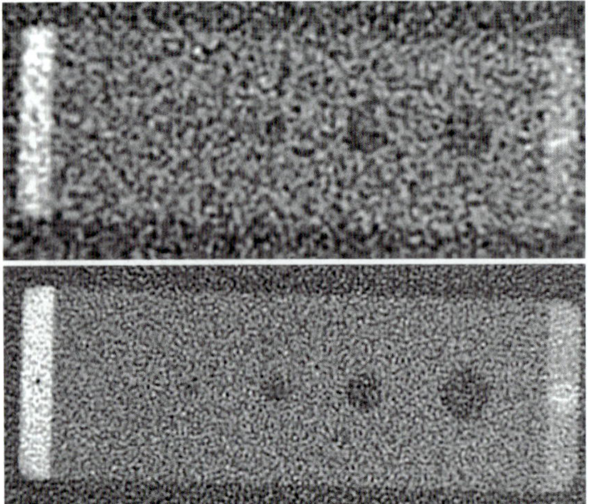
**FIGURE 9-31** Illustration of NPS impact. Both images have identical standard deviations.

and fundamental limitation of physics. In a typical commercial CT system, an image is reconstructed from more than one million independent projection samples. The contribution of each projection reading, on the other hand, is not limited to an isolated point in the reconstructed image as a result of the convolution and back-projection process discussed in Chapter 5. This is a radical departure from conventional radiographic imaging, in which each measured sample affects only the value of a single pixel in the resulting image. As a result, the probability of an artifact for CT is significantly higher compared with the conventional radiograph. Given the numerous sources of artifacts and the complexity of the artifact manifestation, it is impossible to cover this topic in a short section. Instead, this chapter focuses on the most important artifacts in routine clinical applications. Interested readers can refer to Hsieh (2009) for more comprehensive coverage on this topic.

## Types and Causes

Artifacts in CT can be classified according to cause and appearance. Classifying artifacts on the basis of their appearance in the image, four major categories can be identified: streaks, shadings, rings and bands, and "miscellaneous" factors such as the basket weave and moiré patterns (Fig. 9-32; Table 9-2). Streak artifacts may appear as intense straight lines across an image, which may be caused by improper sampling of the data (aliasing), partial volume averaging, motion, metal, beam hardening, noise, spiral/helical scanning, and mechanical failure or imperfections. Streak artifacts are often caused by errors of isolated projection readings (isolated channels and views). These discrepancies are enhanced by the convolution process and manifested into lines during the back-projection, as shown in Figure 9-32, *A*.

Ring or band artifacts are produced when the projection readings of a single channel or a group of

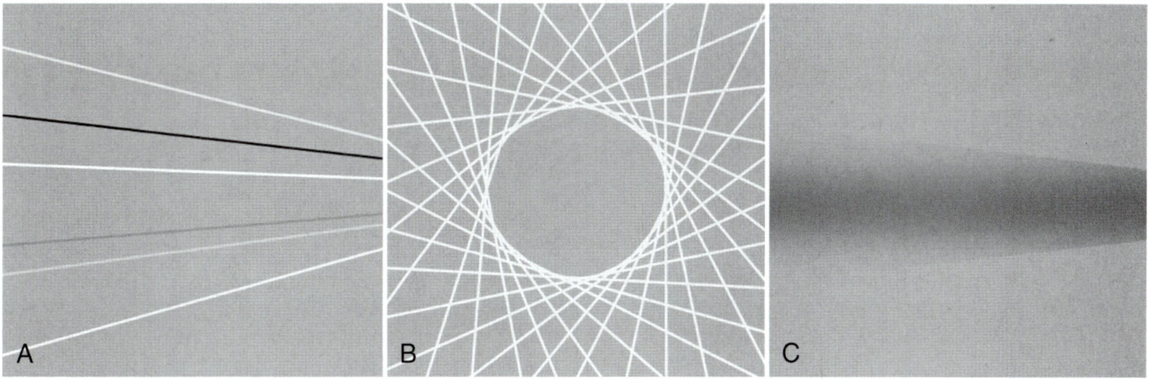


**FIGURE 9-32** Different appearances of artifacts. **A,** Streak. **B,** Ring. **C,** shading.

**TABLE 9-2 Classification of Artifacts on the Basis of Appearance**

| Appearance | Cause |
|---|---|
| Streaks | Improper sampling of data, partial volume averaging, patient motion, metal, beam hardening, noise, spiral/helical scanning, mechanical failure |
| Shading | Partial volume averaging, beam hardening, spiral/helical scanning, scatter radiation, off-focal radiation, incomplete projections |
| Rings and bands | Bad detector channels in third-generation CT scanners |

channels consistently deviate from the truth. They can be the result of defective detector cells or DAS channels, deficiencies in system calibration, or a suboptimal image-generation process. This is predominately a third-generation CT scanner phenomenon. Because a detector channel reading is always mapped to a straight line that is at a fixed distance to the isocenter of the system, a defective reading forms a ring pattern during the back-projection process, as illustrated in Figure 9-32, *B*.

Shading artifacts often appear near objects of high densities and can be caused by beam hardening, partial volume averaging, spiral/helical scanning, scatter radiation, off-focal radiation, and incomplete projections. They are formed by the gradual deviation of a group of projection readings over a limited range of views, as shown in Figure 9-32, *C*.

## Common Artifacts and Correction Techniques

### Patient Motion Artifacts

Patient motion can be voluntary or involuntary. Voluntary motion is directly controlled by the patient, such as swallowing or respiratory motion. Involuntary motion is not under the direct control of the patient, such as head motion with injury, peristalsis, and cardiac motion, as shown in Figures 9-33, *A*, and 9-34, *A*. Both voluntary and involuntary motions appear as streaks that are usually tangential to high-contrast edges of the moving part. Additionally, motion artifacts can arise from movement of oral contrast in the gastrointestinal tract.

The appearance of streaks results from the inability of the reconstruction algorithm to deal with data inconsistencies in voxel attenuation arising from the edge of the moving part. There are several methods to reduce CT artifacts from motion. For patient movements such as breathing and swallowing, it is important to immobilize patients and use positioning aids to make them comfortable and to ensure that patients understand the importance of remaining still and following instructions during scanning. Another useful motion artifact-reduction technique is to shorten the scan time, as discussed earlier in this chapter. Correction of motion artifacts can also be accomplished with **software** such as underscan weighting, as shown in Figures 9-33, *B*, and 9-34, *B* (Hsieh, 2009), and physiological gating such as ECG-gating in cardiac imaging, as demonstrated in Figure 9-22.

### Metal Artifacts

The presence of metal objects in the patient also causes artifacts. Metallic materials such as prosthetic devices, dental fillings, surgical clips, and electrodes give rise to streak artifacts on the image (Fig. 9-35, *A*). As shown in the figure, the metal object is highly attenuating to the radiation, which results in significant error in projection profiles. This error is often the combined effects of signal under-range, beam hardening, partial volume, and limited **dynamic range** of the acquisition and reconstruction systems. The loss of information leads to the appearance of

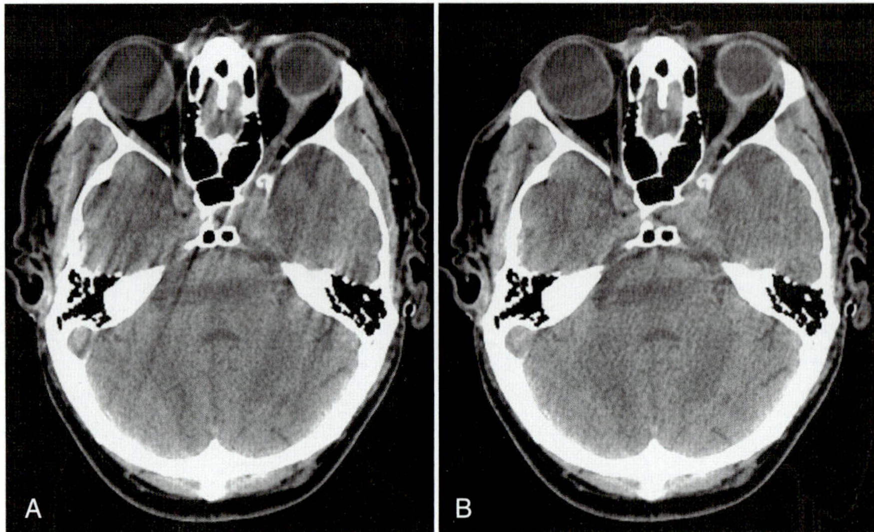


**FIGURE 9-33** Illustration of patient involuntary head motion. **A,** Without compensation. **B,** With correction.

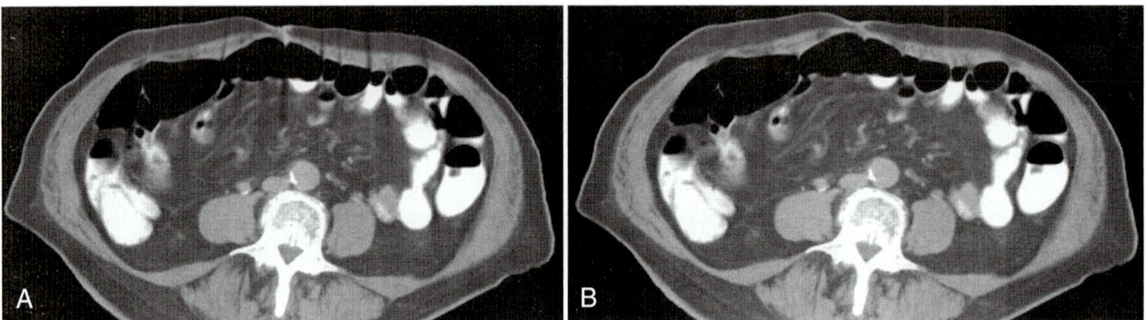


**FIGURE 9-34** Patient peristaltic motion. **A,** Without compensation. **B,** With correction.

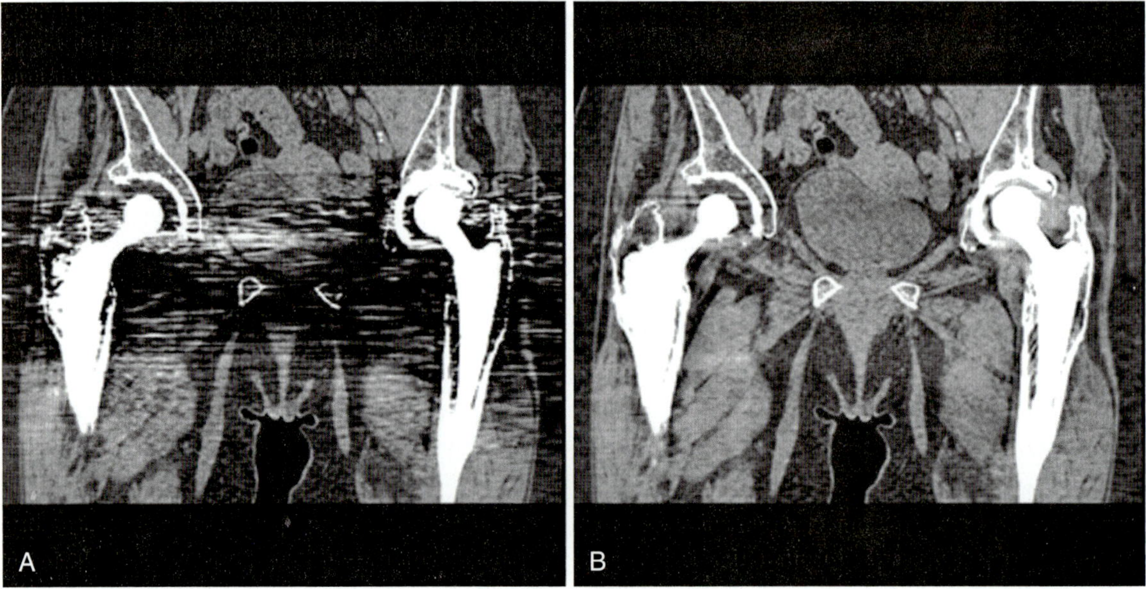


**FIGURE 9-35** Coronal images of a patient with bilateral hip implant **(A)** original image **(B)** with MAR algorithm.

typical star-shaped streaks. It should be pointed out that patient motion is often a major culprit in exacerbating the appearance of artifacts, as illustrated in Figure 9-36 with a pacemaker lead in a patient's heart.

Depending on the dominating causes of metal artifacts, the correction methodology can be significantly different. For example, if the artifact is caused mainly by the beam-hardening effect, DECT can be used by generating monochromatic images at higher keVs. The blooming artifact associated with the stents or other small metal objects (the intensity of the object "bleeds" through the neighboring voxels and makes the object larger than reality) can be significantly reduced when the images are generated at a high keV (e.g., 110 keV). When the artifacts are dominated by photon starvation or signal under-range, the measured projection samples become unreliable. The best approach to combat such artifact is to replace the corrupted projection samples with estimated projection samples, assuming the metal object is removed. This approach often involves techniques such as projection inpainting (a technique to compensate for the missing or deteriorated projection measurements). Images reconstructed with the modified projections are likely free of metal artifacts, and the final images can be produced by replacing metal objects generated with the original reconstruction, as shown in Figure 9-35, *B* (Pal et al., 2013).

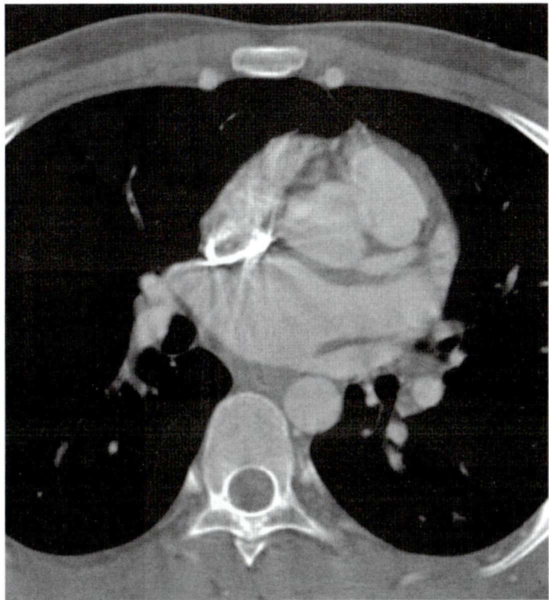

**FIGURE 9-36** Illustration of the impact of patient motion on metal artifacts.

## Beam-Hardening Artifacts

**Beam hardening** refers to an increase in the mean energy of the x-ray beam as it passes through the patient. As the object size increases, the mean energy shifts higher because lower energy photons are absorbed preferentially as the beam passes through the object. The original x-ray tube spectrum, the spectrum after traversing 15 cm water, and the spectrum after traversing 30 cm water are depicted in Figure 9-37. For each graph, the number of detected x-ray photons is kept to one million. The x-ray spectrum modification will lead to changes in the CT numbers if proper compensation is not rendered. Additionally, because radiation beams have different path lengths through the object (Fig. 9-38), the x-ray beam spectrum becomes channel dependent. The top portion of Figure 9-38 shows a short and a long path length, which results in different degrees of beam hardening.

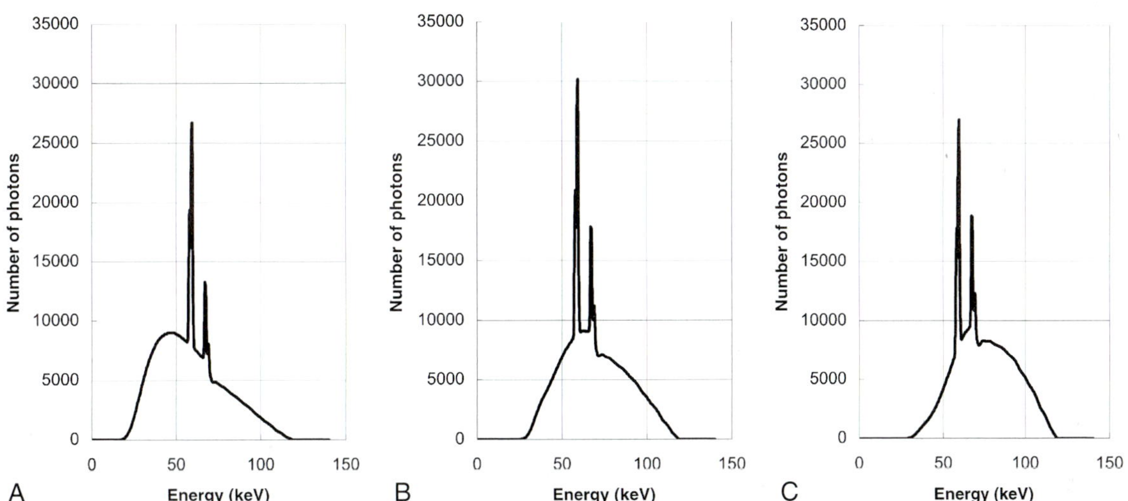


**FIGURE 9-37** Effect of beam hardening as the x-ray beam traverses different object sizes. **A,** Original spectrum. **B,** After traversing 15 cm water. **C,** After traversing 30 cm water.

There is less beam hardening at the periphery of the object, where the radiation path is short, compared with the center of the object, where the radiation path is longer. The bottom portion of Figure 9-38 depicts the intensity profiles of the reconstructed images. Ideally, the intensity should be constant for a uniform object shown by the thick solid line. Because of the beam-hardening effect, errors in CT numbers increase gradually from the periphery to the center of the object depicted by the dotted line. This artifact can be corrected by performance of a polynomial mapping of the measured projections before the reconstruction (Hsieh, 2009). Figure 9-39 shows two reconstructed images of a 35-cm water phantom with (*B*) and without (*A*) beam-hardening correction.

The beam-hardening effect is material dependent. When dense bones or contrast agents are present in the beam path, dark shading artifacts can occur because the beam-hardening correction applied to soft tissue does not work well for bones. This effect is demonstrated in Figure 9-40, *A*. Note the dark banding connecting the temporal bones. It has been shown that iterative correction is effective in combating such artifacts, as shown by Figure 9-40, *B* (Joseph & Ruth, 1997).

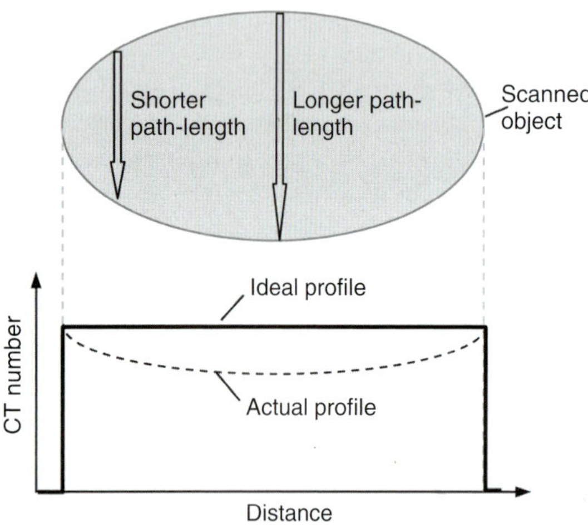


**FIGURE 9-38** Illustration of beam-hardening effect.

## Partial Volume Artifacts

CT numbers are based on the linear attenuation coefficients for a voxel of tissue. If the voxel contains only one tissue type, the calculation will not be problematic. For example, if the tissue in the voxel is gray matter, the CT number is computed at around 43. If the voxel contains three similar tissue types in which the CT numbers are close together—for example, blood (CT number 40), gray matter (43), and white matter (46)—then the CT number for that voxel is based on an average of the three tissues. This is known as **partial volume averaging.**

When the voxel contains multiple materials that are significantly different (e.g., soft tissue and bone), partial volume averaging can lead to partial volume artifacts (Heuscher & Vembar, 1999). In Figure 9-41, *A*, the detector measures x-ray intensity transmitted from the bone, $I_1$, and soft tissue, $I_2$, at the same time. Mathematically, the total intensity is measured as $I_1 + I_2$. To convert from intensities to line integrals for reconstruction, it is necessary to perform the logarithmic operation. Because of the nonlinear nature of the operator, it is clear that:

$$\ln(I_1 + I_2) \neq \ln(I_1) + \ln(I_2) \qquad \textbf{(9-6)}$$

These inaccuracies result in partial volume artifacts in the image, which appear as bands and streaks

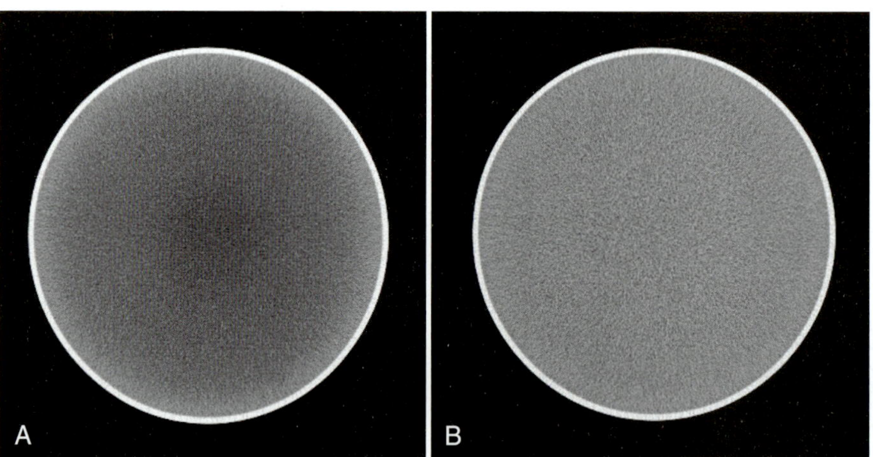


**FIGURE 9-39** Reconstructed images of a 35-cm water phantom. **A,** Without beam-hardening correction. **B,** With beam-hardening correction.

(Fig. 9-42, *A*). Note that a 7-mm detector aperture was used for data acquisition so that partial volume artifacts induced by the sharp bony structure can be easily observed.

Partial volume artifacts can be reduced with thinner slice acquisitions and computer algorithms (Hsieh, 1995). It is interesting to note that the thin-slice data acquisition comes naturally with the multislice CT. When the two intensities, $I_1$ and $I_2$, are measured with two separate detector cells, as shown in Figure 9-41, *B*, the object within each **slice width** is uniform and logarithm operation is performed on the two intensities

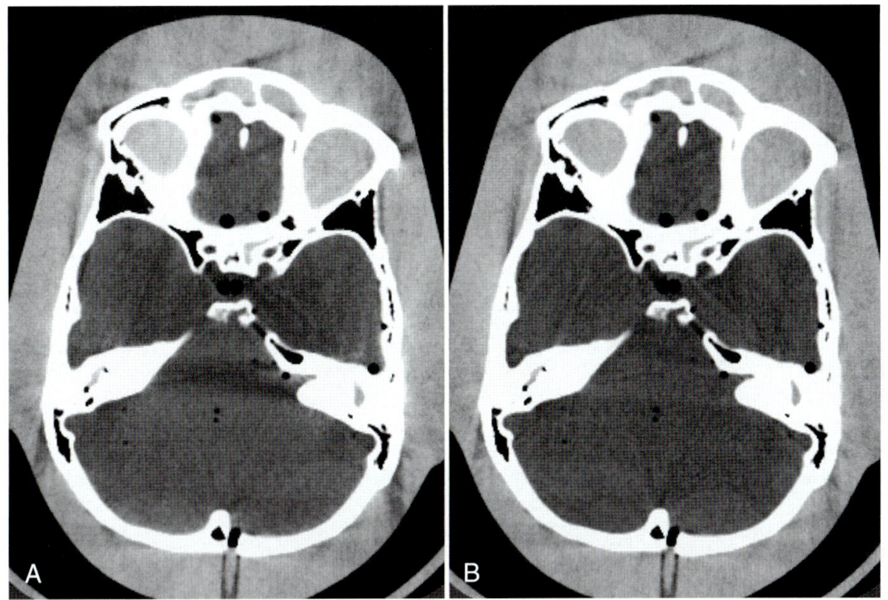


**FIGURE 9-40** Illustration of bone beam hardening with a human skull phantom. **A,** Without correction. **B,** With correction.

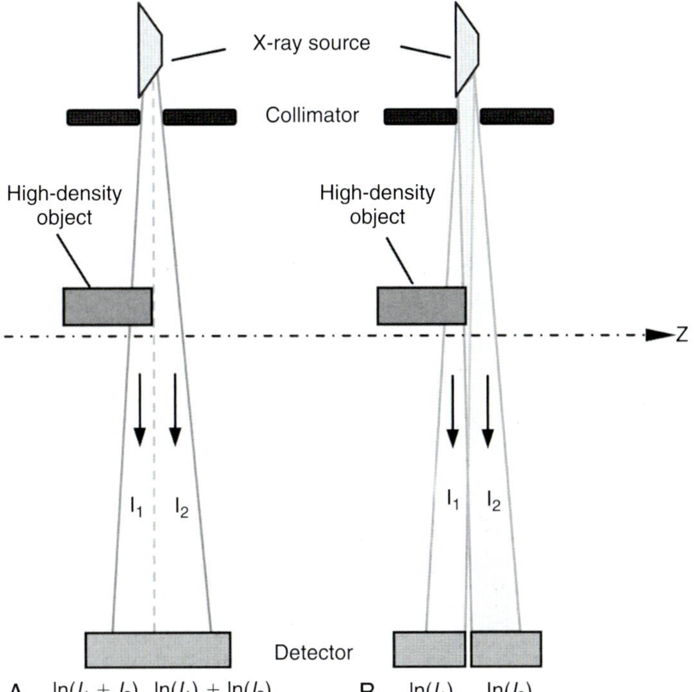


**FIGURE 9-41** Cause and correction for partial volume effect. **A,** Nonlinear operation of logarithm. **B,** Thin-slice scanning.

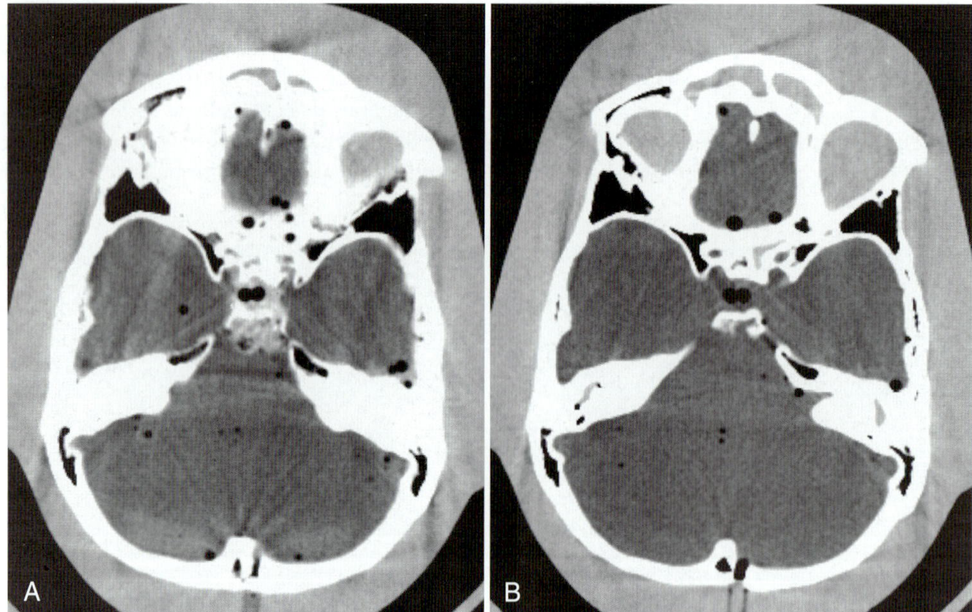


**FIGURE 9-42** Partial volume effect. **A,** 7-mm detector aperture. **B,** 1-mm detector aperture.

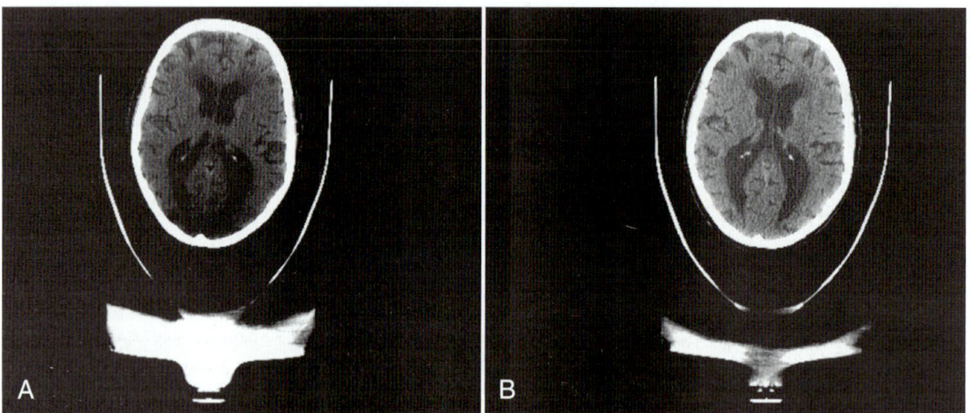


**FIGURE 9-43** Partial volume artifacts induced by foreign objects. **A,** Slice at the transition between thicker and thinner part of the holder. **B,** Slice at the thinner part of the holder.

individually. Figure 9-42, *B*, shows the same phantom scanned with a thinner detector aperture; the partial volume artifacts are nearly eliminated.

It is worth pointing out that partial volume artifacts can occur even with thin-slice acquisition if special attention is not paid to other **accessories** near the patient. As an example, Figure 9-43, *A*, shows a patient head supported by a high-density extension that ends abruptly at the mid brain location. Because of the sharp structure of this particular device, even a 1-mm slice thickness is insufficient to avoid partial volume artifacts, as demonstrated by the severe shading at the lower portion of the brain. Adjacent slice (Fig. 9-43, *B*), which is located 1 mm apart, is free from such artifacts because the supporting structure becomes homogeneous within this slice.

## Aliasing Artifacts

The sampling theorem states that to faithfully represent a continuous signal (e.g., intensity profile of a patient), the sampling frequency $f_N$ (the number of rays/cm in the fan beam) must be at least twice the highest frequency content in the signal, $f_H$. Mathematically, this can be expressed as follows:

$$f_N \geq 2f_H \quad (9\text{-}7)$$

If the Nyquist criterion is not met, aliasing artifacts (streaks) can result after the reconstruction process.

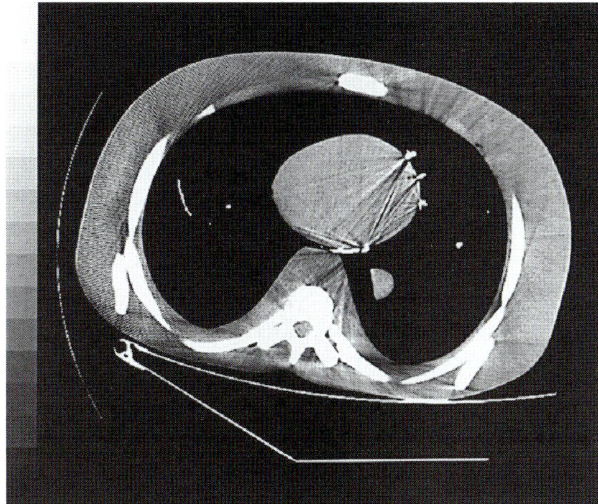

**FIGURE 9-44** View aliasing artifacts resulting from 50% of the normal number of views used to scan this torso phantom. The artifacts are apparent at the periphery of the phantom.

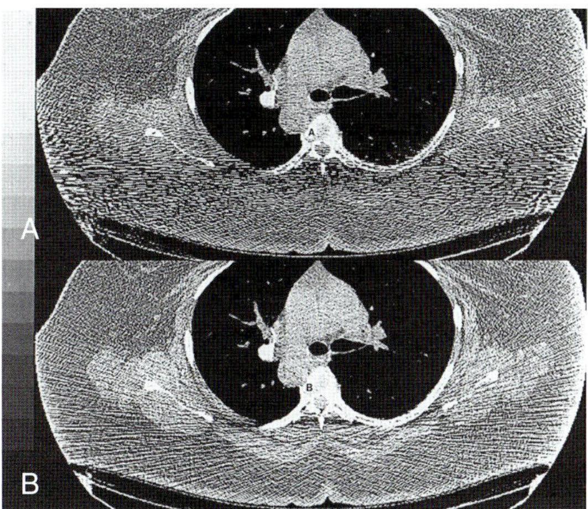


**FIGURE 9-46** **A,** Streak artifacts can arise from an increase in noise resulting from reduced photons at the detector. **B,** Correction of the streaks by adaptive filtering.

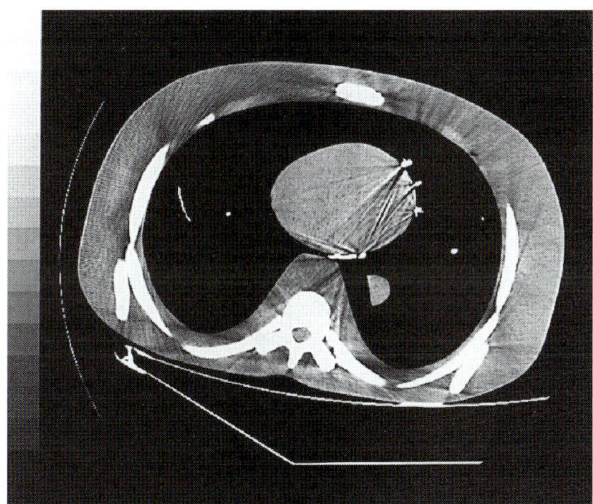

**FIGURE 9-45** Scanning the same torso phantom shown in Figure 9-44 at the Nyquist criterion can reduce view aliasing artifacts.

During CT data acquisition, the original continuous signal is sampled to a discrete form both spatially (each projection is sampled by multiple detector channels) and temporally (each data acquisition is divided into multiple views). Consequently, aliasing artifacts can arise from insufficient projection sampling or from insufficient view sampling. Figure 9-44 shows a torso phantom that was scanned with half the normal number of views.

Various methods are available to minimize aliasing artifacts. In some cases the number of views or number of **ray** samples per view can be increased (Fig. 9-45) to meet the Nyquist requirements. The **convolution kernel** used in the reconstruction can also be modified so that only frequencies below the Nyquist frequency are allowed into the filtered projection. In this case, a trade-off is made between the aliasing artifact reduction and spatial resolution of the reconstructed image.

## Noise-Induced Artifacts

Noise is influenced partially by the number of photons that strike the detector. Photon starvation can occur as a result of poor patient positioning in the scan FOV and poor selection of exposure techniques (kV, peak mA), scan speed, and limitations of the CT scanner such as maximum tube power. More photons mean less noise and a stronger detector signal, whereas fewer photons result in more noise and a weaker detector signal. When it is combined with the electronic noise and the logarithmic operation, photon starvation often leads to severe streak artifacts, as shown in Figure 9-46, *A*.

The technologist should optimize patient positioning, scan speed, and exposure technique factors to minimize streak artifacts. These artifacts can also be reduced with adaptive filtering algorithms (Fig. 9-46, *B*). These algorithms dynamically adjust the amount of smoothing operation on the basis of the x-ray flux level at each projection channel. By selectively smoothing only the channels that contribute to the streaking artifacts and by varying the degree of smoothing on the basis of the noise level of the signal, the technologist can achieve the objectives of simultaneously reducing the streak artifacts in the images and preserving the spatial resolution of the system (Hsieh, 1998).

Another type of noise-induced artifact is related to noise nonuniformity. When the noise within the

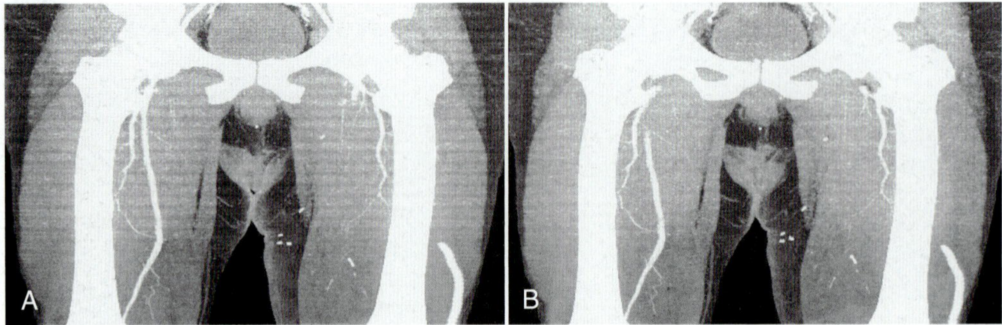


**FIGURE 9-47** Slab MIP images of 87.9 mm of a runoff study. **A,** Original. **B,** With correction.

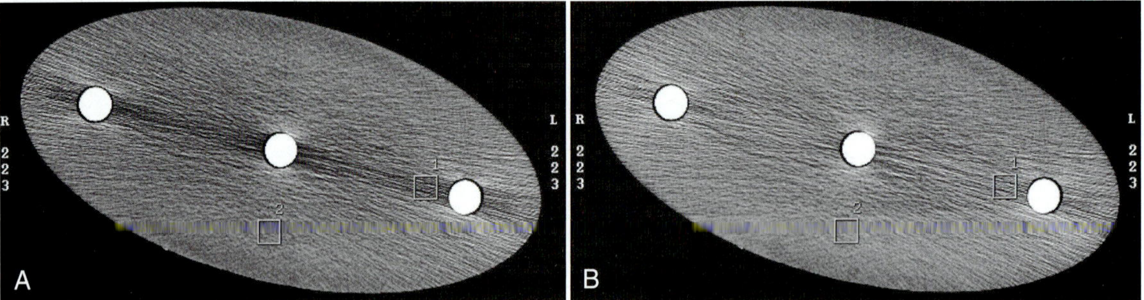


**FIGURE 9-48** Impact of scattered radiation. **A,** Without correction. **B,** With correction.

reconstruction FOV is highly heterogeneous, it can produce bright and dark horizontal strips in the MIP or VR images, as shown in Figure 9-47, *A*. This type of artifact can be reduced with either an improved reconstruction algorithm or advanced **image processing.** Both approaches produce a more uniform noise pattern in the final image (Fig. 9-47, *B*).

## Scatter

Scattered radiation is a fundamental phenomenon associated with the interaction between x-ray photons and matter. It reduces the object contrast in conventional radiography and produces artifacts in CT. Scattered radiation has been controlled effectively in the past by placing a postpatient collimator in front of the detector to reject any photons that do not follow the straight-line path between the x-ray source and the detector cell. With the introduction of multislice and volumetric CT, the volume exposed to the x-ray radiation increases significantly while the detector aperture reduces. As a result, the scatter-to-primary ratio (ratio of the scattered signal versus true signal) increases. The 1D collimator plates are no longer sufficient, as demonstrated in Figure 9-48, *A*. Note the dark shading artifacts connecting the dense rods.

Scatter-induced artifacts can be corrected with algorithms by carefully measuring or estimating the scatter distribution in the projection. The estimated scatter can then be removed from the measured intensities to arrive at the true signals that represent the line integrals of the scanned object. Figure 9-48, *B*, depicts the same scan reconstructed with a software scatter correction. A uniform background is restored.

## Cone-Beam Artifacts

The **cone-beam** artifact is a complicated subject and it is impossible to cover this topic in a subsection. At a very high level, cone-beam artifacts are caused by incomplete or insufficient projection samples as a result of the cone-beam geometry of multislice CT. Understanding the subject involves discussions of the cone-beam reconstruction theory. Given the limited scope of this section, this chapter only provides a specific example of the cone-beam artifact produced with one of the popular reconstruction algorithms: FDK algorithm (Feldkamp et al., 1984). For illustration, a simulation of an oval phantom is scanned in step-and-shoot mode with a 64 × 0.625 mm detector configuration (Tang et al., 2005). The comparison of a relatively centered slice (Fig. 9-49, *A*) and an edge slice (Fig. 9-49, *B*) shows that cone-beam artifacts

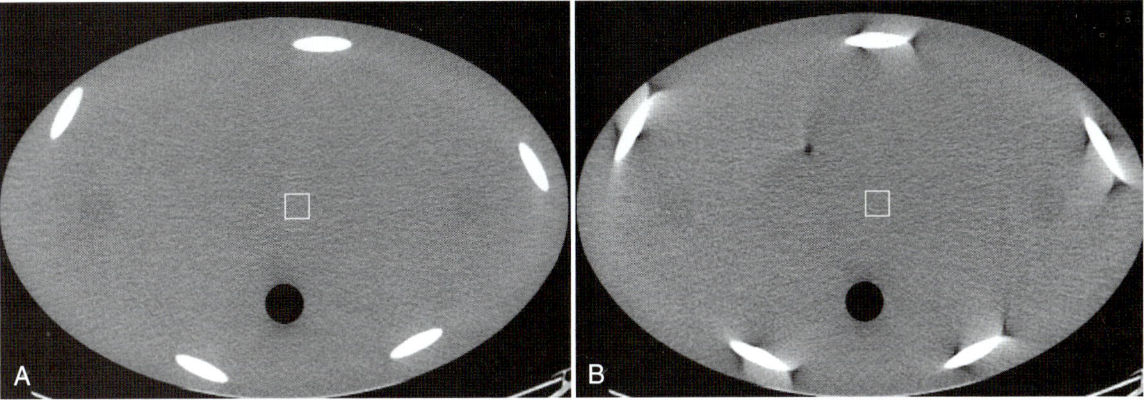


**FIGURE 9-49** Images of a helical body phantom reconstructed with FDK algorithm. **A,** 12.8 mm from the center plane. **B,** 17.8 mm from the center plane.

increase quickly as we move from the center to the edge. Note that the artifact is nearly absent in Fig. 9-49, A, and both distortions of the dense oval objects as well as shading artifacts nearby are quite severe in Fig. 9-49, B. The dense oval objects are ellipsoids positioned at a steep angle with respect to the patient's long axis to accentuate the artifacts. Reduction and elimination of cone-beam artifacts have been the focus of intense investigations in recent years, and this research will likely continue for years to come.

## QUALITY CONTROL

Quality control is an integral part of equipment testing and maintenance programs in hospitals. Quality control ensures the optimal performance of the CT scanner through a series of daily, monthly, and annual tests for spatial resolution, contrast resolution, noise, slice width, peak kV waveform, average CT number of water, standard deviation of CT numbers in water, and radiation scatter and leakage. These tests constitute a general quality control program for CT scanners and need to be documented.

## REVIEW QUESTIONS

Answer the following questions to check your understanding of the materials studied.

1. Which of the following determines image quality?
   1. spatial and contrast resolution
   2. noise
   3. artifacts
   4. radiation dose
   - A. 1 only
   - B. 1 and 2
   - C. 1, 2, and 3
   - D. 1, 2, 3, and 4
2. The unit for spatial resolution of a CT scanner is:
   - A. line pairs per cm (lp/cm).
   - B. lp/inch.
   - C. lp/mm.
   - D. lp/meter.
3. The capability of the CT scanner to discriminate small differences in tissue contrast is called:
   - A. spatial resolution.
   - B. contrast resolution.
   - C. noise.
   - D. cross-field uniformity.
4. Spatial resolution of the FBP algorithm is affected by all of the following ***except***:
   - A. detector cell width
   - B. size of the focal spot
   - C. slice thickness
   - D. photon flux
5. Slice thickness can be measured by _______
   - A. shallow-angled slice ramp
   - B. uniform water phantom
   - C. uniform oval phantom
   - D. Cone phantom
6. The pixel size in CT is equal to:
   - A. FOV – matrix size.
   - B. FOV + matrix size.
   - C. matrix size × FOV.
   - D. FOV ÷ matrix size.
7. CT number fluctuation from pixel to pixel in the image for a scan of water phantom is referred to as:
   - A. noise.
   - B. linearity.
   - C. spatial resolution.
   - D. cross-field uniformity.

8. To reduce noise (standard deviation) by a factor of 2, the dose must be increased by a factor of:
   A. 2.
   B. 8.
   C. 4.
   D. 6.
9. Which of the following produces a streak artifact?
   1. aliasing
   2. metal objects
   3. motion of the patient
   A. 1 only
   B. 2 only
   C. 1 and 2
   D. 1, 2, and 3
10. Ring artifacts in CT arise from:
   A. beam hardening.
   B. the patient's necklace.
   C. one or more bad detector cells.
   D. a depression in the table.

## REFERENCES


Barnes, G. T., & Lakshminarayanan, A. V. (1981). Computed tomography: physical principles and image quality considerations. In J. K. Lee, et al. (Ed.), *Computed tomography with MRI correction* (2nd ed.). New York: Raven Press.

Bhagalia, R., Pack, J. D., Miller, J. V., & Iatrou, M. (2012). Nonrigid registration-based coronary artery motion correction for cardiac computed tomography. *Medical Physics*, *39*(7), 4245–4454.

Blumenfeld, S. M., & Glover, G. (1981). Spatial resolution in computed tomography. In T. H. Newton, & D. G. Potts (Eds.), *Radiology of the skull and brain: technical aspects of computed tomography* (Vol. 5). St. Louis, MO: Mosby.

Bushong, S. (2009). *Radiologic science for technologists* (9th ed.). St. Louis, MO: Mosby.

Chandra, N., et al. (2011). Gemstone detector dual energy imaging via fast kVp switching. In T. Johnson, et al. (Ed.), *Dual energy CT in clinical practice*. New York: Springer.

Curry, T. S., Christensen, E. E., Dowdey, J. E., et al. (1990). *Christensen's physics of diagnostic radiology* (4th ed.). Philadelphia, PA: Lea & Febiger.

Feldkamp, L. A., Davis, L. C., & Kress, J. W. (1984). Practical cone-beam algorithm. *Journal of the Optical Society of America*, *1*, 612–619.

Goodenough, D. J., Weaver, K. E., & Davis, D. O. (1977). Development of a phantom for evaluation and assurance of image quality in CT scanning. *Optical Engineering*, *16*, 52–65.

Hanson, K. M. (1981). Noise and contrast and discrimination in computed tomography. In T. H. Newton, & D. G. Potts (Eds.). *Radiology of the skull and brain: technical aspects of computed tomography* (Vol. 5). St. Louis, MO: Mosby.

Heuscher, D. J., & Vembar, M. (1999). Reduced partial volume artifacts using spiral computed tomography and integrating spiral interpolator. *Medical Physics*, *26*, 276–287.

Hounsfield, G. N. (1973). Computerized transverse axial scanning (tomography). 1. Description of system. *British Journal of Radiology*, *46*, 1016–1022.

Hounsfield, G. N. (1978). Potential uses of more accurate CT absorption values by filtering. *American Journal of Roentgenology*, *131*, 103–106.

Hsieh, J. (1995). Image artifacts, causes and correction. In L. W. Goldman, & J. B. Fowlkes (Eds.), *Medical CT and ultrasound: current technology and applications*. College Park, MD: American Association of Physicists in Medicine.

Hsieh, J. (1998). Adaptive artifact reduction in computed tomography resulting from x-ray photon noise. *Medical Physics*, *25*, 2139–2147.

Hsieh, J. (2001). Investigation of the slice sensitivity profile for step-and-shoot mode multi-slice CT. *Medical Physics*, *28*, 491–500.

Hsieh, J. (2009). *Computed tomography: principles, design, artifacts, and recent advances* (2nd ed.). Seattle, WA: SPIE Press.

Hsieh, J., et al. (1999). Non-uniform phase coded image reconstruction for cardiac CT. *Radiology*, *213*, 401–406.

Hsieh, J., et al. (2013). Recent advances in CT image reconstruction. In N. J. Pelc (Ed.), *Advances in CT imaging. Current Radiology Reports*. New York: Springer.

Isola, A. A., et al. (2010). Coronary segmentation based motion corrected cardiac CT reconstruction. IEEE Nuclear Science Symposium Conference (NSS/MIC).

Joseph, P. M., & Ruth, C. (1997). Method for simultaneous correction of spectrum hardening artifacts in CT images containing both bone and iodine. *Medical Physics*, *24*, 1629–1643.

Kachelriess, M., Ulzheimer, S., & Kalender, W. A. (2000). ECG-correlated imaging of the heart with subsecond multislice spiral CT. *IEEE Transactions in Medical Imaging*, *19*, 888–901.

Kalender, W. A., & Polacin, A. (1991). Physical performance characteristics of spiral CT scanning. *Medical Physics*, *18*, 910–915.

Li, K., Tang, J., & Chen, G. (2014). Statistical model based iterative reconstruction (MBIR) in clinical CT systems, part II: experimental assessment of spatial resolution performance. *Medical Physics*, *41*, 071911.

Mayo, J. R. (1991). High-resolution computed tomography: technical aspects. *Radiologic Clinics of North America*, *29*, 1043–1048.

McCollough, C., et al. (2011). Dual-energy algorithms and postprocessing techniques. In T. Johnson, et al. (Ed.), *Dual energy CT in clinical practice*. New York: Springer.

McCollough, C. H., & Zink, F. E. (2000). Performance evaluation of CT systems. In L. W. Goldman, & J. B. Fowlkes (Eds.), *Categorical courses in diagnostic radiology physics: CT and US cross-sectional imaging* (pp. 189–207). Oak Brook, IL: Radiological Society of North America.

Morgan, C. L. (1983). *Basic principles of computed tomography*. Baltimore, MD: University Park Press.

Pal, D., Shama, K. S., & Hsieh, J. (2013). Metal artifact correction algorithm for CT. IEEE Nuclear Science Symposium on Medical Imaging Conference (NSS/MIC).

Parker, D. L. (1982). Optimal short scan convolution reconstruction for fan-beam CT. *Medical Physics, 9*, 254–257.

Petersilka, M., et al. (2008). Technical principles of dual source CT. *European J Radiology, 68*(3), 362–368.

Pfeiler, M., et al. (1976). Some guiding ideas on image recording in computerized axial tomography. *Electromedica, 1*, 19–25.

Riederer, S. J., Pelc, N. J., & Chester, D. (1978). The noise power spectrum in computer x-ray tomography. *Physics in Medicine and Biology, 23*, 446–454.

Robb, R. A., & Mortin, R. L. (1991). Principle and instrumentation for dynamic x-ray computed tomography. In M. L. Marcus, et al. (Ed.), *Cardiac imaging: a comparison to Braunwald 's heart disease*. Philadelphia, PA: WB Saunders.

Taguchi, K., Segars, W. P., Fishman, E. K., & Tsui, B. M. W. (2007). *Image-based motion compensated time resolved 4D cardiac CT*. San Diego, CA: SPIE Medical Imaging 2007. 6510–6516.

Tang, X., Hsieh, J., Hagiwara, A., Nilsen, R. A., Thibault, J. B., & Drapkin, E. (2005). A three-dimensional weighted cone beam filtered backprojection (CB-FBP) algorithm for image reconstruction in volumetric CT under a circular source trajectory. *Physics in Medicine and Biology, 50*, 3889–3905.

Thorsten, R. C., et al. (2011). Physical background. In T. Johnson, et al. (Ed.), *Dual energy CT in clinical practice*. New York: Springer.

# 10

# Radiation Dose in Computed Tomography

## OUTLINE



## LEARNING OBJECTIVES

On completion of this chapter, you should be able to:

1. state two reasons why the dose in CT is of importance to the CT technologist.
2. explain what is meant by exposure, absorbed dose, and effective dose.
3. explain what is meant by stochastic effects and deterministic effects of radiation exposure, and provide examples of each class of bioeffects.
4. describe the characteristics of the CT beam geometry that affect the dose distribution in a patient.
5. state the function that describes an arbitrarily shaped dose intensity along the patient axis.
6. state several methods for measuring the dose in CT.
7. describe what is meant by the CTDI, MSAD, and DLP.
8. describe the characteristics of CT scanner dosimetry phantoms.
9. describe briefly the basic steps of the CT dose measurement procedure.
10. outline the factors affecting dose in CT and explain various dose reduction methods.
11. describe the basic principles of automatic tube current modulation.
12. state what is meant by iterative reconstruction algorithms.
13. explain the meaning of the term "dose optimization."
14. explain what the CT Dose Index Registry is.
15. explain the Image Wisely® and Image Gently® campaigns.

## KEY TERMS TO WATCH FOR AND REMEMBER

The following key terms/concepts are important to your understanding of this chapter

**absorbed dose**
**as low as is reasonably achievable (ALARA)**
**automatic exposure control (AEC)**
**automatic tube current modulation (ATCM)**
**constant milliamperage-seconds (mAs)**
**CT dose index (CTDI)**
**deterministic effects**
**distance**
**dosimeters**
***D*(*z*)**
**dose distribution**
**dose-length product (DLP)**
**dose optimization**
**effective dose**
**effective milliamperage-seconds (mAs)**
**electrometer**
**exposure**
**longitudinal tube current modulation (z-axis TCM)**
**pitch**
**shielding**
**stochastic effects**
***z*-axis**

## CT USE AND DOSE TRENDS

Since its introduction in the early 1970s, **computed tomography (CT)** has played a significant role in the detection and management of human diseases in medicine. The technical evolution of CT has been dynamic, ranging from the first-generation, single-slice "stop-and-go" technique to multislice **volume CT scanning.** The growth of volume CT scanners continues at a rapid rate (Goldberg-Stein, et al., 2011; NCRP, 2009), from 16- to 64-slice systems, including the 320-slice CT scanner. These developments have created a wide variety of clinical applications such as CT colonography, cardiac CT imaging (Litmanovich et al., 2014), **CT screening** (Brenner, 2006; Liedenbaum et al., 2008), and virtual reality imaging, for example. Furthermore, there has been an increase in CT use worldwide (Amis et al., 2007; Lee et al., 2007; Mukundan et al., 2007). For example, in the United States alone it has been estimated that the number of CT scans increased from 40 million in 2000 to 65 million in 2004, and it is expected to increase to 100 million in 2010 (Baker & Tilak, 2007). In association with the expanding use of CT in medicine, one other major concern receiving increasing attention in the literature relates to the potential for high radiation doses to be delivered by CT scanners (Amis et al., 2007; Baker & Tilak, 2007; Cody & McNitt-Gray, 2006; Colang et al., 2007; ECRI, 2007; FDA, 2010; Frush, 2006; Goldberg-Stein et al., 2011; Goodman & Brink, 2006; Gosling et al., 2011; Martin & Semelka 2007; Moore et al., 2006; NCRP 2009; Pantos et al., 2011; Siegel, 2006), and the potential risks of CT scanning (Brenner & Elliston, 2004; Brenner & Hall, 2007; Brenner et al., 2001).

All individuals working in CT, such as radiologists, technologists, medical physicists, physicians, and manufacturers, should ask three central questions: Why are the doses in CT so high? What is the dose to the patient at my institution? What can be done to reduce the high exposures in CT to protect both patients and personnel?

There are several reasons why these questions are important; however, the most important reason for understanding radiation dose in CT relates to radiation risks (Brenner, 2006; Huda & Vance, 2007). The dose for a CT examination may have to be estimated to make decisions regarding the benefits versus the risks of the procedure. CT manufacturers are now required by law to provide a dose table that shows the doses delivered to patients from their CT scanners.

The purpose of this chapter is to outline the fundamental concepts of radiation dose in CT. In particular, topics such as radiation quantities and their units; factors affecting dose in CT; and CT dosimetry, including **dose descriptors,** phantoms and measurement concepts, **automatic exposure control (AEC)** in CT, dose reduction technology, **dose optimization** strategies, and **radiation protection** considerations are described.

## RADIATION QUANTITIES AND THEIR UNITS

The literature on radiation dose in CT reports the dose in CT using various radiation quantities (exposure, absorbed dose, and effective dose) and their associated units: Roentgens, rads, and rems (old units), respectively, or coulombs per kilogram, Grays, and Sieverts (International System of units = SI units), respectively (Bushberg et al., 2012; Bushong, 2013; Cody and McNitt-Gray, 2006; Seeram, 2001, 2014). For this reason, a brief review of these quantities and units is necessary. The radiation quantities of relevance to this chapter are exposure, absorbed dose, and effective dose. For a more detailed description, the interested reader may refer to a report by Huda (2006).

## Exposure

The radiation quantity, **exposure,** refers to the concentration of radiation at a particular point on the patient. Exposure is easy to measure with an ionization chamber positioned at the point of measurement. Radiation falling on the chamber ionizes the air in the chamber to produce ion pairs (charges). Exposure is a measure of the amount of ionization produced in a specific mass of air by x rays or gamma radiation. The ionization indicates the amount of radiation to which a patient is exposed.

The unit of exposure is the Roentgen (R), the conventional unit, or the coulomb per kilogram (C/kg), the SI unit. One Roentgen produces $2.58 \times 10^{-4}$ C/kg of air at standard temperature and pressure. Exposure is reported in the literature in milliroentgens (mR), a much smaller unit (1 R = 1000 mR) or in microcoulombs/kilogram (μC/kg) where 1 R = 258 μC/kg.

## Absorbed Dose

The **absorbed dose,** or radiation dose as it is popularly referred to, is the amount of energy absorbed per unit mass of material (patient). Any risk associated with radiation is related to the amount of energy absorbed, and this quantity is particularly important in radiation protection.

The old unit of absorbed dose is the rad (r), which is equal to an energy absorption of 100 erg/g of absorber. The SI unit of absorbed dose is the Gray (Gy), so named in honor of Louis Harold Gray, a British radiobiologist who devised ways to measure the absorbed dose. One Gray is equal to 1 joule per kilogram (J/kg) or 1 r is equal to 0.01 Gy or 100 r is equal to 1 Gy. Relevant submultiples of the Gray are 1 centigray (cGy), which equals 1 r and 1 milligray (mGy), which equals 100 millirads (mrads). For the sake of simplicity, 1 r is approximately equal to 0.01 Gy.

## Effective Dose

The quantity **effective dose,** *E*, previously referred to as the effective dose equivalent, is used to quantify the risk from partial-body exposure to that from an equivalent whole-body dose. The term is used to take into account the type of radiation (because different types of radiation can produce varying degrees of biological damage) and the radiosensitivity of different tissues (because some tissues are more sensitive than others).

As described by McNitt-Gray (2002), *E* is a "weighted average of organ doses" and can be expressed mathematically as follows:

$$E = \sum_{T} (D_{T,R} \cdot W_T \cdot W_R)$$

where $D_{T,R}$ is the absorbed dose to the tissue (*T*), $W_T$ is the tissue-weighting factor, $W_R$ is the radiation-weighting factor, and the symbol $\sum$ is the "sum of." These factors can be obtained from previously calculated tables (Bushong, 2009).

Although the old unit of effective dose is the rem, the SI unit is the Sievert (Sv), where 1 Sv = 100 rem. The effective dose relates exposure to risk. As noted by Brenner (2006), "… relevant organ doses for CT examinations are on the order of 15 mSv or less." Brenner also notes that "… there is good epidemiologic evidence of increased cancer risk for children exposed to acute doses of 10 mSv (or more) and for adults exposed to acute doses of 50 mSv (or more)."

To put this into perspective, Huda (2006) emphasized that "the total amount of radiation that a patient receives in any radiographic examination is best quantified by the effective dose, which is related to the risk of carcinogenesis, and with the induction of genetic effects. Effective doses with radiographic imaging are smaller than natural background (3 mSv per year). Effective doses from common fluoroscopic and CT examinations are comparable to natural background and may be much higher with interventional radiology procedures."

It is interesting to recall that the dose limits for occupationally exposed individuals (radiologists and technologists, for example) are given in mSv. The International Commission on Radiological Protection (ICRP) dose limit for radiation workers is 20 mSv per year. Although the dose limits for radiation workers in the United States is 50 mSv per year, it is 20 mSv per year for workers in Canada (Bushong, 2009).

# RADIATION BIOEFFECTS

One of the reasons technologists and radiologists should have a clear understanding of the dose in CT relates to radiation bioeffects. These effects are classified as stochastic and deterministic (nonstochastic). It is not within the scope of this chapter to describe the details of these effects; however, for the sake of relating these effects to dose in CT, a brief review is necessary. For a more detailed account of the risks, the interested reader should refer to the paper by Hendee and O'Connor (2013).

## Stochastic Effects

**Stochastic effects** are those effects for which the probability (rather than the severity) of the effect occurring depends on the dose. The probability increases with increasing dose, and there is no threshold dose for these effects. The linear no threshold (LNT) dose–response model is the radiation risk model most favored by radiobiologists in estimating the risk of exposure in radiology (Bushong, 2013). Medical radiation protection standards, guidelines, and recommendations are based on this model.

The LNT dose–response model states that the radiation risk increases as the dose increases and there is no threshold dose. Hendee and O'Connor (2013) stated that the LNT model is more commonly used because it is a simpler and conservative approach, which is more likely to overestimate cancer risk at low doses than to underestimate risk of cancer induction. The authors further stated, however, that because medical imaging doses are so low, there is no evidence that the no-threshold model is effective at estimating cancer induction risk.

Furthermore, even a small dose has the potential to cause a biological effect. There is no risk-free dose. If harm occurs, the damage generally becomes apparent years after exposure; therefore, stochastic effects also are called *late effects*. Examples of stochastic effects include cancer, leukemia, and hereditary effects. Stochastic effects are considered a risk from exposure to the low levels of radiation used in medical imaging, including CT examinations.

The interested reader should refer to the report by Brenner et al. (2001) for a thorough review of the increased risk of certain cancers from CT exposures, most notably in children. Additionally, Brenner (2006) provided the imaging community with a report dealing with the radiation risks in diagnostic radiology.

## Deterministic Effects

**Deterministic effects** (nonstochastic effects) are those effects for which the severity of the effect (rather than the probability of the effect) increases with increasing dose and for which there is a threshold dose. Below the threshold dose, these effects are not observed. Threshold doses are considered to be relatively high doses that can kill cells and cause degenerative changes in tissues that have been exposed to radiation. Deterministic effects are also referred to as *early effects* and involve high exposures that are unlikely to occur in medical imaging examinations.

Examples of deterministic effects include skin erythema, epilation, and pericarditis for example. A study by Huda and Vance (2007) on radiation doses from CT in children and adults showed that "representative organ absorbed doses in CT are substantially lower than threshold doses for the induction of deterministic effects."

As patients undergo several examinations, it may be possible to reach the threshold dose for certain deterministic effects.

# PATIENT EXPOSURE PATTERNS IN RADIOGRAPHY AND CT

It is clearly apparent that the geometry of the x-ray beam and the way in which the patient is exposed to the beam is different in radiographic imaging and in CT imaging, as shown in Figure 10-1. In radiography, the **x-ray tube** is typically above the patient in a fixed **position** as the examination is conducted, and the shape of the beam is a cone. This shape is sometimes referred to as open-beam geometry. Although the entrance exposure is 100%, it is sometimes used to represent risk; however, this is an overestimation because the dose decreases as it passes through the patient. Such decrease is due to **attenuation** and the inverse square law. The dose distribution for radiographic imaging is illustrated in Figure 10-1, *A*.

In CT, the exposure pattern is somewhat different from that of radiography because of the geometric aspects of the beam and the scanning procedure. In general, the beam is well collimated to describe a fan-shaped beam that rotates around the patient at least for 360 degrees. The x-ray tube is not fixed as in radiography but assumes several positions during one complete revolution around the patient. In modern multislice CT scanners, the fan-shaped beam has now become a cone-shaped beam (see Chapter 11). The dose distribution pattern is more uniform in CT (Fig. 10-1, *B*) compared with radiography because the x-ray beam is rotating 360 degrees around the patient's body. Typical dose values for a 16-cm

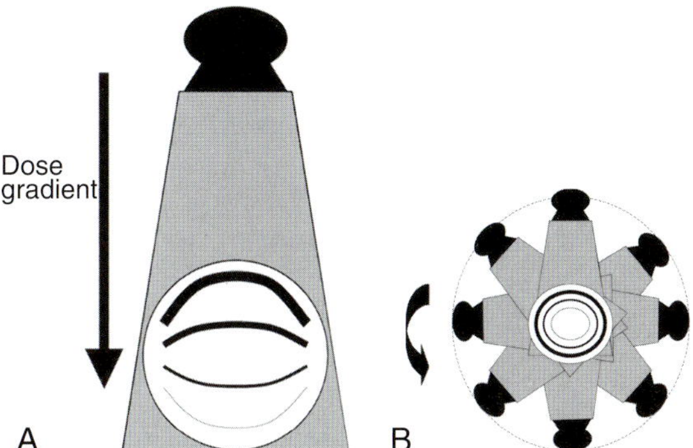


**FIGURE 10-1** **A,** The typical dose distribution for radiographic imaging. The entrance skin dose is greater than the exit skin dose, as illustrated by the thickness of the lines, where the thicker lines denote a higher dose. **B,** The typical dose distribution for CT imaging showing that the dose is greater at the entrance surface of the patient (thick lines) and decreases toward the center of the patient (thin lines). (From McNitt-Gray, M. F. (2002). *Radiographics, 22,* 1541-1553. Reproduced by permission of Radiological Society of North American and the author.)

diameter head phantom and a 32-cm diameter body phantom are given in Figure 10-2, respectively.

## CT SCANNER X-RAY BEAM GEOMETRY

The term ***beam geometry*** refers to the size and shape of the x-ray beam emanating from the x-ray tube and passing through the patient to strike a set of detectors that collects radiation attenuation data. The beam geometry and scanning process of CT imaging are shown in Figure 10-3, in which a fan-shaped x-ray beam and an array of detectors rotate 360 degrees around the patient to collect attenuation data. The table moves during the scanning process, and the x-ray tube traces a spiral or helical beam path around the patient.

Figure 10-4, *A*, shows the same fan-shaped x-ray beam viewed from the side with the thickness exaggerated for clarity. If the longitudinal (cranial–caudal) axis of the patient is defined as the **z-axis,** then in theory the intensity of the radiation beam along that axis can be graphed. Ideally the radiation intensity measured along the *z*-axis would have equal intensity everywhere inside the beam and would have no intensity on either side. Figure 10-4, *B*, shows this ideal rectangular intensity profile of the radiation beam. In reality, the radiation intensity measured along the *z*-axis has smoother edges and appears as a bell-shaped curve. The dose distribution is almost always wider than the nominal **slice width** (SW).

The **dose distribution** is given by the function **D(z),** which describes an arbitrarily shaped dose intensity along the patient axis. In general, the shape of *D*(*z*) varies among CT scanners. *D*(*z*) is extremely important to dose in CT because it is the dose distribution measured. The instrumentation and methods used to measure patient dose from a CT scanner is referred to as CT dosimetry, and it is uniquely different compared with the dosimetry of **projection** radiographic imaging.

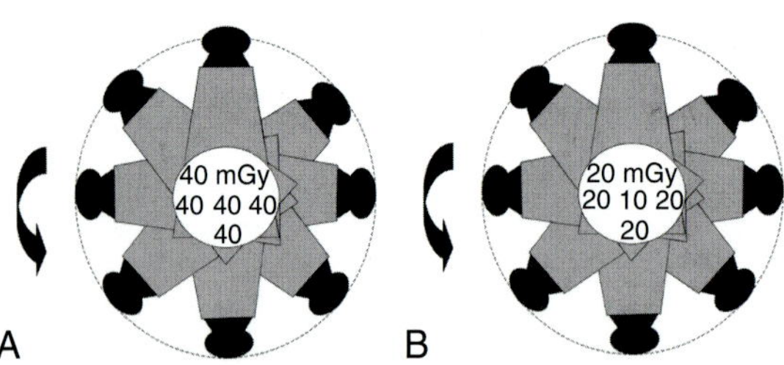


**FIGURE 10-2** Typical dose values for a 16-cm diameter head phantom **(A)** and a 32-cm diameter body phantom **(B)**. (From McNitt-Gray, M. F. (2002). *Radiographics, 22*, 1541-1553. Reproduced by permission of Radiological Society of North America and the author.)

## CT DOSIMETRY CONCEPTS

CT dosimetry is an important concept for CT technologists for several reasons. First, technologists can compare their hospital CT doses with the national average to find out whether their radiation protection efforts are comparable to those of others. Second, technologists can participate effectively in informing both the public and other hospital personnel (physicians and nurses, for example) about the dose in CT. Third, and perhaps more important, CT technologists can assist the medical physicist with not only performing the actual dose measurements (this has been identified as one of the duties of a certified medical physicist by the American College of Radiology) but also being a more integral part of CT acceptance

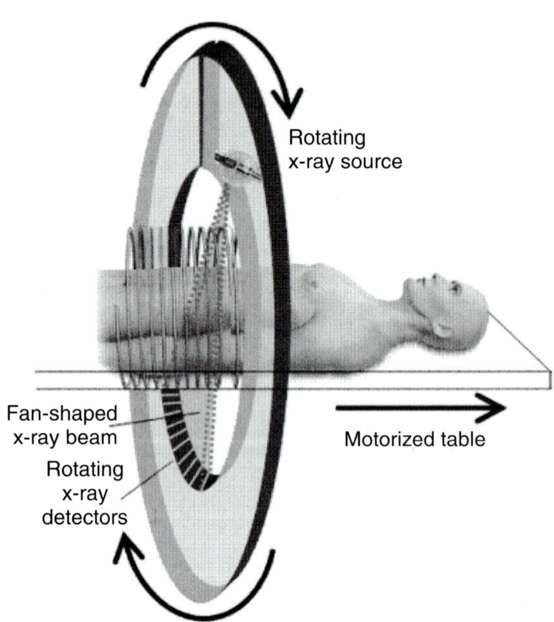


**FIGURE 10-3** The scanning principles of CT imaging in which the x-ray beam and detectors rotate 360 degrees around the patient to collect attenuation data used to build up the image. In this diagram, a fan-shaped beam is used and the table moves during data acquisition to trace a spiral or helical beam path around the patient. This process is referred to as spiral or helical CT scanning. (From Brenner, D. (2006). Radiological Society of North America: *categorical course in diagnostic radiology physics: from invisible to visible—the science and practice of x-ray imaging and radiation dose optimization*, pp 41-50. Chicago, IL: Radiological Society of North America. Reproduced by permission of Radiological Society of North America and the author.)

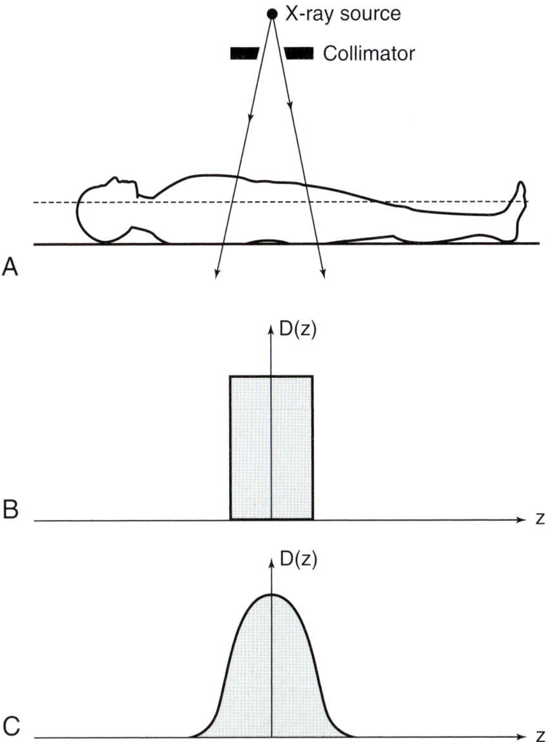


**FIGURE 10-4 A,** The width of the x-ray beam is viewed from the side. The collimator near the x-ray source (the width is exaggerated for clarity) determines the beam width. **B,** An ideal dose distribution along the *z*-axis is shown. It has a flat top and steep sides and is the same width as the x-ray beam. **C,** A more realistic bell-shaped dose distribution curve is typical of most CT scanners.

testing and continuing quality control procedures. Finally, a knowledge of CT dosimetry will assist the technologist in conducting dose measurements in cases where there is no medical physicist to perform this task.

The nature of CT dosimetry is complex and challenging because of the continuous technological evolution of CT scanners. Dosimetry involves the measurement of the dose to the patient and is characterized by several metrics. These metrics refer to radiation dose quantities and their associated units.

It is not within the scope of this text to describe how to conduct the actual dose measurements and how to estimate the radiation doses to patients because these are topics within the domain of medical physicists. It is important, however, to highlight several important and essential concepts, including types of dosimeters used to measure CT doses, CT dosimetry phantoms, and dose descriptors specific to CT.

## Types of Dosimeters

In the past, several types of **dosimeters** were used to measure the dose in CT. These include film dosimeters, thermoluminescent dosimeters (TLDs), and specially designed ionization chambers. In 1981, the Bureau of Radiological Health (BRH), now the Center for Devices and Radiological Health (CDRH), introduced what could be noted as a significant step toward CT dose measurement. The method suggested by the CDRH uses a pencil ionization chamber. Solid-state metal oxide semiconductor field effect transistors (MOSFET) are now used in CT dosimetry studies because they are more sensitive than TLDs, they provide an instant readout, and they can be reused immediately. For further details, the interested reader may refer to Mukundan et al. (2007), which used MOSFET dosimetry to assess the dose to the orbits in pediatric CT imaging. In addition, those interested in the use of the TLD in CT dosimetry may refer to Moore et al. (2006).

Although many dose measurement methods are available, only the pencil ionization chamber method, or what the CDRH referred to as the CT dose index (CTDI) method, is described in this chapter. The ionization chamber method is the easiest and probably the most accurate, and it is used almost exclusively to report dose.

### Ionization Chamber

An ionization chamber is an instrument used to accurately quantify radiation exposure. The ionization chamber shown in Figure 10-5 consists of a small air-filled container with thin walls that allow radiation to pass through easily. As the high-energy photons (x rays) collide with air molecules enclosed within the ionization chamber, some of the molecules are "ionized" (i.e., one or more electrons are knocked from some molecules). These free electrons can be collected on a conducting wire or plate and measured as electric charge. The amount of collected charge is proportional to the amount of ionization, which is proportional to the amount of radiation that passes through the chamber. The charge is removed from the ionization chamber and measured with a very sensitive instrument known as an **electrometer.** The total electric charge generated by an x-ray beam is represented by $Q$ and measured in coulombs (1 coulomb = $6.24 \times 10^{18}$ electrons).

## Phantoms for CT Dose Measurement

To standardize the measurement of the dose and provide a clinically realistic geometry, the BRH researchers suggested that the ionization chamber be placed in one of two cylindrical phantoms during the

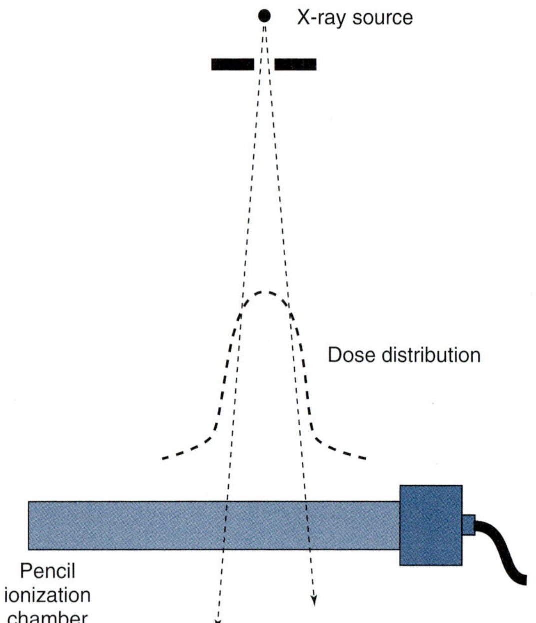


**FIGURE 10-5** An ionization chamber effectively performs the integral in Equation 10-2 by intercepting the radiation beam and sensing the dose from all parts of the dose distribution curve. The charge emitted from the chamber is proportional to the area-under-the-dose-distribution curve.

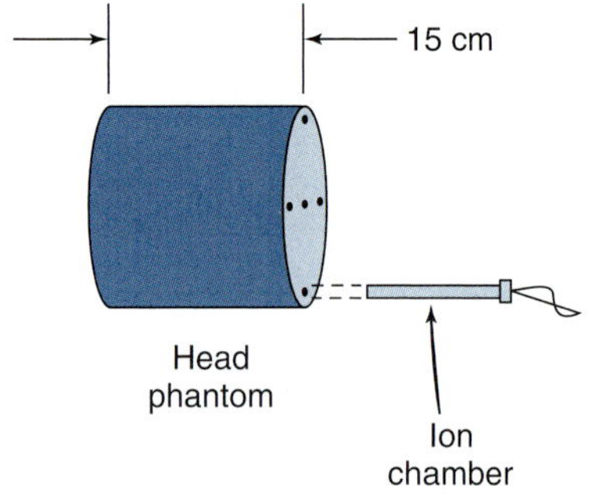


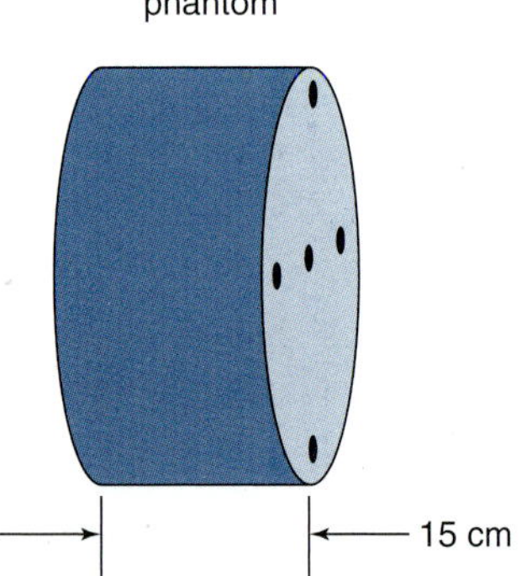


**FIGURE 10-6** The "head" and "body" CT scanner dosimetry phantoms are solid acrylic with holes placed strategically to receive a pencil ionization chamber. Although the phantoms differ in diameter, they are both 15 cm long.

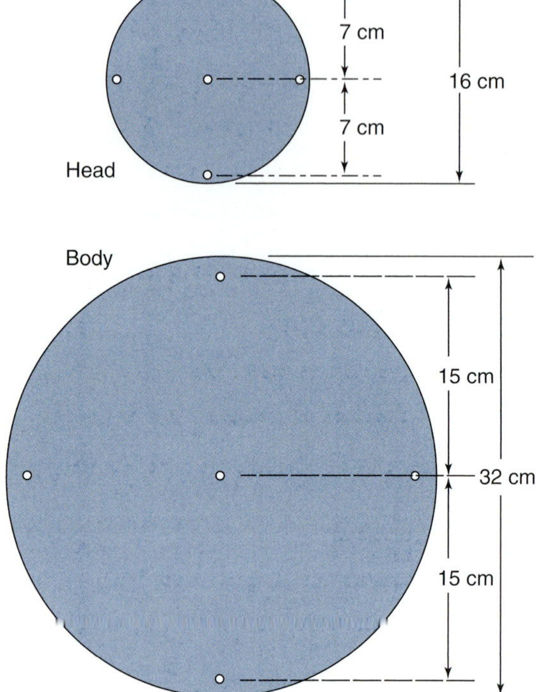


**FIGURE 10-7** A view of the face of a "head" phantom (*top*) and a "body" phantom (*bottom*). Dimensions and location of the ionization chamber holes are shown. Diameters of the holes are typically 1 cm and should be drilled to match the outer diameter of the ionization chamber.

radiation measurement. The smaller phantom simulates a patient's head and the larger phantom simulates a "body" or torso (Fig. 10-6). Both phantoms are 15 cm in length. The diameter of the "head" phantom is 16 cm, and the diameter of the "body" phantom is 32 cm. Both phantoms are solid acrylic with holes drilled through the phantom at specified locations to accommodate the pencil ionization chamber (Fig. 10-7). Acrylic plugs are placed in the holes unoccupied by the ionization chamber. Figure 10-8 shows a pencil ionization chamber about to be inserted into a CT scanner dosimetry phantom. The holes that are not used for the ionization chamber are filled with acrylic plugs. Careful examination of the plug reveals a small hole that can be seen through its diameter. This hole is centered end to end in the plug and is visible in the CT image of the dosimetry phantom if the x-ray beam is centered on the phantom and passes through the hole. The appearance of the hole in the image verifies that the x-ray beam is striking the center of the phantom.

The procedure for measurement is to place the ionization chamber in one of the phantom holes, take a scan, and record the amount of charge emitted

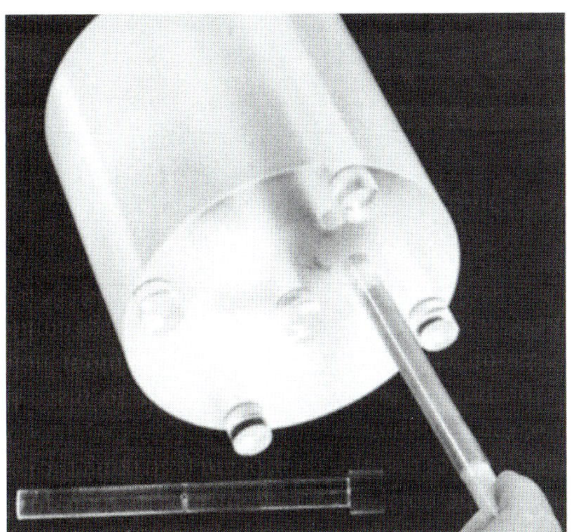

**FIGURE 10-8** A pencil ionization chamber about to be inserted in a "head" CT scanner dosimetry phantom. The holes that are not used for the ionization chamber are filled with acrylic plugs (*bottom*). The appearance of the hole in the image verifies that the x-ray beam is striking the center of the phantom.

from the chamber. Then the chamber is moved to the next hole, the plug is placed in the original chamber hole, and the procedure is repeated. Moving the chamber to another hole (e.g., from the anterior to the posterior) allows the dose to be determined at a variety of locations within the phantom. Generally, the dose varies among locations, even when the same technique is used. For example, the dose at the anterior location of the phantom differs from the dose at the posterior location, which differs from the dose on the patient's right side, and so on. It is usually prudent to measure the dose at several locations for a given technique.

## Display of CT Dose Metrics on the Scanner

In general there are three CT dose metrics (to be described subsequently) commonly used in CT, two of which are shown on the dose report that displays on the CT scanner console. These include the **CT dose index (DI)** and the **dose-length product (DLP).** The third dose metric of importance in CT, and in any imaging modality using ionizing radiation, is the effective dose. The International System of Units quantity for the CTDI and the DLP is expressed in milligrays; it is expressed in millisieverts (mSv) for the effective dose. The effective dose relates the radiation exposure to risk and is considered the best method available to estimate stochastic radiation risk (Wolbarst, 2013). Still, effective dose is an estimate only, based on weighting factors applied to the body's tissue or the organ being irradiated (Hermann et al., 2014).

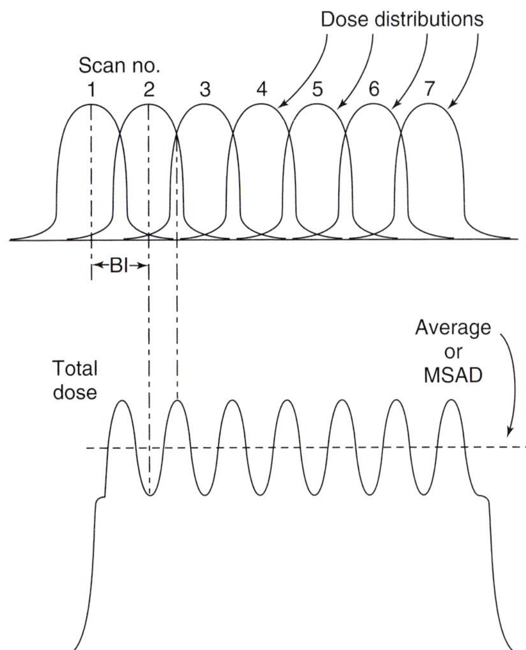


**FIGURE 10-9** A series of seven scans spaced (bed indexing) apart along the *z*-axis disburses seven bell-shaped dose distribution curves (*top*). When the doses from this series are summed, the resultant total dose appears as the bottom curve. The total dose curve has peaks where the bell-shaped curves overlap. The dotted line through the total dose curve is the multiple scan average dose.

## CT Dose Metrics and Calculation

The earlier dose studies reported CT doses by using various terms to describe the absorbed dose in a CT examination. These included single-scan peak dose, multiple-scan peak dose, dose profile, and others such as multiple-scan average dose (MSAD). These results led the CDRH to introduce and recommend the use of CTDI and MSAD in the Federal Performance Standard as the dose descriptors specific to CT. For example, because the early CT examinations consist of a series of stop-and-go scans (slices), the MSAD was the dose descriptor for use in a clinical situation at that time. The MSAD concept will be highlighted for historical reasons only.

Additionally, another dose descriptor, the DLP, has been identified and used in some studies; it is available for CT scanners and is linked to the CTDI (Cody & McNitt-Gray, 2006; McNitt-Gray, 2002).

### Multiple-Scan Average Dose

The MSAD was the first CT dose descriptor to be identified (Cody & McNitt-Gray, 2006; McNitt-Gray, 2002). To use the MSAD, a series of CT scans is performed on a patient (Fig. 10-9). Between each scan, the patient is moved a bed index (BI) distance. Each slice delivers the characteristic bell-shaped dose represented by the curves at the top of Figure 10-9. If the doses from all scans are summed, the resulting total patient dose resembles the oscillating curve at the bottom of Figure 10-9. In the regions where the bell curves overlap, the resultant dose is higher than that from just one scan. If the total dose distribution curve is known (bottom curve), the MSAD (dotted straight line) can be calculated by mathematically **sampling** the peaks and valleys of the multiple scan dose curve. This can be written as follows:

$$\text{MSAD} = \text{CTDI} \times \text{SW/BI} \qquad \textbf{(10-1)}$$

where SW is slice width in millimeters and BI is bed index or slice spacing.

## CT Dose Metrics and Calculation

The CTDI was the next CT dose descriptor after the MSAD. It was developed by the U.S. Food and Drug Administration (FDA) and was therefore labeled $\text{CTDI}_{\text{FDA}}$ (Boone, 2007). $\text{CTDI}_{\text{FDA}}$ has evolved to its present form with several notable changes. These are highlighted in this subsection.

The $\text{CTDI}_{\text{FDA}}$ is defined as follows:

$$\text{CTDI}_{\text{FDA}} = \frac{\text{I}}{\text{n.SW}} \int_{-7}^{+7} D(z)\, dz \qquad \textbf{(10-2)}$$

where $n$ is the number of distinct planes of data collected during one revolution, $SW$ is the nominal slice width in millimeters, $D(z)$ is the dose distribution, and $z$ is the dimension along the patient's axis. For axial (non-spiral/helical) CT scanners and spiral/helical CT scanners with a single row of detectors, $n = 1$. For multislice CT scanners, $n$ is the number of active detector rows ($n = 16$) during the scan.

The $\text{CTDI}_{\text{FDA}}$ represents the mean absorbed dose in the scanned object volume; therefore, the unit of the CTDI is Gy with relevant submultiples such as cGy and mGy.

This equation is not as complicated as it appears. The integral sign ($\int$) merely instructs the user to determine the area under a single curve $D(z)$. Figure 10-10 demonstrates the value of this integral by shading the area under a typical dose distribution curve. If this area is divided by the number of slices times the slice width [$(n)(SW)$], the result is the $\text{CTDI}_{\text{FDA}}$.

This definition, which was accepted by the International Electrotechnical Commission (IEC, 2001), is good for essentially all shapes of dose distribution curves $D(z)$ that are emitted by CT scanners. Note that increasing the area under the curve can increase

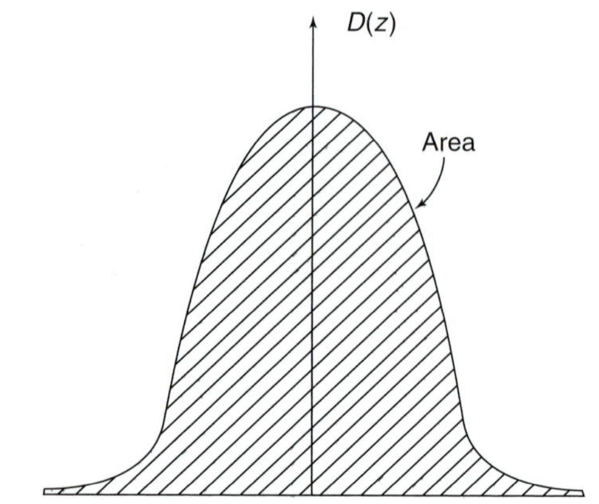


**FIGURE 10-10** The integral in equation 10-2 is numerically equal to the area (shaded region) of the dose distribution curve.

the $\text{CTDI}_{\text{FDA}}$. The area can be increased by either increasing the intensity of radiation, which raises the height of the curve, or by widening the curve, usually by opening the x-ray collimators near the x-ray tube. Either case increases the $\text{CTDI}_{\text{FDA}}$ and ultimately increases the radiation dose to the patient.

For axial CT scanners, as the slice spacing increases, there is a greater likelihood that relevant tissue will be "missed" (it falls between the slices) in the scan sequence, thus limiting the amount that the BI can be increased. Conversely, when the BI is made smaller, the slices become closer together, more overlap of adjacent dose distributions occurs, and the average dose increases. When the SW equals the BI, the MSAD is numerically equal to the $\text{CTDI}_{\text{FDA}}$.

The $\text{CTDI}_{\text{FDA}}$ has evolved from its initial stage of measurement for 14 contiguous slices where the integration would be from –7 to +7. The fixed length of the pencil ionization chamber "meant that only 14 sections of 7-mm thickness could be measured with that chamber alone. To measure $\text{CTDI}_{\text{FDA}}$ for thinner sections, sometimes lead sleeves were used to cover the part of the chamber that exceeded 14 section widths" (Cody & McNitt-Gray, 2006; McNitt-Gray, 2002).

This shortcoming was solved by introducing another dose index, the $\text{CTDI}_{100}$, which "relaxed the constraint on 14 sections and allowed calculation of the index for 100 mm along the length of the entire pencil ionization chamber, regardless of the nominal slice width being used" (McNitt-Gray, 2002). The index is given by the equation

$$\text{CTDI}_{100} = (1/\text{nT}) \int_{-50}^{50} D(z)\, dz \qquad \textbf{(10-3)}$$

where nT is the nominal collimated **slice thickness.**

The next major change in the CT dose descriptor is the introduction of the weighted CTDI ($\text{CTDI}_{\text{W}}$)

to account for the average dose in the *x-y* axis of the patient instead of the *z*-axis. This can be done using a phantom where the pencil ionization chamber is positioned in the center ($CTDI_{center}$) and at the periphery ($CTDI_{periphery}$) of the phantom (Fig. 10-7). In this case the following algebraic expression can be used to calculate the $CTDI_W$ (as provided by Cody & McNitt-Gray [2006] and McNitt-Gray [2002]):

$$CTDI_W = (1/3)\,(CTDI_{100})_{center} + (2/3)\,(CTDI_{100})_{periphery} \quad \textbf{(10-4)}$$

Several early examples of the $CTDI_W$ for head and body dose phantoms at 120 kilovolts (kV) for five CT scanners are given in a report by Huda and Vance (2007). They stated that for the following scanners, LightSpeed Plus (GE Healthcare), Mx8000 IDT (Philips Medical Systems), Sensation 16 (Siemens Medical Solutions), 7000 TS (Shimadzu Corporation), and the Aquilion Multi (Toshiba Medical Systems), the $CTDI_W$ (mGy/milliampere [mA]) for the head were 0.180, 0.130, 0.190, 0.180, and 0.190, respectively. For the body, the $CTDI_W$ were 0.094, 0.066, 0.069, 0.103, and 0.105, respectively.

To consider the dose in the *z*-axis, yet another dose descriptor was developed. This is the $CTDI_{volume}$, which can be calculated with the following relationship for spiral/helical CT imaging:

$$CTDI_{volume} = CTDI_W/Pitch \quad \textbf{(10-5)}$$

It is important to note that the term *pitch* has been defined by the IEC as a ratio of the distance the table travels per revolution (in millimeters) to the total nominal beam **collimation** (in millimeters). For a pitch of 1, the $CTDI_{volume}$ is equal to the $CTDI_W$; for a pitch of 1.5, the $CTDI_{volume}$ is equal to $CTDI_W/1.5$.

The literature is replete with studies of the $CTDI_{volume}$. Two examples include a study by Israel et al. (2010) and another by Pantos et al. (2011). Israel et al. (2010) showed that

> the average volume CT dose index for a 60-kg patient was approximately 11 mGy, which increased to approximately 22 mGy for an 80-kg patient and to approximately 33 mGy for a 100-kg patient. The corresponding average liver doses for 60-kg patients was approximately 16 mGy, which increased to approximately 25 mGy for 80-kg patients and to approximately 34 mGy for 100-kg patients. For this patient cohort, the median doses to the colon, stomach, and liver were approximately 25 mGy; to the bladder, 31 mGy; and to the red bone marrow, 16 mGy. The 90th percentile organ doses were generally three to four times that of the corresponding 10th percentile organ doses.

Pantos et al. (2011) showed that

> considerable variation of reported values among studies was attributed to variations in both examination protocol and scanner design. Median weighted CT dose index (CTDI(w)) and dose length product (DLP) are below the proposed DRLs; however, for individual studies the DRLs are exceeded. Median reported effective doses for the most frequent CT examinations were: head, 1.9 mSv (0.3-8.2 mSv); chest, 7.5 mSv (0.3-26.0 mSv); abdomen, 7.9 mSv (1.4-31.2 mSv); and pelvis, 7.6 mSv (2.5-36.5 mSv).

## Dose Length Product

As mentioned earlier, the DLP is yet another dose descriptor used in CT dose studies and reported in the literature and on CT scanners. Although the $CTDI_{volume}$ provides a measurement of the exposure per slice of tissue, the DLP provides a measurement of the total amount of exposure for a series of scans. The DLP can be calculated if the length of the irradiated volume (scan length) and the $CTDI_{volume}$ are known by using the following relationship:

$$DLP = CTDI_{volume} \times \text{Scan length} \quad \textbf{(10-6)}$$

It is important to note that, although the $CTDI_{volume}$ is not dependent on the scan length, the DLP is directionally proportional to the scan length (Fig. 10-11). DLP is expressed in mGy-cm.

An interesting study by Brady et al. (2012) on the "Assessment of paediatric CT dose indicators for the purpose of optimization" showed that

> The LDRLs across all age categories were 18-45 mGy (CTDI(vol)) and 250-700 mGy cm (DLP) for brain examinations; 3-23 mGy (CTDI(vol)) and 100-800 mGy cm (DLP) for chest examinations; and 4-15 mGy (CTDI(vol)) and 150-750 mGy cm (DLP) for abdomen/pelvis examinations. Effective dose estimates were 1.0-1.6 mSv, 1.8-13.0 mSv and 2.5-10.0 mSv for brain, chest, and abdomen/pelvis examinations, respectively.

In summary, McNitt-Gray (2002) informed the radiologic community that

> these CTDI descriptors are obviously meant to serve as an index of radiation dose due to CT scanning and are not meant to serve as an accurate estimate of the radiation dose incurred by an individual patient. Although the phantom measurements are meant to be reflective of an attenuation environment somewhat similar to a patient, the homogeneous polymethyl methacrylate phantom does not simulate the different tissue types and heterogeneities of a real patient.

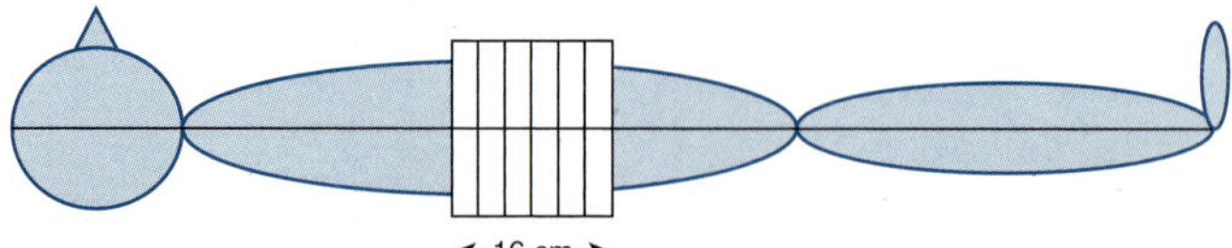


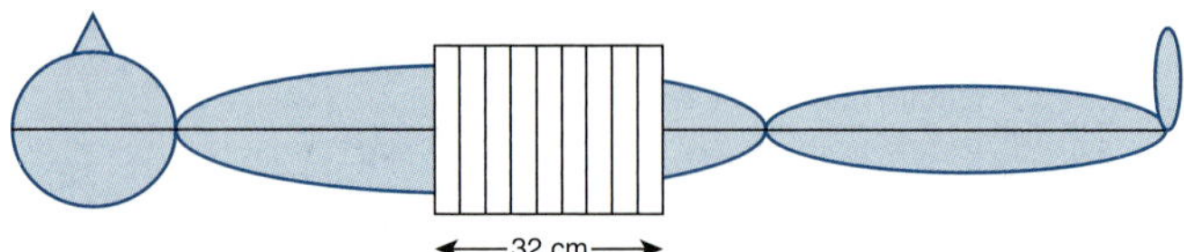


**FIGURE 10-11** Hypothetical DLP values for 2 CT scans of the abdomen. **A,** The scan length is 16 cm, and the DLP is 160 mGy-cm. **B,** The scan length is 32 cm, and the DLP is 320 mGy-cm. The DLP is directly proportional to the scan length. (From Seeram, E. (2014). *Radiologic Technology, 85* (6), 665-675. Reproduced by permission of the ASRT.)

## Effective Dose

The next stage in this area of patient dose assessment is to address the risk of a CT examination. This requires the use of the effective dose. Effective dose is used in radiation protection to relate exposure to risk, and it takes into account that different tissues have different radiosensitivities and the absorbed dose to specific organs. For example, the gonads are more radiosensitive than the brain (Bushong, 2013). Because only parts of the body (rather than the entire body) are exposed in medical diagnostic imaging, risk of stochastic radiation response is proportional to the effective dose rather than to the tissue dose. The effective dose is expressed by the following:

$$E=\sum_{T}(W_T \cdot W_R \cdot D_{T,R}) \quad \textbf{(10-7)}$$

where $W_T$ = tissue weighting factor, $W_R$ = radiation weighting factor, and $D_{T,R}$ = average absorbed dose to tissue $T$. The tissue and radiation weighting factors are available from tables provided by the ICRP and the NCRP.

The SI unit for E is the Sievert; while the old unit is the rem.

$$1\ \text{Sv} = 100\ \text{rem}$$

$$(1\ \text{rem} = 10\ \text{mSv})$$

For simplicity, the effective dose is obtained by multiplying the DLP by constants referred to as *k values*, which have been previously established. For example, the *k* value (mSv/mGy-cm) for a CT scan of the head is 0.0021; the *k* value is 0.015 for a CT scan of the pelvis (McNitt-Gray, 2002). Knowing these *k* values enables calculation of the effective dose as follows:

$$ED = k \times DLP \quad \textbf{(10-8)}$$

The effective dose allows for a comparison of the dose received from CT scanning with the dose received from natural background radiation. For example, Bushong (2013) noted that while the annual effective dose from natural background radiation is reported to be 3 mSv, it is 1.5 mSv for CT and 3 mSv for medical imaging (CT scanning, radiography, and interventional, nuclear medicine).

## Measuring the CT Dose Index

It is not within the scope of this book to describe the details of how to measure the CTDI because this is a task for the medical physicist. However, the following steps are noteworthy, using the phantoms and pencil ionization chamber described earlier:

1. The pencil ionization chamber is placed into one of the holes in the phantom, perpendicular to the fan of the radiation beam (i.e., the chamber is placed parallel to the longitudinal axis of the patient; Fig. 10-5), and the other holes are plugged with acrylic plugs.
2. An exposure is made for a single scan, and the chamber measures the exposure (not dose). The chamber intercepts the entire narrow width of the x-ray beam. The x-ray beam must be positioned in the center of the chamber.
3. The chamber converts the x rays into charge. This charge represents the integral in Equation 10-2.

4. The ionization chamber receives radiation from all parts of the dose distribution $D(z)$ because of its length. The total charge from the ionization chamber is proportional to the integral in the CTDI definition. Mathematically, this is expressed as follows:

$$Q = \frac{1}{C_f} \int_{-\infty}^{+\infty} D(z)\,dz \qquad \textbf{(10-9)}$$

where $Q$ is the total charge collected during a single scan and $C_f$ is the calibration factor of the ionization chamber. Because the ionization chamber measures exposure and not the dose, a conversion factor (the f factor) must be included in $C_f$, which converts exposure (in Roentgens, R) to dose (cGy; recall that 1 cGy = 1 rad). The value of the f factor at CT scanner x-ray energies is approximately 0.94 cGy/R.

An interesting point to note about the CTDI is that the integration range is restricted to single-slice CT scanners collimated to beam widths of 10 mm and less (Boone, 2007) and to 100 mm for the $CTDI_{100}$. As pointed out by Cody and McNitt-Gray (2006),

> with the advent of multidetectors scanners with beam widths from 25 to 40 mm (and a prototype that has a nominal collimated beam width of 128 mm) (Mori et al., 2006a), the 100 mm pencil chamber will not be able to capture all of the primary and scatter radiation in the CTDI phantoms. In addition, CTDI is measured in a single transverse scan so that the pencil chamber can integrate the radiation dose profile, assuming a contiguous transverse scanning protocol; approximations are made to calculate dose when helical scanning is performed....therefore, methods are being developed to measure radiation dose better for multidetector CT (and also for cone beam CT) as well as to measure estimated actual radiation dose to patients.

For example, the nominal beam width for the 256-slice CT scanner is 128 mm; therefore, the integration range has increased to 300 mm for an accurate measurement of the dose from this CT scanner (Mori et al., 2006b). These investigators have developed what they call the dose profile integral. In addition, in a letter to the editor of *Medical Physics*, Dixon (2006) proposed that a Farmer ion chamber be used to measure the dose with a phantom "using the exact protocol that would be used for patients, instead of a single transverse scan, removing the need to make approximations or corrections for helical scanning" (Cody & McNitt, 2006). Other investigators have used MOSFET technology as well to assess dose in CT (Dixon, 2003; Muhundan et al., 2007).

These measurement and dose estimation methods are not described further in this text; however, the interested reader should refer to the reports by Dixon (2003, 2006).

## FACTORS AFFECTING DOSE IN CT

Several factors affect the dose in CT. These fall into two categories, namely, those that have a direct effect on the dose and those that have an indirect effect on the dose (Cody & McNitt-Gray, 2006; Kalra et al., 2004a; McNitt-Gray, 2002). Although the direct factors are those factors that increase or decrease the dose to the patient and are under the direct control of the technologist, the indirect factors are those that "have a direct influence on image quality, but no direct effect on radiation dose; for example, the reconstruction filter" (McNitt-Gray, 2002). It is beyond the scope of this chapter to describe all of these factors; however, only the factors that have a direct effect on the dose to the patient, and those which the technologist has some degree of control, are reviewed. These include the exposure technique factors, x-ray beam collimation, pitch, patient centering, number of detectors, and over-ranging, also referred to as *z*-overscanning, and iterative reconstruction.

### Exposure Technique Factors

Exposure technique factors are characterized by the tube potential defined by the kilovoltage; tube current, defined by the milliamperage; and the exposure time in seconds. The product of the milliamperage and the exposure time is the milliamperage-seconds (mAs). The technologist can select these factors manually or they can be selected by using AEC, which uses a technique known as automatic tube current modulation and is described later in the chapter.

#### Constant Milliamperage-Seconds

The term **constant mAs** refers to the selection of milliamperage and time (in seconds) separately or mAs on some scanners before the scan begins, keeping all other technical factors constant. The mAs determines the quantity of photons (dose) incident on the patient for the duration of the exposure. The dose is directly proportional to the mAs, and if the mAs is doubled, the dose will be doubled. The results of different amounts of mAs on the dose (mGy and mGy/mAs) using a phantom and a 64-slice CT scanner are provided in Table 10-1. It is clearly apparent that as the mAs increases, the dose increases proportionally. For example, the $CTDI_w$ (mGy) for a 32-cm diameter body phantom using 110 mAs and 220 mAs is 7.4 and 15 mGy, respectively, when all other technical scanning factors remain constant (Cody & McNitt-Gray, 2006).

**TABLE 10-1 Changes in $CTDI_w$ in a 32-cm Diameter Body Phantom as a Function of Tube Current-Time Product for Both Constant Rotation Time Settings and Constant Current Settings**

| Tube Current (mA) | Rotation Times (s) | Tube Current-Time Product (mAs) | $CTDI_W$ (mGy) | $CTDI_W$/mAs (mGy/mAs) | % $CTDI_W$/mAs Difference 220 mAs |
|---|---|---|---|---|---|
| 220 | 0.5 | 110 | 7.4 | 0.068 | 0.0 |
| 440 | 0.5 | 220 | 15 | 0.068 | — |
| 580 | 0.5 | 290 | 19.8 | 0.069 | +1.5 |
| 440 | 0.33 | 1459 | .940 | .068 | 0.0 |
| 440 | 0.375 | 165 | 11.3 | 0.068 | 0.0 |
| 440 | 1.0 | 440 | 30.2 | 0.069 | +1.5 |

From Cody, D., & McNitt-Gray, M. (2006). *CT image quality and patient radiation dose: definitions, methods, and trade-offs.* Chicago, IL: Radiological Society of North America. Reproduced by permission of Radiological Society of North America and the authors.

Note: All other factors were held constant at 120 kVp with 20 channels and 1.2-mm channel width (20 × 1.2 mm).

**TABLE 10-2 Changes in $CTDI_w$ in a 32-cm Diameter Body Phantom as a Function of Tube Potential (kV)**

| Peak Voltage (kVp) | $CTDI_W$ (mGy) | $CTDI_W$/mAs (mGy/mAs) | % Difference from 120-kVp Setting |
|---|---|---|---|
| 80 | 18.0 | 0.073 | −63.6 |
| 100 | 32.3 | 0.131 | −34.6 |
| 120 | 49.4 | 0.200 | — |
| 140 | 68.2 | 0.276 | +38.2 |

From Cody, D., & McNitt-Gray, M. (2006). *CT image quality and patient radiation dose: definitions, methods, and trade-offs.* Chicago, IL: Radiological Society of North America. Reproduced by permission of Radiological Society of North America and the authors.

Note: All other factors were held constant at a 0.75-second rotation time, 330 mA, collimation of 12 channels with 1.5-mm channel width (12 × 1.5 mm), and head bowtie filtration.

## Effective Milliamperage-Seconds

The **effective mAs** is a term used for multislice CT scanners that denotes the mAs per slice. This is given by the following relationship:

$$\text{Effective mAs} = \text{True mAs/pitch} \quad \textbf{(10-10)}$$

This expression simply implies that, to keep the effective mAs constant, as the pitch increases, the true mAs must be increased as well (Cody & McNitt-Gray, 2006). For example, increasing the pitch from, say, 1 to 2, increases the mAs per rotation from 100 to 200 while the relative $CTDI_{vol}$ remains the same (Lewis, 2005).

## Peak Kilovoltage

The peak kilovoltage (kVp) determines the penetrating power of the photons coming from the x-ray tube. Higher kVp means that the photons have higher energies and can penetrate thicker objects compared with lower kVp x-ray beams. In CT generally, for adult imaging, high kVp techniques are used, such as 120 kVp. The radiation dose is proportional to the square of the kVp (Bushberg et al., 2012). This means that the quantity of photons increases by the square of the kVp. A 72-kVp technique will have fewer photons than a kVp of 82, all factors held constant.

The results of different amounts of kVp on the dose (mGy and mGy/mAs) with a 64-slice spiral/helical CT scanner are provided in Table 10-2. It is clearly apparent that as the kVp increases, the dose increases. For example, the $CTDI_w$ (mGy) for a 32-cm diameter body phantom using an 80 kV and a 140 kVp beam is 5.2 and 24.9 mGy, respectively, when all other technical scanning factors remain constant (Cody & McNitt-Gray, 2006).

## Collimation (*Z*-Axis Geometric Efficiency)

In CT, the collimation is used to define the beam width for the examination. Collimation schemes are different between single-slice (single detector row along the *z*-axis) and multislice (multidetector rows along the z-axis) CT scanners. The collimation reflects the efficient use of the x-ray beam at the detector, as shown in Figure 10-12. The shaded portion

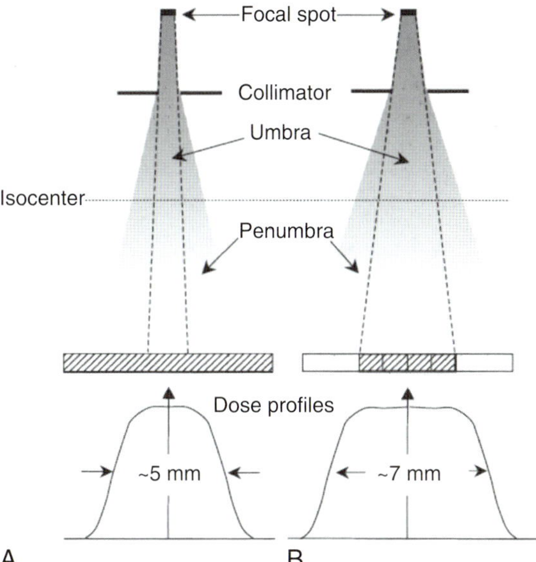


**FIGURE 10-12** The implications of focal spot penumbra on dose. **A,** The geometry of a single-slice scanner collimated to a nominal slice width of 4 mm is illustrated. The umbra and all the penumbra contribute to image formation, resulting in a dose profile of 5 mm that, when corrected to the isocenter, closely corresponds to the nominal slice width of 4 mm. **B,** The geometry for a multislice scanner collimated to a nominal 4 × 1-mm beam width may be compared. The collimators must be opened to ensure that each of the four 1-mm wide detector rows receives similar umbral radiation. The penumbral radiation is not used in the image reconstruction, and the resulting dose profile is approximately 7 mm in width. (From Heggie, J.C., et al. (2006). *Australasia Radiology, 50,* 278-285. Reproduced by permission of Blackwell Publications, Oxford, England.)

represents the penumbra caused by the finite size of the x-ray tube focal spot. It is clearly apparent that on a single-slice CT scanner the entire beam width plus the penumbra fall on the detectors. The penumbra, however, is not used to produce the image, but it does affect the patient dose.

On multislice CT scanners, the beam width, including the penumbra, would fall on a finite set of detectors depending on the scanner, but the penumbra would not be used to produce the image (because the intensity of the beam at the penumbra regions is less than the intensity at the center of the beam). To address this problem, the beam width (collimation) is increased so that the penumbra extends beyond the active detectors that will receive the central beam intensity (Lewis, 2005). The ratio of the area under the *z*-axis dose profile falling on the active detectors to the area under the total *z*-axis dose profile is referred to as the *z*-axis geometric **efficiency** (IEC, 2001).

Cody and McNitt-Gray (2006) showed that for a 32-cm diameter phantom, as beam widths increase from 18.0 mm, 19.2 mm, 24.0 mm, and 28.8 mm, the $CTDI_w$ (mGy) changes from 15.7 mGy, 16.8 mGy, 15.0 mGy, and 13.9 mGy, respectively (all other technical factors held constant). Additionally, Lewis (2005) indicated that

> scanners that acquire a greater number of simultaneous slices have an advantage in terms of z-axis geometric efficiency. This is because for narrow slice widths a wider total collimation can be used.…On multislice scanners z-axis geometric efficiencies are generally in the range of 80-98% for collimators of 10 mm and above, and about 55-75% for collimators of around 5 mm. For collimators around 1-2 mm z-axis geometric efficiencies are as low as 25% on some systems, although in dual slice mode, they can be much higher. Therefore the reduced geometric efficiency of multislice scanners, for wider collimators most commonly used, leads to dose increases around 10% when compared with single slice systems. However, very narrow collimations can result in a tripling, or more, in dose.

## Pitch

The term **pitch** is one common to spiral/helical CT scanners, sometimes called *spiral pitch* or *helical pitch*, depending on the manufacturer of the scanner. As defined by the IEC, pitch is a ratio of the distance the table travels per rotation to the total collimated x-ray beam width. The relationship between the absorbed dose and pitch is as follows:

$$\text{Dose} \propto \text{l/pitch} \qquad \textbf{(10-11)}$$

Therefore if the pitch increases by 2, the dose will be reduced to one half. It is important, however, to note that this relationship only holds true when the pitch changes and all other factors remain constant. For constant mAs (100 mAs per rotation), if the pitch changes from 1 to 2, the relative $CTDI_{vol}$ decreases from 1.0 to 0.5 mGy (Lewis, 2005).

## Number of Detectors

In a study comparing the dose from multislice CT scanners, Moore et al. (2006) demonstrated that the measured radiation dose is inversely proportional to the number of detector rows. They showed that there is a trend that as the number of detector rows increases from 4 to 8 to 16 detector rows, the dose decreases with both standard and near identical technique

## Over-Ranging (*Z*-Overscanning)

In spiral/helical CT scanning, it is important to realize that to image the planned length of tissue required

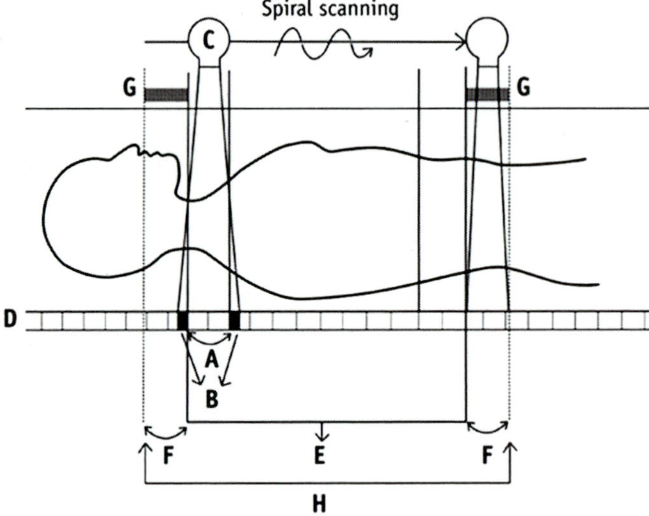


**FIGURE 10-13** Graphic illustration of the concepts of overbeaming, over-ranging, and adaptive section collimation technology during spiral scanning. (Reprinted with permission from Goo, H. W. (2012). *Korean Journal of Radiology, 13* (1), 1-11.)

for the examination and of interest to the radiologist, additional rotations before and after the planned length are essential for the **image reconstruction** process. This is referred to as over-ranging or *z*-overscanning (Tzedakis et al., 2007; Van der Molen and Geleijns, 2007), of which the components and definitions developed by Van der Molen and Geleijns (2007) are clearly illustrated in Figure 10-13. It is clear that there are two definitions of over-ranging:

1. Definition 1: This refers to the difference between the planned and exposed scan length.
2. Definition 2: This refers to the difference between the imaged and the exposed scan length.

Over-ranging increases the dose to the patient, which is validated in studies conducted by Tzedakis et al. (2007) on **pediatric patients** and by Van der Molen and Geleijns (2007). For example, Tzedakis et al. (2007) concluded that "in all cases normalized effective dose values were found to increase with increasing z-overscanning. The percentage differences in normalized data between axial and helical scans may reach 43%, 70%, 36%, and 26% for head-neck, chest, abdomen-pelvis, and trunk studies, respectively." Van der Molen and Geleijns (2007), for example, concluded that "overranging is reconstruction **algorithm** specific, and its length generally increases with collimation and pitch, while the effect of section width is variable. Over-ranging may lead to substantial but unnoticed exposure to radiosensitive organs."

## Patient Centering

Another factor affecting the dose to the patient under the control of the technologist is that of patient centering. The patient must be centered in the **gantry** isocenter for accurate imaging of the anatomy. Inaccurate patient centering (miscentering), as shown in Figure 10-14, degrades the image quality and increases the dose to the patient, especially with the use of AEC in CT (Li et al., 2007; Toth et al., 2007). Additionally, the use of bowtie filters in CT scanners is intended to serve basically two purposes: to shape the beam intensity within the scan field of **view** (SFOV) and to produce a more uniform beam at the detectors (Chapter 4). The x-ray beam is filtered; therefore, the bowtie filter actually plays a small role in reducing the dose to the patient, because the low-energy photons are removed and thus the beam becomes harder, that is, the mean energy of the beam increases. Improper centering of the patient in the gantry isocenter as shown in Figure 10-14 can lead to an increase in surface dose as well as the peripheral dose to the patient (Li et al., 2007; Toth et al., 2007).

In a study on the effect of patient centering on CT dose and image **noise,** Toth et al. (2007) showed that, for a 32-cm CTDI body phantom, a miscentering

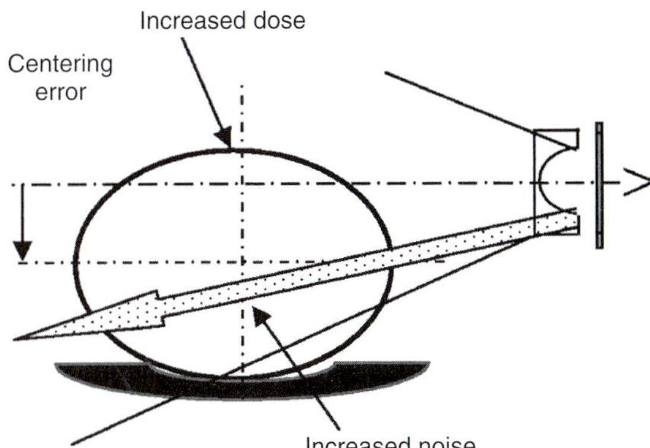


**FIGURE 10-14** A patient who is miscentered in the scan field of view can be expected to have degraded bowtie filter performance with an undesired increase in both dose and noise. (From Toth, T., et al. (2007). *Medical Physics, 34*, 3093-3101. Reproduced by the American Association of Physicists in Medicine.)

of about 3 cm and 6 cm can result in an increase in doses by 18% and 41%, respectively. Similar results were obtained by Li et al. (2007). Furthermore, a miscentering in elevation by 20 mm to 60 mm with a mean position 23 mm below the isocenter can result in a dose increase of up to 140% "with a mean dose penalty of 33% assuming that the tube current is increased to compensate for the increased noise due to miscentering" (Toth et al., 2007).

These findings are positive proof that technologists should always center the patient accurately in the gantry isocenter to avoid image noise problems and reduce the dose to the patient.

### Automatic Tube Current Modulation

AEC is now commonplace on CT scanners. AEC uses a technique referred to as automatic tube current modulation (ATCM) to optimize the dose to the patient while maintaining constant image quality, regardless of the size of the patient, in the *z*-axis and the attenuation changes in the *x-y* axis (Brisse et al., 2007; Toth et al., 2007). ATCM has been hailed as "the most important technique for maintaining constant image quality while optimizing radiation dose" (Li et al., 2007). For this reason, ATCM is described in detail in the next section.

## AUTOMATIC TUBE CURRENT MODULATION

ATCM is a technical development in CT based on the fundamental principles of AEC. AEC is not a new concept for radiologic technologists, for it is used extensively in radiography and fluoroscopy. The purpose of AEC in radiography, for example, is to provide a level of image quality (expressed as optical density for film-based radiography) in which there is consistent optical density for any examination (e.g., chest x ray) regardless of the thickness (small, medium, and large) of the patient. This level of image quality (optical density) is controlled by varying the duration of the exposure on the basis of the size of patient being imaged. For example, although the duration of the exposure will be shorter for smaller patients, it will be longer for larger patients, and therefore images of the same body parts on these patients will all have a consistent level of optical density.

### Problem with Setting Manual Milliamperage Techniques

In CT, the exposure technique factors (mAs and kVp) do not have a direct effect on the image density and contrast, respectively (as they do in film-based radiography), because CT is a digital-imaging modality. The dose to the patient is directly proportional to the mA, and in the past, CT technologists selected the mA values for patients manually. Lewis (2005) explained one of the problems with setting the mA values manually. She noted

> the attenuation of the x-ray beam increases with the thickness of material in its path, and for approximately every 4 cm of soft tissue, the x-ray beam intensity halves. In order to achieve the same transmitted x-ray intensity, and thereby the same level of image noise, changing from a 16 cm to a 20 cm diameter phantom requires a doubling of the mA. Changing from a 32 cm to a 48 cm phantom, the mA should in theory, be increased by a factor of 16. Systems which automatically adapt the overall tube current based on actual patient attenuation remove the guesswork from selecting the appropriate mA setting.

### Definition of Automatic Tube Current Modulation

In CT, **Automatic Tube Current Modulation (ATCM)** refers to the automatic control of the mA in two directions of the patient (the *x-y* axis and the *z*-axis) during **data acquisition** (scanning process) by use of specific technical procedures that take into consideration the patient size and the attenuation differences of the various tissues. The overall goal of ATCM is to provide consistent image quality despite the size of the patient and the tissue attenuation differences and to control the dose to the patient (Brisse et al., 2007; Kalra et al., 2004b; Li et al., 2007; McCollough et al., 2006; Toth et al., 2007) compared with manual mA selection techniques. Although the automatic control of the tube current (mA) in the *x-y* axis (in-plane) is referred to as angular modulation, changing the tube current automatically in the *z*-axis (through-plane) is referred to as *z*-axis modulation or longitudinal modulation. When used together, that is, angular-longitudinal tube current modulation, AEC is the result (Goodman & Brink, 2006).

The use of angular-longitudinal modulation can reduce the dose by as much as 52% compared with use of only the angular modulation technique (Goodman & Brink, 2006).

## Historical Background

ATCM techniques can be traced back to 1981, when Haaga et al. (1981) suggested its use as a dose reduction strategy in CT that did not compromise the needed image quality to make a diagnosis. This was followed by efforts from General Electric (GE) Medical Systems in 1994 and researchers such as Kalender et al. (1999), who published two reports describing dose reductions as much as 40% with ATCM techniques (McCollough et al., 2006). Later in 2001, a number of CT manufacturers such as GE Healthcare, Philips, Siemens, and Toshiba introduced ATCM techniques referred to by several names. For example, angular modulation systems are referred to as Smart Scan (GE Healthcare), DOM-Dose Modulation (Philips), and CareDose (Siemens). In addition, different names are used for both angular-longitudinal modulation systems, such as Smart mA (GE Healthcare), Z-DOM (Philips), CareDose 4D (Siemens), and Sure Exposure (Toshiba).

## Basic Principles of Operation

In CT AEC, the tube current (mA) is adjusted in real time during the scanning of a patient on the basis of differences in radiation attenuation in the transverse or *x-y* direction (in-plane) and the *z*-axis or longitudinal direction (through-plane) during the rotation of the tube and detectors. In addition, these tube current modulation techniques require some knowledge of the attenuation characteristics of the patient, and second, the operator must first set up the defined level of image quality (image noise target value) needed for the examination (Cody & McNitt-Gray, 2006; Lewis, 2005; McCollough et al., 2006). Each of these will be described briefly.

### Longitudinal (*Z*-Axis) Tube Current Modulation

**Longitudinal (z-axis) tube current modulation (z-axis TCM)** is based on differences in attenuation among body parts. For example, thicker body parts such as the abdomen and pelvis will attenuate the radiation more than thinner body parts, such as the head, neck, and chest regions. The technique of *z*-axis TCM is designed (using a specific computer algorithm) to change the mA automatically as the patient is scanned from, say, head to toe (along the *z*-axis) while maintaining a constant (uniform) noise level (image noise target values) for different thicknesses of body parts examined. This is clearly shown in Figure 10-15.

### Angular (*X-Y* Axis) Tube Current Modulation

Angular (*x-y* axis) tube current modulation (*x-y* axis TCM) is based on the fact that the radiation attenuation varies from the anteroposterior (AP) projection (low attenuation) to the lateral projection (high attenuation) as the tube rotates around (gantry rotation) the patient. Although the high-attenuation projections will require higher mA values, the low-attenuation projections will require lower mA values, as illustrated in Figure 10-16. The *x-y* axis TCM algorithm ensures that a constant (uniform) noise level is maintained during the scanning process.

### Angular-Longitudinal Tube Current Modulation

Figure 10-17 illustrates a method where both *x-y* axis and *z*-axis modulation can be used together to provide the "most comprehensive approach to CT dose reduction because the x-ray dose is adjusted according to the patient-specific attenuation in all three planes" (McCollough et al., 2006).

### Approaches to Obtaining Attenuation Characteristics of the Patient

The attenuation characteristics of the patient are one of the first pieces of information required to use AEC systems in CT imaging (that is, vary the mA during the scanning process and keep the image noise constant, regardless of the gantry rotation and the *z*-axis position). Such information is currently obtained by two different schemes. Although the first approach uses a CT scanned projection radiograph (SPR), the typical "scout view" (also referred to as ScoutView, Topogram, or the Scanogram, depending on the CT vendor), the second approach makes use of "on-line" data "from the preceding 180° of rotation to modulate the mA" (Lewis, 2005).

### Defined Level of Image Quality in CT Automatic Exposure Control

The second requirement when AEC is used in CT imaging is that operators must set up the defined level of image quality on their respective CT scanners. The approaches from four CT vendors include

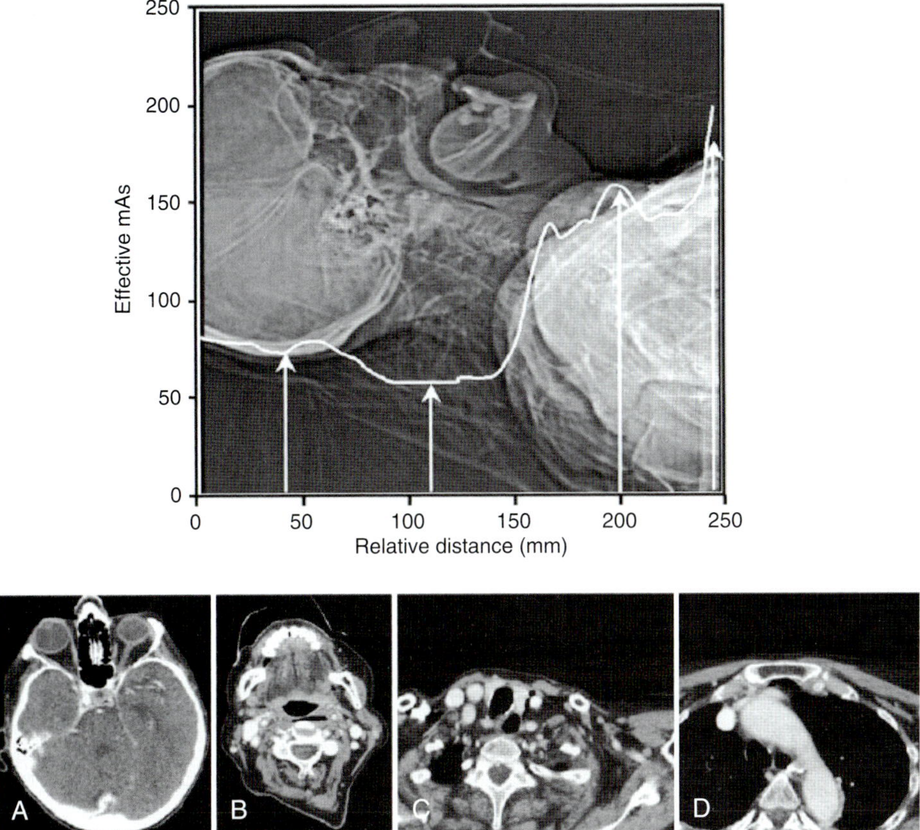


**FIGURE 10-15** The *z*-axis tube current modulation during CT of the neck. On the basis of the attenuation measurements made during the acquisition of the scan projection radiograph, the scanner software adjusts the effective mAs on the fly during the acquisition of the axial images. Axial images shown through orbits **(A)**, midcervical vertebrae **(B)**, the apex of the lung **(C)**, and the aortic arch **(D)** require 75 mAs, 58 mAs, 160 mAs, and 200 mAs, respectively, at 120 kVp. (From Heggie, J. C., et al. (2006). *Australasian Radiology, 50*, 278-285. Reproduced by permission of Blackwell Publications, Oxford, England.)

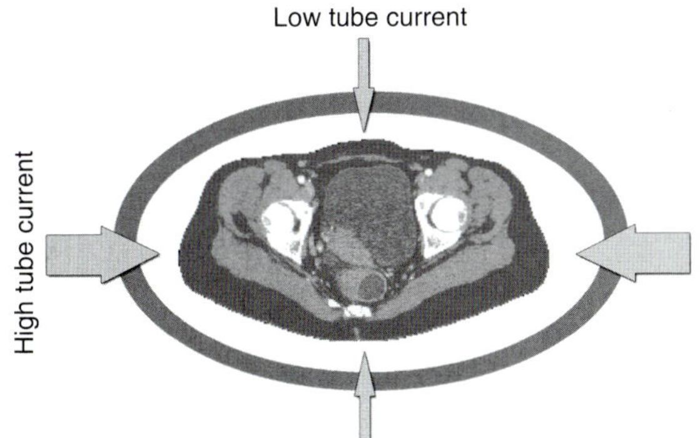


**FIGURE 10-16** Angular modulation with CareDose (Siemens Medical Solutions) ATCM technique. Online modulation of tube current is performed at different projections in the *x-y* plane within each 360-degree x-ray tube rotation. Thin arrows indicate reduction of tube current relative to higher tube current (*thick arrows*). (From Kalra, M., et al. (2004b). *Radiology, 233*, 649-657. Reproduced by permission of the Radiological Society of North America and the authors.)

a noise index (GE Healthcare), a reference image (Philips), a quality reference mAs (Siemens), and the standard deviation of **CT numbers** or an image quality level (Toshiba). Each of these is briefly described in Table 10-3. Essentially, the fundamental basis for these methods, as outlined in Table 10-1, rests on several important points:

1. A CT projection radiograph is required from which attenuation data are obtained.
2. An image quality index is prescribed (prescription of the mA). This index is related to the noise level (standard deviation of the CT numbers in a water phantom; Lewis, 2005).
3. A referenced image is selected (from previous examinations) that has the image quality required and the mA is adjusted to produce the same level of image quality as the referenced image when scanning other patients.
4. These methods are based on the use of proprietary algorithms.

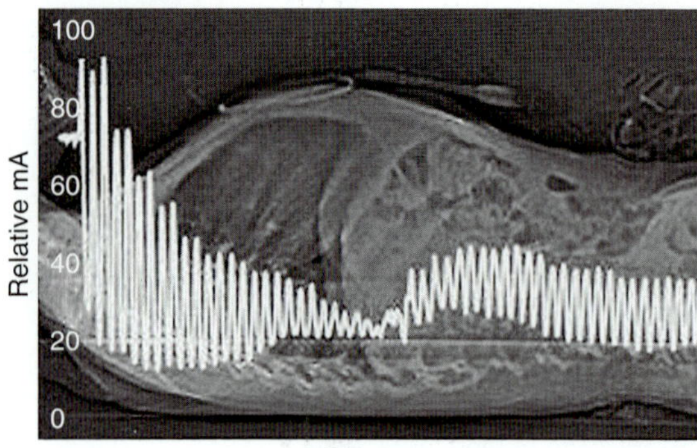


**FIGURE 10-17** Graph of tube current (mA) superimposed on a CT projection radiograph shows the variation in tube current as a function of time (and, hence, table position along the *z*-axis) at spiral CT in a 6-year-old child. An adult scanning protocol and an AEC system (CareDose 4D, Siemens Medical Solutions) were used with a reference effective tube current-time product of 165 mA. The mean effective tube current-time product for actual scanning was 38 mA (effective tube current-time product = tube current-time product/pitch). (From McCollough, C. H., Bruesewitz, M., R., & Kofler, J. M., Jr. (2006). *Radiographics, 26,* 503-512. Reproduced by permission of the Radiological Society of North America and the authors.)

## ITERATIVE RECONSTRUCTION ALGORITHMS

**Iterative reconstruction (IR)** algorithms in CT were described in detail in Chapter 6 in terms of a technical overview as well as their influence on image quality and dose. In summary, the primary advantages of iterative image reconstruction algorithms are to reduce image noise and minimize the higher radiation dose inherent in the filtered **back-projection** algorithm. All major CT manufacturers offer IR algorithms as of 2014.

In general the IR approach uses the filtered back-projection CT image data, referred to as the *measured projections*, to create *simulated projections,* which are then compared with the initial measured projections. These comparisons are done to determine differences in image noise. Once this difference is obtained, it is applied to the simulated projection to correct for inconsistencies. A new CT image is subsequently reconstructed and the process repeats until the difference between the measured and simulated projections are minor enough to be acceptable (Kaza et al., 2014). IR algorithms produce images with reduced noise and **artifacts,** Maldjian and Goldman (2013) and Kaza et al. (2014) showed reductions in radiation dose using IR that vary from 30% to 50%. The studies cited have included dose reductions in pediatric studies, CT abdominal examinations, and **CT angiography.** For more studies on the use of IR algorithms, the interested reader should refer to Chapter 6 for a more thorough discussion.

## IMAGE QUALITY AND DOSE: OPERATOR CONSIDERATIONS

It is clear from the foregoing discussion that image quality and dose are closely related. Image quality includes **spatial resolution,** contrast resolution, and noise. Although spatial resolution depends on geometric factors (such as focal spot size, slice thickness, and **pixel size,** for example), contrast resolution and noise depend on both the quality (beam energy) and quantity (number of x-ray photons) of the radiation beam. Several mathematical equations have been derived to express the relationship between dose and image quality (Bushong, 2009). For CT operators, the following mathematical expression is important:

$$\text{Dose} = \text{Intensity} \times \text{Beam energy}/\text{Noise}^2 \times \text{Pixel size}^3 \times \text{Slice thickness}$$

where intensity and beam energy depend on mA and kVp, respectively, and noise depends on the number of photons detected. This expression is read as follows: dose is directly proportional to the product of mA and kVp and inversely proportional to the product of noise squared, pixel size cubed, and slice thickness.

The expression also implies the following about dose and image quality:

1. To reduce the noise in an image by a factor of 2 requires an increase in the dose by a factor of 4.
2. To improve the spatial resolution (pixel size) by a factor of 2 (keeping the noise constant) requires an increase in the dose by a factor of 8.
3. To decrease the slice thickness by a factor of 2 requires an increase in the dose by a factor of 2 (keeping the noise constant).
4. To decrease both the slice thickness and the pixel size by a factor of 2 requires an increase in the dose by a factor of 16 ($2^3 \times 2 = 2 \times 2 \times 2 \times 2$).
5. Increasing mA and kVp increase the dose proportionally. For example, a twofold increase in mA increases the dose by a factor of 2. Additionally, doubling the dose will require an increase by the square of the kVp. For example, in 2006, Cody and McNitt-Gray found that by scanning a 32-cm body phantom at 220 mAs with a rotation time of 0.5 second, the $CTDI_W$ was 7.4 mGy, and

**TABLE 10-3 Image Quality Paradigms to Help the Computed Tomography Operator Select the Desired Level of Image Quality in Automatic Exposure Control in Computed Tomography**

| CT Vendor | Image Quality Paradigm | Description* |
|---|---|---|
| GE Healthcare | Noise index | The noise index is referenced to the standard deviation of CT numbers within the region of interest in a water phantom of a specific size. A look-up table is then used to map the patient-specific attenuation values measured on the CT projection radiograph (scout image) to tube current values for each gantry rotation according to a proprietary algorithm. The algorithm is designed to maintain the same noise level as the attenuation values change from one rotation to the next. Different noise indices may be required for patients of different sizes. |
| Philips | Reference image | In a process that the manufacturer calls automatic current setting, the user selects an acceptable patient examination, and the system saves the image (including the raw CT projection data and the CT projection radiograph, or "surview") as the reference data for comparison with the CT projection radiograph and data obtained from other patients in examinations for the same diagnostic task. The comparison is performed with the use of a proprietary algorithm and on a protocol-by-protocol basis (i.e., for a given examination type) to enable the automated selection of the appropriate tube current values by the scanner. |
| Siemens | Quality reference mAs | For each examination type (i.e., protocol) the user selects the effective tube current-time product (tube current-time product/pitch) typically used for a CT in a patient with a weight of approximately 80 kg. (For pediatric protocols the effective tube current-time product that should be selected is that typically used for a CT in a 20-kg patient.) The noise target (standard deviation of the CT numbers) is varied on the basis of patient size by using an empirical algorithm; thus, image noise is not kept constant for all patients but is adjusted according to an empirical impression on image quality. CT projection radiography ("topograms") for each patient is used to predict the tube current curve (with variations along the *x-y* and *z*-axes) that will yield the desired image quality, given the patient's size and anatomy. An on-line feedback system fine-tunes the actual tube current values during scanning to precisely match the patient-specific attenuation values at all angles (as opposed to the attenuation values estimated on the basis of one angle of the CT projection radiograph). |
| Toshiba | Standard deviation of CT numbers<br>Image quality level | Both methods are referenced to the standard deviation of CT numbers measured in a patient-equivalent water phantom. Data from the patient's CT projection radiograph (scanogram) are used to map the selected image quality to tube current values. |

*McCollough, M. C., Bruesewitz, M. R., & Kofler, J. M., Jr. (2006). *Radiographics, 26*, 503-512.

at 440 mAs with a rotation time of 1 second, the $CTDI_W$ was 30.2 mGy. These results are consistent with those reported by McNitt-Gray (2002) using a single-detector CT scanner.

Recall that the dose is proportional to the square of the kilovolt peak ($kVp^2$). This relationship often causes some difficulty for technologists in practice. As described by Reid et al. (2010) the power (2) can vary from 2.5 to 3.1 and depends on the patient's size. Maldjian and Goldman (2013), reported that decreasing the kilovolt peak from 140 kVp to 120 kVp, reduced the dose by 28% to 40% for a typical phantom. The authors reported that further decreasing to 80 kVp reduces the dose by approximately 65%. Precise adjustment of dose should not be obtained solely through manipulation of peak kilovoltage.

## CT DOSE OPTIMIZATION

In this chapter so far, two points have been made clear. First, CT is rapidly expanding in its use in medicine. Second, a major concern that is receiving

TABLE 10-4 A Summary of Important CT Dose Parameters

| Dose Parameter | Definition | Effects on Radiation Dose | Unit |
|---|---|---|---|
| Tube potential or voltage | X-ray beam energy | Proportional to square of tube voltage change | kV |
| Product of tube current and time | Photon fluence; number of photons in defined exposure time | Directionally proportional to radiation dose | mAs |
| Pitch | Ratio of table feed per gantry rotation | Inversely proportional to radiation dose | — |
| $CTDI_W$ | Average radiation dose in scan volume measured in standard CT phantoms; 1/3 CTDI center + 2/3 CTDI periphery | Directly proportional to radiation dose in unit volume, influenced by pitch factor | mGy |
| DLP | $CTDI_{vol}$ × scan length (cm) | Directly proportional to total scanned radiation dose | mGy cm |
| Effective dose | Overall risk-related radiation exposure; Σ $W_T$ (tissue weighting factor) × $H_T$ (tissue equivalent factor) | Directly proportional to total scanned radiation dose and overall risk of irradiated tissue | mSv |

Reprinted with permission from Goo, H. W. (2012). *Korean Journal of Radiology, 13* (1), 1-11.

increasing attention in the literature relates to the potential for high radiation doses delivered by CT scanners and the potential biological risks of CT scanning (Brenner & Elliston, 2004; Brenner et al., 2001). With these notions in mind, there have been increasing efforts to reduce the dose to the patient without compromising the image quality needed to make a diagnosis. One such significant approach is that of dose optimization, and to date various strategies have been devised to help CT users reduce the dose to the patient while maintaining optimal image quality (Heggie et al., 2006; Kalra et al., 2004a; Lewis, 2005; McCollough et al., 2006).

## What Is Dose Optimization?

**Dose optimization** is a radiation protection principle intended to ensure that doses delivered to patients are kept **as low as is reasonably achievable (ALARA).** Essentially, the principle of optimization refers to reducing radiation dose while maintaining the required image quality needed to make a diagnosis. Dose optimization is especially important for digital imaging modalities such as computed radiography and CT, for example, where the potential for high doses exists (Brenner & Hall, 2007).

## Early Dose Optimization Strategies

As described in this chapter, a number of factors affect the dose to the patient in CT. These include the **scan parameters** such as exposure technique factors (constant and effective mAs and kVp), collimation (*z*-axis geometric efficiency), pitch, number of detectors, over-ranging (*z*-overscanning), patient centering, ATCM, and iterative image reconstruction. A summary of important CT dose parameters is provided in Table 10-4. To effectively reduce the dose and maintain the needed image quality (Table 10-5), users must have systematic approaches or strategies to CT dose optimization.

Several authors have described various dose optimization strategies in CT, especially in multislice CT (Frush, 2004; Heggie et al., 2006; Kalra et al., 2004a; Kanal et al., 2007; Lai & Frush, 2006; Lewis, 2005; McCollough et al., 2006; Winkler, 2003; Winkler & Mather, 2005). It is not within the scope of this chapter to describe details of these strategies; however, it is noteworthy to highlight the essential guiding principles. Several strategies that emerge as common themes relate to the mAs, kVp, collimation, slice thickness, scanned volume, pitch, and the use of ATCM techniques. Heggie et al. (2006) discussed CT dose optimization and provided a summary of the main items to consider, as listed in Box 10-1.

Dose optimization has received increasing attention in pediatric CT. Lai and Frush (2006) and Goodman and Brink (2006), for example, presented excellent overviews on this topic, examining not only trends and patterns of CT use, radiation risks from CT, and how radiologists can manage CT dose but they also focused on the technical factors for dose management such as controlling tube current and voltage, the influence of gantry cycle time, choice of pitch and detector width, and finally the use of tube current modulation techniques. For example,

## TABLE 10-5 Relationship of Four CT Image Quality Parameters to Radiation

| Image Quality Parameter | Definition | Relationships with Radiation Dose Parameters | Calculation Method |
|---|---|---|---|
| Image noise | Random variation of CT numbers | Inversely proportional to square root of radiation dose; inversely proportional to tube voltage; inversely proportional to fourth power of spatial resolution; influenced by section thickness and reconstruction algorithm | Standard deviation of measured CT numbers |
| Contrast-to-noise resolution | Ability to distinguish between different CT numbers | Not significantly changed at different tube voltages in most of materials except for some with high atomic numbers such as iodine (increased at low tube voltage); low-contrast resolution greatly influenced by image noise level | $(S_A - S_B)/\sigma$, where $S_A$ and $S_B$ are CT attenuation measured in structures A and B and $\sigma$ is measured image noise |
| Spatial resolution | Ability to distinguish small details of object | Inversely proportional to focal spot size, detector collimation; influenced by reconstruction algorithm | Voxel size; line pairs per centimeter; point or line spread function; modulation transfer function |
| Artifacts | Unwanted structures degrading CT image quality | Photon starvation artifacts—inversely proportional to radiation dose; physiologic motion artifacts—inversely proportional to temporal resolution; other artifacts—no direct relationships with radiation dose parameters | — |

Reprinted with permission from Goo, H. W. (2012). *Korean Journal of Radiology, 13* (1), 1-11.

## BOX 10-1 Optimization Technique

Use sequential as opposed to helical techniques for head scans.
Avoid transferring scan protocols applicable to one scanner to another without due consideration to differences in scanner filtration and geometry.
Keep scanned volume to minimum and scan in one large block rather than multiple smaller blocks. See text for possible exceptions.
Use widest x-ray beam collimation consistent with clinical requirements.
Consider using a lower tube potential for CT angiography.
Keep the effective mAs, which is defined as the mAs/pitch, as low as clinically indicated.
Use tube current modulation technology with an appropriately selected reference effective mAs or noise index. For optimum performance of modulation technology, the SPR that is of clinical relevance must be acquired over the full length of the patient by using the same kVp that will be subsequently used for the axial image acquisition.
Minimize use of multiphasic examinations.

From Heggie et al. (2006). *Australasian Radiology, 50,* 278-285. Reproduced by permission Blackwell Publishing Limited, Oxford, England.

Lai and Frush (2006) emphasized the importance of the radiologist to ensure that all examinations ordered should be justified and that the need for **communications** between ordering physicians and radiologists is vital as a first step to CT dose reduction. Additionally, they pointed out that the CT protocols used must include various technical parameters that optimize the dose to the patient without compromising the needed image quality. In this regard, they state that increasing the detector width from 0.625 to 1.25 for a 16-slice CT scanner while holding all other factors constant will result in a reduced dose to the patient. Finally, they also advocate the use of age- or weight-adjusted CT protocols and the use of ATCM techniques. In addition, an interesting study on optimizing image quality and radiation dose in CT pulmonary angiography showed that by decreasing the peak kilovoltage from 120 kVp to 100 kVp, the dose to the patient is reduced significantly without loss of objective or subjective image quality (Heyer et al., 2007).

A more recent checklist for dose optimization, published in 2012, is provided in Table 10-6. The table's checkup items are not evaluated based on their influence on image quality. An interesting exercise would be to compare the checklist in Box 10-1 with Table 10-6 and identify common elements that have not changed through the years.

**TABLE 10-6 Checklist for Dose Optimization**

| Checkup Items | Recommendations |
|---|---|
| Body size-adapted CT protocol | ✓ Traditionally based on body weight or body mass index<br>✓ Based on cross-sectional dimensions and/or body attenuation for better dose adaptation to individually varied body habitus<br>✓ Use best-fit equation rather than dose table or chart |
| Tube current modulation | ✓ Always turn on if applicable<br>✓ Set up appropriate reference image quality index<br>✓ Check how much modulated tube current reaches to maximal limits ("tube current saturation") and adjust parameters such as tube voltage and scan speed to obtain maximal dose reduction by tube current modulation |
| Optimal tube voltage at equivalent radiation dose | ✓ Select most dose-efficient tube voltage<br>✓ Consider lower tube voltages for contrast-enhanced examination, higher tube voltages for examinations requiring lower noise (e.g., unenhanced brain CT), and for examinations detecting low-contrast lesions (e.g., micro-abscesses in liver or ground-glass opacity in lung) |
| Longitudinal scan range | ✓ Adjust to minimal range as required for clinical indications, desirably by using clear anatomic landmarks |
| Repeated scanning | ✓ Reduce number of repeated scanning<br>✓ Omit precontrast examination if possible |
| Scan modes | ✓ Use low-dose scan mode to maximize benefit-risk ration of CT examination (e.g., prospectively ECG-triggered sequential or high-pitch dual-source spiral scanning in cardiac CT) |
| Noise-reducing image reconstruction algorithms | ✓ Use noise-reducing, spatial resolution-reserving algorithms (e.g., IR algorithms) at lower radiation dose |

Reprinted with permission from Goo, H. W. (2012). *Korean Journal of Radiology, 13* (1), 1-11.

## Research on Dose Optimization and Image Quality[1]

Dose optimization in CT based on image quality requires a thorough understanding of CT dose parameters and CT image quality parameters. CT image quality has been described in terms of high-contrast spatial resolution, **low-contrast resolution, temporal resolution,** CT number accuracy and uniformity, image noise, and image artifacts.

Research has continued to determine the best methods for lowering radiation dose in CT examinations without compromising the diagnostic quality of images. These studies often are complex so they can follow precise scientific methods, including identifying the problem, performing a literature review, stating the goals regarding investigation of the problem, and designing a methodology to find a solution to the problem. Scientific methods also include data collection, analysis and interpretation of the data, and dissemination of the study findings (Cresswell, 2008).

In general, research on optimizing dose and image quality involves various methodologies to demonstrate dose reduction without a loss of image quality. To determine optimal image quality, McCollough et al. (2006) stressed that studies must involve quantitative metrics such as image noise and observer performance.

In a special issue of the journal *Radiation Protection Dosimetry* dedicated to optimization strategies in medical imaging for fluoroscopy, radiography, **mammography,** and CT, several studies identified at least four important requirements for dose and image quality optimization research (Mattsson, 2005):

1. Ensure patient safety.
2. Determine the level of image quality required for a particular diagnostic task.
3. Acquire images at various exposure levels from high to low and in such a manner that accurate diagnosis can still be made.
4. Use reliable and valid methodologies for the dosimetry, image acquisition, and evaluation of image quality using human observers, remembering the nature of the detection task.

[1]From Seeram, E. (2014). Computed tomography dose optimization. *Radiologic Technology, 85* (6), 655-675. Reproduced by permission of the American Association of Radiologic Technologists.

To accomplish these requirements, CT dose and image quality optimization studies generally must ensure that the following minimum essential elements are considered:

1. The CT **imaging system** is calibrated to ensure consistent and reliable performance.
2. The dosimeters used to capture dose levels are calibrated.
3. Researchers use appropriate phantoms (anthropomorphic phantoms and phantoms for determining objective image quality parameters [Zarb et al., 2010]) and acceptable dose measurement methodology of acquiring scans at different exposure levels.
4. Images are assessed in two phases:
   A. Expert observers evaluate image quality based on a defined and specific criterion (such as the appearance of image noise) to establish an optimized dose level.
   B. The same set of observers is used to assess images obtained at various dose levels, including an optimized dose level, using established, valid, and reliable observer performance methods. Observer performance methods include receiver-operating characteristic (Zarb et al., 2010) and visual grading analysis (Tingberg et al., 2005) methods. The task of pathology detection requires a different observer performance test than that of detecting normal anatomic structures.

Receiving-operator characteristic is the most common observer performance method. Under this method, a study's observers determine whether an image contains a lesion or pathology. The observer assigns a grade on a scale (e.g., 1 to 5) that rates the observer's level of confidence in the decision (Tingberg et al., 2005).

A visual grading analysis assigns a grade to the image's quality based on comparison with a reference image. Visual grading analysis is based on the assumption that an observer's ability to see and evaluate normal anatomy correlates to the ability to evaluate pathology, or abnormal findings (Tingberg et al., 2005).

### Findings from CT Dose Optimization Studies

Some studies that reduce patient dose markedly by reducing kilovolt peak, changing pitch, adjusting beam width, or collimation, or by using iterative image reconstruction, do not address the important consideration of optimizing image quality while reducing dose. For the most part, the studies did not include observer performance methods to evaluate image quality at these reduced exposures. One of the fundamental problems with this approach to dose management is that the dose may be so low that the diagnostic quality of the image is compromised, thus endangering the integrity of the clinical diagnosis and necessitating repeat examinations.

Other research in CT, however, has included methods of dose and image quality optimization, which include valid and reliable dosimetry, observer image quality assessment, and statistical analysis of results. Examples include the following:

- Sohaib et al. (2001) examined the effect of reducing mAs on image quality and patient dose in sinus CT examinations. The authors reported a dose reduction from 13.5 mGy at 200 mAs to 3.1 mGy at 50 mAs ($P < 0.05$) without loss of image quality. The study used an observer performance method that involved visual grading analysis.
- Russell et al. (2008) examined dose image quality in neck volume CT and showed that ATCM reduced the CTDI by 20% with the noise index set at 11.4 and by 34% with the noise index set at 20.2. The dose reductions were made without compromising image quality significantly.

## RADIATION PROTECTION CONSIDERATIONS

The dose optimization strategies described so far focus on methods to reduce the dose to the patient. What about the protection of personnel in CT scanning? Radiation protection of both patients and personnel in medicine is guided by two triads that are intended to ensure that medical radiation workers work within the ALARA philosophy of the ICRP. One triad deals with radiation protection actions, and the other triad addresses the radiation protection principles (Seeram, 2001).

### Radiation Protection Actions

Radiation protection actions include the use of time, shielding, and distance, which are intended to protect both patients and personnel in radiology. For example, because dose is proportional to the *time of exposure*, to protect personnel in CT, it is essential to minimize the time spent in the CT scan room during the exposure.

**Distance,** on the other hand, is a major dose reduction action because the dose is inversely proportional to the square of the distance. This means that the further one is away from the radiation source, the less the dose received. In CT, because the patient is the main source of scatter, technologists should stand back as far away from the patient as possible if is necessary to be in the scan room during scanning. This implies that a power injector that can be controlled from outside the scan room is recommended. If a hand injector is used, then long tubing should be included.

**Shielding** is intended to protect not only patients (gonadal, breast, eyes, and thyroid) but also personnel and members of the public. Patients are often concerned about the exposure of their gonads during a CT examination. Because most of the gonadal exposure will come from internal scatter and not from the primary beam (unless the gonadal region was being examined), there is no need for this concern. Technologists, however, could place gonadal shielding on the patient because it may alleviate any fears about the risks of exposure to radiation. Shields can also be used to protect the eyes, breast, and thyroid of patients undergoing CT examinations (DeMaio et al., 2014; Fricke et al., 2003; Kennedy et al., 2007; McCollough et al., 2012). Although some of the shields are made of flexible, nonlead (bismuth) composition, lead may also be used (Kennedy et al., 2007) to provide significant dose reduction to these critical organs.

The use of *bismuth shields* in CT discussed in the literature (DeMaio et al. 2014; McCollough et al. 2011, 2012) has sparked some debate among academics and practitioners, and various studies have shown advantages in dose reduction as well as problems imposed by these shields during the examination. This has led the American Association of Physicists in Medicine (AAPM) to issue the following Position Statement on the Use of Bismuth Shielding for the Purpose of Dose Reduction in CT scanning (AAPM, 2014). The following statement is "policy text":

> Bismuth shields are easy to use and have been shown to reduce dose to anterior organs in CT scanning. However, there are several disadvantages associated with the use of bismuth shields, especially when used with automatic exposure control or tube current modulation. Other techniques exist that can provide the same level of anterior dose reduction at equivalent or superior image quality that do not have these disadvantages. The AAPM recommends that these alternatives to bismuth shielding be carefully considered, and implemented when possible.

The AAPM also provides a description of the reason for this policy, and lists the following disadvantages of using bismuth shields. These include:

1. "Applying bismuth shielding together with automatic exposure controls (AEC) systems, such as tube current modulation (TCM), leads to unpredictable and potentially undesirable levels of dose and image quality.
2. The shields can degrade image quality and accuracy.
3. The shields waste some of the patient's radiation exposure."

Furthermore the AAPM also provides "Alternative methods for reducing dose to peripheral organs in CT scanning" and lists 14 references of relevance to the use of bismuth shielding in CT. The interested reader should refer to this AAPM document.

When personnel are expected to be present in the CT scan room during the exposure, lead aprons should be worn (for the same reason that gonadal shields are placed on patients) because of the presence of scatter (Bushong, 2009). For a more detailed account of shielding in CT, the interested reader should refer to the paper by DeMaio et al. (2014) titled "Shielding in Computed Tomography: An Update" in which they "... outline the literature-supported best practices for each method and will attempt to clarify common misconceptions about proper use of shielding during CT procedures.

Because scatter radiation is present during a CT examination and strikes the walls of the CT room, these walls should be shielded to protect members of the public or other radiation workers who are present outside the room. The use of minimum shielding in the form of thick plate-glass control room viewing windows and gypsum wall board with no lead content can sometimes provide the minimum required shielding.

## Radiation Protection Principles

Radiation protection principles deal with justification, optimization, and dose limitation principles vital to radiation protection regulation.

Justification involves the concept of net benefit, that is, there must be a benefit associated with every exposure. This requirement is intended for referring physicians and is one effort to reduce doses to patients undergoing x-ray examinations.

Optimization is a principle that is intended to ensure that doses delivered to patients are kept ALARA, with economic and social factors taken into account. In implementing ALARA, technologists should always apply all relevant technical radiation protection practices to ensure that the dose is optimized and that image quality is not compromised, as discussed earlier in the chapter.

The concept of dose limitation is a major integral component of regulatory guidance on radiation protection. This concept addresses the dose that an individual receives annually or accumulates over a working lifetime. These doses should be within the limits established by international organizations such as the ICRP and other national bodies such as the National Council on Radiation Protection. These recommended limits are intended to reduce the probability of stochastic effects and to prevent detrimental deterministic effects. These dose limits are beyond the scope of this chapter.

### The Role of the CT Technologist

The technologist must always keep the ALARA principle when conducting CT examinations, and must play a significant role in optimizing the dose in CT for several reasons, such as acquiring the images from the patient and paying attention to all aspects of the examination, including patient communication, patient positioning and care, radiation protection, and so on.

Seeram (2014) provided a list of factors to which the technologist must pay careful attention when optimizing the image quality and dose in CT. These include:

1. The risks of radiation and CT dose in particular.
2. Current technical advances in CT.
3. CT dose metrics, particularly $CTDI_{vol}$, the DLP and effective dose, and associated units.
4. CT image quality metrics such as spatial resolution, contrast resolution, noise, and artifacts.
5. The technical factors affecting patient dose in CT, including exposure technique factors ([kVp and mAs], AEC, pitch, effective mAs, slice thickness, SFOV, beam collimation, noise-reducing algorithms [IR algorithms], anatomical coverage, overbeaming and over-ranging, patient centering, and noise index).
6. Scan protocols and reviewing the protocols with the radiologist on an ongoing basis with the goal of optimizing dose and image quality.
7. The prescan and postscan display of CT dose reports showing the $CTDI_{vol}$, the DLP, and effective dose.
8. How to get involved with the development or implementation of a CT dose-monitoring or dose-tracking system for the technologist's CT department. Monitoring and tracking should include items such as dose capture, conversion of absorbed dose to effective dose, patient-specific storage, dose analytics, dose communication, and data export.
9. How to participate in research on CT patient dose and image quality optimization. This requires a fundamental knowledge of CT equipment and dosimeter calibration, image acquisition details, observer performance measures, and appropriate statistical tools.
10. How to ensure continuous professional development through relevant continuing education activities.

## CT DOSE INDEX REGISTRY

### What Is the Dose Index Registry?

The American College of Radiology (ACR; http://www.acr.org/Quality-Safety/National-Radiology-Data-Registry/Dose-Index-Registry) describes the Dose Index Registry (DIR) as:

> ... a data registry that allows facilities to compare their CT dose indices with regional and national values. Information related to dose indices for all CT exams is collected, anonymized, transmitted to the ACR, and stored in a database. Institutions are then provided with periodic feedback reports comparing their results by body part and exam type to aggregate results.

The ACR also lists a number of documents to help facilities understand and record the CT dose indices. Examples of these documents include: Standardized DIR Report User Guide, DIR Measures, DIR 5 Million Examinations Update, DIR Overview and Instructions for Use, DIR Data Dictionary, DIR Mapping Tool User Guide, DIR Sample Report, DIR Pediatric Sample Report, Scanner Models that Have Successfully Transmitted Files to DIR, and the American Board of Radiology (ABR) Practice Quality Improvement (PQI) Project Description.

In "Radiation Exposure from CT Scans: How to Close our Knowledge Gaps, Monitor and Safeguard Exposure—Proceedings and Recommendations of the Radiation Dose Summit," Boone et al. (2011) noted that the CTDIR began in 2011, with the goal of collecting dose index values such as the CTDI and the DLP from several sites for the purpose of comparison, using dose-structured reports. As noted by Boone et al. (2011),

> Participating institutions are provided with periodic feedback consisting of reports that compare their data with aggregate results from other institutions. For the purpose of comparison, the concept of Diagnostic Reference Level (DRL) was introduced. The DRL is the radiation dose level for a typical-sized patient and a particular radiologic procedure. Now, with the use of DRLs, it is possible to identify situations in which the patient dose is unusually high.

## IMAGE WISELY AND IMAGE GENTLY

Image Wisely (2015) and Image Gently (2015) are two website resources that provide essential elements of radiation safety in adult and pediatric imaging, respectively. Specifically, Image Wisely is as follows:

> The American College of Radiology and the Radiological Society of North America formed the Joint Task Force on Adult Radiation Protection to address

> concerns about the surge of public exposure to ionizing radiation from medical imaging. The Joint Task Force collaborated with the American Association of Physicists in Medicine and the American Society of Radiologic Technologists to create the Image Wisely campaign with the objective of lowering the amount of radiation used in medically necessary imaging studies and eliminating unnecessary procedures.
>
> Image Wisely offers resources and information to radiologists, medical physicists, other imaging practitioners, and patients (http://www.imagewisely.org).

Image Wisely also includes participating organizations such as ACR, the Radiological Society of North America (RSNA), American Society of Radiologic Technologists (ASRT), and AAPM.

Image Gently, on the other hand, is the Alliance for Radiation Safety in Pediatric Imaging, whose mission is:

> ... to improve the safety and effectiveness on the imaging care of children worldwide. This is achieved through increased awareness, education and advocacy on the need for the appropriate examination and amount of radiation dose when imaging children. The ultimate goal of the Alliance is to change practice locally to improve the health and safety of the child (http://imagegently.org).

## REVIEW QUESTIONS

Answer the following questions to check your understanding of the materials studied.

1. Which of the following best describes the beam geometry for single-slice spiral/helical CT scanners?
   A. pencil beam
   B. a square beam
   C. a fan-shaped beam
   D. all are correct
2. The dose distribution in CT for a single slice is given by the function:
   A. *D* (*z*).
   B. *D* × *Z* × constant.
   C. *Z* (*d*).
   D. *D* (*z*) *a*
3. The easiest and probably the most accurate method of measuring the dose in CT is:
   A. film dosimetry.
   B. thermoluminescent dosimetry.
   C. pencil ionization method.
   D. all are correct.
4. The average dose to the patient from a series of scans is the:
   A. *D*(*z*).
   B. MSAD.
   C. CTDI.
   D. dose equivalent.
5. The area under typical dose distribution profile for a single scan divided by the slice width is the:
   A. CTDI.
   B. CTID.
   C. MSAD.
   D. effective dose area.
6. The quantity measured by the pencil ionization chamber technique is the:
   A. slice width.
   B. absorbed dose.
   C. MSAD.
   D. CTDI.
7. The dose to the patient in CT is affected by:
   1. noise.
   2. slice thickness and pixel size.
   3. kVp and mAs.
   4. linear attenuation coefficient (μ).

   A. 1 only
   B. 1 and 2
   C. 1, 2, and 3
   D. all are correct
8. The dose to the patient is increased if:
   1. noise decreases.
   2. slice thickness decreases.
   3. pixel width decreases.
   4. mAs is increased and kVp is decreased.

   A. 1 only
   B. 1 and 2
   C. 1, 2, and 3
   D. 1, 2, 3, and 4
9. Which of the following will decrease the MSAD to the patient in a CT examination?
   A. decreasing the width of the dose distribution curve
   B. increasing the bed indexing
   C. reducing the mAs
   D. all are correct
10. Which of the following concept/principle/action deals with the intelligent use of radiation as a radiation protection measure?
    A. time
    B. shielding and distance
    C. justification
    D. optimization

## REFERENCES

American Association of Physicists in Medicine (AAPM). (2004). *AAPM Position Statement on the Use of Bismuth Shielding for the Purpose of Dose Reduction in CT scanning.* <http://www.aapm.org/publicgeneral/Bismuth Shielding.pdf> Accessed on 14.01.02.

Amis, E. S., Butler, P. F., Applegate, K. E., et al. (2007). American College of Radiology white paper on radiation dose in medicine. *Journal of the American College of Radiology, 4,* 272–284.

Baker, S. R., & Tilak, G. S. (2006). CT spurs concern over thyroid cancer. *Diagnostic Imaging, 51,* 25–27.

Boone, J. M. (2007). The trouble with the $CTDI_{100}$. *Medical Physics, 34,* 1364–1371.

Boone, J. M., Hendee, W. R., McNitt-Gray, M. F., & Seltzer, S. E. (2011). Radiation exposure from CT scans: how to close our knowledge gaps, monitor and safeguard exposure—proceedings and recommendations of the Radiation Dose Summit, sponsored by NIBIB, February 24-25, 2011. *Radiology, 265*(2), 544–554.

Brady, Z., et al. (2012). Assessment of paediatric CT dose indicators for the purpose of optimisation. *British Journal of Radiology, 85*(1019), 1488–1498.

Brenner, D. J. (2006). It is time to retire the computed tomography dose index (CTDI) for CT quality assurance and dose optimization. *Medical Physics, 33,* 1189–1191.

Brenner, D. J., & Elliston, C. D. (2004). Estimated radiation risks potentially associated with full body CT screening. *Radiology, 232,* 735–738.

Brenner, D. J., & Hall, E. J. (2007). CT—an increasing source of radiation exposure. *New England Journal of Medicine, 22,* 2277–2284.

Brenner, D. J., Elliston, C., Hall, E., & Berdon, W. (2001). Estimated risks of radiation-induced fatal cancer from pediatric CT. *American Journal of Roentgenology, 176,* 289–296.

Brisse, H. J., Madec, L., Gaboriaud, G., et al. (2007). Automatic exposure control in multichannel CT with tube current modulation to achieve a constant level of image noise: experimental assessment on pediatric phantoms. *Medical Physics, 34,* 3018–3032.

Bushberg, A. T., Seibert, J. A., Leidholdt, E. M., Jr., & Boone, J. M. (2012). *The essential physics of medical imaging* (3rd ed.). Philadelphia, PA: Lippincott-Williams.

Bushong, S. (2013). *Radiologic science for technologists* (10th ed.). St. Louis, MO: Mosby-Year Book.

Cody, D., & McNitt-Gray, M. (2006). *CT image quality and patient radiation dose: definitions, methods, and trade-offs.* Chicago, IL: Radiological Society of North America.

Colang, J. E., Killion, J. B., & Vano, E. (2007). Patient dose from CT: a literature review. *Radiologic Technology, 79,* 17–26.

Creswell, J. W. (2008). *Educational research: planning, conducting, and evaluating quantitative and qualitative research* (2nd ed.). Upper Saddle River, NJ: Pearson Education.

DeMaio, D. N., Turk, J., & Palmer, E. (2014). Shielding in computed tomography: an update. *Radiologic Technology, 85*(5), 563–670.

Dixon, R. L. (2003). A new look at CT dose measurement: beyond CTDI. *Medical Physics, 30,* 1272–1280.

Dixon, R. L. (2006). Restructuring CT dosimetry—a realistic strategy for the future requiem for the pencil chamber. *Medical Physics, 33,* 3973–3976.

ECRI. (2007). Radiation dose in CT. *Health Devices, 36,* 41–63.

FDA. (2010). *Initiative to Reduce Unnecessary Radiation Exposure from Medical Imaging. Center for Devices and Radiological Health.* U.S. Food and Drug Administration.

Fricke, B. L., et al. (2003). In-plane bismuth breast shields for pediatric CT: effects on radiation dose and image quality using experimental and clinical data. *American Journal of Roentgenology, 180,* 407–411.

Frush, D. P. (2004). Review of radiation issues for computed tomography. *Seminars in Ultrasound, CT, and MRI, 25,* 17–24.

Frush, D. P. (2006). Pediatric CT quality and radiation dose: clinical perspective. In *Radiological Society of North America: Categorical course in diagnostic radiology physics: from invisible to visible—the science and practice of x-ray imaging and radiation dose optimization* (pp. 167–182). Chicago, IL: Radiological Society of North America.

Goldberg-Stein, S., Liu, B., Hahn, P. F., & Lee, S. I. (2011). Body CT during pregnancy: utilization trends, examination indications, and fetal radiation doses. *American Journal of Roentgenology, 196*(1), 146–151.

Goo, H. W. (2012). *Korean Journal of Radiology, 13*(1), 1–11.

Goodman, T. R., & Brink, J. A. (2006). Adult CT: controlling dose and image quality. In *Radiological Society of North America: Categorical course in diagnostic radiology physics: from invisible to visible—the science and practice of x-ray imaging and radiation dose optimization* (pp. 157–165). Chicago, IL: Radiological Society of North America.

Gosling, O. E., Iyengar, S., Loader, R., et al. (2011). Radiation doses trends from cardiac CT using a cardiac specific conversion factor: system understanding & an optimisation strategy significantly reduces the dose to the patients in a clinical service. *Heart, 97,* A65–A66.

Haaga, J. R., Miraldi, F., MacIntyre, W., LiPuma, J. P., Bryan, P. J., & Wiesen, E. (1981). The effect of mAs variation upon computed tomography image quality as evaluated by in vivo and in vitro studies. *Radiology, 138,* 449–454.

Heggie, J. C., Kay, J. K., & Lee, W. K. (2006). Importance of optimization of multi-slice computed tomography scan protocols. *Australasian Radiology, 50,* 278–285.

Hendee, W. R., & O'Connor, M. K. (2013). Radiation risks in medical imaging: separating fact from fantasy. *Radiology, 264*(2), 312–320.

Hermann, T. L., Fauber, T. L., Gill, J., et al. (2014). *Best practices in digital radiography.* <http://asrt.org/docs/default-source/whitepapers/asrt12_bstpracdigradwhp_final.pdf?sfvrsn=4> Accessed April 9, 2014.

Heyer, C. M., Mohr, P. S., Lemburg, S. P., Peters, S. A., & Nicholas, V. (2007). Image quality and radiation exposure at pulmonary CT angiography with 100- or 120-kVp protocol. *Radiology, 245*, 577–583.

Huda, W. (2006). Medical radiation dosimetry. In *Radiological Society of North America Categorical course in diagnostic radiology physics: from invisible to visible—the science and practice of x-ray imaging and radiation dose optimization* (pp. 29–39). Chicago: Radiological Society of North America.

Huda, W., & Vance, A. (2007). Patient radiation doses from adult and pediatric CT. *American Journal of Roentgenology, 188*, 540–546.

Huda, W., Ravenel, J. G., & Scalzietti, E. M. (2003). How do radiographic techniques affect image quality and patient doses in CT? *Seminars in Ultrasound, CT, and MRI. 23*, 411–422.

Image Gently. (2015). *The Alliance for Radiation Safety in Pediatric Imaging.* <http://imagegently.org> Accessed January 2015.

Image Wisely. (2015). *Radiation Safety in Adult Medical Imaging.* <http://www.imagewisely.org/> Accessed January 2015.

International Electrotechnical Commission (IEC). (2001). *Particular requirements for the safety of x-ray equipment for CT* (2nd ed.). 60601-2-44.

Israel, G. M., Cicchiello, L., Brink, J., & Huda, W. (2010). Patient size and radiation exposure in thoracic, pelvic, and abdominal CT examinations performed with automatic exposure control. *American Journal of Roentgenology, 95*(6), 1342–1346.

Kalender, W., Wolf, H., & Suess, C. (1999). Dose reduction in CT by anatomically adapted tube current modulation. II. Phantom measurements. *Medical Physics, 26*, 2248–2253.

Kalra, M. K., Maher, M. M., Toth, T. L., Hamberg, L. M., et al. (2004a). Strategies for CT radiation dose optimization. *Radiology, 230*, 619–628.

Kalra, M. K., Maher, M. M., Toth, T. L., Schmidt, B., et al. (2004b). Techniques and applications of automatic tube current modulation for CT. *Radiology, 233*, 649–657.

Kanal, K. M., Stewart, B. K., Kolokythas, O., & Shuman, W. P. (2007). Impact of operator-selected image noise index and reconstruction slice thickness on patient radiation dose in 64-MDCT. *American Journal of Roentgenology, 189*, 219–225.

Kaza, R. K., Platt, J. F., Goodsitt, M. M., et al. (2014). Emerging techniques for dose optimization in abdominal CT. *Radiographics, 34*(1), 4–17.

Kennedy, E. V., Iball, G. R., & Brettle, D. S. (2007). Investigation into the effects of lead shielding for fetal dose reduction in CT pulmonary angiography. *British Journal of Radiology, 80*, 631–638.

Lai, K. C., & Frush, D. P. (2006). Managing the radiation dose from pediatric CT. *Applied Radiology, 35*, 13–20.

Lee, C., Staton, R. J., Hintenlang, D. E., Arreola, M. M., et al. (2007). Organ and effective doses in pediatric patients undergoing helical multislice computed tomography examination. *Medical Physics, 34*, 1858–1873.

Lewis, M. (2005). *Radiation dose issues in multi-slice CT scanning.* London: St. George's Hospital.

Li, J., Udayasankar, U. K., Toth, T. L., Seamans, J., et al. (2007). Automatic patient centering for MDCT: effect on radiation dose. *American Journal of Roentgenology, 188*, 547–552.

Liedenbaum, M. H., et al. (2008). Radiation dose in CT colonography–trends in time and differences between daily practice and screening protocols. *European Journal of Radiology, 18*(10), 2222–2230.

Litmanovich, D. E., Tack, D. M., Shahrzad, M., & Bankier, A. A. (2014). Dose reduction in cardiothoracic CT: review of currently available methods. *Radiographics, 34*, 1469–1489.

Maldjian, P. D., & Goldman, A. R. (2013). Reducing radiation dose in body CT: primer on dose metrics and key CT technical parameters. *American Journal of Roentgenology, 200*(4), 741–747.

Martin, D. R., & Semelka, R. C. (2007). Health effects of ionizing radiation from diagnostic CT imaging: consideration of alternative imaging strategies. *Applied Radiology, 36*(6), 20–29.

Mattsson, S. (2005). Optimization strategies in medical x-ray imaging. *Radiation Protection Dosimetry, 114* (1-3), 1–3.

McCollough, C. H., Bruesewitz, M. R., & Kofler, J. M., Jr. (2006). CT dose reduction and dose management tools: overview of available options. *Radiographics, 26*, 503–512.

McCollough, C. H., Wang, J., & Berland, L. L. (2011). Bismuth shields for CT dose reduction: do they help or hurt? *Journal of American College of Radiology, 8*(12), 878–879.

McCollough, C. H., Wang, J., Gould, R. G., & Orton, C. G. (2012). The use of bismuth breast shields for CT should be discouraged. *Medical Physics, 39*(5), 2321–2324.

McNitt-Gray, M. F. (2002). Radiation dose in CT. *Radiographics, 22*, 1541–1553.

Moore, W. H., Bonvento, M., & Olivieri-Fitt, R. (2006). Comparison of MDCT radiation dose: a phantom study. *American Journal of Roentgenology, 187*, W498–W502.

Mori, S., Endo, M., Nishizawa, K., Murase, K., Fujiwara, H., et al. (2006a). Comparison of patient doses in 256-slice CT and 16-slice CT scanners. *British Journal of Radiology, 79*, 56–61.

Mori, S., Nishizawa, K., Ohno, M., & Endo, M. (2006b). Conversion factor for CT dosimetry to assess patient dose using a 256-slice CT scanner. *British Journal of Radiology, 79*, 888–892.

Mukundan, S., Jr., Wang, P. I., Frush, D. P., et al. (2007). MOSFET dosimetry for radiation dose assessment of bismuth shielding of the eye in children. *American Journal of Roentgenology, 188*, 16–48.

National Council on Radiation Protection (NCRP). (2009). Ionizing radiation exposure of the United States, NCRP Report No. 160.

Pantos, I., Thalassinou, S., Argentos, S., Kelekis, N. L., et al. (2011). Adult patient radiation doses from non-cardiac CT examinations: a review of published results. *British Journal of Radiology, 84*(1000), 293–303.

Reid, J., Gamberoni, J., Dong, F., & Davros, W. (2010). Optimization of kVp and mAs for pediatric low dose simulated abdominal CT: is it best to base parameter selection on object circumference? *American Journal of Roentgenology, 195*(4), 1015.

Russell, M. T., Fink, J. R., Rebeles, F., Kanal, K., et al. (2008). Balancing radiation dose and image quality: clinical applications of neck volume CT. *American Journal of Neuroradiology, 29*(4), 727–731.

Seeram, E. (2001). *Tech guide to radiation protection*. Boston, MA: Blackwell Science.

Seeram, E. (2014). Computed tomography dose optimization. *Radiologic Technology, 85*(6), 665–675.

Siegel, E. (2006). Primum non nocere: a call for a re-evaluation of radiation doses used in CT. *Applied Radiology, April, 6*, 8.

Sohaib, S. A., Peppercorn, P. D., Horrocks, J. A., et al. (2001). The effect of decreasing mAs on image quality and patient dose in sinus CT. *British Journal of Radiology, 74*(878), 157–161.

Tingberg, A., et al. (2005). Evaluation of image quality of lumbar spine images: a comparison between FFE and VGA. *Radiation Protection Dosimetry, 114*(1–3), 53–61.

Toth, T., Ge, Z., & Daly, M. P. (2007). The influence of patient centering on CT dose and image noise. *Medical Physics, 34*, 3093–3101.

Tzedakis, A., Damilakis, J., Perisinakis, K., et al. (2007). Influence of z overscanning on normalized effective doses calculated for pediatric patients undergoing multidetector CT examinations. *Medical Physics, 34*, 1163–1172.

Van der Molen, A. J., & Geleijns, J. (2007). Overranging in multisection CT: quantification and relative contribution to dose—comparison of four 16-section CT scanners. *Radiology, 242*, 208–216.

Winkler, M. L. (2003). Knowledgeable use of MDCT minimizes dose. *Diagnostic Imaging*.

Winkler, M., & Mather, R. (2005). CT risk minimized by optimal system design. July *Toshiba Medical Systems*, 18–23.

Wolbarst, A. B., Capasso, P., & Wyant, A. R. (2013). *Medical imaging: essentials for physicians*. Hoboken, NJ: Wiley-Blackwell.

Zarb, F., Rainford, L., & McEntee, M. F. (2010). Image quality assessment tools for optimization of CT images. *Radiography, 16*, 147–153.

# 11

# Multislice Computed Tomography: Physical Principles and Instrumentation

## OUTLINE



## LEARNING OBJECTIVES

On completion of this chapter, you should be able to:

1. discuss the controversy surrounding the use of the terms "spiral" and "helical" in volume CT.
2. outline the scanning sequence of conventional CT and list its principal limitations.
3. list the requirements for volume data acquisition.
4. outline the physical principles, data acquisition, and image reconstruction technique for single-slice spiral/helical CT.
5. describe the major equipment components of a single-slice spiral/helical CT scanner.
6. define and explain briefly each of the following:
   - pitch
   - volume coverage
   - collimation and table speed
   - scan time
   - reconstruction increment.
7. describe the essential elements of image quality and radiation dose for single-slice spiral/helical CT.
8. state the advantages and limitations of single-slice spiral/helical CT.
9. briefly explain three major technical advances in volume CT scanning.
10. describe the essential characteristics of multi-slice detectors.
11. state the limitations of single-slice volume CT scanning.

## LEARNING OBJECTIVES—cont'd

12. trace the evolution of multislice volume CT scanners.
13. compare and contrast data and image reconstruction for single-slice and multislice volume CT, including cone-beam algorithms.
14. describe the essential features of each of the following equipment components:
    - data acquisition components
    - multislice detectors
    - slice thickness selection
    - data acquisition system
    - patient table
    - computer system.
15. define and explain the goals of isotropic imaging.
16. describe the main technical aspects of the 320-slice dynamic volume CT scanner.
17. outline the major technical components of the dual-source CT scanner.
18. state the advantages of multislice spiral/helical CT.
19. list the clinical application of MSCT.
20. identify potential applications of MSCT.

## KEY TERMS TO WATCH FOR AND REMEMBER

The following key terms/concepts are important to your understanding of this chapter.

**adaptive array detector**
**cone beam**
**fixed array detector**
**interscan delay time (ISD)**
**isotropic**
**multirow detector designs**
**multislice CT (MSCT)**
**single-slice CT (SSCT)**
**slice-to-slice misregistration**
**slice thickness**
**slice width**

In 1990 the first **computed tomography (CT)** scanner to perform **volume data acquisition** was introduced (Kalender, 1995). This scanner was invented to overcome the problems imposed by conventional (slice-by-slice axial sequential **scanning**) CT scanners. Furthermore, the scanners provide shorter scan times to subsecond levels and improvement in 3D imaging. These scanners are referred to as *single-slice spiral/helical CT scanners* or **volume CT** *scanners* on the basis of the **beam geometry** (spiral/helical) used during the data acquisition process. The term **single-slice CT (SSCT)** will be used in this chapter to refer to CT scanners that acquire a volume dataset by scanning a volume of the patient's anatomy using a 1D detector array, as opposed to the conventional CT scanner that obtains a single dataset using a 1D detector array. Subsequent developments and advances in CT technology have led to the introduction of multislice CT (MSCT) scanners that now acquire volume datasets (much faster than SSCT scanners) using 2D detector arrays. MSCT scanners are now commonplace and have replaced SSCT scanners. It is important to note that some authors prefer to use the term **multidetector CT (MDCT)** on the basis of the design of the 2D detector arrays. The acronym MSCT will be used throughout this text.

The purpose of the chapter is twofold. First, the language of SSCT scanning will be introduced followed by a description of the fundamental principles and concepts of spiral/helical data acquisition, **image reconstruction,** major system components, basic **scan parameters,** and the advantages and limitations of SSCT scanners. Second, the evolution of MSCT scanners will be highlighted, followed by a description of the physical principles and technology of MSCT scanners.

The technical principles and concepts of SSCT scanners described in this chapter lay the foundations necessary for a good understanding of MSCT scanners.

## SSCT: HISTORICAL BACKGROUND

An early pioneer in the development of the technique of **volume scanning** in CT was Dr. Willi A. Kalender (see Chapter 1) of the Institute of Medical Physics at the University of Erlangen, Germany. Kalender started work on spiral CT in 1988 with Peter Vock from Switzerland, and in 1989 he described the technical details and clinical applications of spiral CT to the Radiological Society of North America (RSNA) meeting in Chicago. Other early investigators included Mori (1987), various Japanese researchers, and Bresler and Skrabacz (1993).

### Terminology Controversy

Kalender and Vock's presentation at the RSNA in 1989 resulted in a flurry of activities related to volume scanning. An interesting debate that surfaced in the early literature was about what terminology best describes the method of volume data acquisition. Should volume scanning be called spiral CT or helical CT? In a letter to the editors of the *American Journal of Roentgenology* (*AJR*), Towers (1993) used an illustration (Fig. 11-1) to describe the fundamental differences between spiral CT and helical CT. Towers noted that the term *helical* describes a cylindrical configuration, whereas *spiral* refers to both cylindrical and conic configurations. He therefore recommended the use of the term *spiral CT*.

In another letter to the editors of *AJR*, Silverman et al. (1994) argued that the term *helical CT* "best describes this new CT technology." Dr. Mark Bahn of the Mallinckrodt Institute of Radiology offered mathematical definitions to support this **view.** He pointed out that mathematical dictionaries (Baker, 1961; James & James, 1976) provide more technical definitions of these two terms: a **spiral** describes a curve on a plane surface; a **helix** describes a curve in 3D space.

In response, Kalender (1994a) submitted a letter (Appendix A) to the editors of *Radiology* to support use of the term *spiral CT*, which convinced the editors to accept either term for CT papers published in in their journal. This book uses both terms as synonyms, as suggested by Kalender (1994a).

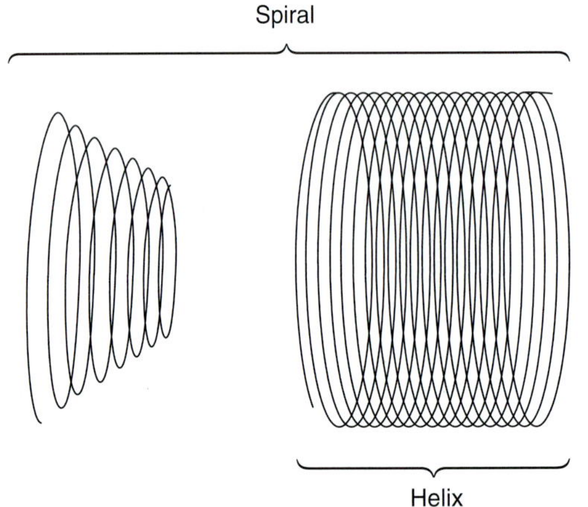


**FIGURE 11-1** Spiral geometries. The helix is one type of spiral. (From Towers, M. J. (1993). *American Journal of Roentgenology, 161*, 901.)

## CONVENTIONAL SLICE-BY-SLICE CT SCANNING

### Scanning Sequence

In conventional CT scanning, the **x-ray tube** rotates around the patient to collect data from a single slice of tissue, followed by table indexing so that the next contiguous slice can be scanned. This process is repeated until data from several contiguous slices have been collected. The scanning sequence for this type of data acquisition consists of four distinct steps (Fig. 11-2).

In the first step, the x-ray tube must be accelerated to a constant speed of rotation. This means that the cables that supply power to the x-ray tube must be long enough to allow for the full 360-degree rotation. During this rotation (step 2), the x-ray tube produces x-rays that are transmitted through the patient to fall on the detectors, which measure the **relative transmission** values (data). At this particular point, the patient holds a breath, and data are collected from a specific axial slice. In step 3, the patient resumes breathing while the x-ray tube slows to a stop. In step 4, it is necessary to unwind the cable because of the 360-degree rotation and to move the patient and table so that the next contiguous slice can be scanned.

This four-step process is repeated until all the required contiguous axial slices have been scanned. The time it takes to accomplish steps 1, 3, and 4 is referred to as the **interscan delay time (ISD).**

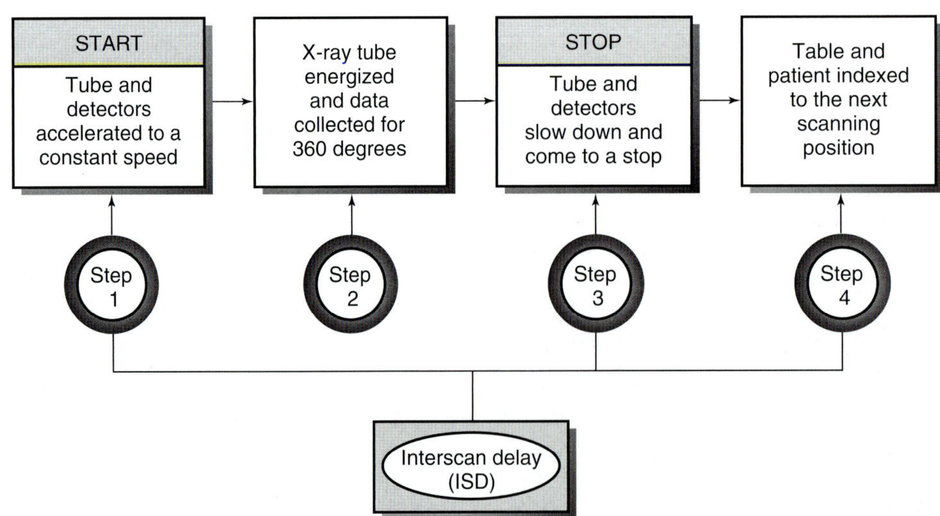


**FIGURE 11-2** Characteristic four-step process of slice-by-slice sequential CT scanning.

Slices are usually collected in groups while the patient holds a breath, with the ISD after each pair of slices. Between two groups of slices is an intergroup delay, and it is at this point that the patient breathes. Additionally, the scan rate is expressed as the following ratio:

$$\text{Scan rate} = \frac{\text{No. of scans per group}}{\text{sum of time to collect slices} + \text{IGD}}$$

If the study requires more slices, its duration would have to be increased. This requirement places an additional burden on the patient to remain still to ensure that images obtained are free of motion **artifacts.**

## Limitations

The limitations imposed by slice-by-slice sequential CT scanning include the following:

1. Longer examination times because of the stop–start action necessary for patient breathing, table indexing, and cable unwinding. This gives rise to the ISD. The cable wraparound and unwinding is shown in Figure 11-3, *A*. This wraparound results from the fixed length of the high-voltage cable, which follows the x-ray tube as it rotates through 360 degrees around the patient. The cable is unwound during the imaging of the next slice. In Figure 11-3, *B*, the cable wraparound process is eliminated through the use of slip-ring technology, which allows the x-ray tube to rotate continuously as the patient moves continuously through the **gantry.** This is spiral/helical CT scanning.
2. Certain portions of the anatomy are omitted because the patient respiration phase may not always be consistent between scans (Fig. 11-4). For example, it has been reported that lesions in the liver smaller than 1 cm may be missed because of inconsistent levels of inspiration. This omission of anatomy is often referred to as **slice-to-slice misregistration.**
3. Inaccurate **generation** of 3D images and multiplanar reformatted images are attributed to the inconsistent levels of inspiration from scan to scan. The result is the appearance of "steplike" contours in 3D images. Figure 11-5 illustrates production of the stairstep artifact and its elimination with spiral/helical CT.
4. Only a few slices are scanned during maximum contrast enhancement when the contrast enhancement technique is used. These problems may be overcome if the scan rate is increased and the ISD is eliminated, both of which are technologically feasible. The scan time can be increased by decreasing the time to accomplish the four steps shown in Figure 11-2. The ISD can be eliminated by having the tube (and detector) rotate continuously around the patient (instead of the start–stop action characteristic of slice-by-slice sequential CT scanning) while simultaneously translating the patient through the gantry aperture at a faster speed. Data are acquired during the patient translation.

This chapter concentrates on methods to remove the ISD with the goal of acquiring the data continuously rather than in slices. This technique is only possible with **continuous rotation** scanners based on slip-ring technology.

## PRINCIPLES OF SSCT SCANNERS

The introduction of CT scanners that can scan rapidly with scan times shorter than 1 second has led to the development of the SSCT scanner. The overall goal of

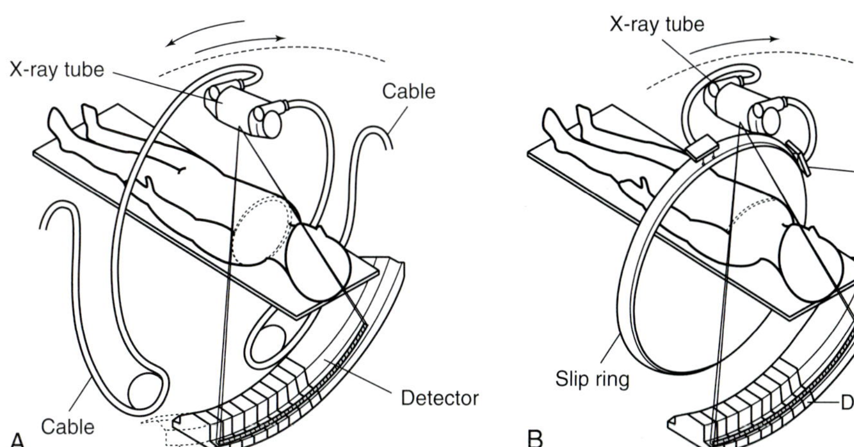


**FIGURE 11-3** One advance in CT technology that facilitates CT fluoroscopy is continuous scanning by using slip-ring technology. The cable wraparound typical of conventional slice-by-slice CT results in a delay that prevents real-time image reconstruction and display. **A,** Reciprocating rotation. **B,** Fast continuous rotation. (From Ozaki, M. (1995). *Toshiba Med Rev, 53,* 12-17.)

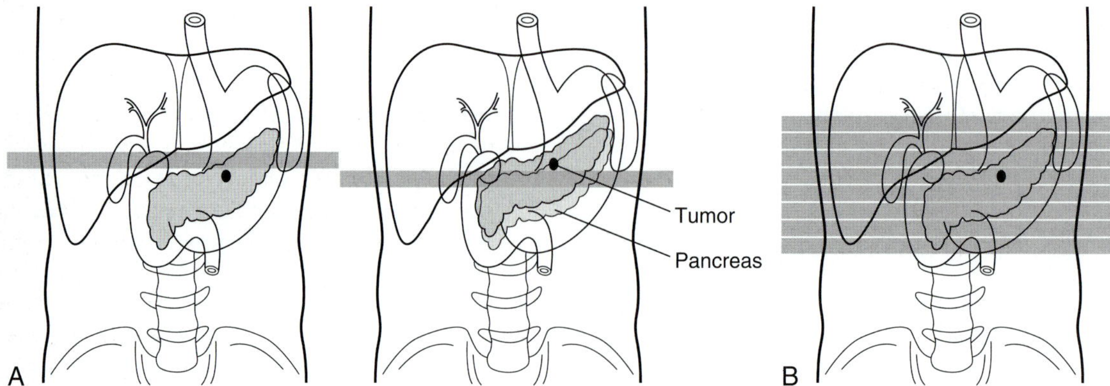


**FIGURE 11-4** Removal of the effects of different levels of respiration. **A,** Conventional scanning. In spiral/helical CT scanning **(B)** there is no shifting of lesions because of different levels of respiration. (Courtesy Toshiba America Medical Systems, Tustin, Calif.)

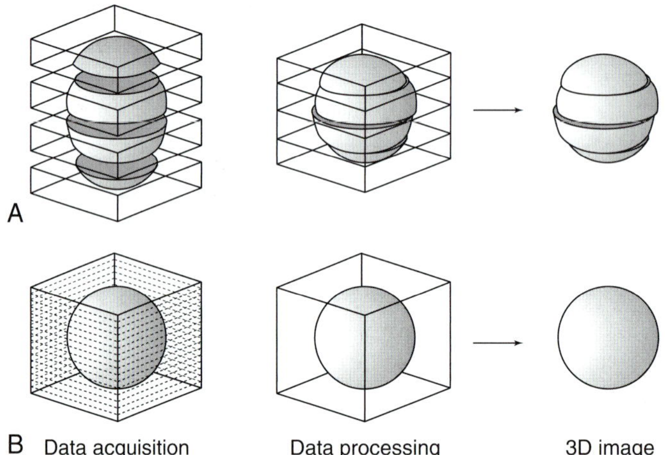


**FIGURE 11-5** Comparison of the accuracy of 3D reconstruction for conventional **(A)** and spiral/helical **(B)** CT scanning. (Courtesy Toshiba America Medical Systems, Tustin, Calif.)

this scanner is to increase the volume coverage speed compared with that of the conventional CT scanner.

To do this efficiently requires that the x-ray tube rotate continuously around the patient while the patient moves through the gantry aperture during the scanning to cover an entire volume of tissue (compared with a single slice characteristic of conventional CT scanners). Rotation of the x-ray tube coupled with patient translation through the gantry aperture traces an x-ray beam path with respect to the patient (Fig. 11-6). The path geometry describes a spiral or helical winding and therefore has been referred to as *spiral/helical* CT. Other terms considered synonymous are *spiral volume* CT and *helical volumetric CT*.

Because a 1D detector array is used, only a single slice is acquired during one rotation of the tube. Because there are several rotations per required length of anatomy imaged (volume of tissue scanned), several slices of tissue and corresponding images can be computer generated for the volume of the anatomy scanned during a single breath-hold.

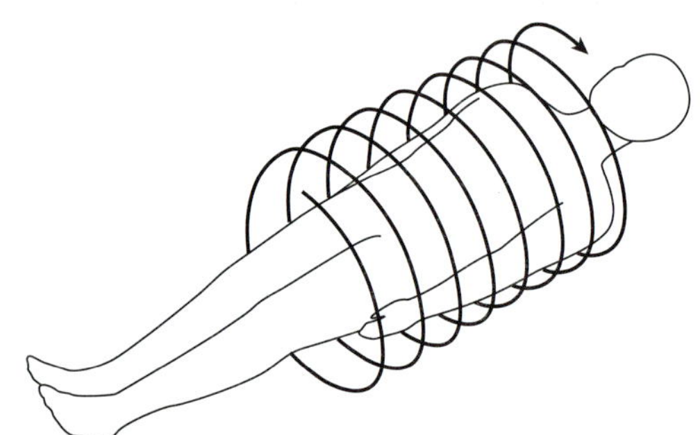

**FIGURE 11-6** The spiral/helical geometry created when the x-ray tube rotates continuously around the patient with simultaneous patient translation.

## Requirements for Volume Scanning

Because the data in spiral/helical CT are collected in volumes rather than slices, the following requirements must be met:

1. Continuously rotating scanner based on slip-ring technology

2. Continuous couch movement
3. Increase in loadability of the x-ray tube, capable of delivering at least 200 mA per revolution continuously throughout the time it takes to scan the volume of tissue
4. Increased cooling capacity of the x-ray tube
5. Spiral/helical weighting **algorithm**
6. Mass memory buffer to store the vast amount of data collected

## Data Acquisition

The first step in volume scanning is data acquisition (Fig. 11-7). The x-ray tube traces a spiral/helical path with a radius equal to the **distance** from the focal spot to the center of rotation. This results in an entire volume of tissue being scanned during a single breath-hold compared with slice-by-slice imaging (Fig. 11-8).

Transporting the patient too quickly leads to image degradation caused by motion artifacts or may cause the patient to feel motion sickness. It is therefore important that the patient moves at a constant speed. In general, patients are moved at a table speed of about 10 mm/s during a continuous 1-second scanning. If a 24-second scan is taken, then the anatomic volume scanned is 240 mm (24 cm). Scanning times differ by manufacturer but average about 32 seconds. In addition the slice thickness may range from 1 cm to 10 cm.

Several problems can result from data acquisition with spiral/helical beam geometry:

1. There is no defined slice, and thus localization of a particular slice is difficult.
2. The geometry of the slice volume is different for spiral/helical scans compared with conventional CT scans (Fig. 11-9). Figure 11-10 explains the origin of the slice volume shown in Figure 11-9, *B*. In conventional slice-by-slice CT, the tube rotates around the patient for 360 degrees to

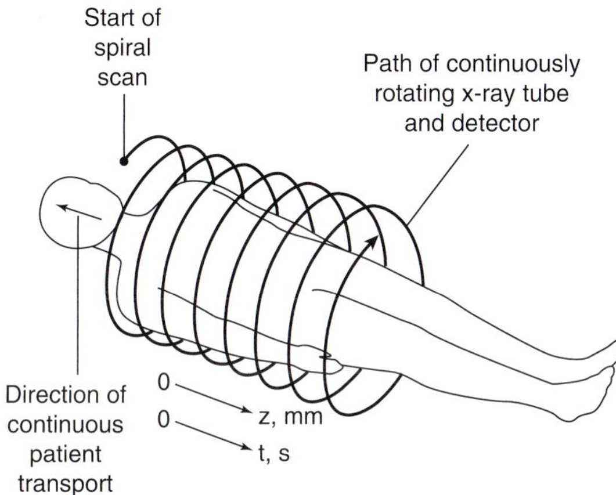


**FIGURE 11-7** First step in spiral/helical CT: data acquisition. As the patient is transported through the gantry aperture, the x-ray tube traces a spiral path around the patient, collecting data as it rotates.

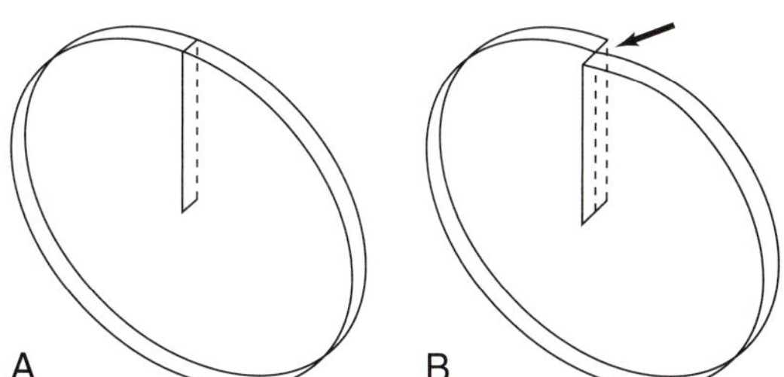


**FIGURE 11-9** Geometry of the slice volume characteristic of conventional CT scanning **(A)** and spiral/helical CT scanning **(B)**.

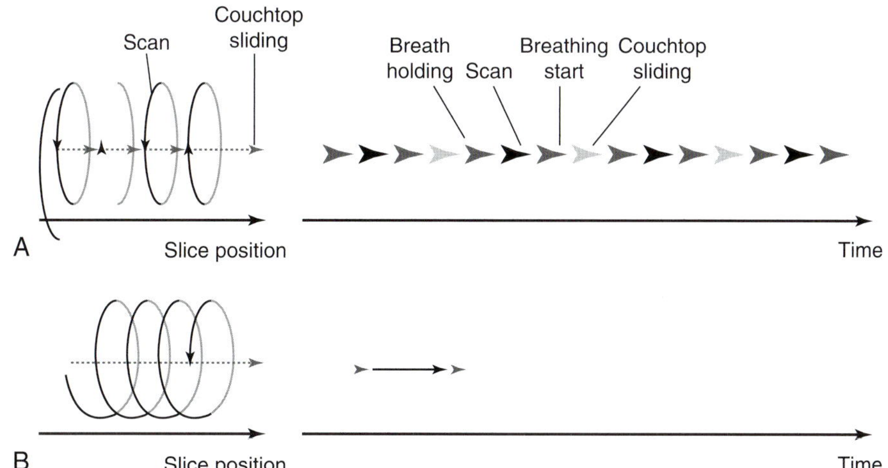


**FIGURE 11-8** Comparison of conventional **(A)** and spiral/helical **(B)** CT scanning sequences. (From Tohki, Y. (1991). *Toshiba Med Rev*, 38, 1-5.)

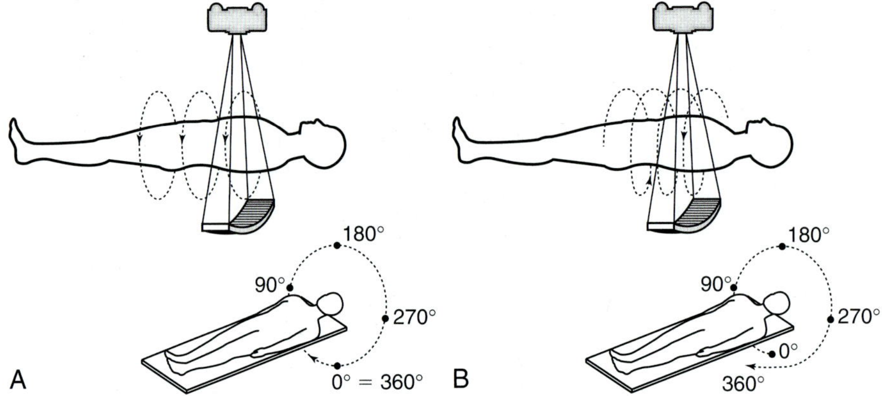


**FIGURE 11-10** Data acquisition geometries for conventional slice-by-slice CT **(A)** and spiral/helical CT **(B)**.

collect a complete set of data in planar geometry for each individual slice shown in Figure 11-9, *A*. This dataset is said to be consistent; that is, it is collected from one slice or plane. In spiral/helical volume CT scanning, the x-ray tube rotates continuously as the patient moves through the gantry continuously as well. In this situation, data are now collected in nonplanar geometry, resulting in the diagram shown in Figure 11-9, *B*. These data are collected from different regions of the volume and not through a particular plane.

3. The effective slice thickness increases because it is influenced by the width of the fan beam and the speed of the table.
4. Because of the absence of a defined slice, the projection data are inconsistent (consistent projection data are needed to satisfy the standard reconstruction process).
5. When inconsistent projection data are used with the standard reconstruction process, streak artifacts akin to motion artifacts are clearly apparent on the image.

These problems can be solved through the use of special postprocessing techniques. One such method involves a "dedicated reconstruction algorithm that synthesizes **raw data** representing a perfectly planar slice from the original spiral data by **interpolation**" (Kalender, 1995). Interpolation is a mathematical technique in which an unknown value can be estimated given two known values on either side (see Chapter 5). Interpolation and extrapolation are illustrated in Figure 11-11.

## Image Reconstruction

Inconsistent data obtained from 360-degree spiral/helical scan rotation are used directly in the image reconstruction process. Motion artifacts are apparent

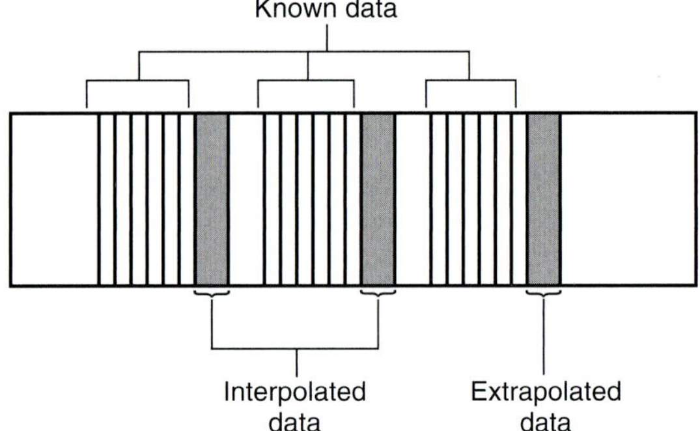


**FIGURE 11-11** A comparison of interpolated and extrapolated data.

as shown in Figure 11-12, for phantom images, and in Figure 11-13, for patient images.

To eliminate these motion artifacts arising from the continuous movement of the patient during scanning, two steps are needed:

1. Calculation (using interpolation) of a planar dataset from the tissue volume dataset for every image (Fig. 11-14). The planar dataset (the image plane in Fig. 11-14) approximates the transverse axial section as with conventional CT. Within the volume scanned, a slice can be selected anywhere between the start and end positions in addition to the spacing and the number of slices (Fig. 11-15).
2. Reconstruction of images similar to conventional CT by use of the filtered **back-projection** algorithm. The results of these two processes are free of blurring as shown in Figure 11-13, *B*.

A number of interpolation algorithms are used to produce the planar dataset, and linear interpolation (LI) represents the "simplest approach" (Kalender, 1995). Two interpolation algorithms for SSCT are the 360-degree LI algorithm and the 180-degree LI algorithm.

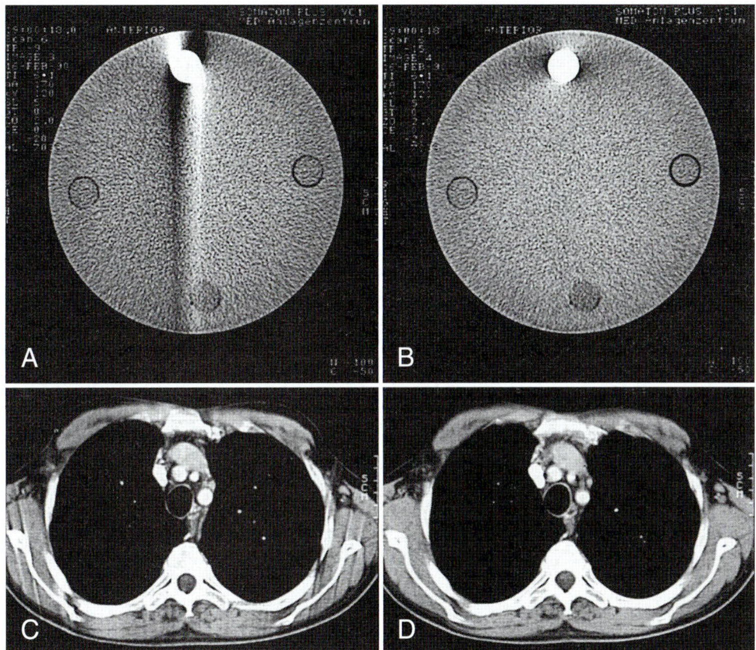

**FIGURE 11-12** Comparison of image quality using direct reconstruction of the spiral data **(A, C)** as opposed to reconstruction using the interpolation algorithm **(B, D)** for phantom **(A, B)** and mediastinal **(C, D)** studies. The streak artifacts are removed when the interpolation algorithm is used. (From Kalender, W. A. (1990). Spiral CT scanning for fast and continuous volume data acquisition. In W. A. Fuchs (Ed.), *Advances in CT.* New York: Springer-Verlag.)

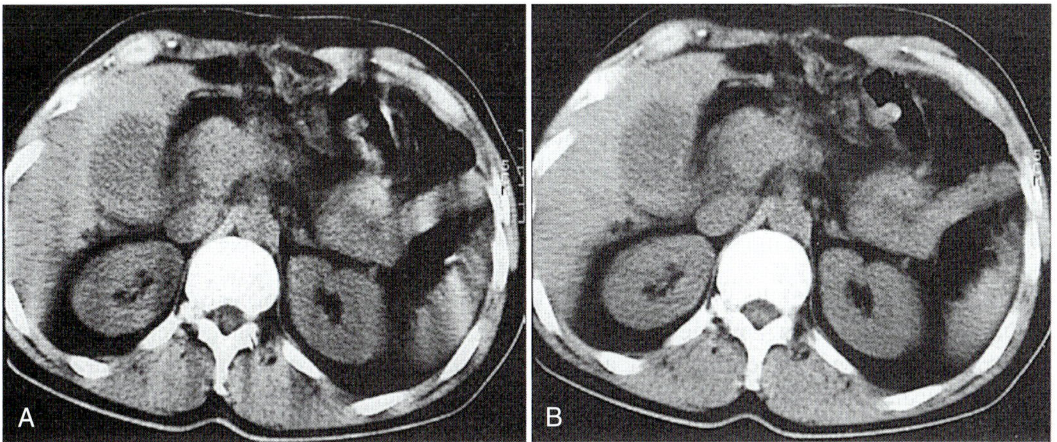

**FIGURE 11-13** Image reconstruction principles in spiral/helical CT. **A,** Direct reconstruction of an image from a 360-degree spiral segment results in motion artifacts. **B,** Image reconstruction from a planar dataset calculated by slice interpolation from the spiral dataset results in images free of artifacts. (From Kalender, W. (1995). Principles and performance of spiral CT. In L. W. Goldman, & J. B. Fowlkes (Eds.), *Medical CT and ultrasound: current technology and applications.* College Park, MD: American Association of Physics in Medicine.)

### 360-Degree Linear Interpolation Algorithm

The 360-degree LI algorithm was the interpolation algorithm used during the initial development of spiral/helical CT scanners (Fig. 11-16). The basis for this algorithm is illustrated in Figure 11-16. The planar slice is interpolated by use of data points measured 360 degrees apart. The fundamental problem with the 360-degree LI algorithm is related to the image quality of the planar slice. This algorithm broadens the **slice sensitivity profile (SSP)** and hence degrades image quality. To overcome this problem, the 180-degree LI algorithm was introduced.

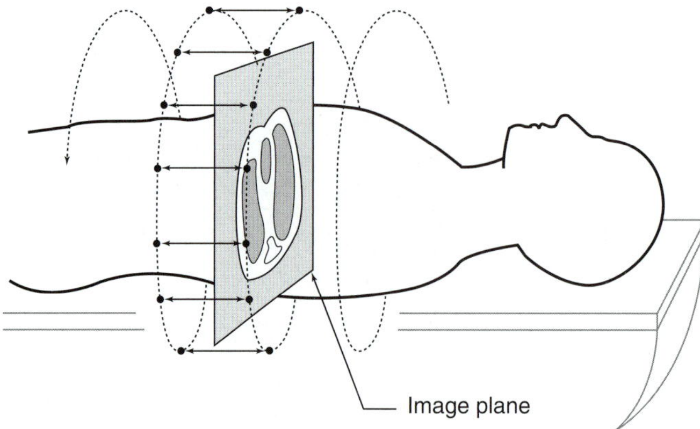


**FIGURE 11-14** The first step to produce an image in spiral/helical CT scanning is to calculate a planar dataset (image plane) from the volume dataset (measured data). This is accomplished by using LI.

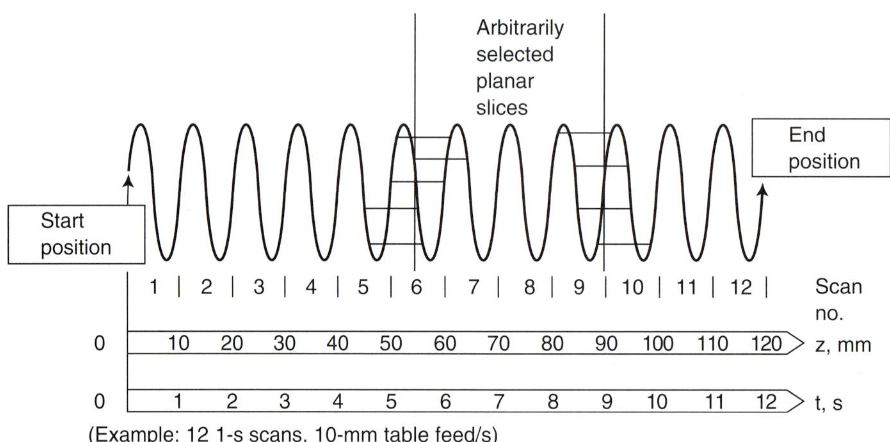


**FIGURE 11-15** The second major step in spiral/helical CT is interpolation. Images of arbitrarily selected slices can be reconstructed with an interpolation algorithm. (Courtesy Siemens Medical Systems, Iselin, NJ.)

### 180-Degree Linear Interpolation Algorithm

The 180-degree LI algorithm improves the image quality of the 360-degree LI algorithm by using points that are closer to the planar slice to be interpolated (Fig. 11-17). The basic difference between the 360-degree and the 180-degree LI algorithms is that a second spiral (the dotted line in Fig. 11-17) is calculated from the measured spiral/helical dataset and is offset by 180 degrees. In this situation, the planar slice can then be interpolated with use of data points that are closer to it compared with the 360-degree LI algorithm. This process improves on the SSP and therefore enhances image quality.

In addition to the algorithms, Kalender (1995) stated that

> higher-order nonlinear interpolation algorithms can be implemented. While they preserve the shape of the sensitivity profiles even better, their influence on **noise** and image quality is not easy to predict and control. On a given scanner, the exact algorithm and above all its implementation, which may have significant influence on image quality and artifact behavior, are not documented as they are considered confidential by the manufacturers in most cases.

These algorithms are not within the scope of this book. The reader should refer to Kalender (2005) for a further description of nonlinear interpolation algorithms.

## INSTRUMENTATION

Spiral/helical CT scanners (SSCT or MSCT; Fig. 11-18) are not different in external appearance from conventional CT scanners. However, there are significant differences in several major equipment components.

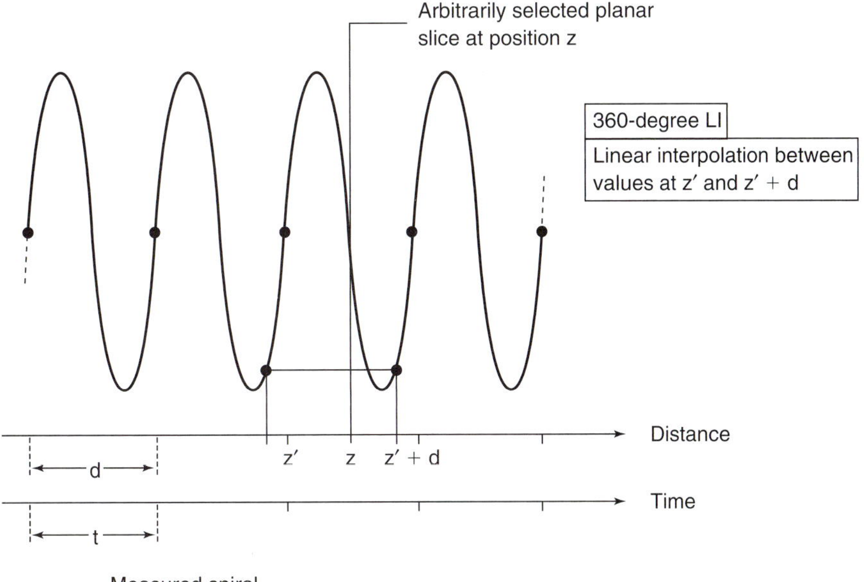


**FIGURE 11-16** The 360-degree LI algorithm. LI between points *Z*′ and *Z*′ + *d* was most commonly used in the early days of spiral/helical scanning to estimate data that would have been obtained in planar geometry for an arbitrarily selected image position *Z*.

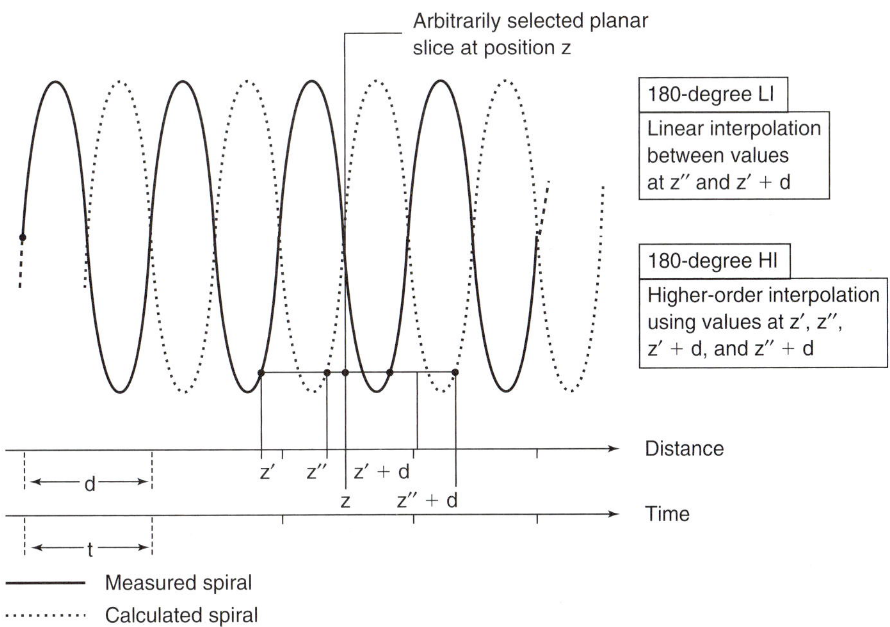


**FIGURE 11-17** The 180-degree LI algorithm. Interpolation between measured data points derived from 180-degree opposite views allows limitation of the scan range used per image. Higher order interpolation schemes can also be implemented.

## Equipment Components

A block diagram of the major equipment components of a spiral/helical CT scanner is shown in Figure 11-19. The most noteworthy feature is the use of *slip rings* to connect the stationary and rotating parts of the scanner.

The rotating part of the system consists of the x-ray tube, high-voltage generator, detectors, and detector electronics (DAS). The stationary part consists of the front-end memory and computer and the first-stage high-voltage component.

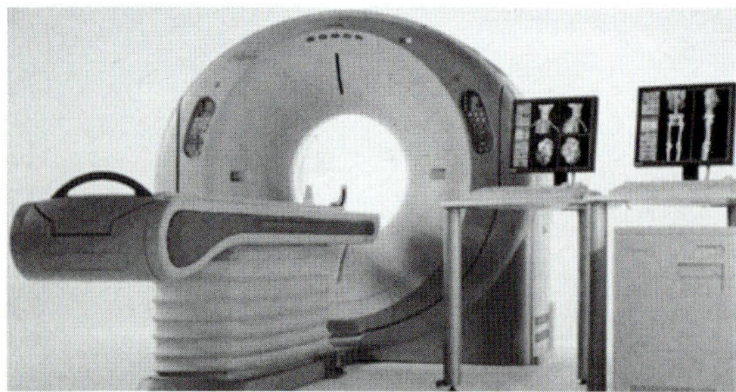

**FIGURE 11-18** The major equipment components (gantry, patient couch, computer, and operator's console) of an MSCT scanner. (Courtesy Toshiba Medical Systems.)

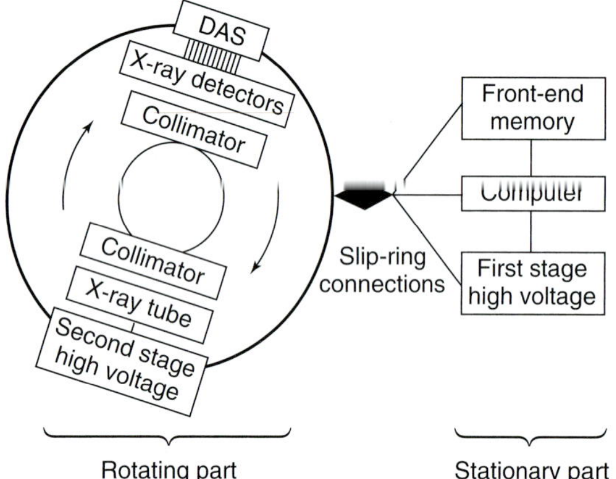


**FIGURE 11-19** The major equipment components of a spiral/helical CT scanner. Connection between the stationary and rotating parts of the scanner is made possible by slip-ring technology.

The x-ray tube and detectors rotate continuously during data collection because the cable wraparound problem has been eliminated by slip-ring technology. Because large amounts of projection data are collected very quickly, increased storage is needed. This is accommodated by the front-end memory, fast solid state, and magnetic disk storage.

In spiral/helical CT scanners (SSCT and MSCT) the x-ray tube is energized for longer periods of time compared with conventional CT tubes. This characteristic requires x-ray tubes that are physically larger than conventional x-ray tubes and have heat storage capacities greater than 3 million heat units (MHUs) and anode cooling rates of 1 MHU/min (Bushong, 2013).

X-ray detectors for single-slice spiral/helical CT scanning are 1D arrays and should be solid state because their overall **efficiency** is greater than gas ionization detectors.

The high-voltage generator for spiral/helical CT scanners is a **high-frequency generator** with a high-power **output.** The high-voltage generator is mounted on the rotating frame of the CT gantry and positioned close to the x-ray tube (Fig. 11-19). X-ray tubes operate at high voltages (about 80 to 140 peak kilovolts) to produce x-rays with the intensity needed for CT scanning. At such high voltages, arcing between the brushes and rings of the gantry may occur during scanning. To solve this problem, one approach is to divide the power supply into a first stage on the stationary part of the scanner, where the voltage is increased to an intermediate level, and a second stage on the rotating part of the scanner, where the voltage is increased to the required high voltages needed for x-ray production and finally rectified to direct current potential (Fig. 11-19; Napel, 1995). Another approach passes a low voltage across the brushes to the slip rings, the high-voltage generator, and then the x-ray tube. In both designs, only a low to intermediate voltage is applied to the brush/slip-ring interface, thus decreasing the chances of arcing.

## Slip-Ring Technology

One of the major technical factors that contribute to the success of spiral/helical CT scanning is slip-ring technology (Fig. 11-19). The purpose of the slip ring is to allow the x-ray tube and detectors (in third-generation CT systems; Fig. 11-19) to rotate continuously so that a volume of the patient, rather than one slice, can be scanned very quickly in a single breath-hold. The slip rings also eliminate the long, high-tension cables to the x-ray tube used in conventional start–stop CT scanners. As the x-ray tube rotates continuously, the patient also moves continuously through the gantry aperture so that data can be acquired from a volume of tissue.

The technical aspects of using slip rings for data acquisition are described in Chapter 4. These include the design and power supply to the rings and a comparison of low-voltage and high-voltage slip-ring CT scanners in terms of the high voltage supplied to the x-ray tube.

# BASIC SCAN PARAMETERS

Several scan parameters for SSCT and MSCT are the same as for conventional CT; however, there are a few parameters and a set of terms associated only with spiral/helical CT. Typical parameters include spiral/helical scan time, table feed per 360-degree rotation, table speed, number of revolutions, scan range or volume coverage, **z-axis** (the axis of rotation of the scanner or the longitudinal axis of the patient), **collimation,** and the reconstruction increment and *z*-interpolation ("calculation of planar **attenuation** data for desired table position interpolation between data points measured for the same projection angle at neighboring *z*-axis positions [synonyms: slice interpolation, section interpolation, *z*-axis interpolation]") algorithms (Kalender, 1995). It is beyond the scope of this chapter to describe all of these parameters; however, important ones such as the **pitch,** beam geometry, collimation, and slice thickness will be described later here.

## LIMITATIONS OF SSCT SCANNERS

Ever since its introduction in 1990, single-slice volume CT has been used successfully in many body CT imaging applications in which speed and volume coverage are important. Volume coverage and speed can be increased by using higher pitch ratios; however, higher pitch ratios in single-slice volume CT scanning degrade image quality (*z*-axis resolution) and produce image artifacts. In SSCT, the volume coverage speed is limited, especially in clinical applications that demand large-volume scanning with critical timing requirements and optimum image quality (*z*-axis resolution and low image artifacts), such as **CT angiography** with 3D, multiplanar reformatting or reconstruction (MPR), and **maximum intensity projection (MIP)** techniques (Hu, 1999a). Single-slice volume CT is based on the use of a single row of detectors (1D detector array). Because the x-ray beam is highly collimated to the size of the detector array, only a small percentage of x-rays emitted by the tube is used in the imaging process. This situation is described as poor geometric efficiency. Also, SSCT uses the 360-degree linear interpolation algorithm (LIA) and the 180-degree LIA to improve the problems imposed by the 360-degree LIA, such as poor image quality and artifact production. However, the 180-degree LIA produces more noise while preserving the detail (slice sensitivity and **spatial resolution**). Additionally, the time duration for covering defined volumes in SSCT (several seconds) is limited by several factors, such as the ability of some patients, particularly those who are critically ill, to maintain a single breath-hold during volume scanning and the heat loading of the x-ray tube.

SSCT is also limited in its ability to meet the needs of time-critical clinical examinations such as multiphase organ dynamic studies and CT angiography, in which both arterial and venous phases are extremely important, with smaller amounts of **contrast media.** The use of higher pitch ratios to solve these problems degrades the slice sensitivity profile (detail). Therefore, other methods are needed to overcome these limitations to improve the performance of SSCT in terms of better use of the x-ray output (improved geometric efficiency) and scan parameters affecting image quality and volume coverage.

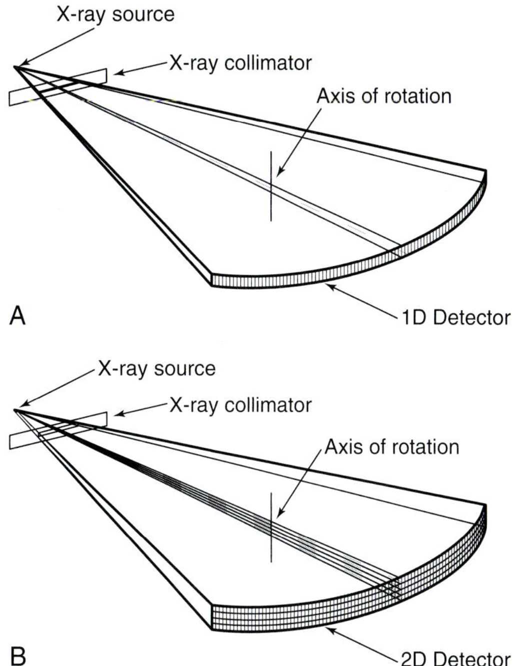


**FIGURE 11-20** One of the most conspicuous differences between an SSCT scanner and an MSCT scanner is the detector design. **A,** A 1D detector is used in single-slice systems. **B,** A 2D detector array is characteristic of MSCT systems.

MSCT offers "substantial improvement of the volume coverage speed performance" (Hu, 1999a). This means that MSCT provides faster scanning and higher resolution for a number of clinical applications (Taguchi & Aradate, 1998). One of the most conspicuous differences between MSCT and SSCT is that the former uses a multiple row of detectors (2D detector array), whereas the latter uses a single row of detectors (1D detector array), as is clearly illustrated in Figure 11-20.

## EVOLUTION OF MULTISLICE CT SCANNERS

### Terminology

Several terms are used in the literature to refer to MSCT, including **multisection CT, MDCT, multidetector row CT,** and **multichannel CT** (Cody & Mahesh, 2007; Douglas-Akinwande et al., 2006). Each of these terms appears to focus on a particular outcome characteristic. For example, although the terms *multislice* and *multisection* focus on images, the terms *multidetector* and *multidetector row* focus on the detectors used during the scanning. Finally, the

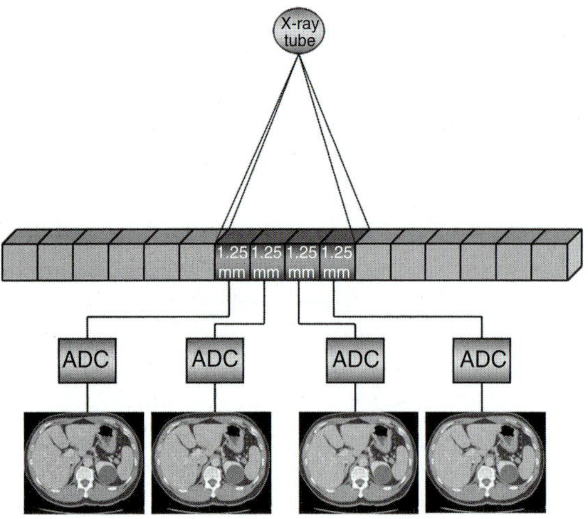


**FIGURE 11-21** A diagrammatic illustration of how the detector elements from an MSCT detector can be electronically combined to create slices of different thicknesses.

term *multichannel* refers to the function of the DAS. In this book, the term **multislice CT (MSCT)** will be used because it has become commonplace not only in the literature but also in clinical practice (Dowsett et al., 2006; Kachelriess et al., 2006; Kalender, 2005).

A CT detector consists of basically two major components: a radiation sensor coupled to suitable electronics, such as photodiodes, and analog-to-digital converters (ADCs; see Chapter 4). Although the radiation sensors convert x-ray photons to light, the photodiodes convert the light into electrical current (signal) that must be digitized before it is sent to a digital computer for processing. The electronics are carefully configured to the sensor elements (cells) of the CT detector and represent the data acquisition channels. As seen in Figure 11-21, the detector consists of 16 elements or cells, each 1.25 mm in size, and the x-ray beam is collimated to fall on four of these cells. Therefore four signals are collected per gantry rotation from each of the four cells and sent to the four ADCs to produce four slices, each 1.25 mm thick. For eight 1.25-mm thick slices, the x-ray beam would fall on eight detector elements. For four 2.5-mm thick slices, the beam would be collimated to fall on eight detector elements, where two 1.25-mm elements would be combined to produce a 2.5-mm thick slice, and so on. This electronic combination (or binning) of detector elements is described in more detail later in this chapter.

The evolution of MSCT technology is outlined in Figure 11-22. Its overall goal is to improve volume coverage speed performance; therefore, scanning is at higher speeds with higher pitch ratios to cover large

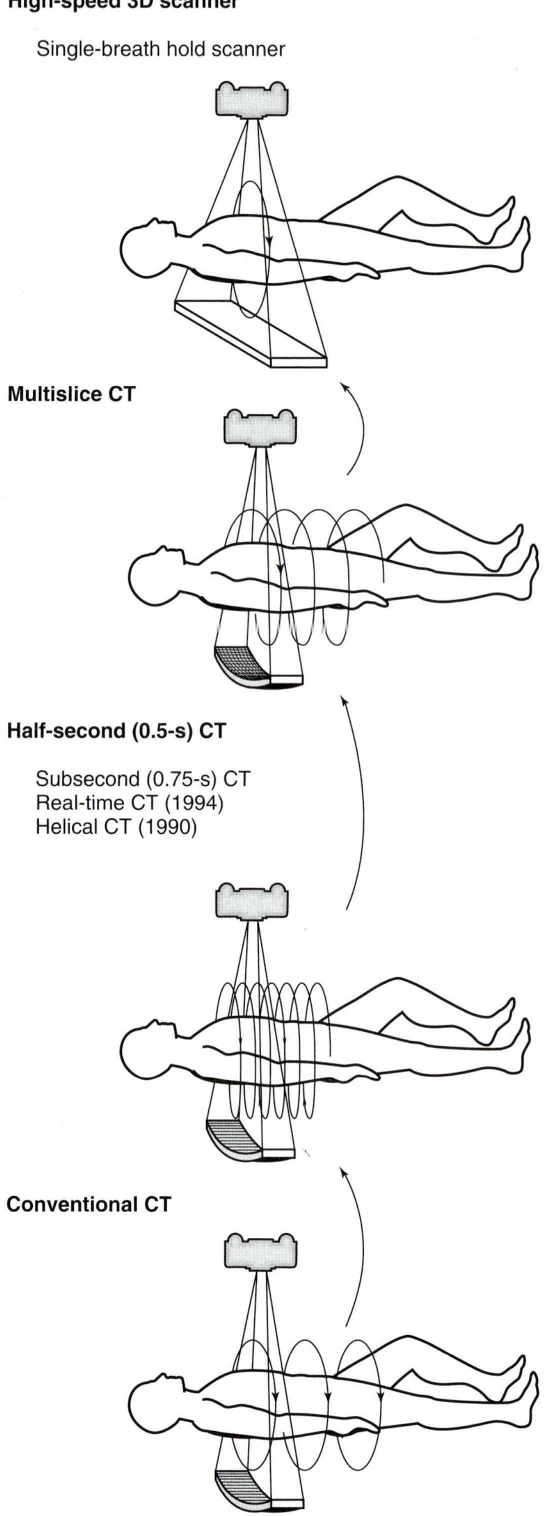


**FIGURE 11-22** The development continuum and milestones for Toshiba's CT scanners.

volumes with equivalent image quality compared with single-slice volume CT scanners introduced in the 1990s. The 256-slice CT scanner was introduced by the Toshiba Corporation Medical Systems Division as a prototype high-speed 3D CT scanner for imaging the entire heart in one complete rotation. The high-speed 3D scanner will use larger area detectors to scan larger volumes at high speeds and subsequently display all images in 3D. Finally, in 2008, Toshiba Medical Systems introduced a new 320-slice CT scanner. These two scanners will be described briefly in a later section.

## Subsecond Scanners

Scanning time continues to decrease from the 5 minutes needed by the original EMI scanner to as low as one half second at present. The engineering barriers to be overcome in reaching this gantry speed are formidable. The acceleration on gantry components such as the tube and generator can reach 13 gravities (Gs), considerably more than experienced by the space shuttle at lift off. Some interesting technological developments have accompanied the design of these **high-speed CT** systems.

To prevent anode movement under the stress of subsecond acceleration, new x-ray tubes have the anode mounted on a shaft that extends along the tube, providing support on both sides of the anode. This design has distinct advantages over the traditional method of supporting a massive anode from the rear only. Other innovative developments in tube design for CT include grounded anodes and a technique to reduce off-focal x rays. Virtually all medical x-ray tubes have applied the potential difference equally between cathode and anode so that the cathode can be at 75 kV while the anode is at 75 kV. This requires a substantial gap between the anode and the tube housing to reduce the possibility of arcs. With all the voltage placed on the cathode and the anode at ground potential, the tube housing can be brought into close proximity to the anode, which facilitates heat transfer and markedly improves anode cooling rate. Recoil electrons, which normally are reattracted to the anode and generate off-focal x rays, can now be collected on a special collimator located near the anode. This eliminates off-focal x rays that can reduce image quality and reduces the anode heat loading by about 30%, thereby reducing tube cooling delays during routine scanning.

The clinical benefits of subsecond scanning include reduced motion artifacts and greater scan coverage. Patient movement during CT scanning, whether by cardiac motion, breathing, or peristalsis, may cause artifacts because filtered back-projection reconstruction combines all the views acquired during the scan rotation to cancel artifacts. Movement of any object in the **field of view (FOV)** during gantry rotation prevents accurate elimination of artifacts with consequent loss of image quality. If the moving object has notably high or low contrast, such as bone, calculi, or air, the artifacts are particularly noticeable. Unfortunately, the left ventricle and pulmonary vessels near the heart move so quickly that scans would have to be completed in less than 20 ms to 25 ms to completely eliminate all blurring. This is a far shorter time than is possible with conventional CT scanners and is even difficult for electron-beam CTs, which are extremely fast. Even so, the half-second scanners, which can acquire "partial" (i.e., less than 360-degree rotation) images in 250 ms to 320 ms, have made it feasible to obtain considerably better images of the heart and chest than is possible with a 1-second system. An example is the ability of these scanners to use gated reconstruction, in which the raw scan data for image reconstruction can be selected on the basis of the patient's electrocardiogram (ECG). Reconstruction of a gated "partial" image during cardiac diastole, when the heart is relatively quiescent, can show fairly sharp ventricular borders and calcium in the coronary arteries.

Prospective gating can also be used in which the patient's ECG triggers the actual scan acquisition. This is a relatively simple technique, although it is not applicable to spiral/helical scanning.

A less dramatic but very practical benefit of subsecond scan times is the increased spiral/helical coverage that can become available. For the same pitch and scan duration, a half-second scanner will cover twice the anatomy that can be acquired with a 1-second scanner.

Alternatively, the half-second scanner could cover the same area by using 50% of the slice thickness, which improves *z*-axis resolution and leads to better image quality in 3D and multiplanar reconstructions. Clinical applications, such as CT angiography (CTA), can benefit from increased patient coverage without increasing pitch. This assumes that the system generator is able to produce enough power to accommodate the faster scans. For example, a 250-mA image of the abdomen requires a tube current of 500 mA in a half-second scanner.

## Dual-Slice CT Scanners

The history of scanning more than one slice at a time (actually two-slice scanners) dates back to one of the early EMI (London, United Kingdom) CT scanners, which became available in 1972, and the Siemens SIRETOM (Siemens Medical Solutions, Germany, personal **communications**) CT scanner, which

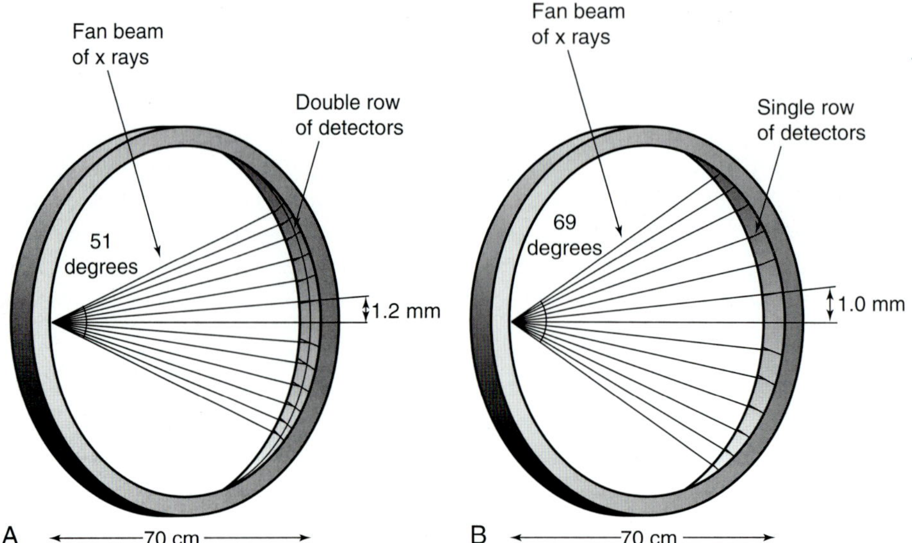


**FIGURE 11-23** **A,** Dual scanner slice geometry based on far beam of x rays falling on two rows of detectors. **B,** SSCT scanner based on far beam of x rays falling on one row of detectors.

appeared in 1974. These scanners used two detectors based on the translate/rotate method of data collection over 180 degrees. The next major step to MSCT scanning appeared in 1993, with the introduction of the first dual-slice volume CT scanner, the Elscint CT-TWIN (Elscint, Hackensack, NJ, personal communications). The most significant difference between the dual-slice volume CT scanner and its single-slice counterpart is shown in Figure 11-23. As can be seen, the dual scanner slice geometry is based on a fan beam of x rays falling on two rows of detectors (Fig. 11-23, *A*) instead of one row of detectors, characteristic of the SSCT scanner beam geometry (Fig. 11-23, *B*).

The dual-slice whole-body fan-beam CT scanner offers improved volume coverage speed performance compared with the single-slice volume CT scanner, reducing the scan time by 50% while maintaining image quality for the same scanned volume.

## Multislice CT Scanners

The dual-slice whole-body fan-beam CT technology paved the way for the development of other MSCT scanners. These scanners were introduced at the 1998 meeting of the RSNA in Chicago. They are based on spiral/helical scanning using multiple detector rows ranging between 8, 16, 32, 40, 64, (Kohl, 2006a), 256 (Mori et al, 2006a), and more recently 320 (Toshiba Medical Systems, 2008, personal communications), depending on the manufacturer. The 256-slice prototype scanner paved the way to the most recent commercially available MSCT scanner, the 320 dynamic volume CT scanner. This scanner is highlighted later in the chapter.

The overall goal of the MSCT scanner is to improve the volume coverage speed performance of both single-slice and dual-slice CT scanners. For example, an MSCT scanner with *N*-detector rows (*N* slices) will be *N* times faster than its single-row (one slice) counterpart. Thus, MSCT opens new avenues and opportunities to improve the quality of care afforded to patients because it now offers a wide range of new clinical applications afforded by recent technological developments.

# PHYSICAL PRINCIPLES

Although the fundamental physics and flow of data are the same as conventional and spiral/helical CT scanners, MSCT scanners introduce several new concepts relating to detector technology, the geometry of data acquisition, slice selection, and multislice image reconstruction algorithms.

## Data Acquisition

Data acquisition is one of two mechanisms that affect image quality in CT (the other is image reconstruction). This section examines data acquisition in MSCT with respect to beam geometry and basic parameters such as collimation, slice thickness, and pitch; but first a brief review of data acquisition in SSCT is in order.

### SSCT

The basic **data acquisition geometry** for SSCT is shown in Figure 11-24. This is a third-generation scheme in which the x-ray tube is coupled to a single-row detector array positioned in the *z*-axis.

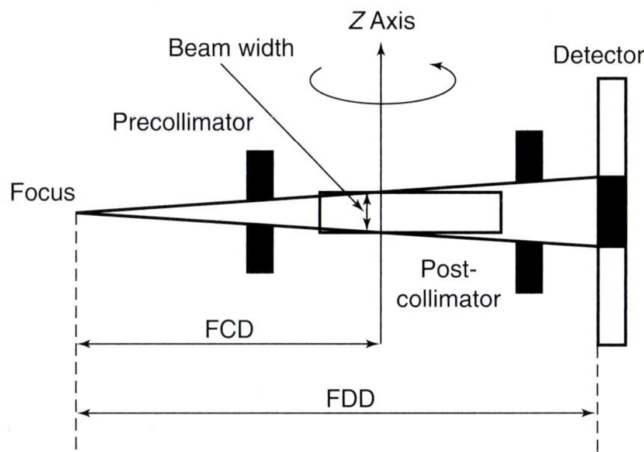


**FIGURE 11-24** A side view of the basic data acquisition geometry for single-slice volume CT scanners. *FCD*, Focus isocenter distance; *FDD*, focus detector distance.

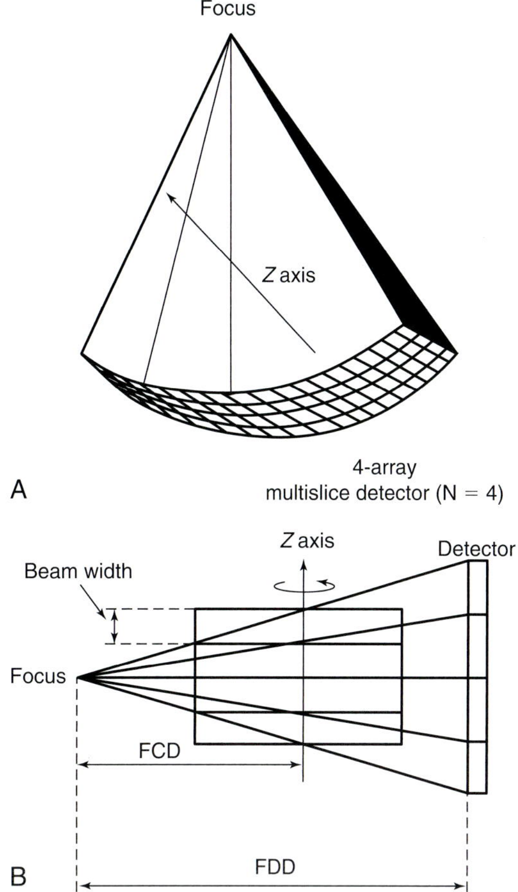


**FIGURE 11-25** Data acquisition geometry for MSCT. **A,** The coordinate system. **B,** A cross section (side view).

***Collimation.*** The x-ray beam collimation system is designed to ensure a constant beam width because the precollimator and postcollimator widths are equal. The beam may or may not be collimated at the detector array. The width of the precollimator defines the slice thickness (*z*-axis resolution or spatial resolution) and affects the volume coverage speed performance. Although thin collimation results in better resolution and takes longer to scan a specified volume, wide collimation results in less resolution but provides better volume coverage speed. The beam width (BW) is measured in the *z*-axis at the center of rotation for a single-row detector array, and it is defined by the precollimator width, which determines the thickness for a single slice. A collimator width of 8 mm falling on a 1D detector array will provide a slice thickness of 8 mm.

***Beam geometry.*** The x-ray beam geometry for SSCT describes a small fan (Fig. 11-24) and is referred to as a *parallel fan-beam geometry*.

***Pitch.*** The pitch for SSCT is defined as the ratio of the distance the table translates per gantry rotation to the BW or precollimator width. As noted by Hu (1999a), "the table advancement per rotation of twice the x-ray beam collimation appears to be the limit of the volume coverage speed performance of an SSCT, and further increase in the table translation would result in clinically unusable images."

***Slice thickness.*** In SSCT, the thickness of the slice is determined by the pitch and the width of the precollimator (which also defines the BW) at the center of rotation (Fig. 11-24).

## MSCT

The data acquisition geometry for MSCT is shown in Figure 11-25. Perhaps the most conspicuous difference between the data acquisition geometry in Figures 11-24 and 11-25 is the multirow detector array (specifically 4) coupled to the x-ray tube to describe a third-generation geometry (Fig. 11-25, *A*). This 2D detector array is what Hu (1999a) referred to as the "enabling component" of an MSCT scanner. Other important and unique features of multislice data acquisition relate to collimation, beam geometry, and pitch.

***Collimation.*** The fundamental collimation scheme is shown in Figure 11-20, *B*. The beam is collimated by a precollimator to fall on the entire multirow detector array. The BW is still defined in the *z*-axis at the center of rotation but now is for a four-row multislice detector array, as shown in Figure 11-25, *B*. This width will be for four slices and is prescribed by the precollimator. A precollimator width of 8 mm that falls on a four-row multislice detector array will produce four slices, each with a thickness of 2 mm (i.e., 8 mm—the total beam width in the *z*-axis at the center of rotation divided by 4). This is unlike the single-slice counterpart, which provides a slice thickness of 8 mm with its 8-mm-wide precollimator. In addition, the four slices are a result of the division of the total x-ray beam into

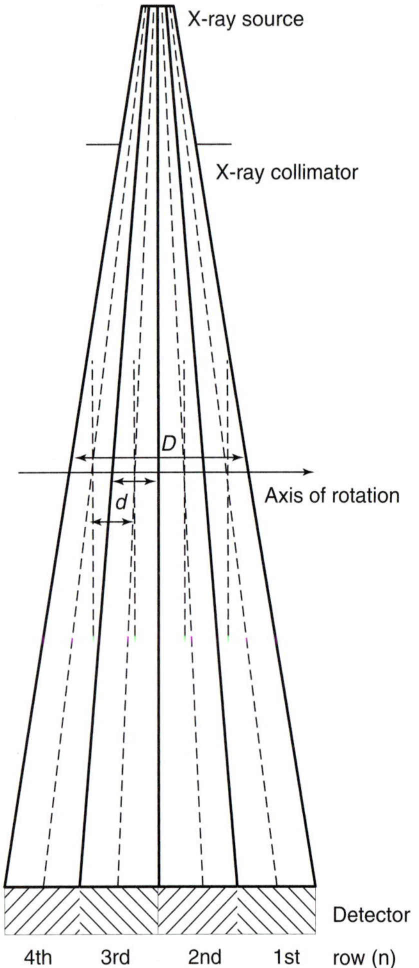


**FIGURE 11-26** A side view or cross section of an MSCT beam geometry from the x-ray tube to a four-row multislice detector array system.

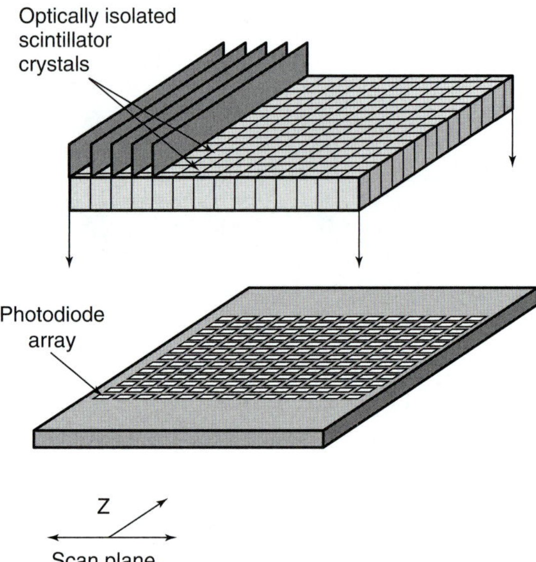


**FIGURE 11-27** A proposed scheme for the use of postcollimation in MSCT to reduce scattered radiation falling on a 2D detector array. The collimators are positioned between detector columns similar to conventional CT single-row detector arrays.

multiple beams, depending on the number of arrays in the 2D detector system. These multiple beams are the result of the detector row collimation or the detector row aperture (Hu, 1999a).

Figure 11-26 is a side view of an MSCT scanner beam from the x-ray tube to the detectors. *D* is the width of the x-ray beam collimator and is measured at the axis of rotation, *N* is the number of detector rows, and *d* represents the detector row collimation. Hu (1999a) explained that, if the gaps between the adjacent detector rows are small and can be ignored, the detector row spacing is equal to the detector row collimation (*d*). The detector row collimation *d* and the x-ray beam collimation *D* have the following relationship:

$$d\,(\text{mm}) = D\,(\text{mm})/N$$

where *N* is the number of detector rows. In SSCT, the detector row collimation equals and is interchangeable with the x-ray beam collimation. "In multislice CT, the detector row collimation is only 1/*N* of the x-ray beam collimation." This makes it possible "to simultaneously achieve high volume coverage speed and high z axis resolution. In general, the larger the number of detector rows *N*, the better the volume coverage speed performance."

For example, if the x-ray prepatient collimation width (x-ray beam collimation) is 20 mm and the scanner has a four-row detector array, the detector row collimation is as follows:

$$d\,(\text{mm}) = D\,(\text{mm})/N$$

in which *d* is the detector row collimation, *N* is the number of detector rows, and *D* is the x-ray beam collimator width (20/4 = 5 mm).

Alternatively,

$$d = 1/N \times \text{X-ray beam collimator width}$$

$$d = 1/4 \times 20$$

$$= 5\ \text{mm}$$

As the beam width increases in the *z* direction to cover the number of rows in the 2D detector system, the amount of scattered radiation increases because a wide area of the patient is scanned. To minimize scattered radiation, antiscatter collimation may be used at the detector array (postcollimation). One such scheme is shown in Figure 11-27. Another scheme is illustrated later.

***Beam geometry.*** As the number of detector rows in a multirow detector array increases, the beam

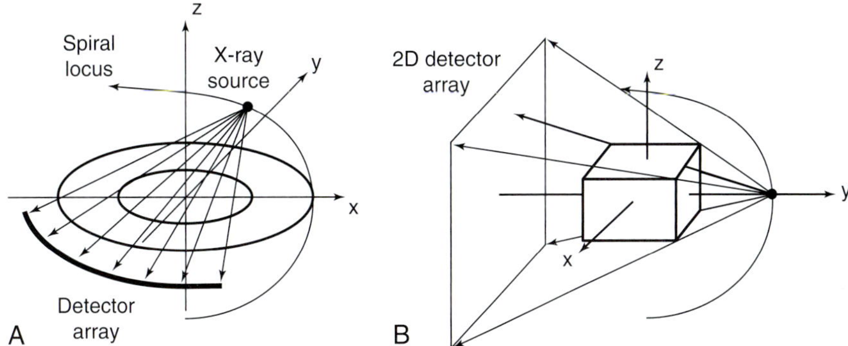


**FIGURE 11-28 A,** The fan-beam geometry of single-row 1D detectors, in which the rays at the detector array are almost parallel and close together. **B,** The concept of cone-beam geometry typical of multirow 2D detectors. The cone beam results in a wider divergence of rays at the detector array than at the fan-beam geometry of single-row 1D detectors.

becomes wider to cover the 2D detector array (Fig. 11-28; see also Fig. 11-26). The beam must cover the length of the detector array. This coverage is influenced by the fan angle of the beam, in which a wider fan angle will cover a longer detector array. The beam must also cover the width of the detector array, which is defined by the number of rows in the detector array. A larger number of rows will result in a wider beam (large cone beam) in the *z*-axis direction.

A **cone-beam** geometry produces more beam divergence along the *z*-axis compared with fan-beam geometry. For this reason, increasing the number of detector rows in MSCT creates a need for a different approach to the interpolation process (compared with single-slice spiral/helical interpolation) because the rays that contribute to the imaging process are more oblique. In addition, the number of detector rows plays an important role in slice thickness selection and volume coverage.

## Pitch—International Electrotechnical Commission Definition

The *pitch* is a term associated with a fastener, and it is actually the distance between the turns on the fastener. In spiral/helical CT, the pitch is defined as the distance (in mm) that the CT table moves during one revolution of the x-ray tube. The pitch is used to calculate the *pitch ratio*, which is a ratio of the pitch to the slice thickness or beam collimation. The pitch ratio is as follows:

$$\text{Pitch} = \frac{\text{distance the table travels during 360-degree revolution}}{\text{Slice thickness or beam collimation}}$$

When the distance the table travels during one complete revolution of the x-ray tube equals the slice thickness or beam collimation, the pitch ratio (simply referred to as *pitch* in the remainder of this text) is 1:1, or simply 1. A pitch of 1 results in the best image quality in spiral/helical CT scanning. The pitch can be increased to increase volume coverage and speed up the scanning process. Pitch is of particular significance because it affects image quality and patient dose and also plays a role in the overall outcome of the clinical examination. A pitch of less than 1 is effectively the same as overlapping slices and imparts a high dose. Conversely, pitches of greater than 1 result in reduced patient dose.

The introduction of multislice detectors resulted in a re-evaluation of the definition of pitch, and in the past, the definition was somewhat varied and controversial. For a discussion of such controversy, the interested reader should refer to Hu (1999a), He (personal communication, 1999), Taguchi and Aradate (1998), and Kalender (2005).

In 1999, the International Electrotechnical Commission (IEC) introduced a definition of pitch, which is stated in the IEC document 60601 regulation for CT, as a means of addressing the variations in definitions offered by different manufacturers (IEC, 1999). The IEC recommends the following:

$$\text{Pitch (P)} = \frac{\text{Distance the table travels per rotation (d)}}{\text{Total collimation (W)}} \qquad \textbf{(11-1)}$$

The total collimation, on the other hand, is equal to the number of slices (*M*) times the collimated slice thickness (*S*). Algebraically, the pitch can now be expressed as follows:

$$P = d/W \text{ or } P = d/M \cdot S \qquad \textbf{(11-2)}$$

For a patient dose comparable to current single-slice scanners at a pitch of 1, a four-slice scanner would require a beam pitch of 1 or a slice pitch of 4. As an example, selection of 4 × 5-mm slices with a table speed of 20 mm per rotation should result in approximately the same patient dose as from a single-slice scanner operated with a 5-mm slice at 5 mm per rotation table speed. Whether this is true in practice depends on the collimator design of the specific scanner.

### Slice Thickness

In MSCT, the slice thickness is determined by the BW (Fig. 11-25), the pitch, and other factors such as the shape and width of the reconstruction filter in the *z*-axis. The details of slice thickness selection for MSCT scanners are described later in this chapter.

## Image Reconstruction

In conventional step-and-shoot CT (conventional CT), a fan-beam geometry and a single-row detector array are used in the data acquisition process, and all rays pass through the image plane (planar section), the slice of interest. With this condition, a fan-beam reconstruction algorithm, specifically, the filtered back-projection algorithm, is used for image reconstruction.

### Single-Slice Spiral/Helical Reconstruction

In SSCT scanners, the fan-beam geometry is maintained and a single-row detector array is used in the data acquisition process. In conventional CT, the patient is stationary during scanning, whereas in SSCT the patient is moving continuously through the gantry aperture during a 360-degree rotation of the x-ray tube and detectors. In this case, all rays do not pass through the image plane. A fan-beam geometry is used, so the fan-beam reconstruction algorithm used in conventional CT is used for image reconstruction. During data acquisition, the fan beam traces a spiral/helical path around the patient, as shown in Figure 11-29. Because all rays do not pass through the image plane (planar section), SSCT requires an additional step of first calculating a planar section. This is done by interpolation, using data points on either side of the section.

The first interpolation algorithm used was 360-degree LI, in which the distance between the two data points used in the interpolation was represented by *s* in Figure 11-29. In an effort to improve the image quality resulting from the 360-degree LI, a different algorithm was developed on the basis of the mathematical fact that a CT view from a specific angle contains the same information as a view in the opposite direction (at 180 degrees). The 180-degree view, when flipped and used for interpolated reconstruction, is referred to as *complementary data*, as opposed to the direct, measured data. With a 180-degree LI, data points are now closer to the image plane. The distance between the two points used for interpolation is now *s*/2. This equation involves calculation of a complementary dataset (*dashed lines*) using the direct fan-beam dataset or measurements (*solid lines*). The distance between the two points used for interpolation is referred to as the *z*-gap (Hu, 1999a). The *z*-gap affects image quality so that the smaller the *z*-gap, the better the image quality. In single-slice spiral/helical CT, increased volume coverage can be achieved with increased pitch; however, as the pitch increases, image quality decreases because the *z*-gap becomes larger. This is one motivating factor for the development of MSCT.

### Multislice Reconstruction

One of the most conspicuous differences between SSCT and MSCT is that the latter uses a new detector technology in which the number of detector rows can vary from 4 to 320. These multiple detector rows result in a large 2D detector array. Because of this, a cone-beam geometry results instead of the fan-beam geometry characteristic of SSCT systems. Cone-beam geometry produces an increase in the beam divergence, which now poses a fundamental problem because all the rays do not pass through the image plane. Rays at the periphery of the beam lie outside the image plane. Approximate cone-beam reconstruction algorithms have been developed for solving this problem (Kudo & Saito, 1991); however, these particular algorithms demand extensive calculations (compared with fan-beam algorithms) and are not suitable for use in medical imaging.

Special fan-beam reconstructions (Hu, 1999a; Taguchi & Aradate, 1998) have been developed for MSCT in its present state. In deriving an algorithm

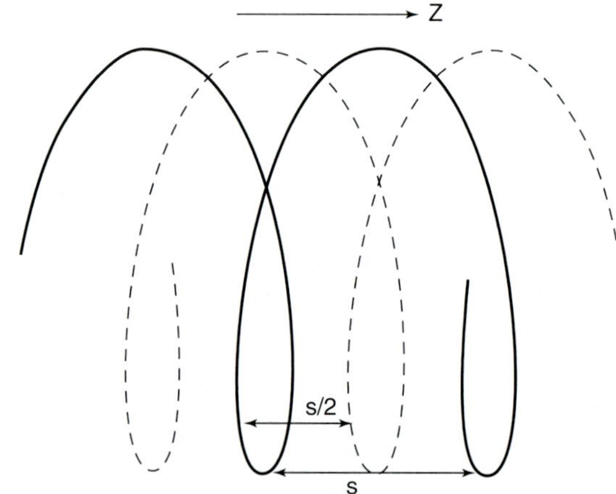


**FIGURE 11-29** The spiral/helical trace of a single-row detector array in single-slice volume CT. The distance of the data points used for 360-degree LI and 180-degree LI is *s* and *s*/2, respectively.

for image reconstruction in MSCT, a logical first step is to extend the principles of 360-degree and 180-degree LI used in SSCT to MSCT. To examine this extension, consider Figure 11-30, which shows the spiral/helical path of a four-row detector array used in MSCT. For a 360-degree LI, the distance between the two points used for interpolation of a planar section is *s*, the same distance as in Figure 11-29 for SSCT. With a 180-degree LI, the distance of the data points is *s*/2 (distance between the solid and dashed lines of the same detector row). The *z*-gap is the same as for SSCT.

***MSCT for up to four detector rows.*** In MSCT, the *z*-gap is determined by the pitch (as in SSCT) and by the detector row spacing, *d*. "As the helical pitch varies, distinctively different z **sampling** patterns and therefore interlacing helix patterns may result in multislice helical CT" (Hu, 1999a). This is illustrated in Figure 11-31 for a four-row detector array for two different pitches. At a pitch of 2:1 (Fig. 11-31, *A*) the distance between the points used for interpolation, the *z*-gap, is *d*, "which is the same as the displacement from one solid helix to the next. This causes a high degree of overlap between different helices, generating highly redundant projection measurements at certain z-positions. Because of this high degree of redundancy (or inefficiency) in z-sampling, the overall z-sampling spacing (i.e., the z-gap of the interlacing helix pattern) is still *d*, not any better than its single-slice counterpart" (Hu, 1999a).

Increased pitch in MSCT from 2:1 to 3:1 (Fig. 11-31, *B*) results in a *z*-gap of *d*/2, a much shorter distance. In this case the volume coverage speed can be increased. In addition, because the *z*-gap is less as the pitch increases, better image quality results. Hu (1999a) pointed out that "the volume coverage

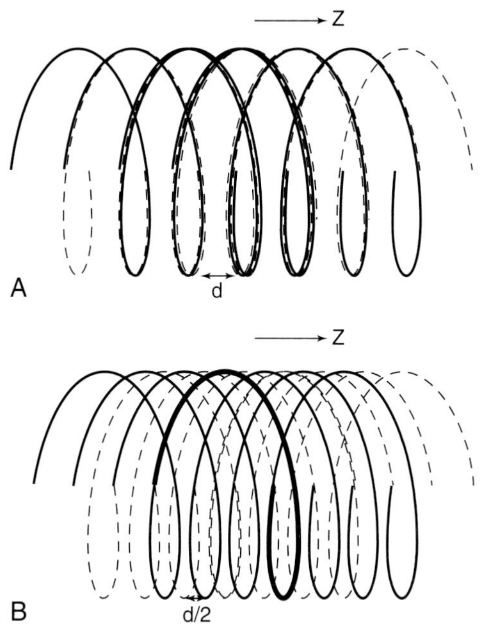


**FIGURE 11-31** Spiral/helical traces for a four-row detector array in MSCT at a pitch of 2:1 **(A)** and a pitch of 3:1 **(B)**.

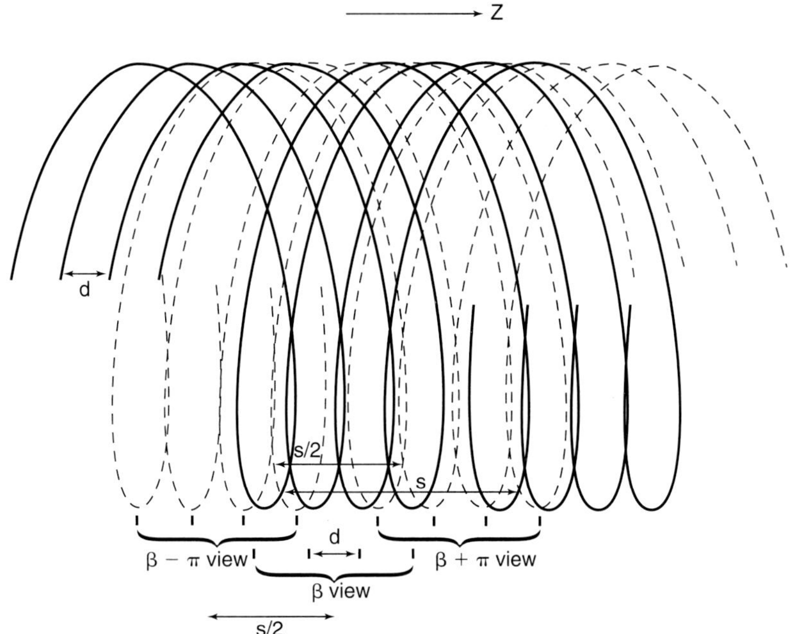


**FIGURE 11-30** The spiral/helical trace of a four-row detector array in MSCT. See text for further explanation.

speed performance of the multislice scanner is substantially better than its single-slice counterpart, and so the selection of helical pitches is very critical to its performance. The pitch selection is determined by the consideration of the z-sampling efficiency and conventional factors such as volume coverage speed (which disfavors very low helical pitch); slice profile; and image artifacts, which disfavor very high helical pitch." The preferred helical pitches are those that represent the preferred trade-offs for various applications.

Alternatively, Figures 11-32 through 11-35 can be used to explain the problem and solution described previously. The unwound helical path for SSCT is shown in Figure 11-32 for both direct and complementary data. The image plane is interpolated using two points from the direct data and the complementary data on either side of it (image plane). Extending the single-slice concept to the multislice case as shown in Figure 11-33 results in a superimposition of the complementary and direct data for each of the detector rows in the four-row array. Note also that the *z*-gap is larger, and this results in image degradation. Additionally, the superimposition does not allow for efficient *z*-sampling. A pitch of 4 is not as preferable as a pitch of 2 because of the redundancy in the data sampling.

Figure 11-34 provides a solution to the problem imposed by Figure 11-33. By separating the direct and complementary data trails, efficient *z*-sampling can be achieved (Saito, 1998). Taguchi and Aradate (1998) referred to this as *optimized sampling scan*. Figure 11-34 is with a pitch of 3.5 less than that of Figure 11-33 (pitch of 4). These figures indicate that a slight compromise in helical pitch (just 0.5) produces amazing improvement in the data sampling pattern.

The detector design for MSCT allows the operator to select variable slice thicknesses on the basis of the requirements of the examination. The new algorithms for MSCT also allow for the reconstruction

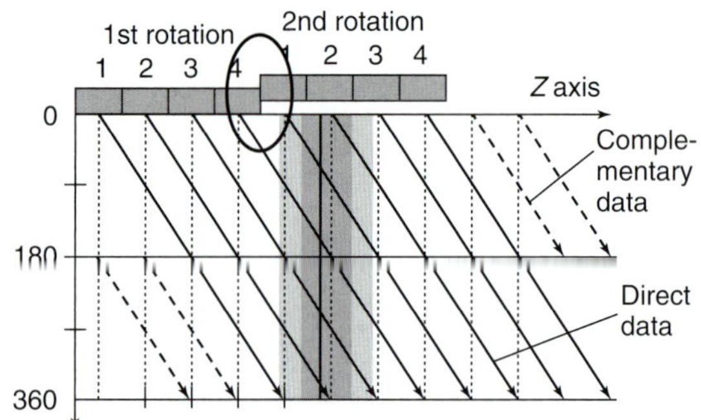


**FIGURE 11-33** Rotation of a multislice detector with an even integer pitch causes the overlap of direct and complementary data from different slices. This duplication reduces the amount of information available for image reconstruction and affects image quality.

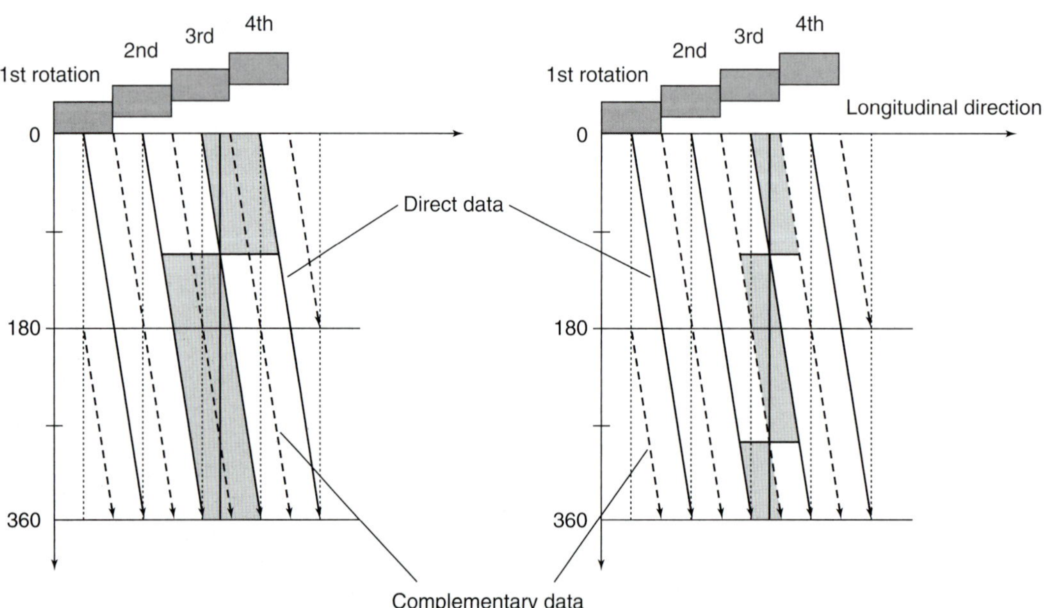


**FIGURE 11-32** Single-slice spiral/helical data are generated from many gantry rotations. Reconstruction of an image in a single plane on the patient axis involves the interpolation of views in front of and behind the image plane. The use of complementary data reduces effective slice thickness but increases noise.

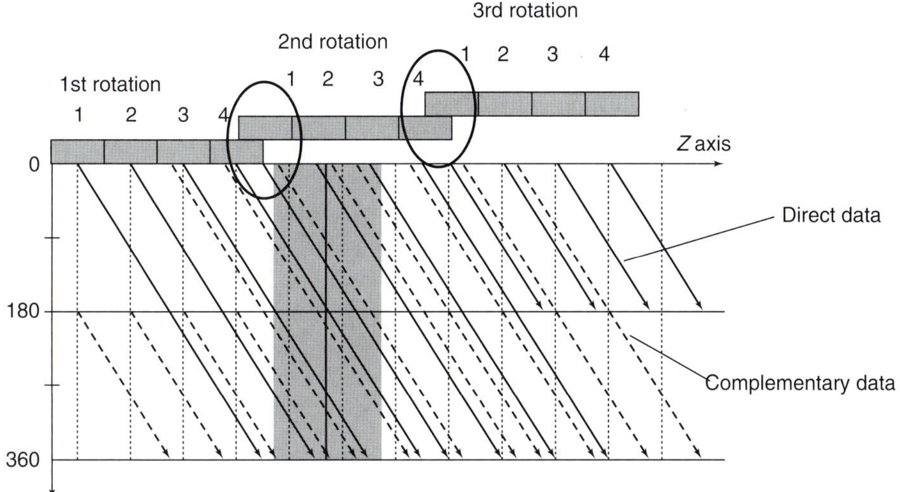


**FIGURE 11-34** Careful choice of multislice pitch avoids the duplication of direct and complementary data so that image quality is not compromised.

of these variable slice thicknesses. These new algorithms address problems (image quality degradation) arising from the increase in speed (hence volume coverage) of the patient moving through the gantry aperture when the pitch is increased. Additionally, these algorithms provide for the selection of the slice thicknesses that meet the needs of the examination.

Two such algorithms were developed by Taguchi and Aradate (1998) and by Hu (1999a). These algorithms are almost identical (including the algorithm developed by Siemens Medical Systems) and are based on the same philosophy (Hu, personal communication, 1999; Taguchi, personal communication, 1999).

In general, these algorithms are based on the following steps:

1. *Spiral/helical scanning by interlaced sampling.* In this step, smaller *z*-gaps are obtained by adjusting or selecting the pitch to separate the complementary data from the direct data.
2. *Longitudinal interpolation by z-filtering.* Another unique aspect of multislice data reconstruction involves averaging data in the *z*-axis direction. Interpolation of spiral/helical data is still needed, but the fact that the density of data points in this dimension is greater than with single-slice scanners is advantageous. One approach to image reconstruction uses a filter in the *z*-axis to select and weight the data points to be used in the averaging (Taguchi & Aradate, 1998; Fig. 11-35). This method uses a filtering process in the longitudinal (*z*) direction. Assuming some range with a width called the *filter width* (FW) in the longitudinal (*z*) direction (Fig. 11-35), all data sampled within that range are processed by weighted summation. The filter parameters (e.g., FW and shape) can control the spatial resolution in the longitudinal direction, the image noise, and the image quality. Again, pitch selection is flexible and should be carefully selected. A practical advantage of this technique is that the size and shape of the filter can be selected by the operator for more control over the effective slice thickness versus noise trade-off. As can be seen in Figure 11-35, the selection of different FWs provides considerably more control over effective slice thickness than has generally been available with single-slice spiral/helical reconstruction. FW can also substantially affect image noise compared with conventional 180- or 360-degree LI.
3. *Fan-beam reconstruction.* This algorithm can be used if the number of detector rows is small. Hu (1999a) used multiple parallel fan beams to approximate the cone-beam geometry characteristic of MSCT. The algorithm used by Taguchi and Aradate (1998) is also based on a fan-beam method. Additionally, Saito (1998) labeled the algorithm multislice cone-beam tomography reconstruction method (MUSCOT). The effect of MUSCOT on image quality is shown in Figure 11-36. Compared with SSCT (180-degree LI), MUSCOT provides good image quality "at a scanning speed that is about three times faster than that for single-slice CT" (Taguchi & Aradate, 1998).

***MSCT for 16 or more detector rows.*** The previous description lends itself to MSCT scanners with up to four detector rows. These scanners use a 2D detector array in which the x-ray beam is now opened in two dimensions to cover the entire detector array. The divergence of the beam describes a cone beam rather than a fan beam, and therefore the scanning geometry is now referred to as a cone beam. The nature and problems of using a cone beam with algorithms designed for fan-beam CT scanning geometries are outlined in Chapter 5. One of the problems, for example, is related to cone-beam artifacts (streaks, for example) that degrade image quality.

The algorithms for four-slice scanners described earlier ignore the cone-beam geometry in four-slice MSCT scanners because these algorithms assume that the measurement rays are parallel and perpendicular to the *z*-axis (longitudinal axis), a condition that satisfies the **filtered back-projection (FBP)** algorithm. Basically, the measurement rays for a planar dataset are obtained by interpolation with 360-degree LI or 180-degree LI algorithms similar to those for single-slice spiral/helical CT scanners (Chapter 11), followed by the well-established and proven FBP algorithm.

As the number of detector rows increases from 4 to 16 to 64 and beyond, the cone beam becomes larger and cone-beam artifacts become more pronounced, especially if the object imaged is not perfectly centered in the isocenter of the CT gantry (Figure 11-37). The outer detectors receive more oblique rays compared with the central set of detectors. The effects of cone-beam geometries on image quality for these 16-slice and beyond MSCT scanners cannot be ignored. The cone-beam angle, for example, increases by up to 16, and previous interpolation algorithms are not useful for these large cone angles (Mather, 2005a). Therefore, cone-beam algorithms are needed to address these increasing cone-beam geometries and minimize cone-beam artifacts.

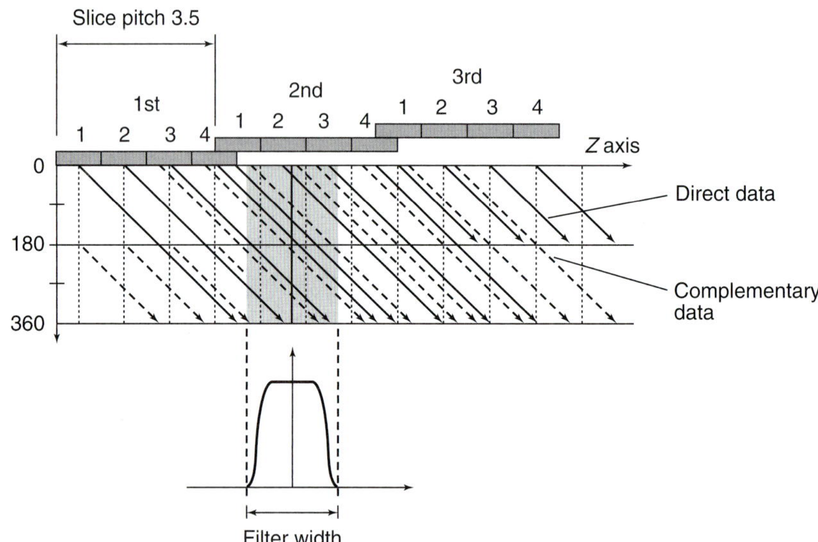


**FIGURE 11-35** Filters may be used to average data along the *z*-axis and provide more trade-off options between effective slice thickness and image noise to the operator.

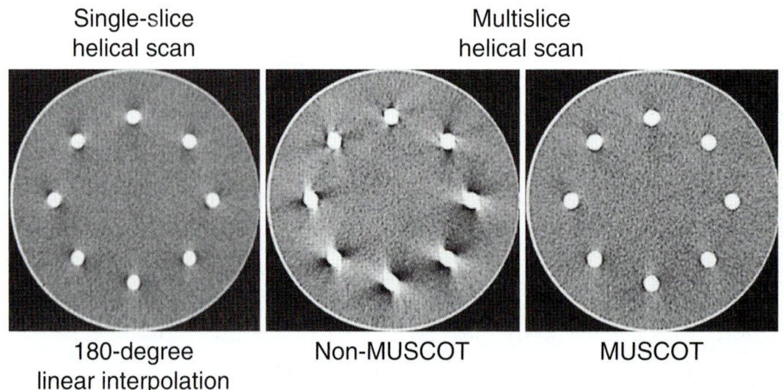


**FIGURE 11-36** The difference in image quality of a ball phantom obtained with a 180-degree LI algorithm (SSCT) and with and without the MUSCOT algorithm used for MSCT imaging. (From Saito, Y. (1998). *Medical Review*, 66, 1-8.)

## Cone-Beam Algorithms: An Overview

Cone-beam algorithms fall into two classes: (1) exact algorithms and (2) approximate algorithms. Although exact algorithms for cone-beam data have not been successful in recent times (Kalender, 2005), they are also "computationally complex and difficult to implement" (Mather, 2005a). For these reasons, they are not described in this book. On the other hand, approximate cone-beam algorithms fall into two categories: 3D and 2D algorithms (Chen et al., 2003). Two such algorithms that have become commonplace in MSCT scanners are as follows:

1. Feldkamp-Davis-Kress (FDK), also simply referred to as the Feldkamp-type 3D algorithm
2. Advanced single-slice rebinning (ASSR) 2D approximate algorithm

### Feldkamp-Davis-Kress Algorithm

The fundamental basis of the FDK algorithm is illustrated in Figure 11-38. As can be seen, the FDK algorithm simply is an extension of the 2D FBP for fan-beam geometry into a 3D FBP for cone-beam geometry (Chen et al., 2003; Kachelriess et al., 2006).

This algorithm is more extensive than the 2D FBP algorithm, and it is more commonplace for use with cone-beam CT scanners (Feldkamp et al., 1984; Hsieh et al., 2013). Although the 2D FBP algorithm filters the acquired data from 1D detectors, followed by a 2D fan-beam back-projection, the FDK algorithm filters the data acquired from 2D detectors (3D dataset) followed by a 3D cone-beam back-projection (Kalender, 2005).

There are several modifications of the FDK algorithm (referred to as Feldkamp-type algorithms) for use in MSCT scanners; however, the principles of these algorithms are beyond the scope of this book. Two examples of these algorithms in use on some MSCT scanners are the true cone-beam tomography Feldkamp-based algorithm developed by Toshiba Medical Systems, which can handle data from large cone angles, and the extended parallel back-projection algorithm developed by Siemens for scanners with more than 64 slices per rotation.

A basic problem with the Feldkamp-type algorithms is that they "cannot incorporate 2D back projection **hardware** already available in conventional medical CT systems" (Chen et al., 2003; Kachelriess et al., 2006). This problem, however, can be solved by 2D approximate algorithms.

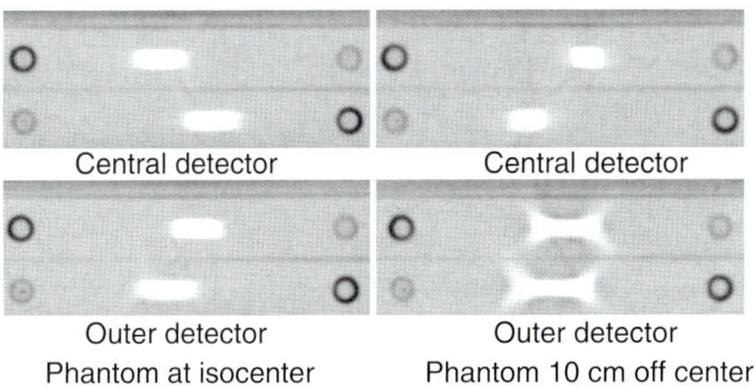


**FIGURE 11-37** The appearance of streaking artifacts that occur with imaging of nonuniform objects in the *z*-axis with a 16-slice (cone-beam) CT scanner. The artifacts are more pronounced for those created by the outer detectors and worsen if the object is not positioned accurately in the isocenter. (Courtesy ImPACT Scan, London, United Kingdom.)

### Two-Dimensional Approximate Algorithm

The main goal of the 2D approximate algorithms "is to provide an image quality close to that of a three-dimensional reconstruction algorithm using two-dimensional and back projection methods" (Chen et al., 2003). This principle is based on the notion of *rebinning*, a term used to describe the resorting of the 3D data collected from the cone-beam acquisition (geometry) to a set of 2D fan-beam projection data and, subsequently, use the conventional 2D FBP algorithm to reconstruct transaxial images, as illustrated in Figure 11-39.

One early rebinning method was the single-slice rebinning (SSR) algorithm; however, it did not produce acceptable image quality for MSCT scanners with large cone angles. Therefore, other methods were developed to solve this problem by use of a technique called tilted plane reconstruction (TPR; Chen et al., 2003). The TPR method requires that the plane

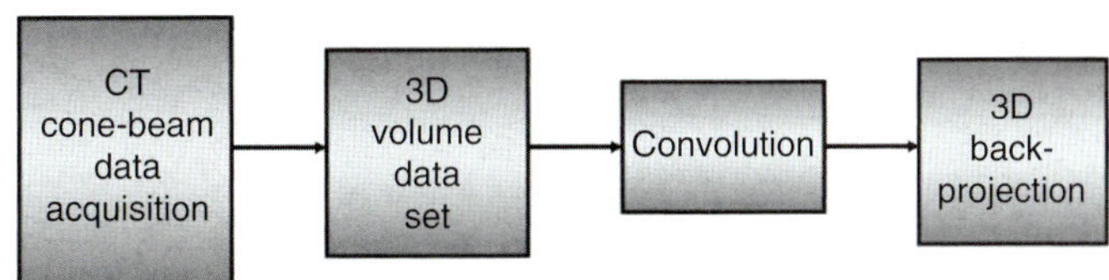


**FIGURE 11-38** The most fundamental representation of the FDK algorithm for cone-beam reconstruction. First, cone-beam projections of the 3D object are obtained, followed by preweighting and filtering (convolution). Finally, 3D back-projection is performed along the identical beam geometry (rays) as used for the initial cone-beam data acquisition.

to be reconstructed is tilted (oblique) to fit the spiral/helical path of the x-ray beam to reduce cone-beam artifacts. One popular TPR algorithm is the ASSR algorithm used by General Electric (GE) Healthcare and by Siemens Medical Solutions.

The fundamental steps of the ASSR algorithm, clearly illustrated in Figure 11-40, are as follows:

1. The image planes to be reconstructed make use of 180-degree segments of the spiral/helical path of the x-ray beam to obtain optimized oblique images (semicircles) because they are tilted to fit the spiral path along the *z*-axis of the patient.
2. The measured cone-beam data are then rebinned (resorted) to produce a large number of overlapping, tilted reconstruction planes that can cover the entire volume of tissue imaged.
3. In the third step, *z*-axis reformation (*z*-axis filtering) is performed to produce axial images by using the conventional 2D reconstruction algorithm on the tilted planes.
4. Finally, step 3 produces an axial image dataset.

One of the fundamental problems with the ASSR algorithm is related to smaller pitch values. To solve this problem, the adaptive multiplane reconstruction (AMPR) algorithm was introduced. The AMPR algorithm is an extension of the ASSR algorithm and determines the *z*-axis resolution by allowing the free selection of pitch values and slice thickness (Flohr et al., 2005).

Another multislice cone-beam reconstruction algorithm somewhat related to the AMPR algorithm is the weighted hyperplane reconstruction algorithm. A hyperplane is a concept in geometry. In a 2D ($x$, $y$) space, a hyperplane is a line, whereas in a 3D ($x$, $y$, $z$) space, a hyperplane is an ordinary plane that separates the space into two halves (Oxford English Dictionary, 2008). Flohr et al. (2005) summarized this algorithm as follows:

> Similar to the AMPR, 3D reconstruction is split into a series of two-dimensional reconstructions. Instead of reconstruction of traditional transverse sections, convex hyperplanes are proposed as the region of reconstruction. The increasing spiral overlap with decreasing pitch is handled by introducing subsets of detector rows, which are sufficient to reconstruct an image at a given pitch value. At a pitch of 0.5625 with a 16-slice scanner the data collected by detector rows one to nine form a complete projection dataset. Similarly, projections from detector rows two to 10 can be used to reconstruct another image at the same z-axis position. Projections from detector rows three to 11 yield a third image and so on.... The final image is based on a weighted average of the sub-images.

For a more detailed treatment of cone-beam algorithms, the interested reader should refer to Kalender (2005) and Flohr et al. (2005).

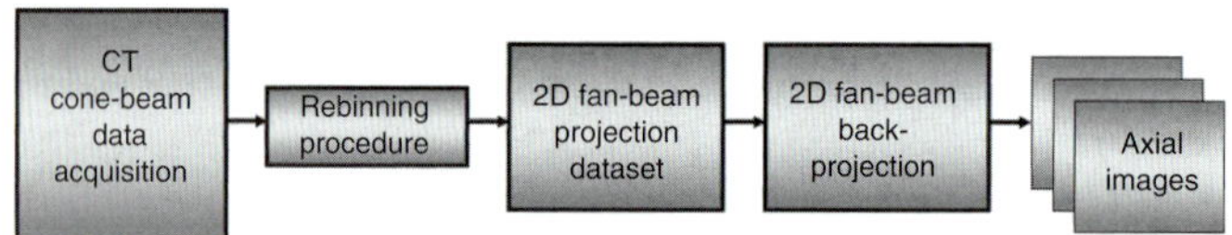


**FIGURE 11-39** The basic steps of the 2D approximate reconstruction algorithm for wide cone-beam CT scanners. The acquired cone-beam data are rebinned into a 2D fan-beam projection dataset that is finally back-projected by use of the 2D fan-beam reconstruction algorithm to create a set of axial images.

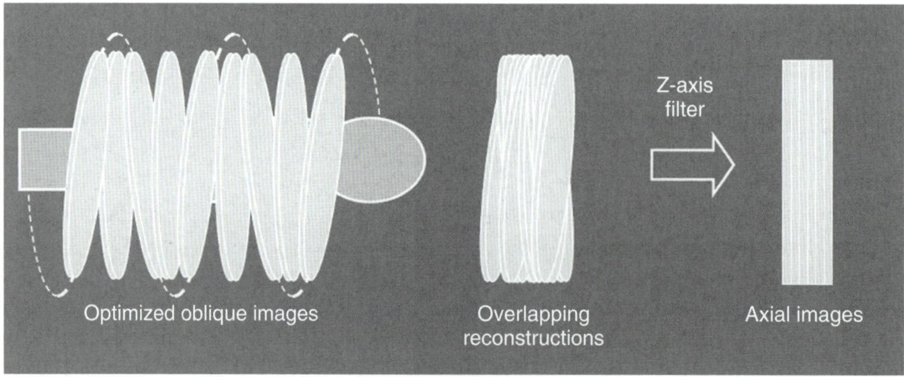


**FIGURE 11-40** The basic steps of the ASSR reconstruction algorithm. See text for explanation. (Courtesy ImPACT Scan, London, United Kingdom.)

## INSTRUMENTATION

In describing the instrumentation for MSCT systems, it is essential to focus on the major components responsible for data acquisition, image reconstruction, image display and manipulation, **image processing,** image storage, recording, and image transmission.

The flow of data in MSCT parallels that of conventional step-and-shoot CT and includes x-ray production and transmission through the patient and conversion of x-rays into electrical signals, which are subsequently converted into digital data for processing by a digital computer. Digital data in the computer are then converted into image data through image reconstruction, to be displayed on a monitor for viewing by an observer. However, the detector technology in MSCT is one of the most significant developments in the evolution of CT. Other components of significance are the DAS and the image reconstruction system for MSCT scanning.

The major equipment components for the MSCT imaging chain are the data acquisition components, patient couch or table, the **computer system,** and the operator console.

### Data Acquisition Components

The MSCT gantry houses the x-ray generator, the x-ray tube, and detectors, as well as the detector electronics (DAS). MSCT scanners are based on the third-generation system design, in which the x-ray tube and detectors are coupled and rotate continuously during continuous patient translation through the gantry aperture. Such data collection strategy is possible through the use of slip-ring technology (see Chapter 4). Today *contactless slip-ring technology* has become available for use in CT scanners. For example, GE Healthcare (personal communication, 2014) reports that the Revolution EVO CT scanner, the next generation volume CT scanner, uses contactless slip ring "to transfer data to and from the rotating side of the gantry to the stationary side through RF technology at 40 Gbps. Induction based, brushless slip ring to reliably transfer high voltage power."

These components (many of which are proprietary in nature and cannot be made publicly available) have improved through the years with the ultimate goal of improving imaging performance such as offering improved spatial resolution and generating images with low noise and reduced artifacts. It is a worthwhile exercise for the interested reader to explore the most recent CT manufacturer websites for state-of-the-art descriptions of the most recent technology, since all new developments cannot be mentioned in this text.

#### X-Ray Generator

The x-ray generator is a compact, lightweight, high-frequency generator that provides a stable high voltage to the x-ray tube to ensure efficient performance such as high instantaneous power output from about 50 kW to 150 kW and high continuous power output. The power output (kW) of these generators varies depending on the manufacturer.

#### X-Ray Tube

The x-ray tube is a rotating-anode tube capable of high heat storage capacity with high anode and tube housing cooling rates. The x-ray beam is usually fan shaped and emanates from either a small or large focal spot. X-ray tubes for MSCTs provide tube voltages ranging from 70 kV to 150 kV in increments of 10 kV, and high tube current (mAs) variation, which is different depending on the manufacturer. In terms of evolution, x-ray tubes for CT scanning are always undergoing refinements to improve the performance output needed to image more sophisticated examinations that demand high x-ray output and short **exposure** times. For example, directly cooled (direct anode cooling) x-ray tubes are currently available from Philips and Siemens. See Chapter 4 for a more detailed description of x-ray tubes, including the most recent design for use with MSCT scanners.

#### Multislice Detectors

Multislice detectors have evolved over time; therefore, they are described in the next subsection of this chapter.

### MSCT Detectors

The first clinical scanner, the EMI Mark 1, and several of its successors recorded two image slices simultaneously in an effort to offset their agonizingly slow scan speeds. In 1992, Elscint introduced the first modern multislice scanner, which used dual-detector banks. A major difference between the EMI Mark 1 and Elscint scanners was that a particular image from the Elscint system could take advantage of data acquired by both detector banks, whereas the old EMI scanner, which predated spiral/helical acquisition, simply generated two independent images.

Detectors capable of providing more than two slices for CT scanners were introduced in 1998. At present, they allow acquisition of up to 320 slices simultaneously, and their design suggests that this number may increase in the future. This dramatic technical advance promises to have a major impact on the way CT is used in clinical practice. The tremendous increase in the rate of data collection will influence routine CT applications and create new areas for CT imaging.

## Types of Detectors

As noted earlier in this chapter, the most significant difference between SSCTs and MSCTs is the detector technology.

There are three types of detectors used in MSCT scanning (Cody & Mahesh, 2007; Dowsett et al., 2006; Kachelriess et al., 2006; Kohl, 2005):

1. Uniform or **matrix** detectors (also referred to as **fixed array detectors** or *linear array detectors*)
2. Nonuniform or variable detectors (also referred to as **adaptive array detectors**)
3. Hybrid detectors

Several different approaches to the construction of these detectors are available (Fig.11-41). As can be seen in Figure 11-41, detector arrays in the *z*-axis can be uniform, with all elements of the same dimensions or nonuniform to reduce the number of elements needed for thicker slices. An advantage of the nonuniform elements is the reduction of dead space (the gap between detector elements to ensure optical isolation). On the other hand, this arrangement offers less flexibility for the future, when slice numbers greater than 320 will be practical. Element dimensions shown are "effective" detector sizes, calculated at the center of gantry rotation where slice thickness is measured. The size and distribution of detector elements in the *x-y* plane are similar to those in current single-slice systems. Consequently, spatial or high-contrast resolution is unlikely to change significantly. Such arrays can involve more than 30,000 individual detector elements.

## Detector Materials

As described in Chapter 4, detectors in CT fall into two categories: gas ionization detectors and solid-state detectors. It is important to note, however, that MSCT scanners do not use gas ionization detectors such as xenon detectors (used in the earlier SSCT scanners) because they have low quantum detection efficiency (<50%) and low x-ray absorption (Dowsett et al., 2006; Kachelriess et al., 2006; Kohl, 2005).

The detector elements of MSCT scanners use solid-state materials (scintillation crystals or ceramics) such as cadmium tungstate and rare earth materials such as gadolinium oxysulfide or yttrium-gadolinium oxide, gadolinium oxide, or ceramics (Dowsett et al., 2006; Kohl, 2005). The detectors are doped with suitable dopants (europium, for example) to decrease **afterglow** below 0.1% at 100 ms (Dowsett et al., 2006).

These materials convert x-ray photons to visible light that is subsequently detected by photodiodes (see Chapter 4).

More recently, CT vendors have improved the design of their **scintillation detectors** for improved performance during imaging by using complex rare earth materials to function as activators in the scintillators used to capture and convert x-ray photos into light. For example, while GE uses a *lutetium (Lu)-based garnet* in their Gemstone CT detector array, Toshiba Medical Systems uses a *praseodymium-activated scintillator* in their PureViSION CT detector array. Furthermore, the more recent design considerations of CT detectors also include miniaturized detector electronics through the use of integrated DAS circuits. The purpose of such design elements is to reduce electronic noise and to reduce power consumption. The reduction in electronic noise results in low image noise with very small signals. Figure 11-42 illustrates the noise comparison between the Siemens Stellar<sup>Infinity</sup> CT detector and a conventional CT detector. A more comprehensive description of CT detectors is provided in Chapter 4.

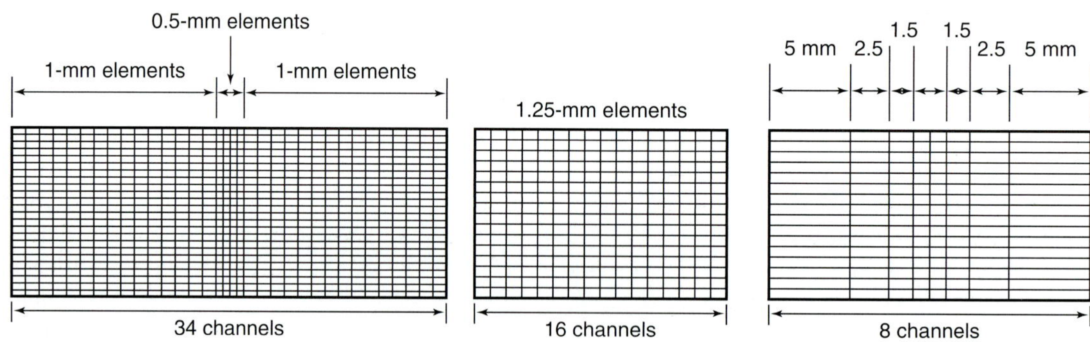


**FIGURE 11-41** Multirow CT detector designs. Detector elements may be uniform or nonuniform. See text for further explanation.

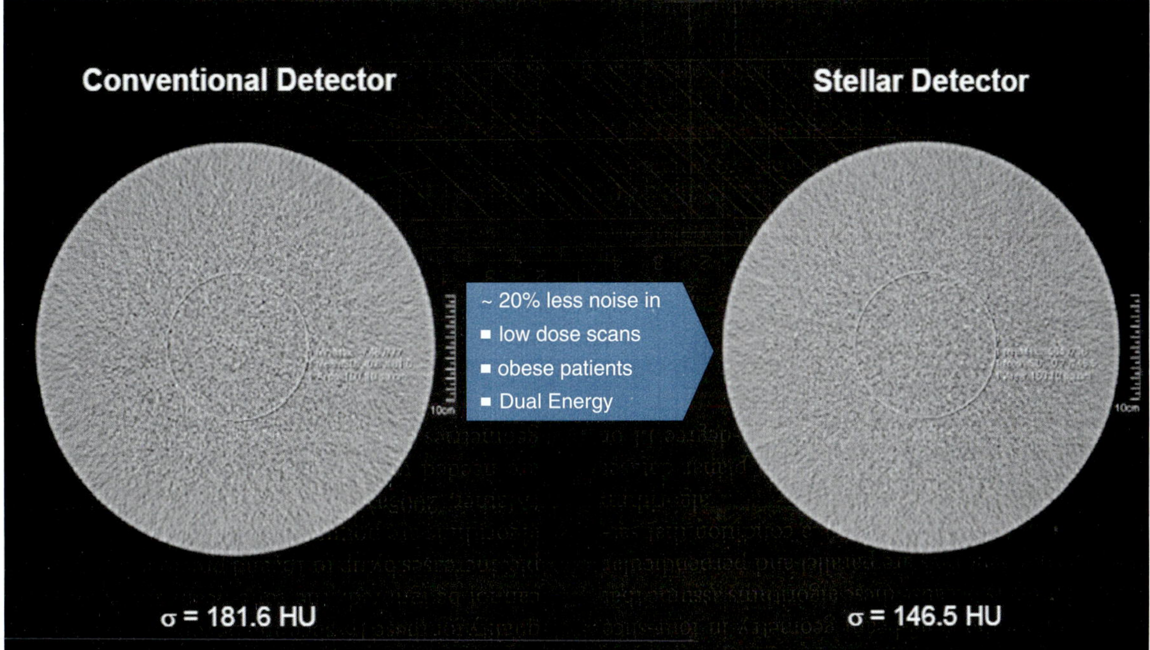


**FIGURE 11-42** The image noise comparison between the Siemens Stellar$^{Infinity}$ detector with a conventional CT detector in a 40-cm water phantom, at 120 kVp and 50 mAs. (Courtesy Siemens Healthcare.)

## Performance Properties of Detectors

It is beyond the scope of this text to discuss the physical performance properties of CT detectors; however, Dowsett et al. (2006) emphasized that detectors for MSCT scanners should have several properties. These include a large **dynamic range,** high quantum **absorption efficiency,** high luminescence efficiency, good geometric efficiency, small afterglow, and high precision machinability. In addition, they noted that all detector elements must have a uniform response. Readers interested in these properties should refer to the work of Dowsett et al. (2006). Several of these properties are described further in Chapter 4.

## Detector Configuration

The term *detector configuration* "describes the number of data collection channels and the effective section thickness determined by the data acquisition system settings" (Dalrymple et al., 2007). MSCT detectors can be configured in several ways by combining various detector elements electronically (or binning) to produce the desired slice thickness required for the examination at the isocenter. Typical slice thicknesses that can be obtained include:

- 2 × 0.5 mm, 4 × 1.0 mm, 4 × 5.0 mm, 2 × 8.0 mm, and 2 × 10 mm for four-slice adaptive array detector
- 16 × 0.5 mm, 16 × 1.0 mm, and 16 × 2.0 mm for a 16-slice fixed array detector
- 40 × 0.625 mm and 32 × 1.25 mm for a 40-slice fixed array detector
- 64 × 0.5 mm and 32 × 1.0 mm for a 64-slice fixed array detector

The reader should consult the manufacturer data sheets for specific slice thicknesses offered by their scanners.

# Slice Thickness Selection

As mentioned earlier, individual slice widths (Fig. 11-43) are generally defined by the number of detector elements grouped (or binned) into each data channel (Dalrymple et al., 2007). The smallest **slice width** available is determined by the smallest single detector element. An exception to this generalization occurs in the nonuniform array shown in Figure 11-43, in which two 0.5-mm slices can be acquired by moving the collimator leaves inward so that only the inner half of the two central 1-mm elements are exposed to the x-ray beam. Similarly, four 1-mm slices are acquired by irradiating the two central elements and two thirds of the adjacent 1.5-mm elements. Slice width is defined at the center of rotation (center of the gantry aperture), so the actual detector dimensions for that slice will be greater because of the magnification produced by beam divergence. The x-ray beam width, as defined by the prepatient collimators, will be approximately four times the slice width.

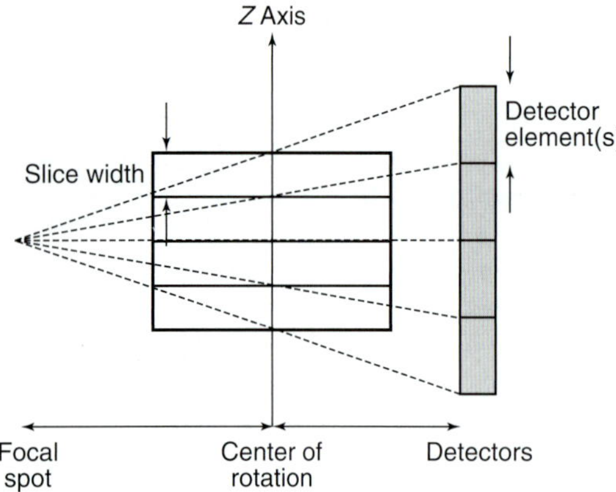


**FIGURE 11-43** Slice geometry in multislice scanners. The number of detector elements grouped together determines the size of the slice. Slice width is defined at the center of gantry rotation.

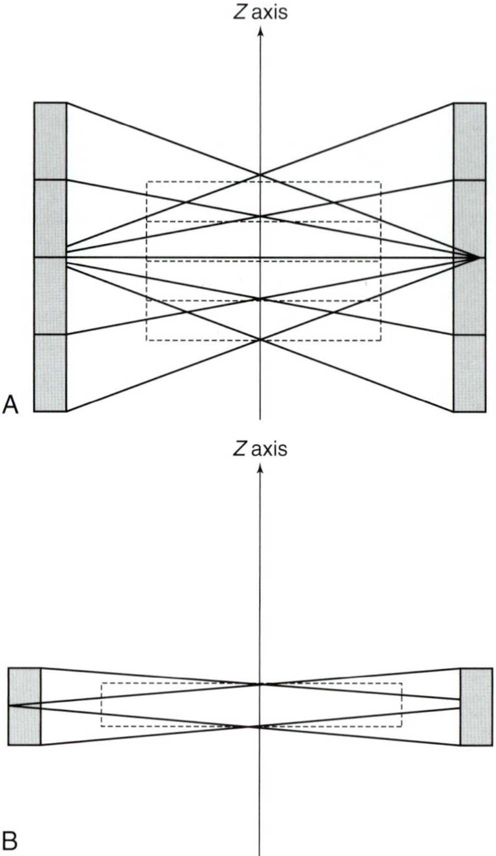


**FIGURE 11-44** Comparison of slice geometry between multislice **(A)** and single-slice **(B)** scanners. The x-ray beams are shown at opposite sides of gantry rotation. Although the diagram is exaggerated, there is more beam divergence with the multislice system.

The slice, as defined by the tissue irradiated during the rotation of a multislice detector, is significantly different from that of a single-detector scanner (Fig. 11-44). This is an extension of the problem with the earlier dual-detector scanners. In this case, however, the outer two slices are considerably more affected by beam divergence than are the inner two slices.

The significance of this geometric nonuniformity may be most severe in the case of conventional scanning. Reconstruction of the CT image involves all views acquired throughout the 360 degrees of data collection. When views from different angles are actually measuring quite different tissue pathways, there will be varying degrees of volume averaging with an increased likelihood of artifact and inaccurate reconstruction. If detector size is increased in future scanners to add more slices, this geometric situation will be further exaggerated. With the x-ray beam fan extended in the *z*-axis, as well as the *x-y* plane, a reconstruction algorithm different than those used for single-slice scanners is needed to process the raw data (Hu, 1999a; Taguchi & Aradate, 1998).

The signals from the individual detector elements are fed to four DASs through a bank of switches that combines the signals from the appropriate number of elements into the slice width selected by the operator (Fig. 11-45).

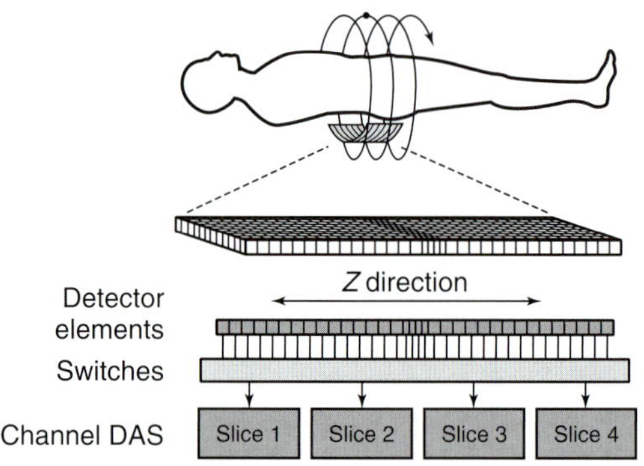


**FIGURE 11-45** Switches group the signal from individual detector elements. The signals are then transferred to one of four DASs that generate the four simultaneous slices. Additional DAS channels can be added in the future.

Detector elements outside the selected slices are switched off and do not contribute any signal to the DAS. Patient dose is controlled by prepatient collimators that restrict the x-ray beam to only those detector elements needed for the four data slices. At present, the slice thickness must be selected before scanning, and it is not possible to narrow the slice width after data collection. Summing slices after scanning to create fewer thicker images is certainly feasible and can have clinical value. In this case, it would be possible to return to the thinner slices if clinically indicated and if the raw data were still available.

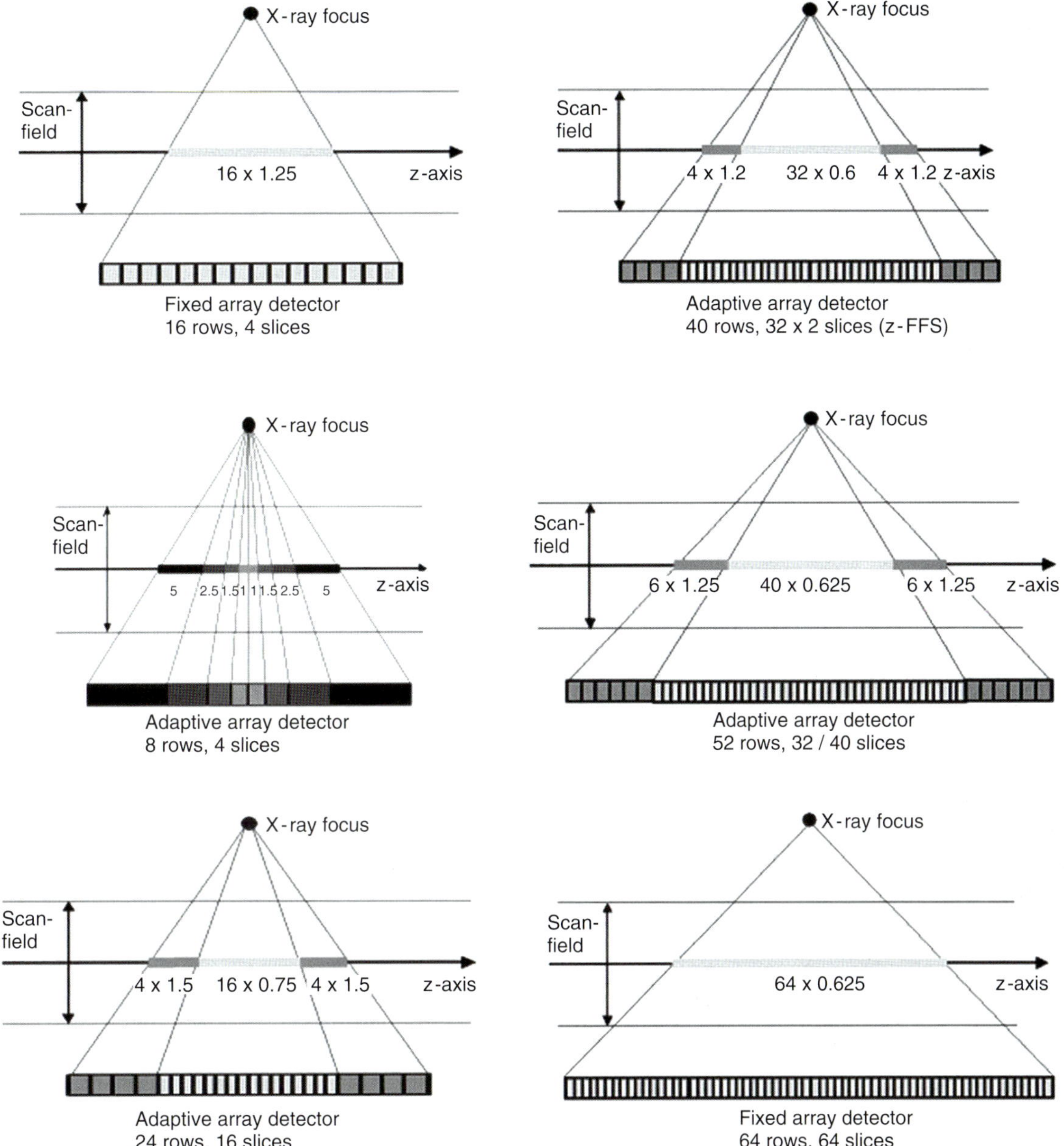


**FIGURE 11-46** Examples of the use of fixed array and adaptive array detectors in MSCT scanners in determining the slice thicknesses to be obtained. (From Kohl, G. (2005). *Proceedings of the American Thoracic Society, 2,* 470-476. Reproduced by kind permission.)

Figure 11-46 provides examples of various combinations of detector elements for both fixed array and adaptive array detectors for MSCT imaging. In addition, the detector module of a 64-slice MSCT scanner (SOMATOM Sensation 64, Siemens Medical Solutions, Germany) together with its antiscatter collimators (diagonally cut) is shown in Figure 11-47.

The design of the multirow detector influences the speed of acquisition of the slices and the resolution of the slices, as shown in Figure 11-48.

## Data Acquisition System

Another major component of the gantry is the DAS, the detector electronics responsible mainly for digitizing the signals from the detectors before they are sent to the computer for processing. Figure 11-48 shows an example of a DAS coupled to the multirow detector array by switches. In this case, four slices are acquired at the same time because of the presence of four DAS systems (four times the electrical circuits compared with SSCT systems; Saito, 1998). Regardless of which four slices are required for the

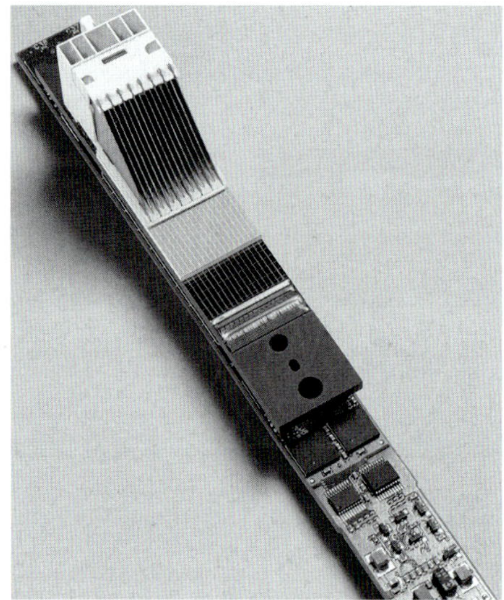

**FIGURE 11-47** Photo of a detector module for the Siemens 64-slice SOMATOM Sensation MSCT scanner showing the electronics and the antiscatter collimators that are cut diagonally (left side of the detector module). (From Kohl, G. (2005). *Proceedings of the American Thoracic Society, 2,* 470-476. Reproduced by kind permission.)

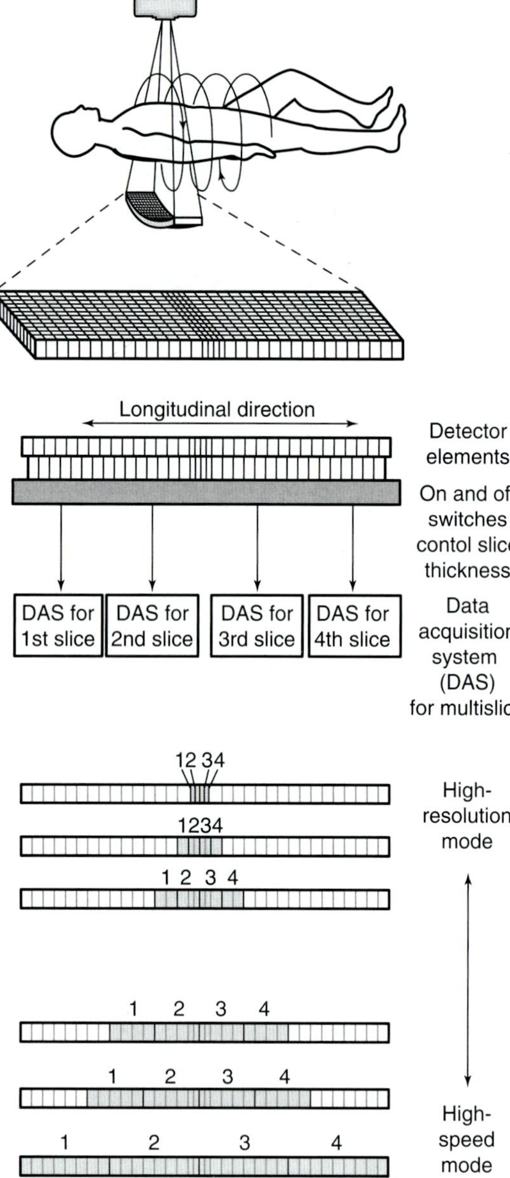


**FIGURE 11-48** The multirow detector allows for various selections of slice thicknesses to meet the needs of the examination. Thinner slice thicknesses are selected in the high-resolution mode, whereas thicker slices are selected in the high-speed mode. The slice thickness is varied by turning the switches "on" or "off."

examination, the switches can be turned on and off to ensure that the appropriate detector segments are exposed to x rays.

## Patient Table

The patient table, or couch, features are essentially similar to those associated with SSCT and conventional step-and-shoot CT scanners. The purpose of the table is to support the patient and to facilitate MSCT scanning through the variable speed of travel of the tabletop and its wide range of movement. The table can be raised and lowered to accommodate positioning of the patient in the gantry aperture and to facilitate easy transfer of the patient from the scanner to a bed or gurney and vice versa. Movement of the tabletop in the longitudinal direction also facilitates patient position in the gantry aperture, with variable scannable ranges.

Patient tables for CT are equipped with a head holder or headrest to ensure patient comfort during the examination. In an emergency during the examination, the movement of the table can be controlled manually to ensure patient safety.

## Computer System

The computer system for MSCT receives data from the DAS and the operator, who inputs patient data and various examination protocols. These systems must be capable of handling vast amounts of data collected by the 2D multirow detector array. These computers have hardware architectures that provide high-speed preprocessing, image reconstruction, and postprocessing operations. Although preprocessing includes various corrections to the raw data, *image reconstruction* refers to the use of multislice reconstruction algorithms for image buildup. On the other hand, postprocessing involves the use of a wide range of image processing and advanced visualization

**software,** such as the generation of 3D and MPR, as well as virtual endoscopic images from the axial dataset stored in the computer.

All MSCT scanners now incorporate *iterative reconstruction algorithms* (see Chapter 6), which play a significant role in CT **dose optimization.** Furthermore, CT **computer architectures** also now include the graphics processing units (GPUs) for the simple reason that they can be used to reduce the processing requirements of the CPU. As reviewed by Pratx and Xing (2011), the GPU is now used in image reconstruction, image processing, dose calculation and treatment plan optimization, radiation treatment planning, and in other applications. Chapter 7 provides a further description of the role of the GPU in MSCT scanners. Furthermore, and as noted in Chapter 6, iterative reconstruction algorithms are now available on all MSCT scanners (Kalender, 2014). This marks what has been described as a "new era" in CT dose optimization, and recent studies have shown improved CT image quality at reduced dose compared with FBP algorithms (Kordolaimi et al., 2013). Buxi et al. (2014) showed that the average dose reduction for the thorax, abdomen/pelvis, and trunk examinations were estimated at 33.2%, 32.45%, and 49.70%, respectively.

The results of computer processing are displayed for viewing by an observer on a monitor. Several characteristics of the monitor are important to the observer, such as the display matrix, bandwidth, display memory, and the gray level and color resolution.

Data storage devices for holding the raw data and image data include hard disks, usually of the Winchester type with high storage capacities, and erasable optical disks of the magneto-optical type.

### Operator Console

The operator console allows the operator to interact with the scanner before, during, and after the examination. Essentially the major components include the keyboard, mouse, monitor, and other controls for the execution of specialized functions.

The operator console controls the entire CT scanner system and facilitates the selection of scan parameters and scan control (automatic or manual), image storage, communication, image reconstruction, image processing, **windowing,** control of the gantry, and x-ray tube rotation. The console allows for communication of images to other parts of the department and hospital and other remote sites through the use of local and wide-area networks. The MSCT console also supports full digital imaging and communication in medicine (DICOM) **connectivity** to other equipment, such as network printers. MSCT consoles also provide for the use of a wide range of software options for image processing, such as 3D imaging, virtual endoscopy, MIP, MPR reconstruction, cardiac applications, and dental CT and bone mineral analysis.

## ISOTROPIC IMAGING

One of the major goals of developing scanners with an increasing number of slices (4, 8, 16, 32, 40, 64, and 320 slices) per rotation of the x-ray tube and detectors around the patient is to achieve **isotropic** imaging.

### Definition

Several technical developments in MSCT scanners have made it possible to perform isotropic imaging. The term *isotropic* is used to refer to the size of the voxels used in a volume dataset. When the slice thickness is equal to the **pixel size,** all dimensions of the voxel ($x$, $y$, $z$) are equal. In other words, the voxel is a perfect cube, and the dataset acquired is said to be isotropic. If, however, all voxel dimensions are not equal, that is, the slice thickness is not equal to the pixel size, the dataset acquired is said to be anisotropic. The geometry of both isotropic and anisotropic data is clearly illustrated in Figure 11-49.

### Goals

One of the major goals of isotropic imaging in CT is to achieve excellent spatial resolution (detail) in all imaging planes, especially in MPR and 3D imaging. There are other benefits as well (Dalrymple et al., 2007; Paulson et al., 2004, 2005), but at the expense of more dose to the patient. Furthermore, the use of narrow collimation increases the scanning time. As noted by Dalrymple et al. (2007), "the parameters that affect the radiation dose and exposure time vary considerably according to scanner design and these variations determine the proportions of the trade-off in increased radiation dose and scanning time relative to the voxel size." Therefore, in MSCT scanning, personnel should have a working knowledge of how voxel size affects not only the spatial resolution but also the radiation dose. Such understanding ensures that personnel work within the ALARA (as low as reasonably achievable) philosophy to optimize the image quality and radiation dose.

### Data Acquisition

Isotropic imaging with 4-, 16-, 40-, and 64-channel MSCT scanners has been described in some detail by Dalrymple et al. (2007). One of the major technical parameters that has an effect on isotropy is the detector configuration, that is, how the detector elements are used together with the effective slice thickness. Although the 4-channel MSCT scanner can achieve near isotropic imaging, the 16-, 32-, 40-, and

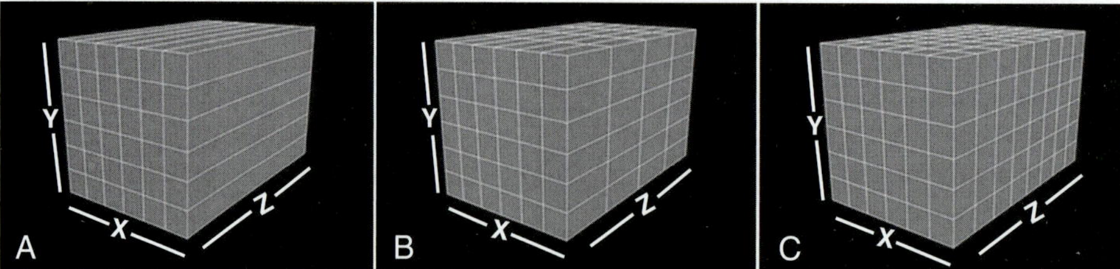


**FIGURE 11-49** Geometry of isotropic and anisotropic acquisitions. Anisotropic data consist of voxels that have a section thickness greater than the *x*-axis and *y*-axis dimensions of the facing pixels. Section thickness along the *z*-axis is four times the size of each pixel in **A** but only twice the size of each pixel in **B.** Although both datasets are anisotropic, there is a significant difference in image quality for 3D applications, with improved longitudinal spatial resolution in **B** compared with that in **A.** When the section thickness is equal to the pixel size, as in **C,** the data are isotropic. (From Dalrymple, N. C., Prasad, S. R., El-Mehri, F. M., & Chintapalli, K. N. (2007). *Radiographics, 27*, 49-62. Figure and legend reproduced by permission of the Radiological Society of North America and the authors.)

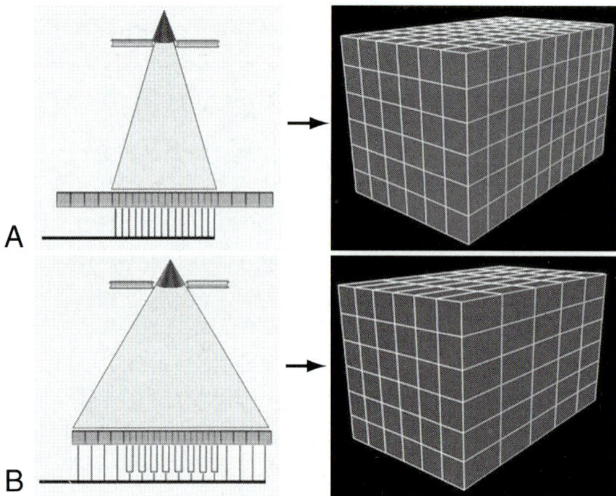


**FIGURE 11-50** Detector configurations and voxel dimensions at 16-channel MDCT. **A,** *Left,* Diagram shows narrow collimation, with exposure of only the central 16 detector elements. Each element functions as a separate unit, and 16 sections with a thickness of 0.625 mm each are acquired per gantry rotation. *Right,* Diagram shows that the reconstructed voxels are isotropic, with about equal length in each dimension. **B,** *Left,* Diagram shows wide collimation, with exposure not only of the central small elements but also to larger elements at the periphery. Central elements function in pairs, and peripheral elements are used individually. As a result, 16 sections with a thickness of 1.25 mm each are acquired per rotation. *Right,* Diagram shows that reconstructed voxels are anisotropic, about twice as long in the longitudinal plane as in the transverse plane. (From Dalrymple, N. C., Prasad, S. R., El-Mehri, F. M., & Chintapalli, K. N. (2007). *Radiographics, 27,* 49-62. Figure and legend reproduced by permission of the Radiological Society of North America and the authors.)

64-channel MSCT scanners can produce isotropic voxels, achieving isotropy. As demonstrated by Dalrymple et al. (2007), the scanners (beyond 4-slice) can also produce voxels that are anisotropic.

The detector configurations and voxel dimensions for isotropic and anisotropic imaging are illustrated in Figure 11-50, *A*, for a 16-channel CT scanner and in Figure 11-51, *A*, for a 64-channel CT scanner. The fundamental principles for isotropic reconstructed voxels are shown in Figures 11-50, *A*, and 11-51, *A*, and anisotropic reconstructed voxels are illustrated in Figures 11-50, *B*, and 11-51, *B*. The effects of isotropic data acquisition and anisotropic data acquisition on 3D volume-rendered images are shown in Figures 11-52 and 11-53 for 16- and 64-channel CT scanners, respectively.

## IMAGE QUALITY CONSIDERATIONS

Image quality in CT is described in detail in Chapter 9. Essentially there are three main parameters: spatial resolution, contrast resolution, and noise. Spatial resolution, the ability of the scanner to image fine detail, is measured in line pairs per centimeter. Contrast resolution (or **low-contrast resolution**) or tissue resolution is the ability of the scanner to discriminate small differences in tissue contrast. Noise, on the other hand, is a fluctuation of **CT numbers** from point to point in the image for a scan of uniform material such as water. Noise degrades image quality and affects the perceptibility of detail. Artifacts can also degrade image quality and cause problems in image interpretation.

In MSCT, these parameters are the same in terms of definition. The purpose of MSCT is to improve on the performance of SSCT in terms of speed and coverage. The volume coverage speed performance in

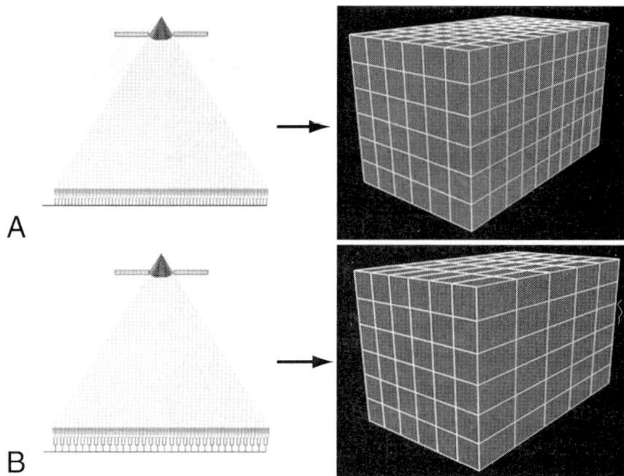


**FIGURE 11-51** Detector configurations and voxel dimensions at 64-channel MDCT. Because the width of the incident beam does not change between detector configurations, the concepts of narrow and wide collimation do not apply. **A,** *Left,* Diagram shows the detector configuration for thin-section acquisitions. With each detector element used individually, 64 sections with a thickness of 0.625 mm each are acquired per gantry rotation, resulting in long-axis coverage of 40 mm. *Right,* Diagram shows that reconstructed voxels in this mode are isotropic, with approximately equal length in each dimension. **B,** *Left,* Diagram shows the detector configuration for acquisition of thicker sections. Although the beam collimation does not change, the data acquisition system pairs the elements for the receipt of data. As a result, 32 sections with a thickness of 1.25 mm each are acquired per gantry rotation, while long-axis coverage remains constant. *Right,* Diagram shows that reconstructed voxels in this mode are anisotropic, approximately twice as large in the longitudinal plane as in the transverse plane. (From Dalrymple, N. C., Prasad, S. R., El-Mehri, F. M., & Chintapalli, K. N. (2007). *Radiographics, 27,* 49-62. Figure and legend reproduced by permission of the Radiological Society of North America and the authors.)

MSCT is better than its counterpart in SSCT without compromising image quality.

In addition, image quality depends on radiation dose. Although the dose in CT has received increasing attention in the literature and has been identified as an increasing source of radiation exposure and may be viewed as "a public health issue in the future" (Brenner & Hall, 2007), there have been increasing technical efforts to reduce this dose not only to adults but to children in particular. One such dose reduction technology is the tube current modulation techniques introduced by manufacturers. Dose in CT is described in detail in Chapter 10.

**Acceptance testing** and research studies will provide verification on image quality parameters and more information on the performance of MSCT scanners in the image quality and radiation dose arenas.

## BEYOND 64-SLICE MSCT SCANNERS: FOUR-DIMENSIONAL IMAGING

### Limitations of Previous MSCT Scanners

The technical evolution of MSCT scanners from 16-slice, 32-slice, 40-slice, and 64-slice CT scanners has resulted in numerous clinical benefits not only for enhancing diagnosis but also for use in radiation therapy and surgical simulation. One such benefit of MSCT imaging is improved 3D imaging of anatomic structures. It is still a problem, however, to obtain dynamic 3D images of the beating heart in cardiac imaging. Dynamic 3D is referred to as 4D imaging (Mori et al., 2004, personal communications). In addition, these MSCT scanners can increase the dose to patients (Brenner & Hall, 2007), create image artifacts especially in cardiac CT imaging as a result of the beating heart, and have limited organ coverage because of the size of the detector (20 mm to 40 mm). The latter implies that two or more rotations are needed to cover the entire organ, such as the heart or lungs. To solve these problems, two other multislice scanners have been developed and are being implemented in clinical practice, the 256-slice and 320-slice CT scanners. The 256-slice scanner is described in the next subsection to lay the foundations for the 320-slice scanner, which is now available commercially.

### The 256-Slice Beta Four-Dimensional CT Scanner

The first model of the 256-slice 4D CT scanner was developed at the National Institute of Radiological Sciences in Japan in 2003 (Mori et al, 2004: personal communications). The major goal of this scanner is to produce 4D CT images with a wide-area detector capable of covering the entire organ (heart or lung) in a single rotation rather than multiple rotations.

The second model of the 256-slice 4D CT scanner (Fig. 11-54, *A*) is based on the design of the first model, and in 2006 and 2007 this model prototype scanner was installed in three centers for clinical beta trials (Fujita Health University, Nagoya, Japan; National Cancer Center, Tokyo, Japan; and Johns Hopkins University, Baltimore, Maryland).

The most conspicuous difference is the use of a wide-area 2D detector mounted on the gantry frame of a 16-slice CT scanner (Aquilion, Toshiba Medical Systems, Tokyo, Japan), as shown in Figure 11-54, *B*. The scanner uses a cone beam with a larger

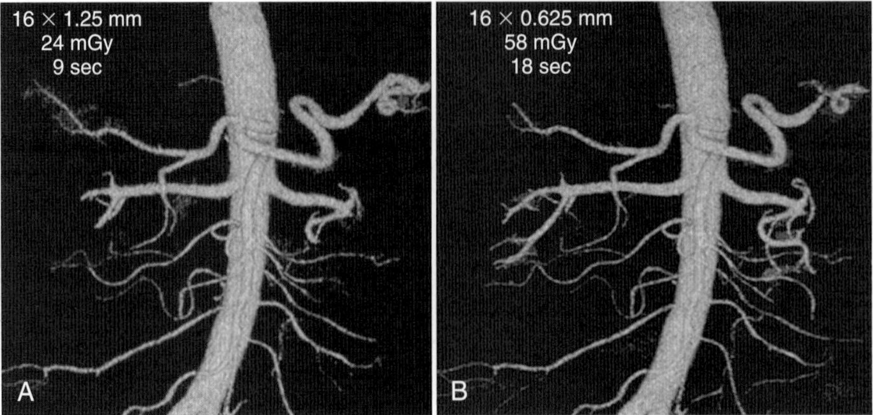


**FIGURE 11-52** 3D volume-rendered images from renal CT angiography with a 16-channel scanner. The first row of data on the images is the detector configuration, the middle row is the volume CT dose index, and the bottom row is the scanning time. **A,** Image reconstructed from anisotropic data provides satisfactory depiction of the aorta and central vessels. **B,** Image reconstructed from isotropic data provides slightly improved definition of smaller vessels. The automated "seed and grow" software program used to create these images provided better depiction of peripheral branches of the renal vessels with the use of isotropic data. (From Dalrymple, N. C., Prasad, S. R., El-Mehri, F. M., & Chintapalli, K. N. (2007). *Radiographics, 27,* 49-62. Figure and legend reproduced by permission of the Radiological Society of North America and the authors.)

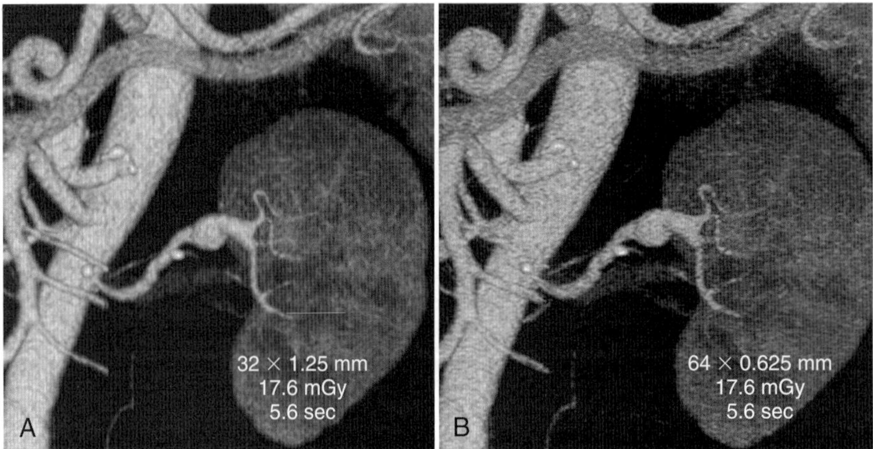


**FIGURE 11-53** Volume-rendered images from 64-channel MDCT. The first row of data on the images is the detector configuration, the middle row is the volume CT dose index, and the bottom row is the scanning time. **A,** Image reconstructed from anisotropic data (section thickness, 1.25 mm; increment, 0.625 mm) clearly depicts a peripheral aneurysm of the left renal artery. **B,** Image reconstructed from isotropic data (section thickness, 0.625 mm; increment, 0.3 mm) provides sharper definition of vessel margins and allows visualization of small lumbar and mesenteric vessel branches. (From Dalrymple, N. C., Prasad, S. R., El-Mehri, F. M., & Chintapalli, K. N. (2007). *Radiographics, 27,* 49-62. Figure and legend reproduced by permission of the Radiological Society of North America and the authors.)

cone angle (about 13 degrees) compared with the previous MSCT scanners to cover a wider FOV. The total beam width is 128 mm, four times the size of the Aquilion 16-slice CT scanner (Toshiba Medical Systems). This wide beam ensures complete coverage of the entire organ (heart) in one complete rotation (Fig. 11-55).

The 256-slice 4D CT scanner has 912 (transverse) × 256 (craniocaudal) detector elements, each approximately 0.5 mm × 0.5 mm at the center of rotation. The 128-mm total BW allows for the continuous use of several collimation sets. The detector element is made of a gadolinium oxysulfide and a single crystal silicon photodiode as used in the current MSCT scanners.

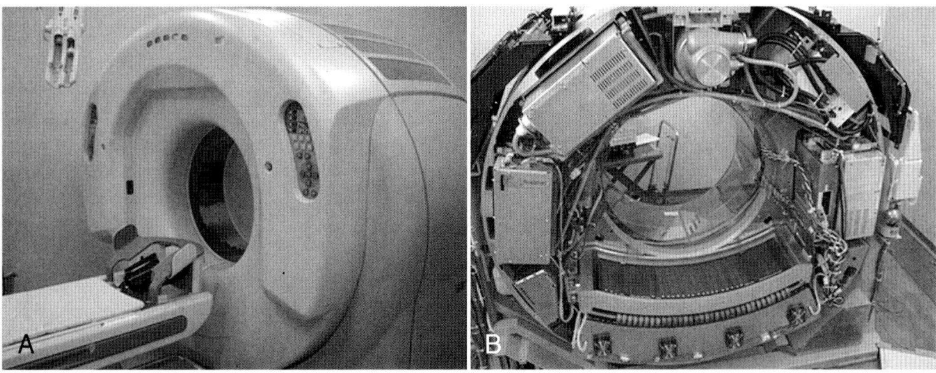


**FIGURE 11-54** The second model of the 256-slice beta 4D CT scanner showing the external gantry and table in **A** and the x-ray tube, wide-area detector, and associated electronics mounted on the rotating frame of the gantry **(B)**. (**A,** Courtesy Shinichiro Mori, Radiological Protection Section, National Institute of Radiological Sciences, Japan. **B,** Courtesy Toshiba Medical Systems.)

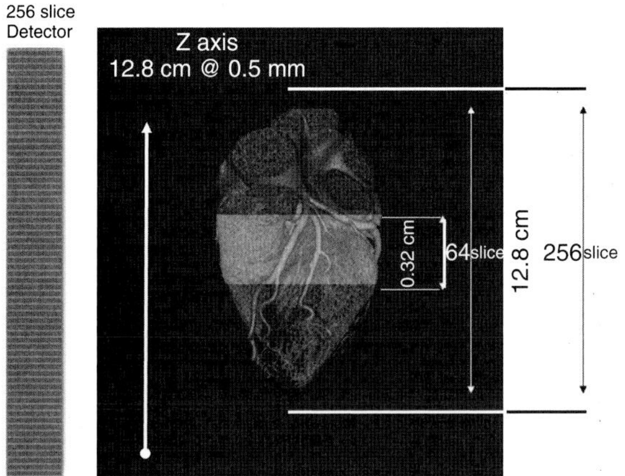


**FIGURE 11-55** The wide-area detector of the 256-slice beta 4D CT scanner ensures coverage of the entire heart with one complete rotation. (Courtesy Toshiba Medical Systems.)

The rotation time is 0.5 seconds per rotation and the dynamic range is 18 bits. The reconstruction algorithm used in this scanner is the Feldkamp cone-beam algorithm. Real-time reconstruction processing is done by 32-field programmable gate arrays (FPGSs-Virtex II Pro, Xilinx, San Jose, Calif.) with a clock speed of 125 MHz. Volumes of 256 × 256 × 128 can be produced.

The clinical beta testing program of the 256-slice CT scanner laid the foundations for the design of a new MSCT scanner designed to image the entire heart in a single rotation. This scanner is Toshiba's 320-slice AquilionONE Dynamic Volume CT scanner (Toshiba Medical Systems), which is described briefly in the next section.

## The 320-Slice Dynamic Volume CT Scanner

In 2007, the 320-slice CT scanner, referred to as the AquilionONE MSCT scanner (Fig. 11-56), was introduced at the RSNA meeting in Chicago. One of the characteristic technical features of this scanner is its wide-area 2D detector, which ensures a field coverage of 160 mm (compared with 128 mm of the 256-slice prototype CT scanner). The detector is designed with a number of detector rows with 320 ultrahigh resolution detector elements. This feature allows for scanning the entire anatomical structures such as the heart, lungs, and brain in a single rotation; therefore, it does not require the spiral/helical scanning principle.

This high-speed volume scanner features a rotation time of 350 ms, which is needed to provide a **temporal resolution** for imaging the entire heart in one heartbeat with excellent spatial and contrast resolution at lower doses (Mather, 2007). In addition, the reconstruction time is fast (less than 10 seconds) and is made possible through the use of specially designed reconstruction processors.

A major challenge in the development of this wide-area detector CT volume scanner is the large cone angle because the beam divergence is much greater than that of the 256-slice scanner. To address this problem, Toshiba developed an FDK-based algorithm called the coneXact reconstruction algorithm, which eliminates any cone-beam image artifacts.

The essential features of the AquilionONE 320-Detector Row Dynamic Volume CT Scanner include the 160-mm wide-area detector, high-speed volume scan, exposure reduction, high-quality images, image reconstruction selectable image slice thickness, improved image workflow functions, high-speed volume data workflow, I-station (display system for patient information), gantry and patient couch operating controls, dual-monitor system, ECG-gated scan and reconstruction (option), and the SUREFluoro (option)

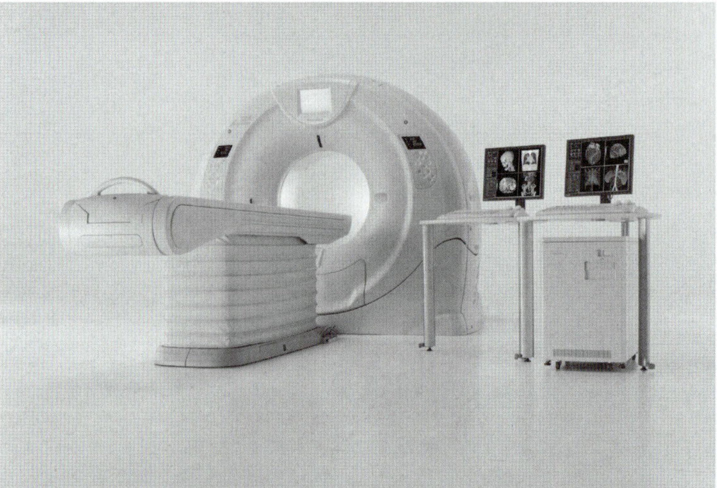

**FIGURE 11-56** The gantry, patient table, and display workstations of the 320-slice dynamic volume CT scanner. (Courtesy Toshiba Medical Systems.)

The 320-slice volume scanner can be used in neurological imaging, including whole-brain CT perfusion studies, to reduce "the chances of misregistration of lesions regardless of location, and makes the selection of the arterial **input** function easy" (Shankar & Lum, 2011), and in perfusion studies (Motosugi et al., 2012), CT angiography (Gang et al., 2012; Luo et al., 2012; Qin et al., 2012; Tatsugami et al., 2012; Tomizawa et al., 2013), cardiopulmonary imaging (Yang et al., 2012), and other applications, such as in pediatric imaging (Sorantin et al., 2013), where entire organs (chest, for example) can be scanned very quickly. Such scanning results in large datasets that will provide more information for the radiologist to use in diagnostic management of the patient.

## BEYOND SINGLE-SOURCE MULTISLICE CT SCANNERS: DUAL-SOURCE CT SCANNER

In 2006, a CT scanner primarily for cardiac imaging (and other applications as well) was introduced at the RSNA meeting. This scanner, the dual-source CT (DSCT) scanner introduced by Siemens Medical Solutions (Forchheim, Germany, personal communications), featured a unique design incorporating two x-ray tubes coupled to two detector systems that provided a scanner with two DASs.

CT imaging of the heart with MSCT scanners dates back to 1999 and, because the heart is in constant motion (beating heart), temporal resolution is essential to avoid motion artifacts. Additionally, for cardiac imaging with CT, it is important to cover the entire heart in a single breath-hold. Although four-slice CT scanners provided acceptable results, problems with respect to motion artifacts, greater heart rates, long breath-hold times, and limited spatial resolution still persisted (Flohr et al., 2006).

The introduction of 16-slice scanners provided improved gains in spatial and temporal resolution compared with four-slice systems. The subsequent arrival and use of 64-slice CT scanners provided further improvements in the technical requirements for cardiac imaging. For example, these scanners provided spatial resolution (by isotropic imaging) and temporal resolution because of the reduction of gantry rotation times to 0.33 ms (necessary to deal with high rates) compared with about 0.375 seconds for 16-slice scanners (Flohr et al., 2006). One of the problems in CT cardiac imaging is removing the need for heart rate control; therefore, efforts are needed to improve temporal resolution below 100 ms at any heart rate.

To solve these problems, other scanners are needed, such as the electron beam CT scanner (see Chapter 4). Although this scanner provided some benefits in imaging (for example, the scanner does not have any moving parts), it did not provide a sufficient signal-to-noise ratio when imaging large patients. Therefore, this scanner "is currently not considered adequate for state-of-the-art cardiac CT imaging or for general radiology applications" (Flohr et al., 2006).

In an effort to further improve the temporal resolution needed for cardiac CT imaging by a factor of 2 (Cody & Mahesh, 2007, and their reference 3), another CT scanner, the DSCT scanner, dedicated to cardiac imaging (developed by Siemens Medical Solutions), was called the Definition (Forchheim, Germany, personal communications). The design concept of the scanner is based on the use of two x-ray tubes coupled to two separate detector systems.

## Major Technical Components

The major system components of the DSCT scanner are illustrated in Figure 11-57. The most noticeable difference between this scanner and other MSCT scanners is that there are two DASs offset by 90 degrees (Engel et al., 2008). Although an acquisition system labeled "Det A" has a scan (FOV coverage of 50 cm in diameter), an acquisition system labeled "Det B" is smaller in size compared with "Det A" and has a smaller scan FOV diameter of 26 cm. This reduction in size of one acquisition system is due to the restricted space in the gantry.

Each x-ray tube is of the STRATON type (Siemens Medical Solutions, Forchheim, Germany, personal communications) that uses the **z-flying focal spot technique** (see Chapter 4) and cone-beam geometry to image two 32-slices (0.6 mm) combined to produce 64 slices per revolution. The detectors are multislice detectors with 40 detector rows of the hybrid design where the central 32 rows would produce a 0.6-mm slice width and the two outer rows provide slice widths of 1.2 mm. In addition, each x-ray tube can be operated separately with regard to the exposure technique (kVp and mA). This feature allows the scanner to perform dual-energy imaging, where one tube can operate at, say, 80 kVp and the other at, say, 140 kVp (Flohr, 2006).

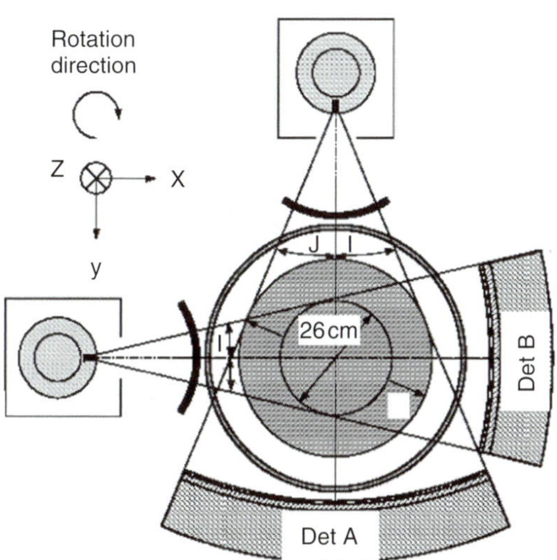


**FIGURE 11-57** The major components of the dual-source CT scanner, which consists of two DASs, that is, two x-ray tubes coupled to two separate detector systems: Det A, which covers the entire scan field of view (scan FOV = 50 cm in diameter), and Det B, which covers a smaller central scan FOV (26 cm in diameter). See text for further explanation. (From Flohr, T. G., McCollough, C. H., Bruder, H., et al. (2006). *European Journal of Radiology, 16*, 256-268. Reproduced by kind permission.)

## Cardiac Imaging with the Dual-Source CT Scanner

The DSCT scanner is primarily "well-suited" for cardiac imaging (Cody & Mahesh, 2007), including coronary angiography, "... the most useful clinical application of DSCT ..." (Ghonge, 2013). One important reason for such specific use is related to the design of the system, which offers excellent temporal resolution compared with other MSCT scanners. Such resolution is needed to reduce motion artifacts created by the beating heart. Although it is not within the scope of this text to describe the details of cardiac CT imaging, the following points (from several experts) about the DSCT scanner are noteworthy:

1. "Because the minimum rotation speed required for a cardiac CT image is equal to just over one-half of a rotation for a conventional MSCT scanner, it is also equal to just over one-fourth of a rotation for a dual-source MSCT scanner" (Cody & Mahesh, 2007).
2. The dual-source CT scanner improves the temporal resolution for cardiac CT imaging by a factor of 2 (Cody & Mahesh, 2007).
3. "In a single detector row spiral CT, noise is independent of pitch. Conversely in non-cardiac multi-detector row CT, noise depends on pitch because the spiral interpolation algorithm makes use of redundant data from different detector rows to decrease noise for pitch values less than 1 and increase noise for pitch values >1. However, in cardiac CT, redundant data cannot be used because such data averaging would degrade the temporal resolution" (Primak et al., 2006).
4. "In addition, linking the heart rate to the pitch (by which a higher rate can be examined by using a higher pitch), effectively reduces the dose to radiation delivered during the examination and can also eliminate the need for additional drugs (e.g., β-blockers) before the cardiac CT examination to reduce the heart rate" (Cody & Mahesh, 2007).
5. "The minimum amount of data required to reconstruct a CT image is 180° plus the angle (in degrees) of the x-ray beam in the plane of the image (known as the fan angle). Hence cardiac algorithms use partial reconstruction technique (180° + the fan angle) to reconstruct an image. These data are collected either during a single cardiac cycle (single segment reconstruction) or during two or more consecutive heartbeats (multi-segment reconstruction). In both cases the

number of photons N contributing to the cardiac reconstruction depends only on the tube current and time it takes the gantry to rotate through 180°° plus the fan angle, and not the pitch" (Primak et al., 2006). Because faster rotation times require lower pitch values in cardiac multidetector row CT, dose is increased without a commensurate decrease in noise (Primak et al., 2006).

6. "Several steps can be taken to reduce the dose, including lowering the tube current as the x-ray beam crosses over certain areas of the body, decreasing the tube current during certain phases of the cardiac cycle, and using a higher pitch" (Primak et al., 2006).

### Other Imaging Applications

Other applications of the DSCT scanner include the following:

1. *Imaging obese patients.* Because the DSCT scanner can operate at a higher power rating (higher kW) compared with the lower kW power rating of a single-source CT scanner by using the power of two x-ray tubes, better image quality for obese patients can be obtained.
2. *Dual-energy imaging.* The DSCT scanner overcomes the problems of dual-energy imaging afforded by the earlier CT scanners. The two x-ray tubes can be operated at two different kVp values, producing images with different tissue characterization, because the absorption of x-rays in tissues depends on the kVp of the beam used. For example, scanning at 80 kVp, the CT numbers for bone and iodine are 670 Hounsfield units (HU) and 296 HU, respectively. At 140 kVp, the CT numbers for bone and iodine are 450 HU and 144 HU, respectively (Siemens Medical Solutions, 2006). This difference is useful in CTA, where it is necessary to separate bone from vessels filled with iodine.
3. Finally, the dual-source CT scanner can perform in a similar manner as a single-source 64-slice CT scanner by using only one acquisition system (one x-ray tube coupled to a detector array; Siemens Medical Solutions, personal communication, 2007).
4. DSCT has been used in abdominopelvic imaging (Coursey et al., 2010), CTA of the supra-aortic arteries (Lell et al., 2010), abdominal imaging (Silva et al., 2011), imaging in the genitourinary tract (Kaza et al., 2012), and more recently in imaging pulmonary hypertension (Ameli-Renani et al., 2014), CT of the abdomen (Marin et al., 2014), and CT colonography (Karcaaltincaba & Ozdeniz, 2014).

## ADVANTAGES OF MSCT

MSCT offers a wide range of both technical and clinical advantages. Since the introduction of MSCT a number of advantages have been outlined by Saito (1998), as well as by Kohl (2005), Kalender (2005), Mather (2005b), Douglas-Akinwande (2006), Kachelriess et al., 2006, and Cody and Mahesh (2007). There are several technical factors in MSCT scanning that combine to improve not only the spatial and contrast resolution of images but also the temporal resolution (fewer motion artifacts). Furthermore, MSCT opens up improved gains in other clinical applications, including CT imaging in emergency and ICU settings, CT imaging in trauma, abdominal and pelvic imaging, pulmonary imaging, cardiovascular imaging, musculoskeletal imaging, neurological and head and neck imaging, and CT-guided **interventional procedures** (Ghonge, 2013). Furthermore, MSCT offers improved MPR images and 3D-rendered images, retrospective creation of thinner or thicker sections from the same raw data, and delivery of intravenously administered iodinated contrast material at faster rates, and so on.

Specifically, these advantages include the following:

1. *Increase in speed and volume coverage.* In MSCT, the increase in pitch and the increase in rotation speed of the x-ray tube and detectors allow for a larger volume of the patient to be scanned in less time. Hu (1999a), for example, showed that a four-slice helical/spiral CT scanner is about two times faster than an SSCT scanner for comparable image quality.
2. *Improved spatial resolution.* MSCT images thin slices with better isotropic resolution. This is sometimes referred to as isotropic imaging (described earlier in the chapter), in which case all the sides (axial, vertical, and horizontal) of the voxels in the slice have equal dimensions compared with SSCT. This advantage provides improved MPR and 3D images with reduced image artifacts.
3. *Efficient use of the x-ray beam.* In MSCT, the x-ray beam width has to be opened to fall on the 2D detector array compared with a single-row detector array characteristic of SSCT scanners. The entire beam is thus used to acquire four slices (images) per 360-degree rotation without wasting any portion of the x-ray beam, as opposed to one slice per 360-degree rotation in the SSCT case, in which a portion of the x-ray beam is wasted during data acquisition. Such use of the beam increases the life of the x-ray tube. The tube can now be used to produce a large number of thin

slices without having to wait for it (x-ray tube) to cool, a problem with SSCT systems. In 1999, Kopecky et al. (1999) noted that with an x-ray tube with a lifespan of 200,000 seconds, a SSCT scanner will provide about 200,000 images (one image per second) compared with 800,000 images for a four-slice MSCT scanner (same conditions are maintained), "or 1.6 million images if the gantry spins at two revolutions per second, or 3.2 million images if two images are created for each full rotation of 0.5 secs."

4. *Reduction of radiation exposure.* The development of new dose reduction technology such as tube current modulation techniques (Kanematsu et al., 2015; McNitt-Gray, 2011) and the recent use of iterative reconstruction algorithms (Buxi et al., 2014; Kalender, 2014; Kordolaimi et al., 2013; Chapter 6) will play a significant role in CT dose reduction.
5. *Improved accuracy in needle placement in* **CT fluoroscopy.** One of the problems with needle placement under CT fluoroscopic control with an SSCT scanner is illustrated in Figure 11-58. The image shows that the needle has hit the target, which is simply not the case. This problem is solved with MSCT scanners that offer CT fluoroscopy because multiple images are obtained. It is apparent in Figure 11-58 that the target has been hit.
6. *Cardiac CT imaging.* MSCT technology has been developed to such a level that "dedicated" CT scanners for imaging the heart such as the DSCT scanner and the 320-slice 4D CT scanner. These scanners can image the heart (and other organ systems) with exceptional spatial, contrast, and temporal resolution, as well as with reduced doses compared with 64-slice CT scanners. Additionally, the use of special cardiac reconstruction algorithms can have an impact on artifact reduction when the beating heart is imaged (Cody & Mahesh, 2007; Dowe, 2006; Flohr, 2006; Flohr et al., 2006; Kachelriess et al., 2006; Mather, 2005b, 2007; Primak et al., 2006).

## TECHNICAL APPLICATIONS

In addition to the routine imaging modes that generate transverse axial images, the volume scanning capability of MSCT opens new dimensions in CT imaging. The vast amount of data collected from the patient volumes, when subjected to appropriate computer processing, has created techniques such as *real-time CT fluoroscopy* (continuous imaging), *3D imaging, CT angiography*, and *virtual reality imaging* or *CT endoscopy*.

Today these technical applications have become more refined and efficient, and they provide

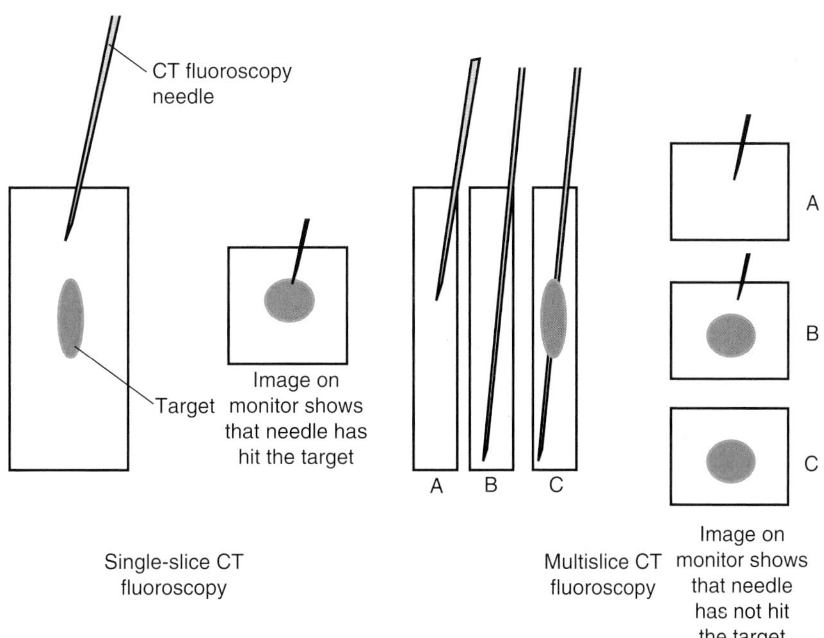


**FIGURE 11-58** A comparison of the accuracy of needle placement in CT fluoroscopy from SSCT and MSCT systems.

additional clinical information for the medical management of the patient. Each of these technical applications of volume CT scanning are described further in Chapter 12 and 13.

## CLINICAL APPLICATIONS

Several clinical applications of MSCT scanning have been identified in this chapter. The immediate advantages of MSCT are the speed of volume acquisition and the reduced loading on the x-ray tube. The same anatomic coverage may be obtained in one fourth the time and at one fourth the anode heating with all other parameters remaining the same. The implications for the x-ray tube are enormous. Not only is it possible to perform many more acquisitions before the necessary pause for tube cooling, but the wear and tear on the tube is also greatly reduced for the same scan volume. For example, a full-body scan from head through the pelvis, which would require more than 95 seconds of data collection in a 1-second, single-slice scanner (excluding interscan delays), could be performed in less than 12 seconds of data collection for a half-second multislice system.

Such amazing speed should have immediate value in examinations of trauma and **pediatric patients.** Better phase differentiation in contrasted studies is now possible, which hopefully will lead to improved diagnostic information. However, just as the introduction of spiral/helical CT emphasized the need for accurate contrast timing, the speed of multislice scanning will make this accuracy even more critical. Accurate contrast tracking techniques, such as those available from continuous imaging technology, will play an even greater role in the optimization of contrast opacity in both routine and special examinations.

As with spiral/helical scanning, speed may be exchanged for improved image quality. With the single-slice scanner, technique selection must balance the volume to be covered against slice thickness and pitch. Multislice systems offer the possibility of extended coverage with thin slices, which improves *z*-axis resolution and reduces **partial volume averaging.** These effects should be particularly noticeable in 3D and MPRs of scan data in CT angiography.

It has been demonstrated that, for example, 0.5-mm slices can be achieved in reasonable scan times, which brings isotropic resolution in 3D reconstructions within reach. This is particularly valuable in cerebral CT angiography for the more accurate visualization of small vessels. Aneurysms and stenoses may be characterized quantitatively to yield better diagnostic information and allow the presurgical preparation of customized stents and other devices for more effective therapy. Similar improvements in CTA of the neck, aorta, and renal vessels are available with these scanners because of the combination of speed and thin slices for high axial resolution. Indeed, examples of peripheral runoff studies are appearing in which superb CT angiograms of the aorta and lower extremities can be completed in 75 seconds with substantially less contrast volume. In addition to more accurate CT angiography, the ability to cover large volumes with excellent spatial resolution should also provide more accurate datasets for the performance of CT endoscopy and the diagnosis of pulmonary embolism.

Another exciting prospect with multislice detectors is the continued development of functional CT imaging (see Chapter 14). Examples of the usefulness of CT in the evaluation of perfusion and other functions in various parts of the body have been reported (Chapter 14). Now that a larger volume of data can be continuously acquired, the potential of CT in functional studies has been fully realized. An application of this technique is the evaluation of brain perfusion through the observation of first-pass contrast flow in patients suspected of acute infarction.

Clinical applications are discussed in detail in Chapters 15–17.

## REVIEW QUESTIONS

Answer the following questions to check your understanding of the materials studied.

1. The limitations of conventional CT are:
    1. poorly created 3D images with stair-step artifacts.
    2. slice-to-slice misregistration.
    3. longer examination times.

    A. 1 only
    B. 2 only
    C. 1 and 2
    D. 1, 2, and 3

2. The shortcomings of single-slice volume CT imaging are:
    1. limited volume coverage speed.
    2. limited time duration for covering larger volumes.
    3. limited in its ability to meet the requirements of time-critical examinations.

    A. 1 only
    B. 2 only

## REVIEW QUESTIONS—cont'd

C. 1 and 2
D. 1, 2, and 3

3. The definition of pitch in a multislice scanner, as defined by the International Electrotechnical Commission, states:
   A. P = distance the table travels per rotation (d) / total collimation (W)
   B. P = distance the table travels per rotation (d) + total collimation (W)
   C. P = distance the table travels per rotation (d) × total collimation (W)
   D. P = total collimation (W) / distance the table travels per rotation (d)
4. Pitch directly relates to:
   1. patient comfort.
   2. patient dose.
   3. volume scanned.

   A. 1 and 2
   B. 2 and 3
   C. 1 and 3
   D. 2 and 3
5. In multislice computed tomography, a ________________ beam geometry results, rather than a fan beam as in single-slice computed tomography scanners.
   A. circular
   B. cone
   C. rectangular
   D. triangular
6. As the pitch increases, the image quality:
   A. increases.
   B. decreases.
   C. does not change.
   D. no direct relationship.
7. In a multislice computed tomography scanner, what type of algorithm can be used if the number of detector rows is small?
   A. cone-beam reconstruction
   B. fan-beam reconstruction
   C. *x*-axis reconstruction
   D. *z*-axis reconstruction
8. All of the following are materials used in solid-state detectors ***except***:
   A. calcium tungsten.
   B. gadolinium oxisulfide.
   C. gadolinium oxide.
   D. yttrium-gadolinium oxide.
9. What term is used to describe the number of data collection channels and the effective section thickness determined by the data acquisition system settings?
   A. detector array
   B. detector configuration
   C. detector geometry
   D. detector set
10. When the slice thickness is equal to the pixel size, the data acquired are said to be:
   A. anisotropic.
   B. dystrophic.
   C. isotropic.
   D. unitropic.

## REFERENCES


Ameli-Renani, S., Rahman, F., Nair, A., et al. (2014). Dual-energy CT for imaging of pulmonary hypertension: challenges and opportunities. *Radiographics, 34,* 1769–1790.

Baker, C. C. T. (1961). *Dictionary of mathematics.* New York: Hart.

Brenner, D. J., & Hall, E. J. (2007). Computed tomography—an increasing source of radiation exposure. *New England Journal of Medicine, 357,* 22.

Bresler, Y., & Skrabacz, C. (1993). Optimal interpolation in helical scan 3D computerized tomography. *National Science Foundation, MIP88-10412,* 1472–1475.

Bushong, S. (2013). *Radiologic science for technologists* (10th ed.). Philadelphia, PA: Mosby.

Buxi, T. B. S., Yadav, A., Singh Rawat, K., & Ghuman, S. S. (2014). Effect of iterative reconstructions in low dose computed tomography. *Journal of Biomedical Graphics and Computing, 4*(3), 1–9.

Chen, L., Liang, Y., & Heuscher, D. J. (2003). General surface reconstruction for cone-beam multislice spiral computed tomography. *Medical Physics, 30,* 2804–2812.

Cody, D. D., & Mahesh, M. (2007). Technologic advances in multi-slice CT with a focus on cardiac imaging. *Radiographics, 27,* 1829–1837.

Coursey, C. A., et al. (2010). Dual-energy multidetector CT: how does it work, what can it tell us, and when can we use it in abdominopelvic imaging? *RadioGraphics, 30*(4), 1037–1055.

Dalrymple, N. C., Prasad, S. R., El-Merhi, F. M., & Chintapalli, K. N. (2007). Price of isotropy in multidetector CT. *Radiographics, 27,* 49–62.

Douglas-Akinwande, A. C., Buckwalter, K. A., Rydberg, J., Rankin, J. L., & Choplin, R. H. (2006). Multichannel CT: evaluating the spine in postoperative patients with orthopedic hardware. *Radiographics, 26,* S97–S110.

Dowe, D. A. (2006). Prospectively gated CTA dramatically reduces dose. *Diagnostic Imaging, 28*, S1–S5.

Dowsett, D., et al. (2006). *The physics of diagnostic imaging*. London: Hodder Arnold.

Engel, K. J., Hermann, C., & Zeitler, G. (2008). X-ray scattering in single- and dual-source CT. *Medical Physics, 35*, 318–332.

Feldkamp, L. A., Davis, L. C., & Kress, J. W. (1984). Practical cone-beam algorithm. *Journal of the Optical Society of America, 1*, 612–619.

Flohr, T. G. (2006). Radiation dose with dual source CT. *Siemens Medical Solutions*, June 94–97.

Flohr, T. G., Schaller, S., Stierstorfer, K., et al. (2005). Multi-detector row CT systems and image reconstruction techniques. *Radiology, 235*, 756–773.

Flohr, T. G., McCollough, C. H., Bruder, H., et al. (2006). First performance of a dual-source CT PSCT system. *European Journal of Radiology, 16*, 256–268.

Gang, S., Min, L., Li, L., Guo-Hing, L., Lin, X., et al. (2012). Evaluation of CT coronary artery angiography with 320-row detector CT in a high-risk population. *British Journal of Radiology, 85*, 562–570.

Ghonge, N. P. (2013). Computed tomography in the 21st century: current status and future prospects. *Journal of the International Medical Sciences Academy, 26*(1), 35–42.

He, H. D. (1999). Personal communication, General Electric Medical Systems, 1999.

Hsieh, J., et al. (2013). Recent advances in CT image reconstruction. *Current Radiology Reports*. Published online. doi: 10.1007/g40134-012-0003-7.

Hu, H. (1999a). Multislice helical CT: scan and reconstruction. *Medical Physics, 26*, 5.

IEC (International Electrotechnical Commission). (1999). *Medical Electrical Equipment-60601 Part 2-44: particular requirements for the safety of x-ray equipment for computed tomography*. Geneva: Switzerland.

James, G., & James, R. (Eds.). *Mathematics dictionary* (4th ed.). New York: Van Nostrand Reinhold.

Kachelriess, M. (2006). Clinical x-ray computed tomography. In W. Schlegel, et al. (Ed.), *New technologies in radiation oncology*. New York: Springer.

Kalender, W. A. (1990). Spiral CT scanning for fast and continuous volume data acquisition. In W. A. Fuchs (Ed.), *Advances in CT*. New York: Springer-Verlag.

Kalender, W. A. (1994a). Spiral or helical CT: right or wrong? *Radiology, 193*, 583.

Kalender, W. A. (1995). Principles and performance of spiral CT. In L. W. Goldman, & J. B. Fowlkes (Eds.), *Medical CT and ultrasound: current technology and applications*. College Park, MD: American Association of Physics in Medicine.

Kalender, W. A. (2005). *Computed tomography: fundamentals, system technology, image quality, applications*. Erlangen, Germany: Publicis Corporate Publishing.

Kalender, W. A. (2014). Dose in x-ray computed tomography. *Physics in Medicine and Biology, 59*, R129–R150.

Kanematsu, M., Kondo, H., Miyoshi, T., & Goshima, S. (2015). Whole-body CT with high heat-capacity X-ray tube and automated tube current modulation—effect of tube current limitation on contrast enhancement, image quality and radiation dose. *European Journal of Radiology* (in press).

Karcaaltincaba, M., & Ozdeniz, I. (2014). Dual-energy CT for diagnostic CT colonography. *Radiographics, 334*, 847–848.

Kaza, R. K., et al. (2012). A. Dual-energy CT with single- and dual-source scanners: current applications in evaluating the genitourinary tract. *Radiographics, 32*(2), 353–369.

Kaza, R. K., Platt, J. F., Cohan, R. H., et al. (2012). Dual-energy CT with single- and dual-source scanners: current applications in evaluating the genitourinary tract. *Radiographics, 32*, 353–369.

Kohl, G. (2005). The evolution and state-of-the-art principles of multi-slice computed tomography. *Proceedings of the American Thoracic Society, 2*, 470–476.

Kopecky, K., Buckwalter, K. A., & Sokiranski, R. (1999). Multislice CT spirals pass single-slice in diagnostic efficacy. *Diagnostic Imaging, 21*, 36–42.

Kordolaimi, S. D., Argento, S., Pantos, I., Kelekis, N. L., et al. (2013). A new era in computed tomography dose optimization: the impact of iterative reconstruction on image quality and radiation dose. *Journal of Computer Assisted Tomography, 37*(6), 924–931.

Kudo, H., & Saito, T. (1991). Helical-scan computed tomography using cone-beam projections. In *IEEE Conf. Record 1991 Nuclear Science Symposium and Medical Imaging Conference* (pp. 1958–1962). Santa Fe, New Mexico.

Lell, M. M., et al. (2010). Dual energy CTA of the supra-aortic arteries: technical improvements with a novel dual source CT system. *European Journal of Radiology, 76*(2), e6–e12.

Liang, Y., & Kruger, R. A. (1996). Dual-slice spiral versus single-slice spiral scanning: comparison of the physical performance of two computed tomography scanners. *Medical Physics, 23*, 205–217.

Luo, Z., Wang, D., Sun, X., Zhang, T., et al. (2012). Comparison of the accuracy of subtraction CT angiography performed on 320-detector row volume CT with conventional CT angiography for diagnosis of intracranial aneurysms. *European Journal of Radiology, 81*(1), 118–122.

Marin, D., Boll, D. T., Mileto, A., & Nelson, R. C. (2014). State of the art: dual-energy CT of the abdomen. *Radiology, 271*(2), 327–342.

Mather, R. (2005b). Patient focused imaging—Aquilion's low dose vision. *Toshiba Med Rev, 17*, July 4–8.

Mather, R. (2005a). Meeting the cone-beam challenge—Aquilion's sureCardio™ and TCOT. Toshiba Med Rev October 15, 16–21.

Mather, R. (2007). *Aquilion ONE—dynamic volume computed tomography*. Toshiba Medical Systems.

McNitt-Gray, M. (2011). Tube current modulation approaches: overview, practical issues and potential pitfalls. *AAPM 2011 Summit on CT dose.* American Association of Physicists in Medicine.

Mori, I. (1987). *Computerized tomographic apparatus utilizing a radiation source.* U.S. Patent No. 4630202.

Mori, S., Endo, M., Tsunoo, T., Kandatsu, S., et al. (2004). Physical performance evaluation of a 256-slice CT-scanner for four-dimensional imaging. *Medical Physics, 31*, 1348–1356.

Mori, S., Endo, M., Komatsu, S., Kandatsu, S., Yashiro, T., & Baba, M. (2006a). A combination-weighted Feldkamp-based reconstruction algorithm for cone-beam CT. *Physics in Medicine and Biology, 51*, 3953–3965.

Motosugi, U., Ichikawa, T., & Sou, H. (2012). Multi-organ perfusion CT in the abdomen using a 320-detector row CT scanner: preliminary results of perfusion changes in the liver, spleen, and pancreas of cirrhotic patients. *European Journal of Radiology, 81*(10), 2533–2537.

Napel, S. A. (1995). Basic principles of spiral CT. In E. D. Fishman, & R. B. Jeffrey, Jr. (Eds.), *Spiral CT: principles, techniques, and clinical applications.* New York: Raven Press.

*Oxford English Dictionary.* (2008). http://oed.com. Accessed September 19, 2008.

Ozaki, M. (1995). Development of a real-time reconstruction system for CT fluorography. *Toshiba Med Rev, 53*, 12–17.

Paulson, E. K., Jaffe, T. A., Thomas, J., Harris, J. P., & Nelson, R. C. (2004). MDCT of patients with acute abdominal pain: a new perspective using coronal reformations from submillimeter isotropic voxels. *American Journal of Roentgenology, 183*, 899–906.

Paulson, E. K., Harris, J. P., Jaffe, T. A., Haugan, P. A., & Nelson, R. C. (2005). Acute appendicitis: added diagnostic value of coronal reformations from isotropic voxels at multi-detector row CT. *Radiology, 235*, 879–885.

Pratx, G., & Xing, L. (2011). GPU computing in medical physics: a review. *Medical Physics, 38*(5), 2685–2687.

Primak, A. N., McCollugh, C. H., Bruesewitz, M. R., Zhang, J., & Fletcher, J. G. (2006). Relationship between noise, dose, and pitch in cardiac multi-detector row CT. *Radiographics, 26*, 1785–1794.

Qin, J., Liu, L. Y., Fang, Y., et al. (2012). 320-detector CT coronary angiography with prospective and retrospective electrocardiogram gating in a single heartbeat: comparison of image quality and radiation dose. *British Journal of Radiology, 85*, 945–951.

Saito, Y. (1998). Multislice x-ray CT scanner. *Medical Review, 66*, 1–8.

Shankar, J. J., & Lum, C. (2011). Whole brain CT perfusion on a 320-slice CT scanner. *Indian Journal of Radiologic Imaging, 21*(3), 209–214.

Silva, A. C., et al. (2011). Dual-energy (spectral) CT: applications in abdominal imaging. *Radiographics, 31*, 1031–1046.

Silverman, P. M., et al. (1993). Helical vs spiral. *American Journal of Roentgenology, 162*, 1247.

Silverman, P. M., et al. (1994). Helical vs spiral. *American Journal of Roentgenology, 162*, 1247.

Sorantin, E., Riccabona, M., Stucklschweiger, G., Guss, H., & Fotter, R. (2013). Experience with volumetric (320 rows) pediatric CT. *European Journal of Radiology, 82*(7), 1091–1097.

Taguchi, K., & Aradate, H. (1998). Algorithm for image reconstruction in multislice helical CT. *Medical Physics, 25*, 550.

Tatsugami, F., Matsuki, M., Nakai, G., Inada, Y., et al. (2012). The effect of adaptive iterative dose reduction on image quality in 320-detector row CT coronary angiography. *British Journal of Radiology, 85*, e378–e382.

Tohki, Y. (1991). The helical scanning technique. *Toshiba Med Rev, 38*, 1–5.

Tomizawa, N., Komatsu, S., Akahan, M., Torigoe, R., et al. (2012). Influence of hemodynamic parameters on coronary artery attenuation with 320-detector coronary CT angiography. *European Journal of Radiology, 81*(2), 230–233.

Toshiba Medical Systems (2008). Personal communications.

Towers, M. J. (1993). Spiral geometries: the helix is one type of spiral. From spiral or helical CT? [letter]. *American Journal of Roentgenology, 161*, 901.

Yang, L., Xu, L., Yan, Z., Yu, W., Fan, Z., et al. (2012). Low dose 320-row CT for left atrium and pulmonary veins imaging—the feasibility study. *European Journal of Radiology, 81*(7), 1549–1554.

# 12

# Other Technical Applications of Computed Tomography Imaging: Basic Principles

## OUTLINE



## LEARNING OBJECTIVES

On completion of this chapter, you should be able to:

1. outline the basic technical aspects of cardiac CT imaging.
2. describe the technical elements of CT angiography and outline its postprocessing techniques and visualization tools.
3. discuss the technical factors involved in CT fluoroscopy.
4. discuss the applications of CT in radiation therapy.
5. define medical image fusion (MIF) and list its application areas.
6. describe the steps of MIF and list the clinical applications of MIF.
7. define flat-detector CT and outline its technical elements.
8. describe the technical components of breast CT.
9. define CT screening and state the rationale for its use.
10. explain briefly the nature of quantitative CT.
11. describe the elements of multislice portable CT.

## KEY TERMS TO WATCH FOR AND REMEMBER

The following key terms/concepts are important to your understanding of this chapter.

**CT angiography**
**CT fluoroscopy**
**flat detector**
**mammography**
**image fusion**
**portable MSCT scanners**
**quantitative CT (QCT)**
**screening**

There are several other technical applications of **computed tomography (CT)** imaging that have been used to image the patient to provide more information to enhance diagnostic interpretation of CT images and also play a role in the medical management of the patient. These applications range from those that have been used successfully in the past, such as subsecond CT **scanning** (see Chapter 11), **CT angiography** (CTA), **CT fluoroscopy,** quantitative CT, and applications of CT in radiation treatment planning, such as CT simulation and **image fusion,** to other developments. These include **CT screening,** breast CT, and more recently improved methods for CT imaging of the heart and portable CT scanners.

This chapter presents a description of these technical applications while setting the stage for further exploration of these topics. Therefore only the essential technical elements will be introduced, and the interested reader should refer to the literature (journal articles and textbooks) dedicated to a more detailed explanation of the various techniques presented later. This chapter begins with a description of cardiac CT imaging and concludes with a brief introduction to portable CT scanners.

## CARDIAC CT IMAGING

The technical advances in CT have provided the motivation for the development of artifact-free cardiac CT imaging. Two of these advances include faster rotation times and multislice **data acquisition** methods at submillimeter **slice thickness** (Blobel et al., 2008; Hsieh et al., 2006). Although the faster rotation times relate to the **temporal resolution** needed to image the beating heart without motion **artifacts,** multislice data acquisition addresses the need to cover the organ in its entirety in a single rotation at high **spatial resolution.** This is necessary to demonstrate the tiny vasculature associated with the anatomy of the heart. The temporal resolution is a measure of the data acquisition time for one image. In addition, multisegment **image reconstruction** can be used to improve the temporal resolution, which is accomplished by using a set of **raw data** from a number of cardiac cycles (Blobel et al., 2008). As introduced in Chapter 1, cardiac CT applications include quantitative assessment of coronary artery calcifications, ventricular function assessment, coronary angiography assessment of pulmonary veins, cardiac masses and pericardial disease, and coronary artery bypass grafts (Prat-Gonzalez et al., 2008).

Although the rotation time for 64-slice **multislice CT (MSCT)** scanners is about 330 ms, the temporal resolution is about 165 ms, which is not fast enough to image a fast-beating heart without motion artifacts (Gupta et al., 2006). In an effort to reduce the temporal resolution, two dedicated cardiac CT scanners were introduced: the dual-source CT (DSCT) scanner (Siemens Medical Solutions) and the more recent AquilionONE (Toshiba Medical Systems), a dynamic **volume CT** scanner.

The AquilionONE scanner features high temporal resolution and covers the entire heart in a single rotation with its wide-area detector. The DSCT scanner, on the other hand, uses two data acquisition systems (two x-ray tubes coupled to two sets of detector arrays) offset by 90 degrees to improve the temporal resolution and scan speed. The characteristic features of these two scanners are described in Chapter 11.

### Physics of Cardiac Imaging with Multiple-Row Detector CT

Cardiac CT imaging is now used almost routinely in large centers throughout the world, therefore, it is essential that users and operators (technologists and radiologists) have a firm understanding of the fundamental physics of cardiac CT. Mahesh and Cody (2007) described such physics comprehensively in a seminal article titled "Physics of Cardiac Imaging with Multiple-Row Detector CT." See Appendix B for a description of the essential technical considerations that should be considered in Cardiac CT imaging.

## CT ANGIOGRAPHY: A TECHNICAL OVERVIEW

### Definition

A significant advantage of spiral/helical CT data acquisition is its application to 3D imaging of vascular structures with an intravenous injection of contrast medium. Such an application is referred to as *CT angiography* (Kalender, 2005; Lell et al., 2006).

During spiral/helical data acquisition, the entire area of interest can be scanned during the injection of contrast. Images can be captured when vessels are fully opacified to demonstrate either arterial or venous phase enhancement through the acquisition of both datasets (arterial and venous). CTA has been applied successfully to a number of examinations investigating vascular anatomy problems and diseases. In particular, CTA techniques have proved useful in imaging the neurovasculature, and in particular stroke, coronary artery disease, the abdominal and thoracic aorta, and renal vasculature and in evaluating the vasculature of the abdominal viscera (Gupta et al., 2006; Pomerantz et al., 2006; Schoepf et al., 2007; Tanenbaum, 2006). Specifically, CTA can provide information regarding carotid artery stenosis, intracranial stenosis, venous thrombosis, vascular malformns, and aneurysms (Lell et al., 2006).

CTA is based on 3D imaging techniques, to display images of the vasculature through intravenous administration of contrast, differing from conventional intra-arterial angiography. In 1995, there were numerous advantages of CTA over conventional angiography, which are highlighted in Table 12-1. At the time, one of the major disadvantages of CTA was its poor spatial resolution (Rawlings, 1995); however, MSCT scanners were developed that featured **isotropic** imaging, where the voxels are perfect cubes (equal dimensions in all three axes, *x*, *y*, and *z*). The 16- to 64-slice scanners can provide isotropic imaging with thin slice images that show a dramatic improvement in the spatial resolution of CTA images (Tanenbaum, 2006). Furthermore, spiral/helical scanning provides increased volume coverage (Fig. 12-1) without the loss of image quality.

**TABLE 12-1 Comparison of the Advantages of Computed Tomographic Angiography and Conventional Angiography**

| Conventional Angiography | CT Angiography |
|---|---|
| Biplane systems can acquire at most two view angles of a given vascular structure per contrast injection. When required, alternate views and examination of additional structures require added x-ray exposure and contrast media. | CTA acquires an entire volume of 3D data with a single injection of contrast agent. Thus, arbitrary views can be retrospectively targeted and reconstructed without the need for additional iodine or x-ray exposure. |
| Because an arterial puncture is made, patients must recover from the procedure with close nursing observation and strict bed rest for a minimum of 6 to 8 hours. An overnight hospital stay may also be required. Thus, recovery time adds significantly to the cost of the examination. | Peripheral intravenous injections permit a true outpatient examination with minimal postprocedure observation. |
| Serious complications from angiography can include reactions to contrast media and thromboembolic complications from catheterization of arteries that can lead to infarctions, strokes, arterial dissections, pseudoaneurysms, and arterial bleeding. Using cerebral angiography as an example, the risk of a neurological complication such as a transient ischemic attack or stroke is about 4% and the risk for development of a permanent neurological deficit from a disabling stroke is about 1%. | Although the contrast agent is the same, peripheral intravenous injections significantly reduce the risk of thromboembolic complications. |
| Conventional angiography is a projection imaging technique that produces two-dimensional images of 3D structures. Therefore, blood vessels and other structures that overlap in the direction of the projection may obscure the site of interest. | CTA is a 3D examination. Overlying structures may be eliminated by postprocessing. |
| Conventional angiography is an intraluminal technique and as such does not display mural abnormalities or true mural dimensions, making percent stenosis and aneurysm size measurements difficult. | CT is a cross-sectional imaging modality that exhibits excellent soft tissue discrimination. As such, it has utility for depicting mural thrombus, calcifications, and true mural dimensions. |

From Napel, S. A. (1995). Principles and techniques of 3D spiral CT angiography. In E. K. Fishman, & R. B. Jeffrey, Jr. (Eds), *Spiral CT: principles, techniques and clinical applications*. New York: Raven Press.

## Technical Requirements

Several authors, such as Lell et al. (2006), Tanenbaum (2006), and Schoepf et al. (2007), have described the techniques for CTA with MSCT scanners, and they generally identify at least four major steps that are crucial to carrying out a CTA examination. Careful execution of these steps will optimize the examination and produce high-quality images that will aid the radiologist in making an accurate diagnosis. Essentially these steps include the following:

1. Patient preparation
2. Acquisition parameters
3. Contrast medium administration
4. Image postprocessing techniques

### Patient Preparation

A successful CTA examination depends on careful **preparation** of the patient before the examination. Such preparation requires that both the technologist and radiologist work together to obtain the appropriate and correct information from the patient and to ensure that the patient understands the procedure, particularly breath-holding techniques. It is not within the scope of this chapter to describe the specifics of patient preparation, because this will differ somewhat from department to department.

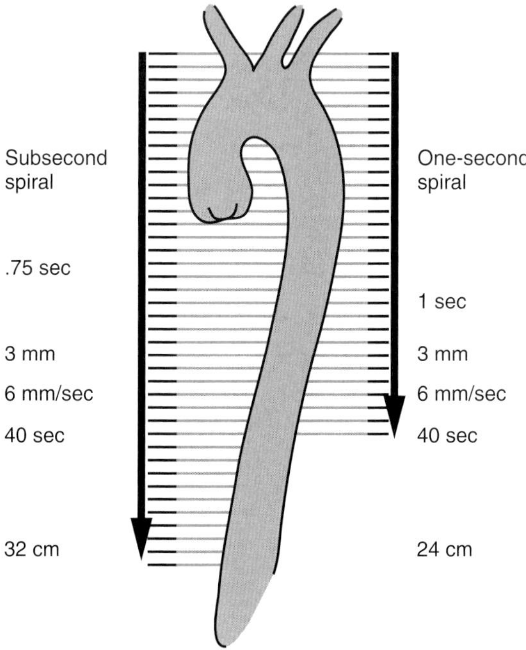


**FIGURE 12-1** In CTA, a subsecond spiral/helical scanner increases volume coverage without a loss of image quality compared with its counterpart 1 second spiral/helical scanner. (From Kuszyk, B. S., & Fishman, E. K. (1998). *Seminars in Ultrasound, CT, and MRI*, 19, 394-404.)

### Acquisition Parameters

The acquisition parameters include the scan speed, the **pitch,** the spatial resolution needed, contrast material administration, and the image reconstruction **algorithm.**

In general, a routine CT examination precedes a CTA examination. The routine examination provides some evidence of the range of anatomy to be scanned. Once the scan distance or scan range, $R$ (in mm), has been determined, a number of parameters must be carefully chosen to optimize both the quality of the 3D images and the accuracy of the CTA examination. These parameters include the total spiral/helical scan time, $T$ (seconds), the slice thickness, $S$ (mm), and the speed of the patient through the **gantry,** that is, the table speed, $d$ (mm/s; Kalender, 2005).

The table speed (or scan speed), can be calculated by using Equation 12-1 or 12-2 (Kalender, 2005):

$$d = R/T \quad \textbf{(12-1)}$$

$$d = S \times P/t \quad \textbf{(12-2)}$$

where $S$ is slice collimation, $P$ is pitch, and $t$ is scan time (seconds) per 360-degree rotation.

The spatial resolution (**z-axis** or longitudinal resolution) of the CTA images is influenced by the **collimation.** To image the basal intracranial arteries, for example, a 100-mm length of tissue coverage is necessary. An early study by Lell et al. (2006) showed that for a four-slice MSCT scanner with a collimated 1-mm section width, a pitch of 1.5, and a gantry rotation time of 0.5 seconds, a 100-mm volume of tissue can be scanned in 9 seconds, while for a 16-slice MSCT scanner with the same pitch and rotation time and at a **slice width** of 0.75 mm, the 100-mm volume can be scanned in 3 seconds.

In addition, the in-plane spatial resolution is important and is affected by not only the detector design (with thin slices such as 0.5 and 0.75 mm on 16- to 64-slice scanners). As noted by Lell et al. (2006), the typical in-plane resolution for a 64-slice scanner with a 0.6-mm detector element is 0.6 mm to 0.7 mm.

Also influencing the quality of the CTA examination is careful selection of peak kilovolt (kVp) and milliampere (mA) values and the image reconstruction intervals. The selection of kVp and mA used in CTA examinations is usually determined by the size of the patient and the level of **noise** in the images. To maintain a good signal-to-noise ratio, mA and kVp must be adjusted accordingly. In this respect,

Lell et al. (2006) and Tanenbaum (2006) point out that 120 kVp is commonly used, mA values selected are based on the size of the patient's body section to be examined, and 140 mAs (effective) is not uncommon. Finally, the role of isotropic imaging (voxels are perfect cubes) has made a significant impact on the quality of CTA images, especially 3D images and reformatted images (Tanenbaum, 2006).

The image reconstruction interval, or increment, refers to the spacing between the center of the slices. Reconstruction intervals are important because they play a role in the quality of the 3D CTA images. Overlapping reconstructions improve the 3D image quality, and a reconstruction increment of 50% to 75% of the slice width can serve as a "reasonable rule of thumb" (Lell et al., 2006). Spatial resolution is also influenced by the reconstruction algorithm used. Lell et al. (2006) pointed out that "the ideal kernel would combine low image noise and sharp edge definition, maintaining good **low-contrast resolution.**" Additionally, although soft kernels decrease noise and smooth images, edge-enhancement kernels improve sharpness but create increased image noise.

### Contrast Medium Administration

Imaging the contrast while it is in the vascular area of interest during the CTA examination is a critical step in the acquisition of images. Contrast injection techniques take into consideration the volume of contrast needed to opacify vascular regions, the contrast injection rate, and the timing between the start of contrast medium injection and the start of the spiral/helical scan. Measuring the contrast circulation times for different patients is important in CTA to ensure that images are recorded when flow-in of contrast is optimum in the vessels. To help with this task, various automated systems have been developed in the past and include SmartPrep (General Electric Medical Systems), Siemens Combined Applications to Reduce Exposure (CARE Bolus), and Toshiba's SureStart, which are all available commercially. These products ensure optimized contrast monitoring in CTA. Figure 12-2

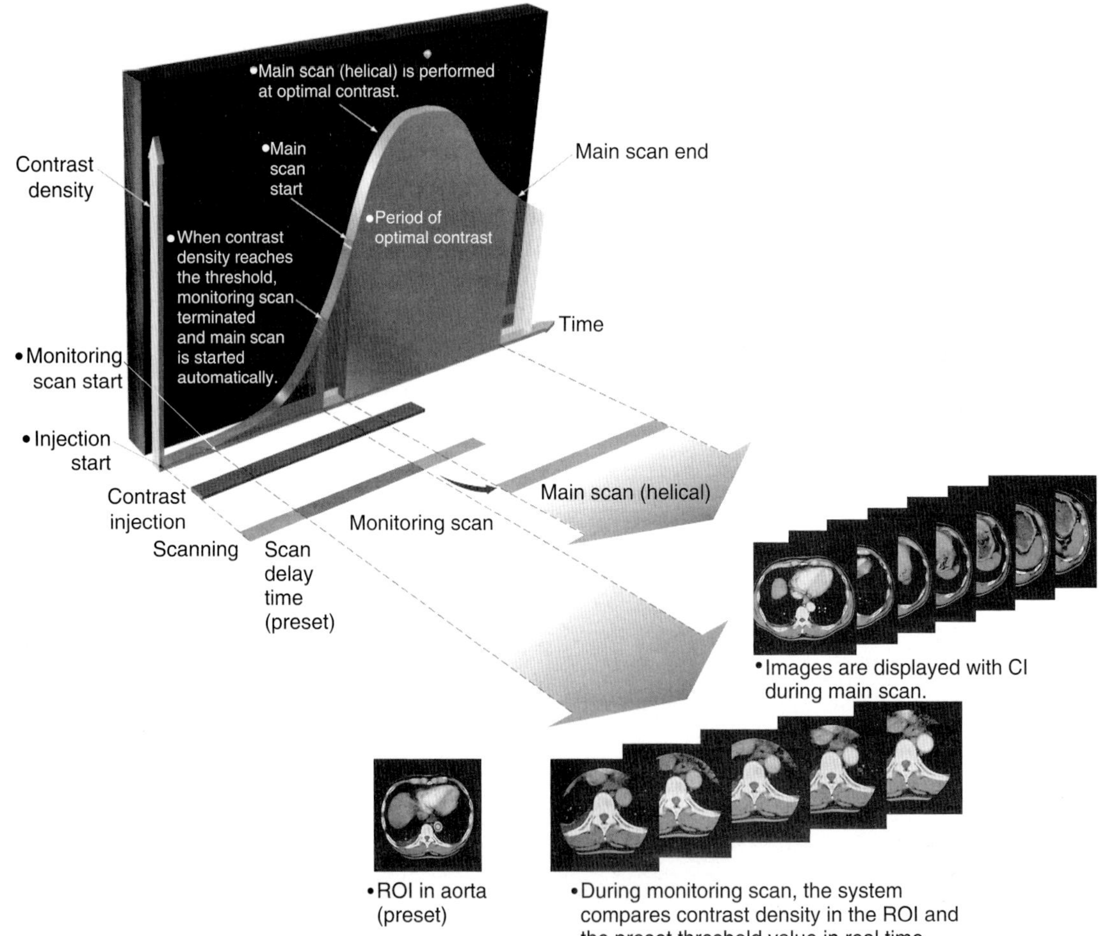


**FIGURE 12-2** Optimization of contrast monitoring for CTA examinations using SureStart, an automated package for optimal scan control for contrast studies. *ROI*, Region of interest. (Courtesy Toshiba America Medical Systems, Tustin, Calif.)

demonstrates such optimization with Toshiba's SureStart package. The change in CT number on the image, which is displayed in real time, is monitored by the monitoring scan. When the contrast reaches a set value (threshold), the monitoring scan ends, and the main scan (helical scan) starts automatically to provide images when contrast flow in the vessels is optimum. Figure 12-3 details the essential steps for operating SureStart. The reader should consult with CT vendors for the most recent updates available.

Consideration must be given to the size of the needle and the site of the injection. Various sized intravenous angiocatheters, such as 18-gauge, 20-gauge, or 22-gauge, are commonly inserted into a medial antecubital vein, using injections at rates from 3 ml/s to 4 ml/s to 5 ml/s (Lell et al., 2006). These injection rates may vary among radiology departments.

## Image Postprocessing Techniques: Volumetric Image Visualization Tools

The algorithms used to display 3D images from the axial dataset are described in detail in Chapter 13. These algorithms are digital postprocessing techniques or volumetric image **visualization tools** (Furlow, 2014; Zhang et al., 2011), which are used quite extensively in CTA. CT volumetric visualization tools include three volume-rendering algorithms such as **multiplanar reconstruction (MPR),**

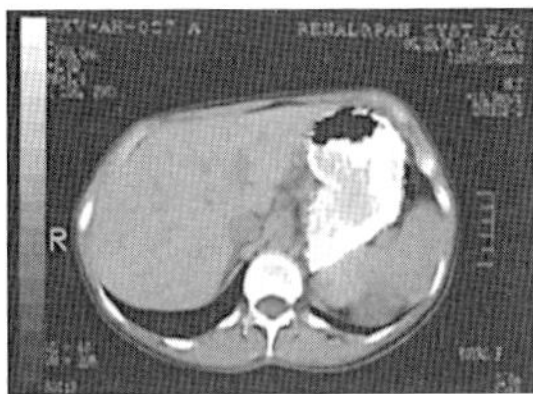


**1 Observe the target vessel**
The operator views an axial image, which includes the structure to be monitored for contrast arrival.

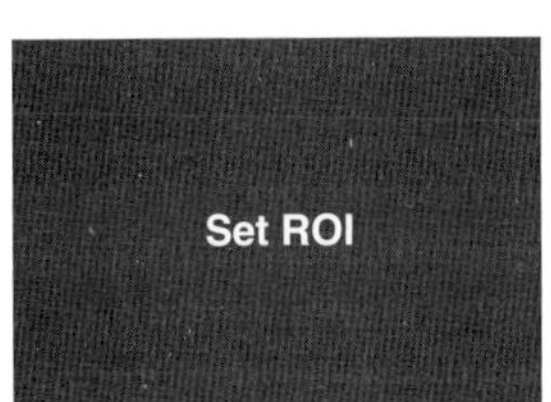


**2 Define an ROI and set target threshold**
A threshold CT value is assigned to the ROI for automatic initiation of the scan. SureStart operating techniques and preset delay times may be selected at this time.

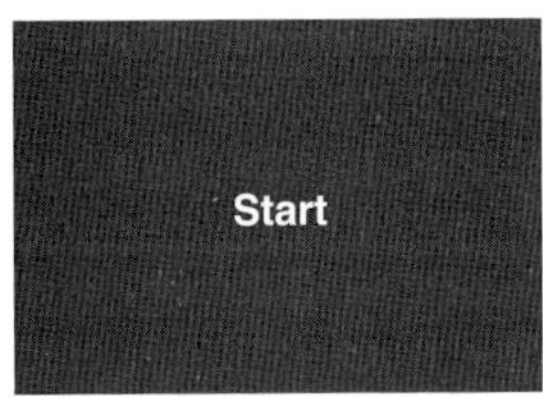


**3 Begin SureStart**
SureStart preparation is selected from the touch panel of the console. The contrast injection is begun, and the START key is pressed. SureStart imaging commences at the end of a preset delay.

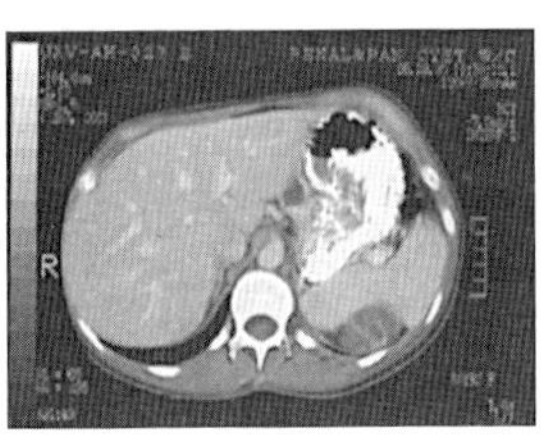


**4 Begin scanning**
When the ROI CT number matches or exceeds the threshold value, or when the NEXT SCAN key is hit, the next scan in the exam plan sequence is initiated.

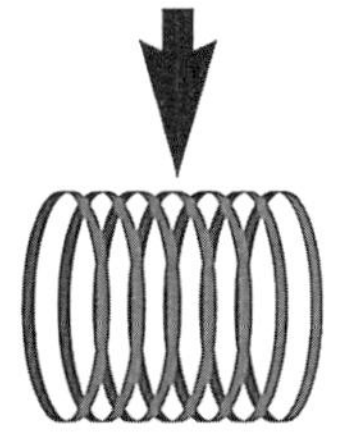

NOTE: SureStart is a selectable element which can be included in any exam plan, and can be followed by helical or dynamic acquisition. SureStart may be interrupted at any time using the ABORT KEY.

**FIGURE 12-3** The four essential steps to operating SureStart, Toshiba's automated system for optimized contrast monitoring in CTA. *ROI*, Region of interest. (Courtesy Toshiba America Medical Systems, Tustin, Calif.)

surface **rendering** (SR), and **volume rendering** (VR; Dalrymple et al., 2005; Fatterpekar et al., 2006; Furlow, 2014; Udupa and Herman, 2000; Zhang et al., 2011). Currently, the following volumetric image visualization tools are commonplace in CTA:

1. MPR, including curved MPR
2. **Shaded surface display (SSD)**
3. **Maximum intensity projection (MIP)**
4. VR
5. Interactive cine

See Lell et al. (2006) for an excellent review of the use of these image **postprocessing operations** in CTA. In addition, the interested reader should refer to Nair et al. (2012) and Furlow (2014) for the advantages and limitations of the use of MPR, curved MPR, MIP, and VR images in CTA.

***Multiplanar reconstruction.*** MPR is the first visualization tool for use in CTA. It is simple and faster to reconstruct than any other 3D technique and enables visualization of the volume dataset in any plane, including curved planes. However, MPR is less useful in a number of applications, such as visualization of complex vessels (circle of Willis) and intracranial arteriovenous malformations. In addition, no editing is required when using MPR in CTA examinations.

The use of isotropic imaging possible with MSCT scanners offering slices from 16 to 320 per revolution provides excellent spatial resolution because the voxels are perfect cubes under certain imaging conditions. Additionally, a variation of the MPR technique, called curved MPR, can be used to demonstrate tortuous structures (Lell et al., 2006).

***Shaded surface display.*** The SSD visualization tool requires little editing to remove overlapping structures obscuring the vessels. It is faster than VR because it uses only a small fraction of the total axial dataset. This characteristic can result in artifact **generation** and images that are not very accurate. SSD images are useful in the display of vascular relationships, vessel origins, and the surface contours of vessels.

***Maximum intensity projection.*** The MIP visualization tool is most frequently used in CTA examinations to display the structure of vessels. It is popular in CT and **magnetic resonance imaging (MRI)** and is more accurate than SSD (Kuszyk & Fishman, 1998). Although MIP has proved useful in CTA, it requires editing to remove unwanted structures, such as bone and calcified plaques, which prevent the observer from viewing intravascular detail. The MIP can be used successfully to separate vascular calcifications, lumen thrombus, and intravascular thrombus.

***Volume rendering.*** Another postprocessing 3D visualization tool popular in CTA is VR. VR uses all the information in the axial dataset to display internal structures (soft tissues and vascular and bony anatomy) and to provide accurate vessel diameters and 3D vascular relationships. In the past, VR was performed only on powerful workstations, but it was expensive and time-consuming.

SSD and MIP processing techniques use data from surface and voxel intensities, respectively. However, VR uses all the data in the axial volume dataset. Therefore, all voxel information is used in the processing. Developments in computer graphics **hardware** now make it possible to process VR images at higher speeds and higher frame rates (5 to 20 frames/s), thus resulting in real-time rendering.

Kuszyk and Fishman (1998) described four VR parameters intended to enhance the "accuracy and the practicality of CT angiography." These parameters include **windowing** (window width and window level), opacity, brightness, and accuracy. Although windowing allows observers to alter the image contrast and density to suit their viewing needs, opacity refers to the degree that structures that are close to the user obscure structures that are farther away. Opacity can be varied from 0% to 100%. Higher opacity values produce an appearance similar to SR, which helps to display complex 3D relationships. Lower opacity values allow the user to "see through" structures and can be very useful for such applications as seeing a free-floating thrombus within the lumen of a vein or evaluating bony abnormalities such as tumors that are located below the cortical surface (Kuszyk & Fishman, 1998).

Brightness, on the other hand, provides the observer with the ability to alter the image appearance from 0% to 100%. Kuszyk and Fishman (1998) reported that a brightness setting of 100% is useful for a wide range of examinations. Finally, VR provides more accurate results for a number of vascular problems (stenosis, e.g.) than do SSD and MIP 3D visualization tools (Johnson et al., 1998; Kuszyk et al., 1998). However, Ebert et al. (1998) showed that VR is not without problems, such as *interobserver variability*.

These 3D visualization tools are described in detail in Chapter 13.

***Use of the graphics processing unit.*** In Chapter 7, the **graphics processing unit (GPU)** was introduced as an innovative piece of computer hardware for use in medical physics and imaging. GPUs offer powerful computing in computer graphics and visualization. (Goodnight et al., 2005). In medical imaging, and in particular CT, the GPU offers an important contribution to **image postprocessing,** such as in volumetric image visualization (i.e., MPR, SR, and VR) (Zhang et al., 2011).

***Interactive cine.*** The developments in **image processing** and display of 3D images have led to interactive cine viewing and display. *Interactive cine* refers to the viewing and evaluation of the images in the axial dataset by panning through the set of images. Because each of these images is separated only slightly in time, the rapid display of the set of axial images provides the effect of motion (much like a cine film). Although axial images can be used to provide a diagnosis, 3D images help to demonstrate anatomic relationships and show vessels that run along the *z*-axis.

## CT FLUOROSCOPY

The basis for continuous CT imaging or real-time CT fluoroscopy depends on slip-ring technology, high-speed processing of the data collected from the patient, and a fast processing algorithm for image reconstruction. CT fluoroscopy has been used as a guidance tool in interventional radiology procedures (Carlson et al., 2001, 2005; Hohl et al., 2008; Inoue et al., 2012; Kalender, 2005; Kataoka et al., 2006; Kloeckner et al., 2013; Paulson et al., 2001; Prosch et al., 2012; Sarti et al., 2012).

This section of the chapter focuses on a basic description of the imaging principles, equipment components, image quality, and radiation dose considerations.

### Conventional CT as an Interventional Guidance Tool: A Limitation

Conventional slice-by-slice CT has been used as a clinical tool for guidance in nonvascular interventional radiologic procedures, including percutaneous interventions such as biopsies and drainage, together with other techniques (e.g., ultrasonography, conventional fluoroscopy, and MRI). A problem with conventional CT-guided interventional procedures, compared with ultrasonography and fluoroscopy, is the lack of real-time display of images, resulting from a time lag between data collection and image reconstruction. Such image display is especially important during needle puncture of the patient. Conventional CT-guided intervention is also limited in imaging body regions where movement is present, such as the respiratory system and the upper abdominal region. The movement associated with these body regions is responsible for shifting and disappearance of lesions of interest, making localization almost impossible (Daly & Templeton, 1999; Froelich et al., 1997). This results in an unsuccessful examination that must often be repeated.

This limitation of conventional CT-guided interventional technique has been overcome by CT hardware and **software** that allow current CT scanners to reconstruct and display images in real time with frame rates that can vary from two to eight frames per second, depending on the scanner. Such improvements facilitated the development of CT fluoroscopy (Katada, 1996).

### CT Fluoroscopy Fundamentals

#### Historic Background

In 1993 Dr. K. Katada of the Fujita Health University, School of Health Sciences, in Japan initiated the idea for real-time imaging with use of a CT scanner. Dr. Katada subsequently approached Toshiba CT Systems Design Group with a proposal for decreasing the image reconstruction time, the image **matrix** size, the number of views, and the field of view (Katada, 1996). This resulted in a modification of one of Toshiba's CT scanners to provide images at a rate of three per second with a time delay of 0.83 seconds. Having conducted preliminary experiments and clinical trials, Katada et al. (1996) reported their early clinical experience with real-time CT fluoroscopy at the Radiological Society of North America (RSNA) meeting in 1994. The first CT scanner capable of real-time imaging was introduced in North America in 1994.

In 1996 the U.S. Food and Drug Administration approved real-time CT fluoroscopy as a useful clinical tool (Daly & Templeton, 1999). Today, several CT scanner manufacturers offer scanners capable of performing real-time CT fluoroscopy, including Toshiba Medical Systems, Siemens Medical Solutions, Philips Medical Systems, and General Electric Healthcare. These scanners feature multiple-image multidetector row CT fluoroscopy compared with the single-image CT fluoroscopy system (Kataoka et al., 2006; Keat, 2001; Paulson et al., 2001).

The evolution of CT fluoroscopy has now made it possible to acquire dynamic CT images in real time (Fig. 12-4), analogous to dynamic images produced in conventional fluoroscopy.

#### Imaging Principles Overview

The fundamental principles of real-time CT fluoroscopy are based on three advances in CT technology that have also led to other innovations in CT. The fundamental imaging principles involved in real-time CT fluoroscopy are illustrated in Figure 12-5, which shows three steps that are based on the initial framework of Ozaki (1995): fast continuous scanning, fast image reconstruction, and continuous image display. Each of these is briefly described.

***Fast continuous scanning.*** Fast continuous scanning was a major technological development in CT, which resulted in spiral/helical scanning. Spiral/helical scanning is made possible by slip-ring technology, which allows for **continuous rotation** of the **x-ray tube** compared with the stop-and-go scanning characteristic of conventional CT systems, which resulted from cable wraparound. Continuous rotation of the x-ray tube speeds up data collection and allows data to be collected for one rotation (360 degrees) per second.

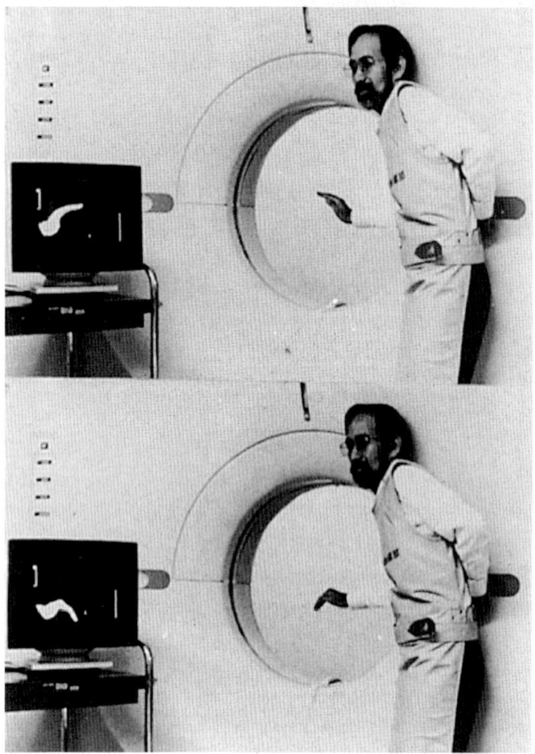

FIGURE 12-4 Real-time CT fluoroscopy is capable of producing dynamic CT images. Images of the hand in both flexion and extension are displayed in real time. (From Katada, K. (1995). *Medical Review, 53,* 1-11.)

An important point to note during data acquisition in CT fluoroscopy is that the patient does not move during continuous rotation of the x-ray tube. The patient remains stationary. When data are collected after one rotation (360 degrees), the first image is displayed on the monitor for viewing. Subsequent images are displayed every time a dataset has been collected for every 60-degree rotation. The dataset for every 60-degree rotation is used to refresh the previous image, which is discarded as new 60-degree datasets are processed. This means that six images per second (360/60) can be displayed as shown in Figure 12-6.

***Fast image reconstruction.*** In real-time CT fluoroscopy, fast image reconstruction is made possible by a set of hardware components dedicated to provide fast computations, together with a new image reconstruction algorithm. An important point to note about CT fluoroscopy is that the **interpolation** algorithm used in spiral/helical CT scanning is not used. The purpose of this algorithm is to compute a planar section from which all other sections can be obtained by interpolation. This process removes artifacts resulting from the simultaneous movement of the patient through the gantry while the x-ray tube rotates continuously during data acquisition.

In CT fluoroscopy motion artifacts are therefore present on the image and appear as streaks; however,

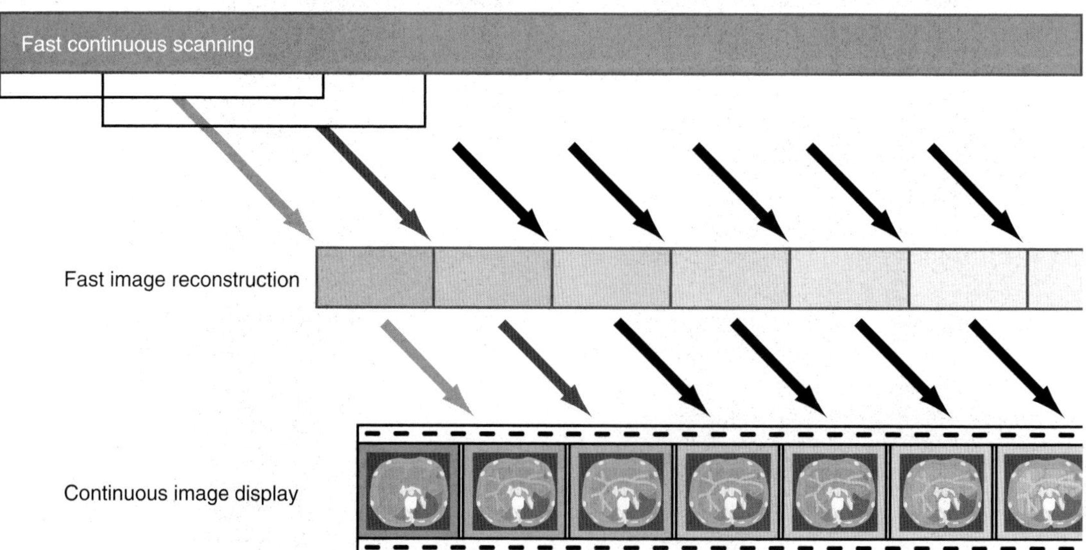


FIGURE 12-5 The principles of real-time CT fluoroscopy are based on three steps: fast continuous scanning, fast image reconstruction, and continuous image display.

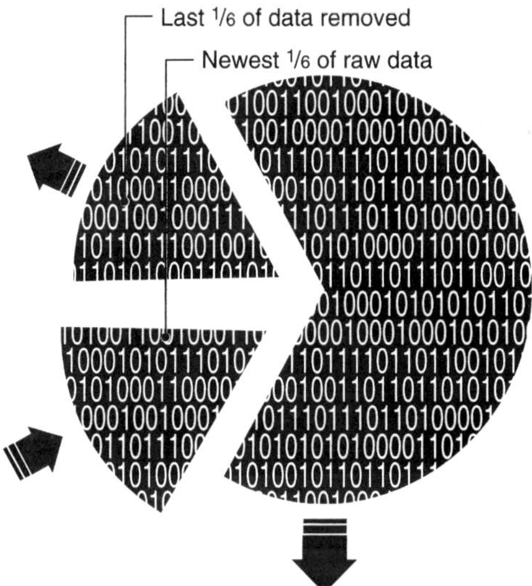


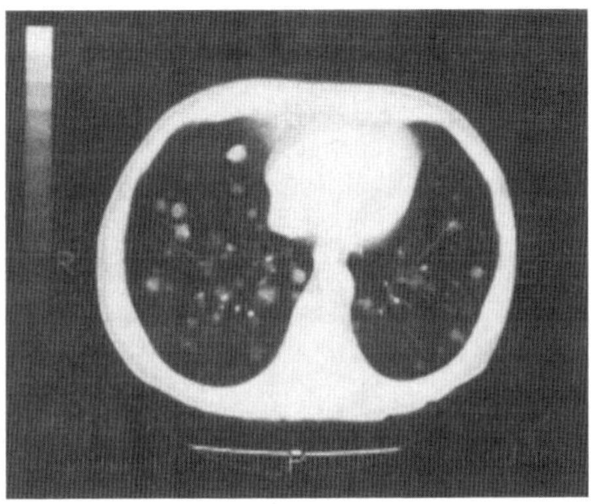

**FIGURE 12-6** A diagrammatic representation of fast image reconstruction and display of images in CT fluoroscopy. During continuous scanning of the patient, images are reconstructed and displayed every 1/6 second. (Courtesy Toshiba America Medical Systems, Tustin, Calif.)

these artifacts do not restrict visualization of relevant structures. The dedicated hardware components include a fast arithmetic unit, high-speed memory, and a **back-projection** gate array. All these components are housed in the image reconstruction unit. **Parallel processing** of the data is an integral element of real-time CT fluoroscopy.

The other key element of a real-time CT fluoroscopic **imaging system** is an image reconstruction algorithm, the fundamental elements of which were described earlier by Ozaki (1995) and Katada et al. (1996). Conceptually, the fast image reconstruction algorithm for CT fluoroscopy processes six images per second (for a 1-second spiral/helical scanner) by first adding the next 60-degree dataset acquired and subsequently subtracting the previously acquired 60-degree dataset from the image as the dataset is acquired continuously (Fig. 12-6).

***Continuous image display.*** As data are collected continuously, they are reconstructed by the fast reconstruction unit on a defined matrix size (256 × 256) and subsequently interpolated to larger matrix sizes 768 × 768 (Paulson et al., 2001) or 1024 × 1024 to provide better resolution. Images are subsequently displayed on a monitor in the cine mode (dynamic display) at frame rates that can vary from two to eight images per second (Carlson et al., 2001).

## Equipment Configuration and Data Flow

The basic equipment configuration of a CT fluoroscopic imaging system consists of a number of acquisition, image processing, image display, and recording components (Fig. 12-7).

The acquisition components include the scanner, which uses a third-generation spiral/helical data collection geometry with slip-ring technology for continuous data acquisition. The gantry aperture will vary with a variable field of **view** (FOV; 18 cm to 40 cm is not uncommon), depending on the type of system. The scanner houses the x-ray generator, x-ray tube, detectors, and associated electronics. The x-ray generator is a **high-frequency generator,** and the x-ray tube is a high-capacity tube capable of very high heat units.

Once the raw data are acquired, they are sent to a **preprocessor** and then to the high-speed memory. The first 360-degree dataset is processed using **convolution** and back-projection, and the reconstructed image is displayed on a monitor for viewing. Subsequent CT fluoroscopic data are acquired and processed with the real-time reconstruction unit (as described earlier). With use of a display interface (I/F), images can be stored and displayed for viewing and interpretation.

The control console for CT fluoroscopy allows the operator to have full control of the table movement through the gantry, to vary height of the tabletop, and to tilt the gantry during the interventional procedure.

## X-Ray Technique Parameters

The x-ray **exposure** parameters can vary depending on the department and the needs of the examination. In general, however, tube currents of 30 mAs to 50 mAs and tube voltages of 80 kVp to 120 kVp are not uncommon. Additionally, in the CT fluoroscopy mode, a special filter is introduced into the dose to the patient. The magnitude of the dose reduction depends on the type of scanner and the exposure parameters used during the examination.

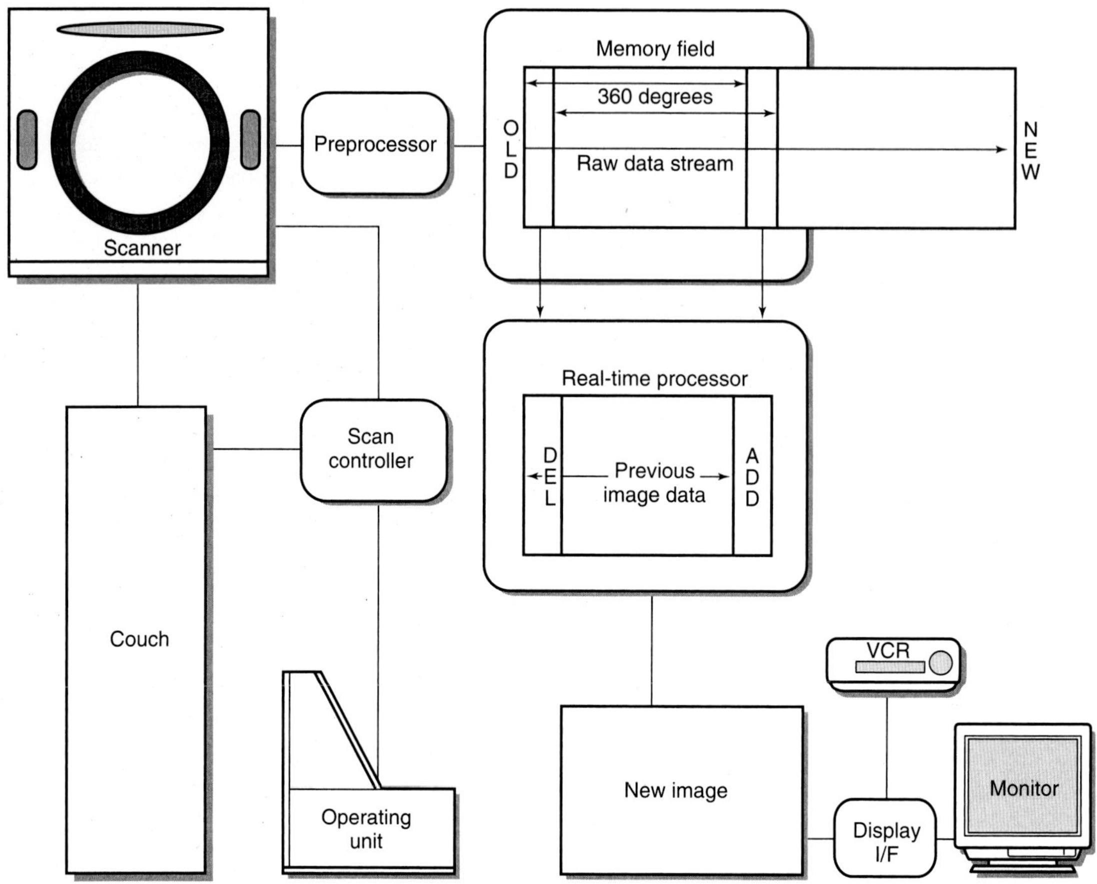


**FIGURE 12-7** The basic equipment configuration for CT fluoroscopy. See text for further explanation. (From Katada, K., Kato, R., Anno, H., et al. (1996). *Radiology, 200*, 851-856.)

Other technique parameters that must be considered in CT fluoroscopy are slice widths (collimator width), the FOV, and the maximum fluoroscopy time. In addition, a choice of slice widths ranging from, say, 1 mm, 2 mm, 3 mm, 5 mm, 7 mm, to 10 mm and FOV of 18 cm, 24 cm, 32 cm, or 40 cm is available to the operator, and the maximum fluoroscopy time for continuous imaging is 100 seconds. This timer must be reset after 100 seconds of fluoroscopy.

## Image Quality and Radiation Dose Considerations

Measuring the parameters that affect image quality and radiation dose ascertains the performance of a CT scanner. In CT fluoroscopy, image quality and radiation assessment are ongoing concerns.

### Image Quality

Image quality parameters in CT fluoroscopy include spatial resolution, density resolution, image noise, and artifacts. As early as 1995, these parameters were examined by Ozaki (1995), who compared spatial resolution, density resolution, and image noise of CT fluoroscopy with that of conventional CT. These early results demonstrate that the image quality parameters measured for CT fluoroscopy are comparable to those of conventional CT. For example, Ozaki (1995) showed that, although the spatial and density resolution for CT fluoroscopy was 6.8 line pairs per centimeter (lp/cm) and 3 mm at 0.45%, respectively, it was 7.5 lp/cm and 3 mm at 0.41%, respectively, for conventional CT. Although the image noise for a 10-mm slice at 50 mA used for CT fluoroscopy was ±3.9 Hounsfield units (HU), it was the same (±3.9 HU) at 150 mA for conventional CT.

### Radiation Dose Considerations

With any new technique that uses x-rays to image the patient, radiation dose is always a primary consideration, because the goal of radiology is to operate within the as low as reasonably achievable (ALARA) philosophy. Furthermore, the dose in CT fluoroscopy is also important because personnel are present in the room during the procedure.

A number of factors influence the dose to the patient and operator in CT (Hohl et al., 2008;

Kataoka et al., 2006; Keat, 2001). One of the important factors is the length of time of the exposure because dose is directly proportional to exposure time. For example, in an early dose assessment study, Daly and Templeton (1999) reported **absorbed doses** in the range of 3.53 rad (35.3 milligrays [mGy]) for 50 seconds of exposure at 80 kVp and 30 mA to 19.81 rad (198.1 mGy) for a similar exposure time at 120 kVp and 50 mA.

In a 2010 study titled "Optimal **scan parameters** for CT fluoroscopy in lung interventional radiologic procedures: relationship between radiation dose and image quality," Yamao et al. (2010) found that

> both the SNR and the CNR improved as the radiation dose increased, leading to improvement in the image quality. Acceptable image quality was achieved in 94% (30 of 32) of patients when the radiation dose was 1.18 mGy/sec (120 kV, 10 mA) and in all patients when it was greater than 1.48 mGy/sec (135 kV, 10 mA). The piecewise linear curve showed rapid improvement in image quality until the radiation dose increased to 1.48 mGy/sec (135 kV, 10 mA). When the radiation dose was increased greater than 1.48 mGy/sec, improvement in the image quality became more gradual.

The authors concluded that these results can assist operators in establishing optimal parameters in lung CT fluoroscopy.

In a retrospective study titled "CT fluoroscopy-guided vs. multislice CT biopsy mode-guided lung biopsies: accuracy, complications and radiation dose," Prosch et al. (2012) showed that "compared to CTF-guided biopsies, chest biopsies using the MS-CT biopsy mode show dramatically lower CTDI levels. Although the diagnostic yield of the procedures does not differ significantly, biopsies using the MS-CT-biopsy mode have a three-fold higher rate of chest tube placement."

Finally, in a study called "Radiation exposure in CT-guided interventions," Kloeckner et al. (2013) analyzed 1576 consecutive CT-guided procedures in 1284 patients performed over 4.5 years and found that "Eighty-five percent of the total radiation dose was applied during the pre- and post-interventional CT series, leaving only 15% applied by the CT-guided intervention itself. Single slice acquisition was associated with lower doses than continuous CT-fluoroscopy (37 mGy cm vs. 153 mGy cm, $p < 0.001$). The third quartile of radiation doses varied considerably for different interventions. The highest doses were observed in complex interventions like radiofrequency and microwave ablations (RFA/MWA) of the liver, followed by vertebroplasty and RFA/MWA of the lung." On the basis of these findings, the authors

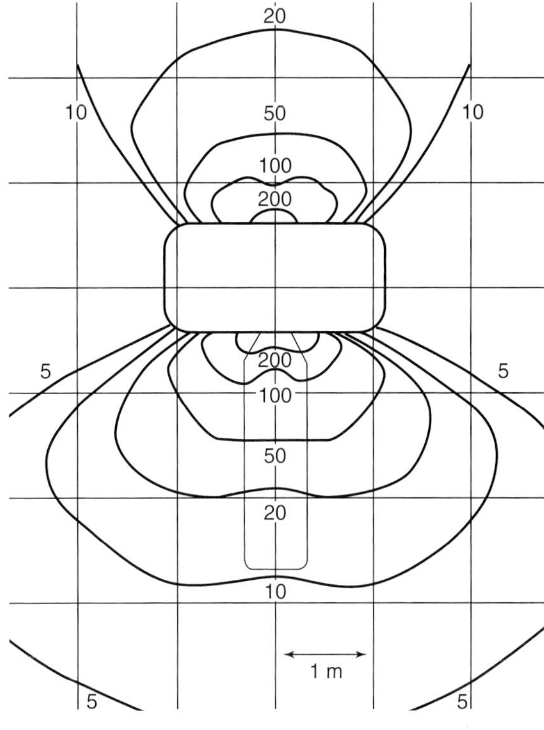


**FIGURE 12-8** Scatter radiation dose distribution at CT fluoroscopy.

recommend that "a multicenter registry of radiation exposure including a broader spectrum of scanners and intervention types is needed to develop definitive reference levels."

During the development and early implementation of CT fluoroscopy, the dose to the hands of the operator was of particular concern because they were directly in the x-ray beam during the procedure. Early studies reported excessively high doses to the operator's hands during the procedure (Katada et al., 1996; Kato et al., 1996). The solution to this problem was the development of needle holders, which are intended to keep the hands of the operator out of the x-ray beam. An early study by Kato et al. (1996) showed that the needle holders reduced the absorbed dose rate to the operator's hands. Additionally, the needle holders do not produce image artifacts. Another concern related to the dose in CT fluoroscopy procedures is that of scatter radiation distribution in the room during the procedure and the dose received by the operator resulting from this scatter. One example of an early scattered radiation dose distribution is shown in Figure 12-8. It is clear that there are two sources of scatter, the patient (who is the main source of scatter) and the scanner itself. In terms of **radiation protection** of personnel, the scanner gantry can be considered a shield in itself, and radiologists and technologists may stand at the side of the CT gantry. Furthermore, for protection from scattered radiation from the patient, personnel should always observe the three radiation protection actions: **distance, shielding,** and time. Use of the inverse square law (distance) and lead and bismuth shielding are effective ways to minimize the personnel exposure. For example, Sarti et al. (2012) found the following:

1. "a lead drape placed over the patient absorbs scattered radiation and decreases operator exposure to radiation by 96%."
2. "Protective bismuth gloves and a lead drape for the patient placed adjacent to, but outside, the scanning area reduce operator exposure to radiation by as much as 97%."
3. "...we use intermittent CT fluoroscopy, which is often referred to as the "quick-check" technique and was first described in the 1990s (12). In intermittent imaging, a single step on the acquisition pedal yields three contiguous images centered on the axial level of choice in one-third of a second of fluoroscopy time. With practice, the quick-check technique may provide excellent results with substantially decreased CT fluoroscopy times; it reduces dose, even during biopsy of small lung nodules, and obviates the need for direct exposure of the operator's hand to radiation."
4. "CT fluoroscopy devices have continued to improve in terms of ergonomic design and workflow, and fluoroscopy exposure times of less than 10 seconds should now be the norm."

Wearing a protective apron during the procedure will certainly reduce the **effective dose** to the operator. Operators standing in the CT room during the procedure must wear protective lead aprons, thyroid shields, and lead glasses or goggles (Daly & Templeton, 1999; Stoeckelhuber et al., 2005). Furthermore, Daly and Templeton (1999) showed that the use of a lead drape can result in 72% scattered radiation dose reduction. Protective apparel must be at least 0.5 mm lead equivalent. Additionally, the use of lead drapes in close proximity will result in a marked reduction of exposure to scattered radiation (Nawfel et al., 2000; Wagner, 2000).

Reducing radiation dose to both patients and personnel is an important goal of radiology. In CT fluoroscopy, one technique incorporated in the design of the equipment to reduce the dose to the patient is the use of a special x-ray filter. In addition, lower tube currents and shorter examination times also play a significant role in reducing patient exposures (Paulson et al., 2001). Another technique, referred to as the quick-check technique, can be used to reduce the dose in CT fluoroscopy. As described by Paulson et al. (2001), the quick-check technique is similar to conventional CT and uses single-section CT fluoroscopic spot images to check the location of the needle and ensure that the correct alignment is obtained.

Another useful method for reducing the dose to the patient and operator is the use of a tungsten antimony shielding drape, which hangs near the scan plane. With a 16-slice volume CT scanner operating in the CT fluoroscopy mode, the dose was measured from adult and pediatric phantoms with a solid-state UNFORS (Billdal, Sweden) dosimeter.

A more recent study by Hohl et al. (2008) investigated the use of angular beam modulation (ABM; see Chapter 10) to reduce the dose in CT fluoroscopy. Their prospective study was done with an Alderson–Rando phantom using thermoluminescent **dosimeters** and a 64-slice volume CT scanner. Their results showed that the ABM technique reduced the effective dose to the patient by 35%, the skin dose by 75%, the breast dose by 47%, and the hand dose by between 27% and 72%. The authors conclude that "ABM leads to significant dose reduction for both patients and personnel during CT fluoroscopy-guided thoracic interventions, without impairing image quality."

## APPLICATIONS IN RADIATION THERAPY: CT SIMULATION

Radiation therapy is an interdisciplinary field based on not only radiation biology but also on physics, mathematics, and engineering. The goal of radiation therapy is to kill tumor cells (tumor volumes) by delivering the maximum radiation dose to these cells with minimum dose to the surrounding healthy tissues, especially those that are highly radiosensitive, such as the gonads, eyes, and thyroid.

Through the years radiation therapy has experienced significant technical developments intended to improve the clinical performance of radiation treatment schemes, including the use of imaging techniques to provide more accurate localization of tumor volumes (Bissonnette et al., 2012; Kessler, 2006; McDermott & Orton, 2010; Newbold et al., 2006; Schlegel et al., 2006) and guidance, such as CT-based image-guided radiation therapy (IGRT; Bissonnette et al., 2012; Mah & Chen, 2008) and target delineation (Ahn & Garg, 2008). One such important milestone was the development of the CT scanner, which became a significant tool in radiation treatment planning in the late 1970s. The fact that the CT scanner produces 3D images paved the way for 3D treatment planning that has now become an integral tool in radiation therapy. With these 3D images from the CT scanner, the tumor volumes can now be accurately localized with respect to the surrounding healthy tissues. In addition, the physical properties such as the electron densities of the tissues can be extracted from the 3D image datasets and are used to calculate radiation treatment doses.

This section of the chapter outlines the elements of the use of the CT scanner in radiation treatment planning through a technique referred to as *CT simulation*. The physical principles and technology of the CT scanner, image quality, quality assurance, and image processing, including 3D imaging techniques, are covered in detail in the rest of this book. It is interesting to note here that CT-based IGRT includes a number of systems, such as kilovolt and megavolt cone-beam CT, fan-beam MVCT, and CT-on-rails (Bissonnette et al., 2012), to help address the challenge of geometry accuracy in radiation therapy. These integrated imaging systems specifically attempt to "improve and facilitate internal patient anatomy visualization, enabling efficient positioning of these anatomical structures relative to the treatment room" (Bissonnette et al., 2012). Furthermore, to ensure and maintain system function with respect to geometric accuracy, image quality (scale and distance accuracy, spatial resolution, low-contrast resolution, uniformity, and noise), image dose, accuracy of **CT numbers,** image registration, the accuracy of remote-controlled CT couch, and daily operational issues, it is of vital importance that departments have a quality assurance (QA) program in place. It is not within the scope of this text to describe QA for CT-based IGRT systems; however, the interested reader should refer to a paper by Bissonnette et al. (2012) for a description of such a QA program.

## CT Simulation Basics

The CT scanner is now used in the radiation oncology department and plays a role in the radiation treatment planning process. It is an integral part of the CT simulation process (Brunetti et al., 2008; Mutic et al., 2003).

### Definition

As defined by Mutic et al. (2003), *CT simulation* "is a geometric simulation process that provides beam arrangements and treatment fields without any dosimetric information." As shown in Figure 12-9, the CT simulator is coupled to the radiation treatment planning system to provide data for radiation dose calculation.

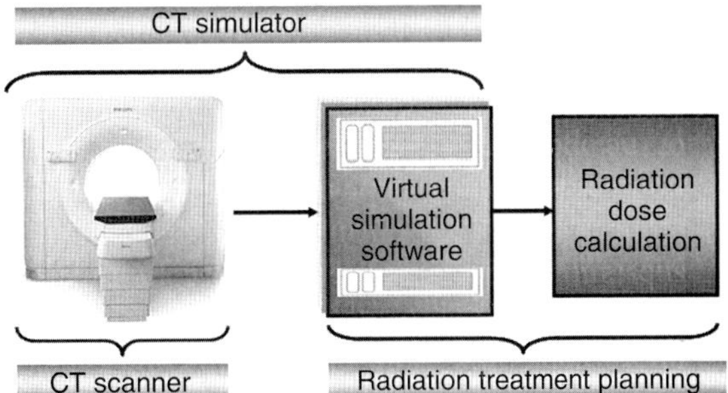


**FIGURE 12-9** The CT simulator is coupled to the radiation treatment planning system to provide data for radiation dose calculation.

### CT Simulator

The CT simulator is a CT scanner characterized by physical devices (hardware) and specialized software.

The hardware is a CT scanner, specifically an MSCT scanner featuring all the major components (x-ray generator, x-ray tube, detector system, e.g.) as described in Chapter 11; however, there are several notable features that are different from a CT scanner used in diagnostic CT examinations. For example, this scanner has a flat tabletop with **immobilization** devices, a large bore (gantry aperture), a registration device, and a laser system. The flat tabletop and immobilization devices ensure that patients are scanned in exactly the same **position** as they would be when they are on the radiation treatment machine, and the large bore (e.g., 85 cm) of the scanner accommodates patients in specific positions on the tabletop and enables the use of a large scan FOV. The registration device, on the other hand, ensures that the immobilization device on the CT scanner can be moved and used in exactly the same manner on the treatment machine. Finally, the laser system is intended to facilitate accurate positioning with the axes of the CT scanner.

The CT simulator also includes specialized software referred to as *virtual simulation* software. While the CT scanner acquires a volumetric dataset from the patient and represents the "virtual" patient (or digital patient), the CT simulation software

> provides virtual representations of the geometric capabilities of a treatment machine. This software can be a special virtual simulation program or it can be a component of a treatment planning system. Often CT simulation is referred to as virtual simulation and the two terms are used interchangeably. Virtual simulation is used to define any simulation based on the software created "virtual simulator" and a volumetric patient scan. The scan does not necessarily have to be a CT and other imaging modalities can be used. A virtual simulator is a set of software which recreates

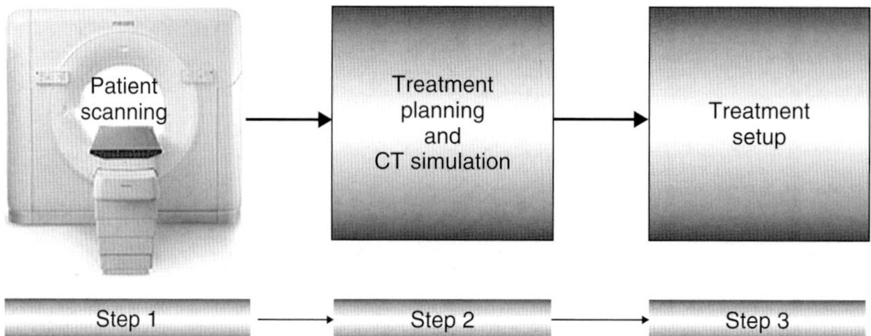


**FIGURE 12-10** The three steps of the CT simulation process. See text for further explanation.

the treatment machine and which allows import, manipulation, display, and storage of images from CT and/or other imaging modalities (Mutic et al., 2003).

### CT Simulation Process

The CT simulation process includes at least three steps (Fig. 12-10) as identified by Mutic et al. (2003). These include the following:

1. *Scan the patient in the CT scanner.* The patient is positioned, immobilized, and scanned in exactly the same position that he or she would be on the treatment machine. The electron densities from the image dataset obtained would be used to compute dose distributions.
2. *Plan the treatment and CT simulation.* This is where the beam placement and the treatment design are executed using the virtual simulation software, which includes "contouring of the target and normal structures, placement of the treatment isocenter and the beams, design of the treatment portal shapes" and the production of digitally reconstructed radiographs, and finally documentation. It is not within the scope of this section to describe these procedures; however, the interested reader should refer to Mutic et al. (2003) for a description of each procedure.
3. *Treatment setup.* In this final step, the CT simulation software results are used to set up the patient in the treatment machine.

### Use of the Graphics Processing Unit in Radiation Therapy

The use of the GPU in medical imaging and therapy was introduced in Chapter 6, subsequently described in Chapter 7, and later noted in Chapters 8 and 13. The GPU is used in image processing and image reconstruction. In radiation therapy, the GPU is used primarily in dose calculation and treatment plan optimization (Pratx & Xing, 2011). Such use is not within the scope of this book and therefore will not be described further. The interested reader should refer to the paper by Pratx and Xing (2011) for a detailed discussion of such use.

## MEDICAL IMAGE FUSION OVERVIEW

### Definitions

*Image fusion* is a branch of computer vision where relevant information from two or more **input** images are combined into one image (Haghighat et al., 2011a), thus making the combined image more useful than any of the input images (Haghighat et al., 2011b).

In diagnostic radiology and radiation treatment planning, image fusion has become popular, and in a recent paper, James and Dasarathy (2014) defined *medical image fusion* as "the process of registering and combining multiple images from single or multiple imaging modalities to improve the imaging quality and reduce randomness and redundancy in order to increase the clinical applicability of medical images for diagnosis and assessment of medical problems."

In diagnostic imaging major imaging modalities including CTA, quantitative computed tomography (QCT), magnetic resonance imaging such as for angiography, nuclear medicine such as single-photon emission computed tomography and positron emission tomography, ultrasound and x-ray imaging such as **mammography,** and several others (James & Dasarathy, 2014) provide input images to be used for image fusion. The overall goal of using these combined images is to enhance the medical management of the radiation therapy patient (Brunetti et al., 2008; James & Dasarathy, 2014; Kessler, 2006; Webb, 2003).

### Medical Image Fusion Areas of Studies

James and Dasarathy (2014) identified three major focused "areas of studies" in medical image fusion, as shown in Figure 12-11. These include:

1. "identification, improvement and development of imaging modalities useful for medical image fusion,
2. development of different techniques for medical image fusion, and

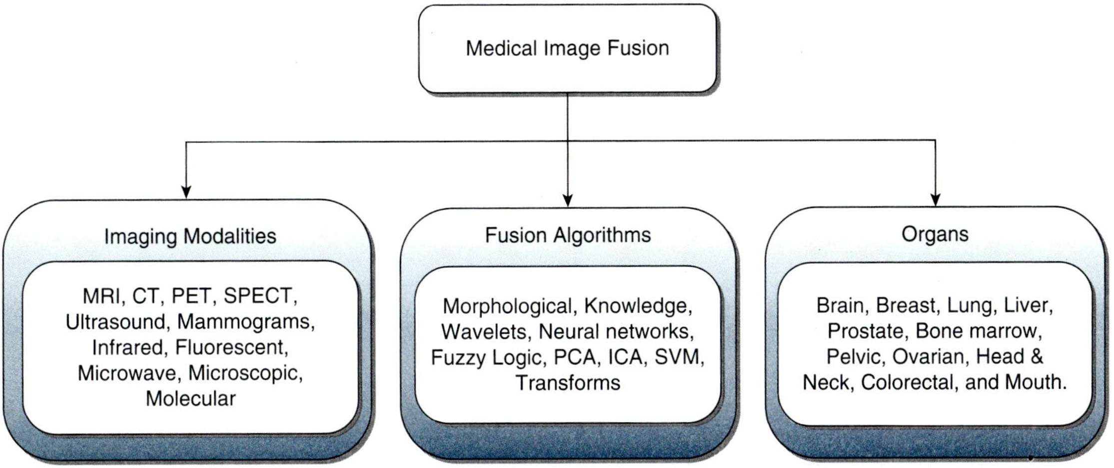


**FIGURE 12-11** A chart showing the nature of modalities, methods, and organs of interest as applied in medical image fusion studies. (From James, A. P., & Dasarathy, B. V. (2014). *Information Fusion, 19*, 4-19. Reproduced by permission.)

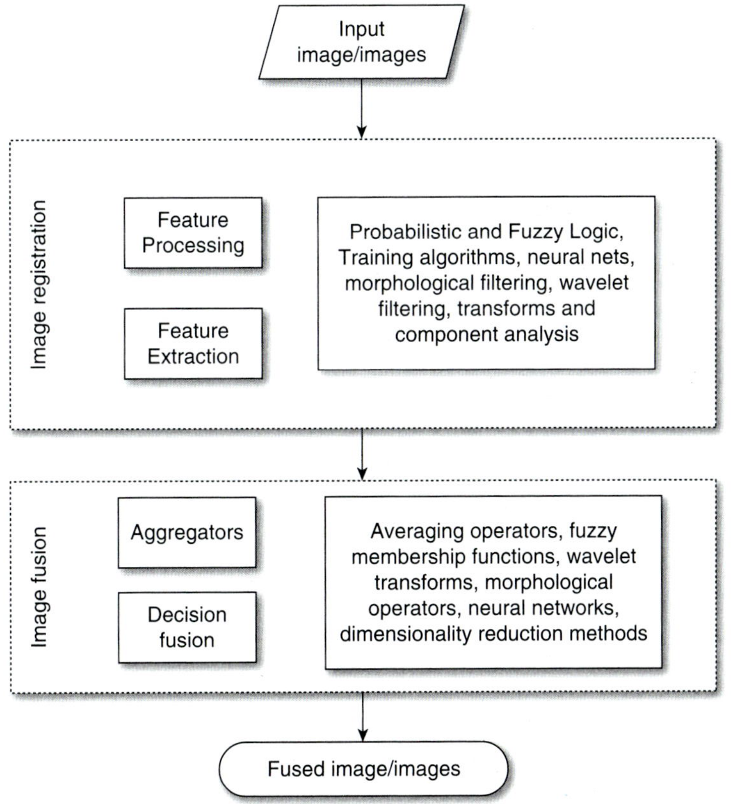


**FIGURE 12-12** The summary of the stages in the image fusion of medical images. The two stage process consists of image registration followed by image fusion. (From James, A. P., & Dasarathy, B. V. (2014). *Information Fusion, 19*, 4-19. Reproduced by permission.)

3. application of medical image fusion for studying human organs of interest in assessments of medical conditions. There exist several image fusion studies that can be directly applied for fusing medical images."

## Steps in Medical Image Fusion

There are essentially two steps in medical image fusion performed on the input image or images, and they are summarized in Figure 12-12. These include *image registration*, followed by *image fusion*. These are complex

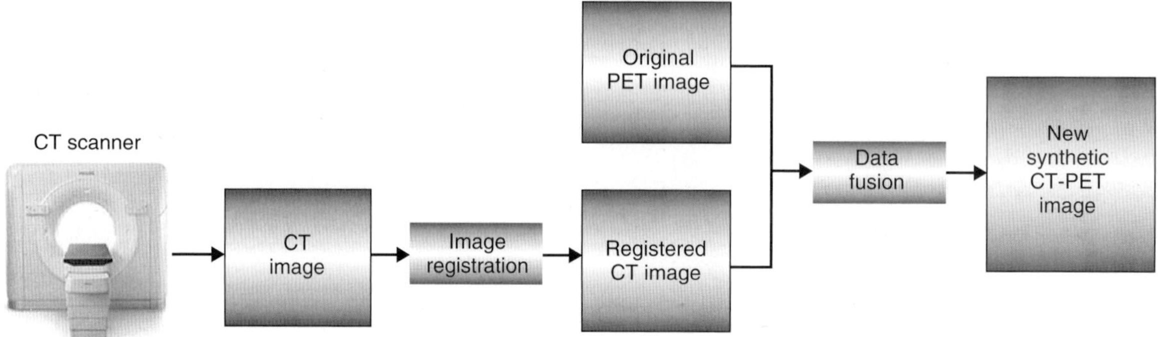


**FIGURE 12-13** The medical image fusion of a CT anatomic image with a functional PET image.

processes and are beyond the scope of this book; however, the following brief points are noteworthy:

1. Image registration involves two stages, feature processing and feature extraction intended "to correct the spatial misalignment between the different image datasets that often involve compensation of variability resulting from scale changes, rotations, and translations" (James & Dasarathy, 2014).
2. The purpose of image fusion, on the other hand, is to identify and select "features with a focus on relevance of the features for a given clinical assessment purpose" (James & Dasarathy, 2014).

The medical image fusion of a CT anatomic image with a functional PET image is illustrated in Figure 12-13.

## Major Medical Image Fusion Algorithms

There are several algorithms used in medical image fusion including morphological methods, knowledge-based methods, wavelet-based methods, neural network-based methods, and methods based on Fuzzy Logic. These methods are far beyond the scope of this book, and the interested reader should refer to James and Dasarathy (2014) and to digital image processing for medical applications textbooks such as by Bourne (2010) and Dougherty (2009).

## Clinical Applications and Conclusion

The clinical applications of medical image fusion range from research studies on organs such as the brain, breast, prostate, lungs, and liver (James & Dasarathy, 2014) to treatment planning and treatment delivery to treatment adaptation and customization (Kessler, 2006). Medical image fusion examples are shown in Figure 12-14.

In conclusion, James and Dasarathy (2014) stated the following:

> The extensive developments in medical image fusion research summarized in this literature review indicate the importance of this research in improving the medical services such as diagnosis, monitoring and analysis. The availability and growth of a wide range of imaging modality have enabled progress in medical image fusion to be useful for clinical deployment. Although, there has been significant progress in the medical image fusion research, the application of the general fusion algorithms is limited by the practical clinical implications as imposed by the medical experts based on the requirements of specific medical studies. In addition to medical reasons, there exist technical challenges in image registration and fusion resulting from image noise, resolution difference between images, inter-image variability between the images, lack of sufficient number of images per modality, high cost of imaging and increased computational complexity with increasing image space and time resolution ... the image fusion in medical imaging has proved to be useful and the trust in these techniques is on the rise. It is expected that the innovation and practical advancements would continue to grow in the upcoming years.

# FLAT-DETECTOR CT

The use of flat detectors or **flat-panel digital detectors** used in digital projection radiography and fluoroscopy is replacing image intensifier-based C-arm imaging systems that are used in a CT-like fashion in interventional and intraoperative medical imaging. A flat-panel C-arm imaging system is shown in Figure 12-15.

## Definition and Use

**Flat-detector CT** (FD-CT) refers to "CT imaging using C-arm systems built for radiography and fluoroscopy which are equipped with an FD and prepared to take **projection** data over an angular range of 180° or more" (Kalender & Kyriakou, 2007).

One of the early applications of using the principle of collecting data over 180 degrees (plus the fan angle of the x-ray beam) was with image

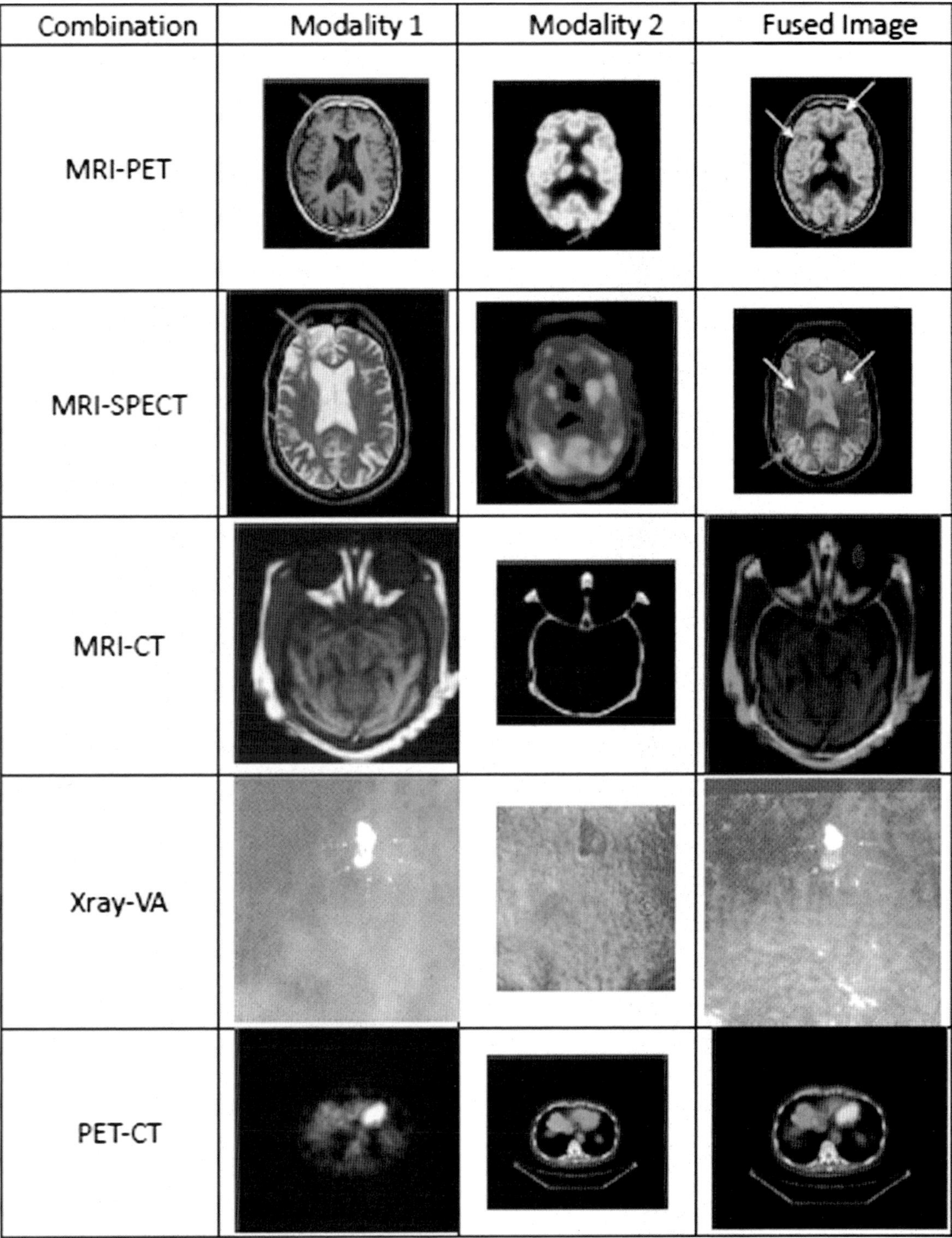


**FIGURE 12-14** Examples of multimodal medical image fusion. The combination of modality 1 with modality 2 using specific image fusion techniques results in improved feature visibility for medical diagnostics and assessments as shown in the fused image column. (From James, A. P., & Dasarathy, B. V. (2014). *Information Fusion, 19*, 4-19. Reproduced by permission.)

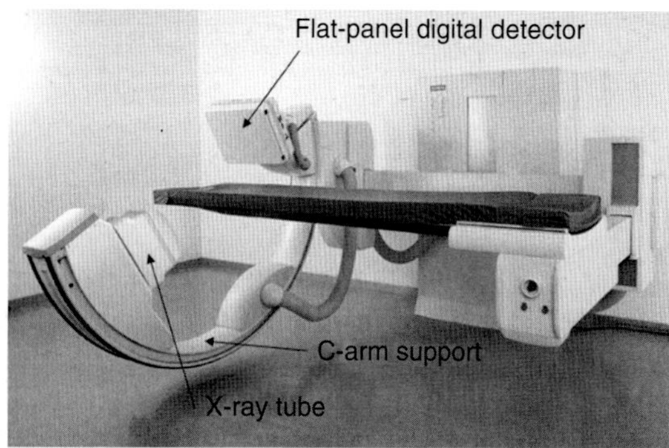


**FIGURE 12-15** A C-arm imaging system using a flat-panel digital detector. The digital detector has replaced the image intensifier tube. (Photo courtesy General Electric Healthcare.)

intensifier-based C-arm units in interventional angiography (Fahrig et al., 2006). Although these units demonstrated high-contrast vascular structures after intra-arterial injection of **contrast media** with good spatial resolution, they failed to show low-contrast resolution characteristic of soft tissues. This limitation provided the motivational factors for replacing the image intensifier tube with the flat-panel digital detector used in digital radiography imaging systems.

FD-CT systems are now used in interventional and intraoperative imaging, radiation therapy, maxillofacial scanning, micro-CT imaging (micro-CT scanners are now used to image small animals), breast CT imaging (Machida et al., 2010), CT brain imaging (Struffert et al., 2010), and in a physical setup where they are incorporated in a standard CT gantry (Kalender & Kyriakou, 2007). It is not within the scope of this chapter to outline the details of these applications, and the interested reader should refer to the works of Kalender (2005) for more information. The use of FD-CT for breast imaging is reviewed briefly at the end of this chapter.

## Technical Elements

Kalender and Kyriakou (2007) presented an excellent technical overview of the major components of FD-CT systems. These include the x-ray tube, the digital detectors, image reconstruction, image quality, artifacts, and radiation dose. In summary they identify the following points as being noteworthy:

1. Table 12-2 presents a comparison of the "typical parameters" between MSCT and FD-CT. It is clear that there is a difference between the two technologies with respect to kVp, mA, generator power, focal spot size, rotation time, detector elements, field of measurement, slice thickness, and data rate.

**TABLE 12-2 Typical Parameters for Multislice and Flat-Detector Computed Tomography**

| | MSCT | FD-CT |
|---|---|---|
| Tube voltage (kV) | 80-140 | 50-125 |
| Tube current (mA) | 10-600 | 10-800 |
| X-ray power (kW) | 20-100 | 10-80 |
| Focal spot size (mm) | 0.6-1.2 | 0.3-0.8 |
| Rotation time (seconds) | 0.33-1 | 5-20 |
| Detector elements | | |
| In fan direction | 512-1024 | 512-2490 |
| In *z*-direction | 16-64 | 512-2490 |
| Field of measurement (mm) | | |
| In fan direction | 500-700 | 100-250 |
| In *z*-direction | 2-40 | 100-200 |
| Minimum slice thickness (mm) | 0.6 | 0.1-0.3 |
| Typical scintillator/ thickness (mm) | $Gd_2O_2S$: 1.4 | CsI: (T1) 0.4-0.8 |
| Data rate (MB/s) | ≤1000 | ≤60 |

From Kalender, W. A., & Kryiakou, Y. (2007). Flat-detector computed tomography (FD-CT), *European Journal of Radiology, 17*, 2767-2779. Reproduced with kind permission of Springer Science and Business Media and the authors.

2. Of the two flat-panel digital detectors (indirect and direct conversion detectors graphically illustrated in Fig. 12-16, *A* and *B*, respectively) used for digital radiography, the indirect conversion flat-panel detector is used in FD-CT systems.
3. The indirect conversion detector (Fig. 12-16, *A*) converts x-ray photons to light by using a cesium iodide (CsI) scintillation phosphor coupled to a photodiode thin film transistor (TFT) array. The photodiode receives the light from the CsI phosphor and converts it into electrical charges that are subsequently stored and read out as an electrical signal **(analog signal)** by the TFT array. This signal is then digitized by the analog-to-digital converters (ADCs) and sent to a digital computer for processing and image creation. As shown in Figure 12-16, *A*, the CsI phosphor is arranged in a needlelike fashion (structured fashion) to reduce the lateral spread of light characteristic of a turbid phosphor. This spread of light (lateral dispersion) destroys the spatial resolution of the image. This problem is solved by the structured phosphor arrangement that improves the spatial resolution of the image.
4. The direct conversion flat-panel digital detector (Fig. 12-16, *B*) converts x-ray photons directly

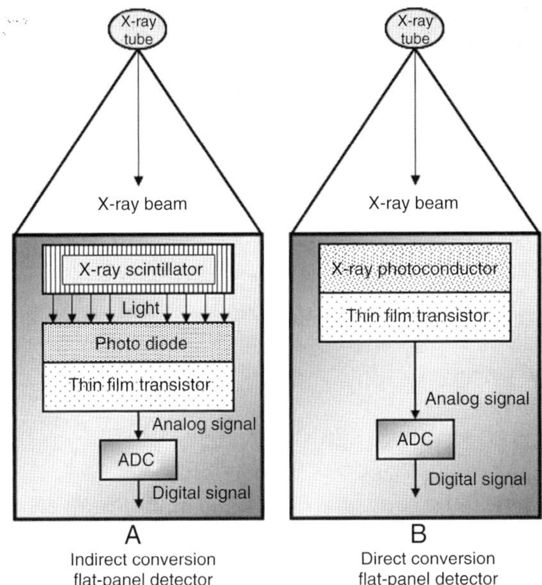


**FIGURE 12-16** The basic design structure of two types of flat-panel digital detectors. The indirect conversion detector is shown in **A** and the direct conversion detector is shown in **B**. See text for further explanation.

into electrical signals by using amorphous selenium (a-Se). There is no light conversion step. The a-Se detector has been used in some research units; however, it has not become commonplace in clinical FD-CT systems only because they "do not provide the necessary temporal resolution characteristics and dynamic capabilities" (Kalender & Kyriakou, 2007).

5. The beam from the x-ray tube that falls on a 2D detector is a cone beam; therefore, a cone-beam algorithm, namely, the Feldkamp algorithm (see Chapter 11), is used in the image reconstruction process.
6. Image quality can be discussed in terms of spatial resolution, noise, and contrast resolution. Although the spatial resolution for MSCT systems is about 1.2 lp/mm to 1.4 lp/mm (in the high-resolution mode), the spatial resolution from FD-CT is about 1.5 lp/mm with a **pixel** binning (where pixels in a region, say $n \times n$, are combined and read out as one to increase frame rates and reduce noise). With no binning, the spatial resolution is 3.0 lp/mm. This is clearly illustrated in Figure 12-17.
7. Compared with MSCT detectors, the FD-CT detector has higher noise and reduced low-contrast resolution for a given dose. This is visually illustrated in Figure 12-18. To improve low-contrast detectability, the dose must be increased.

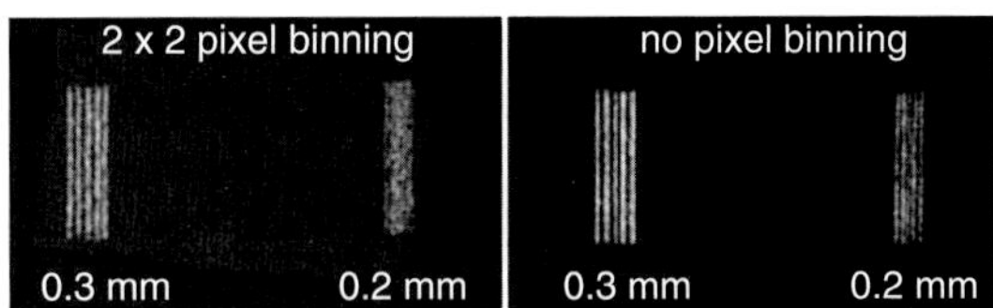


**FIGURE 12-17** The visual effect of combining (binning) the pixels on spatial resolution of the FD-CT detector with bar resolution test pattern. No binning of the pixels results in better spatial resolution (sharper bar patterns). (From Kalender. W. A., & Kryiakou, Y. (2007). *European Radiology, 17*, 2767-2779. Reproduced with kind permission of Springer Science and Business Media and the authors.)

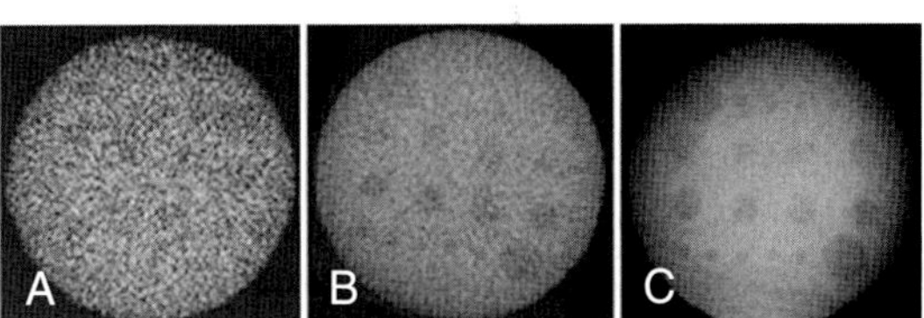


**FIGURE 12-18** The detectability of low-contrast details depends on reconstruction parameters and dose. **A** and **B,** High-resolution and low-resolution reconstructions are associated with high and low noise, respectively. **C,** An increase of dose compared with **A** and **B** leads to lower noise and results in improved low-contrast detectability. (From Kalender, W. A., & Kryiakou, Y. (2007). *European Radiology, 17*, 2767-2779. Figure and legend reproduced with kind permission of Springer Science and Business Media and the authors.)

8. FD-CT is not an artifact-free imaging system. Artifacts can arise from **beam hardening** (see Chapter 9), defective detector elements, and metal present in the patient. Other artifacts such as cupping and truncation artifacts (see Chapter 9) are also possible. These artifacts, however, can be corrected by using suitable correction algorithms.
9. The radiation dose from an FD-CT system is higher compared with that from a clinical CT study for the same image quality because the detection **efficiency** of the FD-CT detector is lower (Kalender & Kyriakou, 2007).

***Use of antiscatter grids.*** A fundamental problem with FD-CT scanners is that of scatter radiation artifacts due to the wide cone-beam geometry (compared to the smaller cone-beam geometry of the conventional CT systems). To address this problem, the use of scattered radiation grids has been considered to improve image quality. A study by Kyriakou and Kalender (2007) evaluated the use of three antiscatter grids on clean-up efficiency and improvement of image quality. The researchers found that

> ... The employment of a grid does not generally provide a significant improvement of the signal-to-noise ratio (SNR). Antiscatter grids led to a significant reduction of cupping artifacts in all cases. There is a trade-off between the SNR and the reduction of the scatter intensity described by the signal-to-noise improvement factor ($SNR_{if}$). For low or medium-scatter conditions the increase in noise caused by the reduced primary transmission through the grid has to be compensated by a higher exposure. For high-scatter conditions $SNR_{if}$ is significantly greater than 1; i.e. a decrease of dose of up to 50% can be reached.

In yet another study addressing scatter radiation and correction of artifacts arising from scatter and in particular, cupping artifacts (Chapter 9) in FD-CT, Meyer et al. (2010) used a fast projection-based algorithm which "combines a **convolution method** to determine the spatial distribution of the scatter intensity distribution with an object-size-dependent scaling of the scatter intensity distributions using *a priori* information generated by Monte Carlo simulation." This optimization approach reduced the cupping artifact down to 0.9%.

***Radiation dose and image quality.*** The radiation dose from FD-CT (DynaCT) was compared to that from an MSCT using a phantom model. In this study, Bai et al. (2012) showed that while the effective doses for the FD-CT system for the head, chest, and abdomen were 1.18 mSv, 7.32 mSv, and 7.48 mSv for a 20-second scan, respectively, they were 3.33 mSv, 7.62 mSv, and 8.42 mSv for the head, chest, and abdomen, respectively, for MSCT. The researchers indicated that "significant difference between the organ doses from DynaCT and from MSCT ($p < 0.05$) was shown. The spatial resolution of 12 lp/cm was achieved and it was able to recognize a 3 mm low contrast object at 0.5% contrast level in DynaCT, which was on the same level as in the MSCT images." This means that the FD-CT scanner "applies significantly less dose to patient and achieves similar spatial resolution and low contrast detectability to standard diagnostic MSCT."

## BREAST CT IMAGING

Mammography is still considered a valuable imaging modality for the early detection of cancer of the breast through its use as a **screening** tool (Boone et al., 2004; Bushong, 2012; Glick et al., 2007). Apart from the screening tool advantage, mammography offers high spatial resolution that is critical in demonstrating microcalcifications and masses located in adipose tissue (Glick et al., 2007), but mammography has some drawbacks. These include its poor performance in imaging dense breasts and the superimposition of structures, which is a common problem in projection imaging where a 3D object (the breast) is projected as a 2D image. Such superimposition can create detection problems for the observer.

A comprehensive article on the evolution of breast imaging to the present day is written by Joe and Sickles (2014), and the interested reader should refer to this article for historic perspectives and developments.

### Early CT Mammography

In the mid-1970s, General Electric Healthcare (formerly General Electric Medical Systems, Milwaukee, Wis.) built two research prototype CT scanners for mammography (CT/M), one of which was installed at the Mayo Clinic and the other at the University of Kansas Medical Center. Researchers at these two facilities conducted clinical efficacy studies of the CT/M systems.

The CT/M unit used a continuously rotating fan beam (26 degrees), a water box, and an array of xenon detectors. Operating at 116 kVp and 30 mA, the absorption values from the breast ranged from −127 to +127, with water assigned the value of zero (Gisvold et al., 1979). The patient was placed in a prone position and the breast inserted into a hole cut into the tabletop. The breast was lowered into the water box and immersed in water for scanning. X-ray transmission readings were recorded, and images were reconstructed by the already established fan-beam algorithms typical of conventional diagnostic CT scanners in clinical use. Reconstructed images were displayed on a 128 × 128 matrix with pixel dimensions of 1.5 mm × 1.5 mm (Gisvold et al., 1979).

Clinical studies conducted by Gisvold et al. (1979) and Chang et al. (1979) showed that "the spatial resolution of CT/M was poor and that the main feature used in interpreting results was the **attenuation**-related measure. With infusion of contrast material, CT/M was capable of revealing clinically and mammographically occult malignancy but was not considered suitable for routine screening of asymptomatic women. The reconstructed images of the original CT/M were prone to artifacts caused by the long scanning time: the lower detectability of small lesions was due to the large slice thickness and poor spatial resolution" (Chen & Ning, 2002).

### Major Technical Components

Interest in developing dedicated breast CT scanners using FD detector technology surfaced as early as

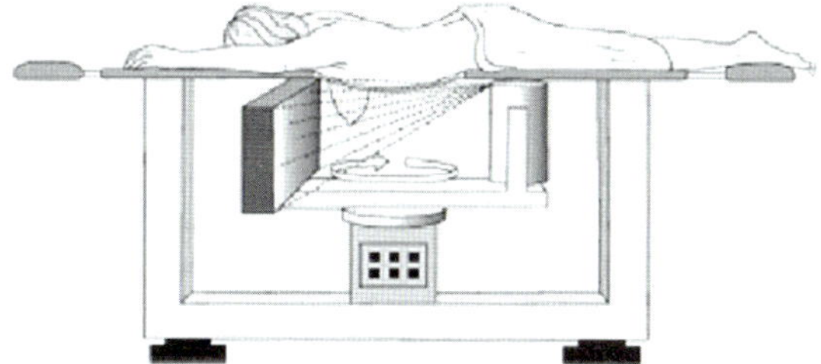

**FIGURE 12-19** The basic design framework for an FD-CT scanner for breast imaging on the basis of pendant geometry. See text for further explanation. (From Glick, S. J., Thacker, S., Gong, X., & Liu, B. (2007). *Medical Physics, 34,* 5-9. Reproduced by permission of the American Association of Physicists in Medicine.)

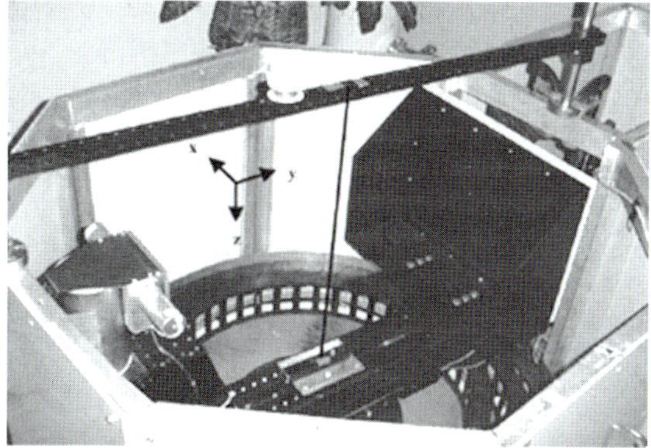


**FIGURE 12-20** An inside view of the flat-panel CsI amorphous silicon TFT digital radiography detector used in the FD-CT scanner for imaging the breast. (From Kwan, A. L. C., Boone, J. M., Yang, K., & Huang, S. Y. (2007). *Medical Physics, 34,* 275-281. Reproduced by permission of the American Association of Physicists in Medicine.)

2001 (Boone et al., 2004). The advantages offered by FD technology such as wide **dynamic range,** high spatial resolution, excellent **linearity,** high detective quantum efficiency, and no geometric distortion provide a good rationale for using them in the design of FD-CT scanners for breast imaging (Chen & Ning, 2002).

The basic design framework for an FD-CT scanner for breast imaging, shown in Figure 12-19, is based on what is referred to as a pendant geometry cone-beam CT imaging system. The major system components include an x-ray tube coupled to a flat-panel digital detector and a tabletop with a hole cut in it. Although the x-ray tube is designed to produce an x-ray beam optimized for breast imaging with appropriate target materials, filters, and beam intensity (lowered kVp and mAs compared with MSCT scanners; Boone et al., 2004; Chen & Ning, 2002; Glick et al., 2007; Shaw et al., 2005), the flat-panel detector in most systems is a CsI amorphous silicon TFT digital radiography detector. The FD-CT scanner for imaging the breast shown in Figure 12-20 uses a 14-bit ($2^{14}$) 40 cm × 30 cm CsI amorphous silicon TFT digital detector.

The patient is placed in a prone position on the tabletop and the breast to be scanned is inserted through the hole to hang during the imaging process by use of a cone beam wide enough to cover the detector, as shown in Figure 12-19. This geometry is referred to as *pendant geometry* (Boone et al., 2004), and it prevents exposure of the chest cavity. The x-ray tube and detector are positioned close to the underside of the tabletop and rotate around the hanging breast. X-ray transmission readings are collected, digitized, and subsequently sent to the computer for image reconstruction with use of the Feldkamp cone-beam algorithm (see Chapter 11).

## Research Studies

A number of research studies have been conducted to evaluate the physical imaging parameters of the FD-CT breast scanner, such as the dose and image quality (Boone et al., 2001, 2004; Chen & Ning, 2002; Glick et al., 2007; Kwan et al., 2007; Shaw et al., 2005). More recently, the technique of digital breast tomosynthesis (DBT) has become available for clinical use, and provides solutions to the shortcomings of conventional mammography (Roth et al., 2014). As noted by Roth et al. (2014):

> With DBT, multiple low-dose x-ray images are acquired in an arc and reconstructed to create a three-dimensional image, thus minimizing the impact of overlapping breast tissue and improving lesion conspicuity. Early studies of screening DBT have shown decreased false-positive callback rates and increased rates of cancer detection (particularly for invasive cancers), resulting in increased **sensitivity** and **specificity.** In our clinical practice, we have completed more than 2 years of using two-view digital mammography combined with two-view DBT for all screening and select diagnostic imaging examinations (over 25,000 patients). Our experience, combined with previously published data, demonstrates that the combined use of DBT and digital mammography is associated with improved outcomes for screening and diagnostic imaging.

It is beyond the scope of this section to elaborate on the results of these studies, and therefore the interested reader should refer to them for details of the findings with respect to each of these parameters.

In conclusion, Shaw et al. (2005) showed that "the 3D nature of the image data may help eliminate interference from overlapping structures and allow lesions to be better defined and localized for biopsy or needle localization procedures. This suggests that cone-beam CT breast imaging is a potentially powerful tool for diagnosis and management of breast cancers."

## CT SCREENING

### Definition

The use of any medical technology for early detection of disease in healthy (asymptomatic) people is referred to as screening. In particular, the use of CT technology for the early detection of diseases in asymptomatic patients is popularly referred to as a CT screening (Beinfield et al., 2005; Brant-Zawadzki, 2002; Brenner, 2006; Furtado et al., 2005; Horton et al., 2004.

### Rationale

Several investigators have provided the rationale for CT screening; it is fundamentally based on the increased prevalence of various types of high-risk diseases that may cause death to the population (Brant-Zawadzki, 2002). The increasing availability and ease of use of CT imaging has also provided a basis for its use as a screening tool.

Although there are those who support the use of CT as a screening tool, there are others who are vehemently opposed to its use in screening asymptomatic individuals. In this regard, CT screening "has generated significant controversy" (Horton et al., 2004), and it is not within the scope of this book to outline the elements of the controversy. The interested reader may refer to the various references cited in this section for an elaboration of the controversy.

### Applications

The literature exploring the use of CT screening continues to increase from 2002 to the present. CT screening has been used in lung cancer screening, colon screening, coronary artery disease screening, and whole-body screening of healthy individuals. Although clinical efficacy studies have been performed on the first three mentioned previously to provide tangible justification for the use of CT screening, the latter (whole-body screening) remains a highly controversial subject (Brenner, 2006). The reason is that no studies have clearly demonstrated that whole-body CT screening has extended the life of individuals (Brenner, 2006).

### Radiation Doses

Personnel working in radiology operate within the ALARA philosophy, which requires that the dose to the patient should be kept as low as possible. To operate effectively within this philosophy, operators are now concerned with dose/image quality optimization, a procedure that ensures that the use of low doses does not compromise the image quality needed to make a diagnosis.

In addressing the dose issues in imaging asymptomatic individuals by CT screening, one notable expert, Dr. David Brenner, PhD, DSc, provided the radiological community with the following statement: "… the radiation exposure issues that relate to CT-based mass screening are unique. It is true, of course, that mammography also involves the use of x-rays, but the radiation doses involved are generally much higher for CT-based screening than for mammography. Thus, in addition to the more general efficacy issues discussed … the potential benefits of any CT-based screening procedure must far outweigh any potential harm from repeated low-dose x-ray exposures" (Brenner, 2006).

A study conducted by the National Lung Screening Trial Research Team (2011) on "reduced lung-cancer mortality with low-dose computed tomographic screening" essentially demonstrated that "screening with the use of low-dose CT reduces mortality from lung cancer."

Finally, the Radiological Society of North America (RSNA) and the American College of Radiology (ACR) (RadiologyInfo.org-http://www.radiologyinfo.org/en/news/newdetarget.cfm?ID=5), in addressing the future of whole-body CT screening as well as the question of whether whole-body CT screening is worthwhile, present the following statement in looking at both sides of this controversial topic:

> *New CT scanners currently under development will reduce the amount of radiation. If screening is limited to persons older than 50 years, exposing children or women of childbearing age will not be an issue. Future scanning may routinely include the use of oral and intravenous contrast material. Results could be reported to a central database so as to better determine the effectiveness of whole-body CT. It might be a good idea to offer whole-body CT along with other exams at comprehensive screening centers. The same people who are likely to opt for screening would tend to be interested in diet, fitness and other health-promoting lifestyle changes, and screening could provide an opportunity to explore these issues. For instance, the desirability of supplementing the diet with vitamins, aspirin or other substances could be addressed. Even without a formal risk reduction program, whole-body CT allows the radiologist or an associate to talk with people about their health-related behaviors. Smoking is an obvious behavior to target.*
>
> *As happens with the invention of any new health-care technology or the discovery of new uses for estab-*

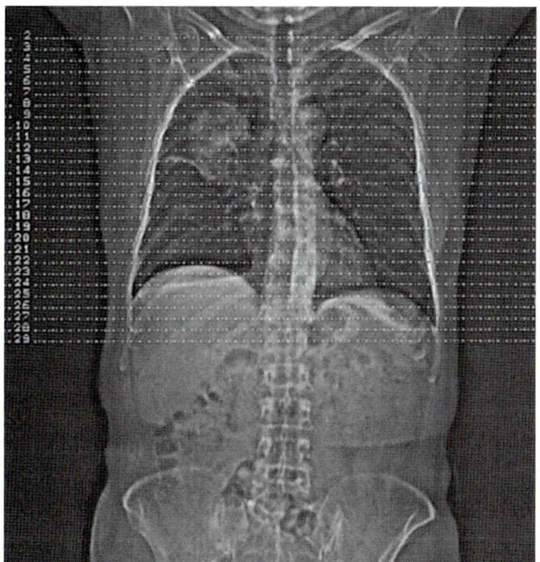

**FIGURE 12-21** Prescan localization image produced when the patient moves continuously through the gantry while the x-ray tube and detectors remain in a fixed position. (Courtesy Siemens Medical Systems, Iselin, NJ.)

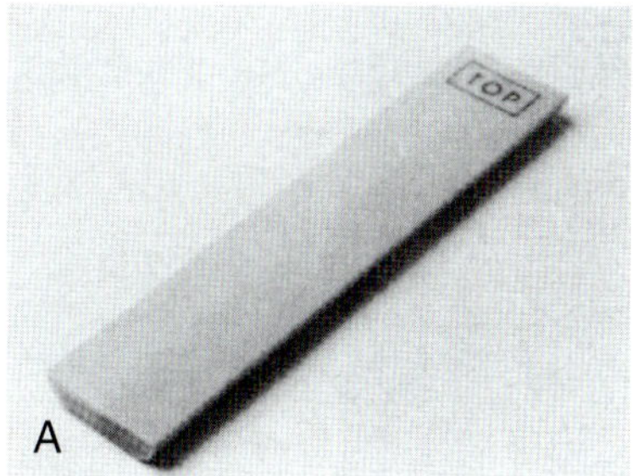


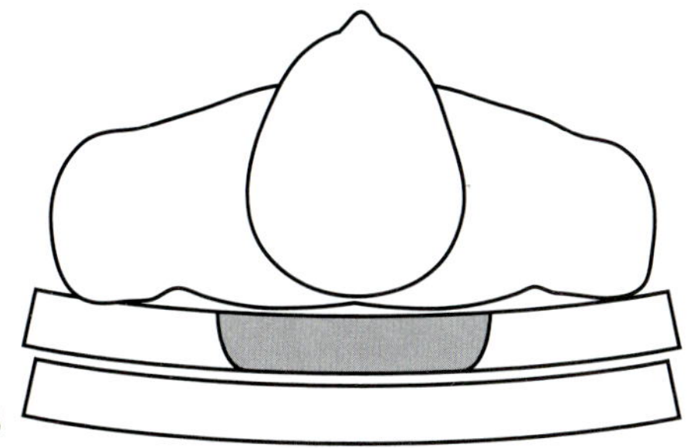


**FIGURE 12-22** Reference phantom **(A)** and its position in relation to the patient **(B)** for QCT.

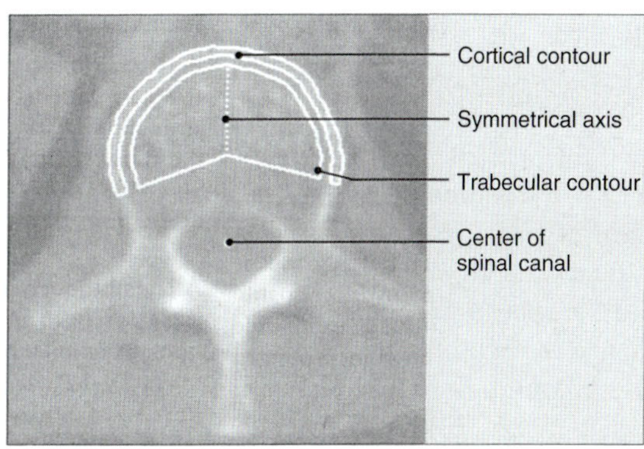


**FIGURE 12-23** Automatic contour tracing of trabecular and cortical regions of interest. (From Nagel, W., et al. (1987). *Electromedica 55*, 104-110.)

*lished technologies, the issues surrounding whole-body CT will continue to be investigated and debated by the scientific and healthcare communities. More research will surely bring new socioeconomic and scientific findings to light prompting further professional discourse. The debate is far from over* (RadiologyInfo.org, 2015).

## QUANTITATIVE CT

QCT is the most sensitive of all x-ray techniques for the measurement of the mineral content of trabecular bone in osteoporosis. This measurement is the bone mineral density (Kalender, 2005). QCT involves at least seven steps, as follows:

1. A prescan localization image is obtained (Fig. 12-21). This is sometimes referred to as a *scout view* (General Electric) or *topogram* (Siemens). The image is obtained as the patient moves through the gantry aperture while the x-ray tube and detector remain stationary. The computer then builds an image that resembles a conventional radiographic image.
2. The slices are selected from the prescan localization image, and the midvertebral planes are examined.
3. Transverse axial images are obtained. At this time, a reference phantom (Fig. 12-22, *A*) that contains water and bone-equivalent parts is positioned and scanned with the patient (Fig. 12-22, *B*).
4. An automatic contour tracing of trabecular and cortical regions of interest (ROIs) is obtained (Fig. 12-23).
5. The computer calculates the mean values of the ROIs.
6. The ROI values are converted to bone mineral density values.
7. An image graphics **output** is obtained, which shows the bone mineral density values plotted as a function of age. The bone mineral content is then determined and compared with normal values.

A study on the "quantitative CT assessment of chronic obstructive pulmonary disease" done by Matsuoka et al. (2010) showed that "CT-based quantitative analyses can help differentiate the COPD phenotype (emphysema-predominant, airway-predominant, or mixed), which is crucial information for determining the appropriate management strategy."

## PORTABLE MULTISLICE CT IMAGING

### Rationale

Several problems are associated with transporting patients to a fixed CT scanner: (1) the risks of transporting unstable patients, (2) the costs associated with the workload of staff who are involved in patient transportation, and (3) the maintenance of the nurse-to-patient ratio in critical care. These problems are solved by using portable CT scanners. These scanners can be transported to critically ill patients in the intensive care unit, for example, to the emergency department, to the operating room, and other areas of the hospital where these patients are cared for. In addition, these scanners can be used in private medical facilities as well, to image ambulatory and other patients seen for various CT examinations.

### Physical Principles

**Portable MSCT scanners** are now commercially available from the NeuroLogica Corporation (Danvers, Mass.) specifically for imaging critically ill patients and other patients in the hospital who cannot be easily transported to the radiology department for examination by fixed CT scanners. The NeuroLogica Corporation has developed a portable multislice (eight slices/revolution) CT scanner called the CereTom, which is specifically designed for imaging anatomy that can fit into a 25-cm scan FOV—namely, the head and neck. More recently the BodyTom has become commercially available. It is battery powered and is a portable, full-body, 32-slice CT scanner with a gantry 85 cm and 60 cm FOV. These scanners therefore have been designed to image the brain; the neck up to the fifth cervical vertebrae (C5); and the ear, nose, and throat; and specific body anatomy. In addition, CT perfusion and xenon CT studies can be done on these portable MSCT scanners.

The CereTom and the BodyTom portable CT scanners are based on the same physical principles as fixed MSCT scanners with up to eight detector rows (see Chapter 11). The goal of the portable CT scanner is to produce diagnostic quality images that are based on x-ray attenuation data collected from the patient and measured by multirow detectors. The detectors convert the x-ray photons into electrical signals (analog data) that are subsequently converted into digital data by the detector electronics (ADCs). The digital data are then sent to the computer for image reconstruction.

### The CereTom Portable Multislice Head and Neck CT Scanner

Portable MSCT scanners are compact, lightweight, high-speed, battery- and wall-powered scanners that can be transported to any point of care. The CereTom portable MSCT scanner is characterized by three major equipment components: a compact CT gantry (Fig. 12-24), a silhouette scan board that is made of carbon fiber, and a laptop computer workstation/cart.

#### System Features

The general system requirements can be described in terms of site requirements (space, room, temperature, and humidity) and installation requirements (power requirements and minimum line current ratings).

The CereTom portable CT scanner does not require any special electrical considerations because it can operate with single-phase alternating current power and 90-V to 260-V wall power outlets operating at 50 Hz to 60 Hz. In case of a power failure, the scanner is equipped with an independent battery power source that can last 2 hours (no scans) when fully charged.

The CereTom portable CT gantry (Fig. 12-24) houses the x-ray tube, generator, detectors, and detector electronics. The detector electronics play an important role in ADC and digital data transmission to the minicomputer system, which is responsible for image reconstruction and image processing.

The gantry characteristics of the CereTom portable CT scanner include the gantry aperture with an opening of 32 cm to accommodate the patient's anatomy. Furthermore, the gantry will not tilt so patient positioning is used to deal with views that require a gantry tilt. As mentioned earlier, the maximum scan FOV is 25 cm to accommodate examinations of the head, face, and neck.

The gantry also houses the x-ray tube with a fixed anode having a focal spot size of 1 mm × 1 mm and a maximum cooling of 2 minutes, and it can operate at tube currents between 1 mA and 7 mA and at 100 kVp, 120 kVp, and 140 kVp. The beam emerging from the x-ray tube is a cone beam because an eight-slice multirow solid-state detector system is used. Therefore, image reconstruction follows that described for cone-beam CT scanners using up to eight detector rows, as described in Chapter 11.

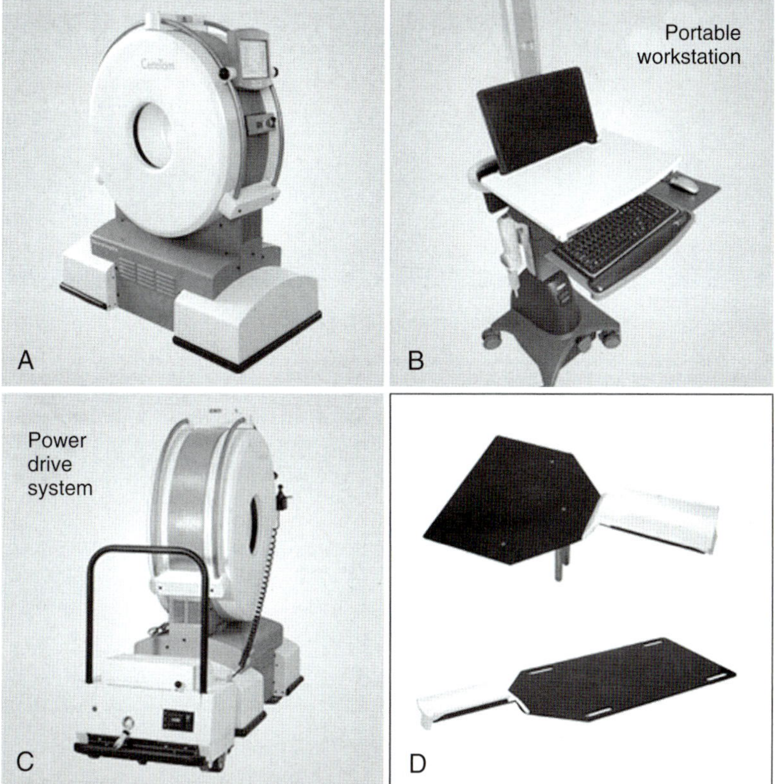


**FIGURE 12-24** The gantry of the portable MSCT scanner. **A,** Typical portable workstation. **B,** Power drive system. **C,** Scan boards to convert the patient's bed into a scanning platform **(D)**. (Courtesy NeuroLogica, Danvers, Mass.)

The CereTom portable CT scanner is based on the third-generation CT design concept, in which the x-ray tube is coupled to the multidetector row system that can provide slice thicknesses of 1.25 mm, 2.5 mm, 5 mm, and 10 mm. Both the x-ray tube and detectors rotate at the same time during data collection.

An integral component of the CereTom portable CT scanner system is the operator's console, which is a digital imaging and communication in medicine (DICOM)-compliant gigabit Ethernet networked laptop computer workstation with wireless **connectivity** to a picture archiving and communication system (PACS). In addition, a 20-inch liquid crystal display monitor is available with a display matrix of 1920 × 1200. The CT number range with this scanner is between −1024 and 3071, featuring both variable and preset windows.

The workstation allows the operator to select scan protocols and window settings optimized from specific protocols. The operator can also perform several image-processing functions such as advanced 3D visualization (targeted, **segmentation,** and MIP) and MPR (sagittal, coronal, axial, curved, and sliding slab) and so on, as shown in Figure 12-25.

## Imaging Performance

The imaging performance of the CereTom portable CT scanner can be described in terms of spatial resolution, contrast resolution, noise, and radiation dose considerations. NeuroLogica provided the data presented later.

***Spatial resolution.*** Spatial resolution refers to the ability of the scanner to image fine detail, measured in lp/cm. Several figures for spatial resolution have been reported for the CereTom portable CT scanner and the user should refer to the manufacturer product data for these numbers. For example, spatial resolution has been reported to be 7.4 lp/cm at 10% **modulation transfer function (MTF)** to 13.0 lp/cm at 10% MTF depending on the reconstruction kernel and the windowing used.

***Contrast resolution.*** Contrast resolution refers to the ability of the scanner to demonstrate small differences in tissue contrast. The contrast resolution of the CereTom portable CT scanner has been measured

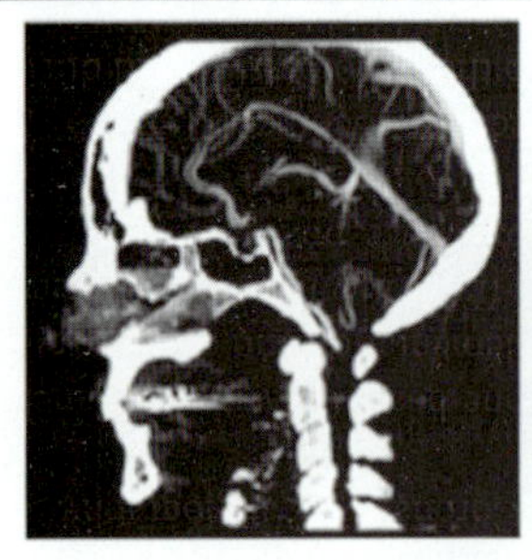
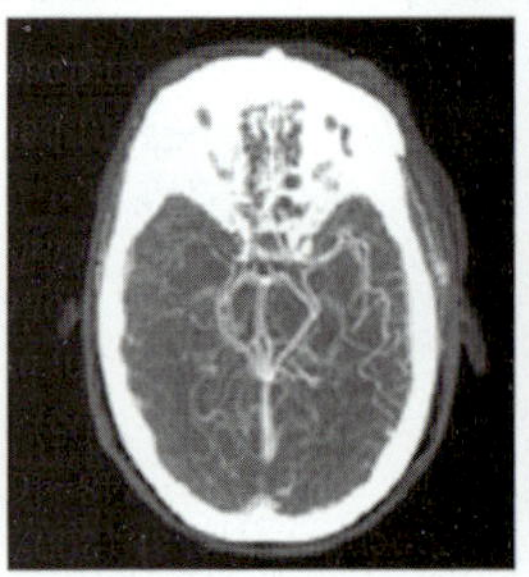
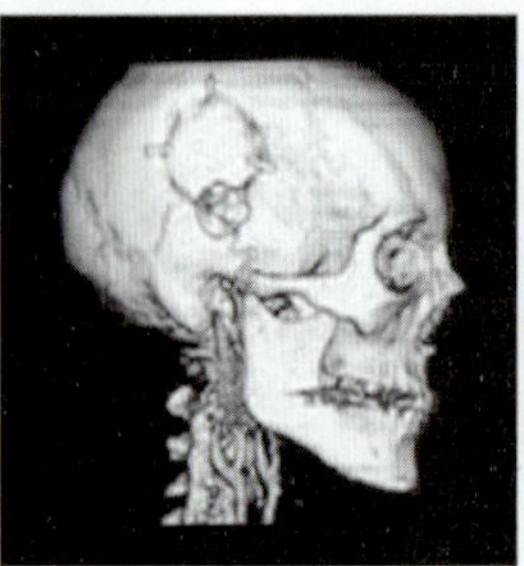
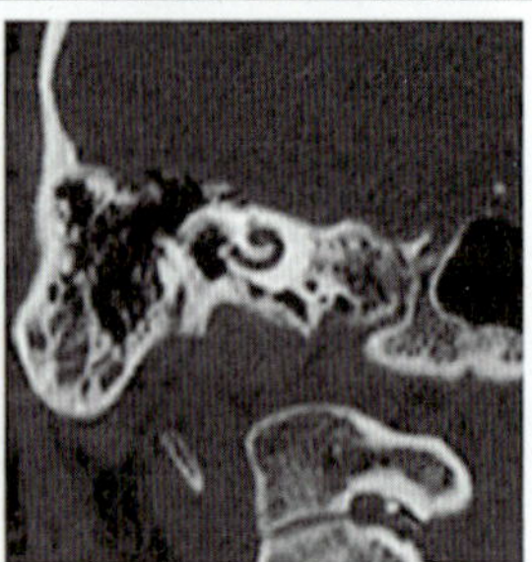

CereTom® portable 8-slice CT scanner—neuro images

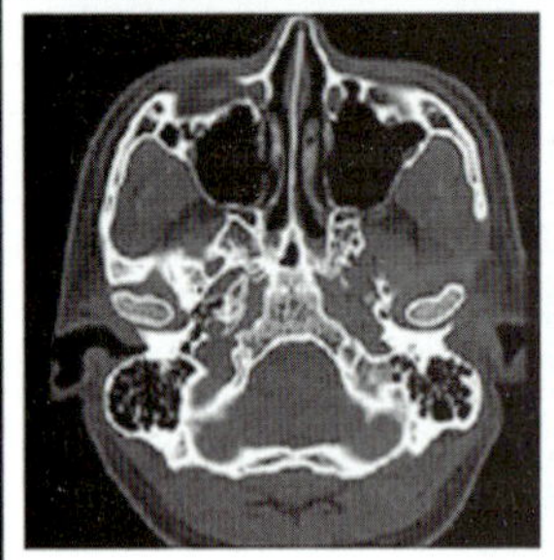
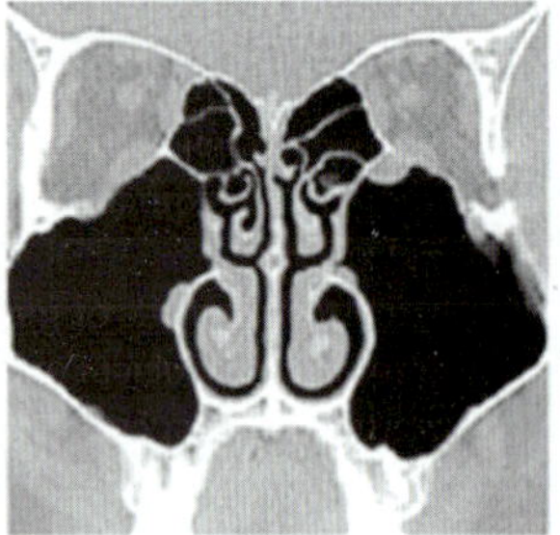
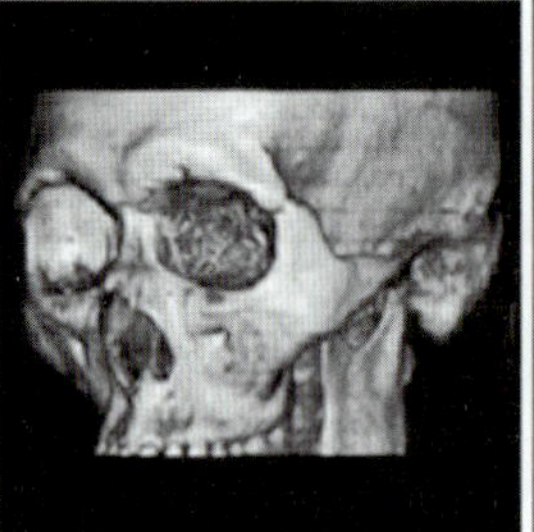
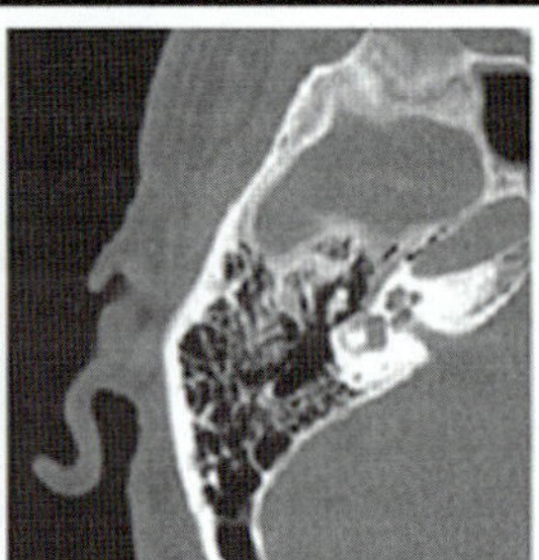

CereTom® portable 8-slice CT scanner—ear, nose, and throat images

**FIGURE 12-25** Images from the CereTom portable eight-slice CT scanner. (Courtesy NeuroLogica, Danvers, Mass.)

by using an 8-inch Catphan phantom with 10-mm slice thickness at 15 mAs and 140 kVp and has been reported to be 3 mm at 0.3%.

***Noise.*** Image quality from the portable CT scanner is also affected by noise. In CT, *noise* refers to the fluctuation of CT numbers between points in the image for a scan of uniform material such as water. The *noise level* is a percentage of contrast in CT numbers. The noise level of the CereTom portable CT scanner is 0.3% at 15 mAs and 140 kVp with a 10-mm slice thickness.

***CT dose index.*** Manufacturers of CT scanners are now required by law to provide the **CT dose index (CTDI)** for their scanners. For the CereTom portable CT scanner, with a head phantom only (because of the small CereTom patient aperture) at 120 kV, 14 mAs, 2-second scan time, and a 10-mm aperture, the CTDI for the center and surface of the head phantom is 35.8 and 46.64 mGy, respectively.

***Scattered radiation considerations.*** As in any portable x-ray imaging procedure, scattered radiation from the portable CT scanner concerns radiation workers and those individuals working in areas in which portable CT examinations are performed. For the CereTom portable CT scanner, the scatter radiation in general at 1 m from the isocenter of the scanner is about 0.2 mR.

## The BodyTom Portable Multislice Body CT Scanner

The BodyTom is a more recent development in NeuroLogica's portable computed tomography systems. It is a portable, full-body, 32-slice CT scanner that can be transported from room to room in a hospital or clinic. This scanner is optimized for imaging in spinal surgery, brain surgery, orthopedics, vascular surgery, thoracic surgery, and several other areas of patient imaging.

### System Features and Imaging Performance

While the portable gantry and workstation are shown in Figure 12-26, the dimensions of this scanner are shown in Figure 12-27. The machine is battery powered with a built-in drive system and internal lead shielding, and can be plugged into a standard wall outlet. Furthermore it is capable of 3D image quality with such features as 32-slice, 32 images per second; 85-cm gantry; 60-cm FOV; 4-cm aperture;

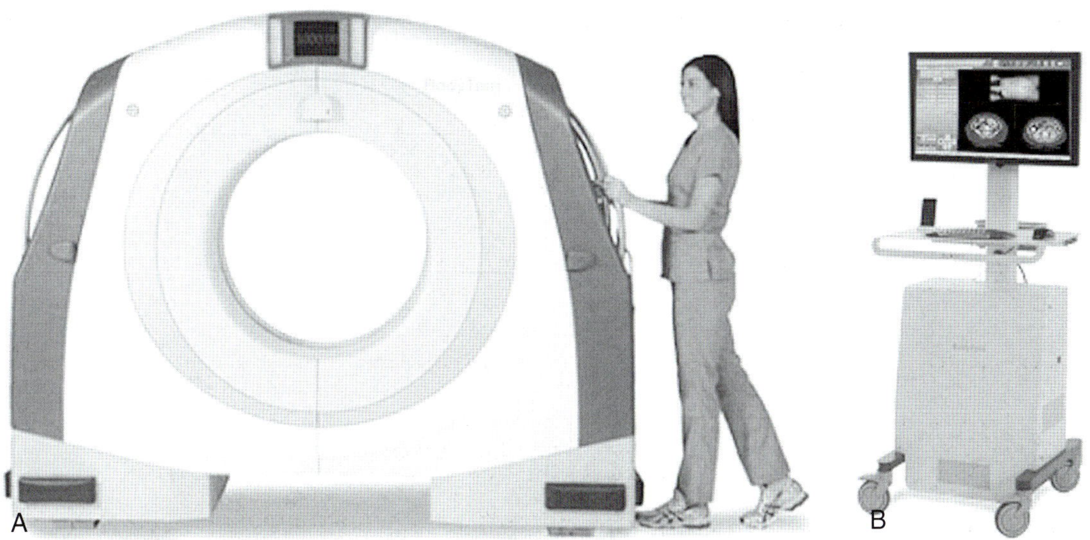


**FIGURE 12-26** The gantry (**A**) and workstation (**B**) of the BodyTom portable MSCT scanner. (Courtesy NeuroLogica, Danvers, Mass.)

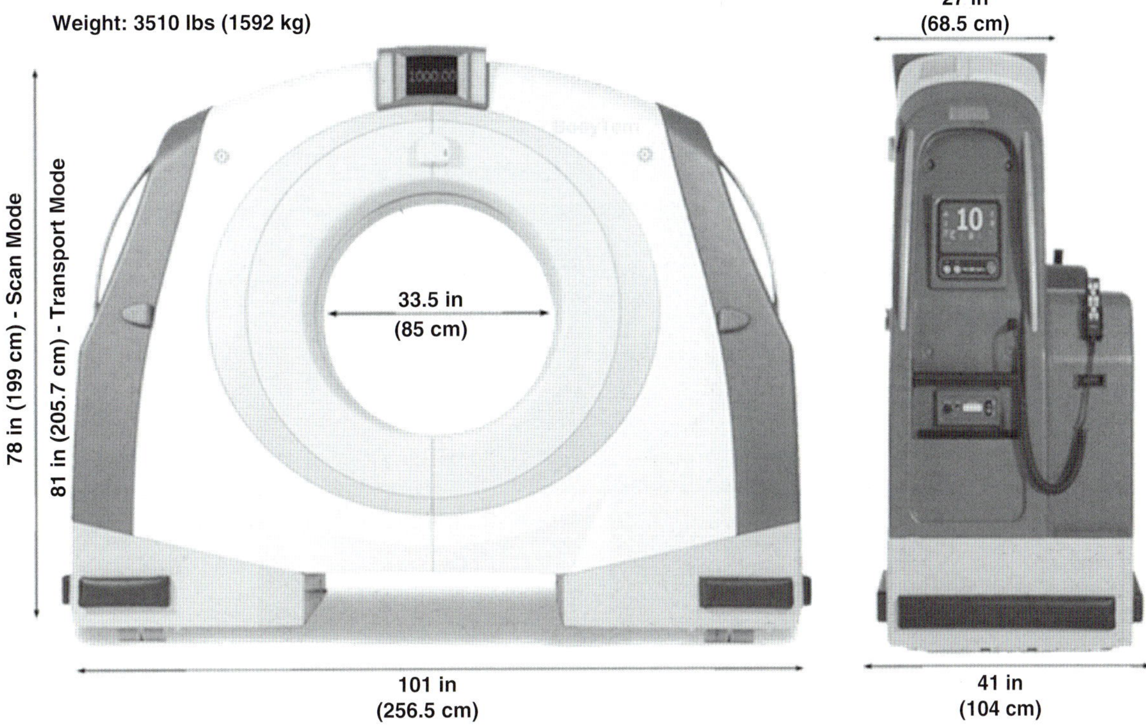


**FIGURE 12-27** The dimensions of the gantry of the BodyTom portable MSCT scanner. (Courtesy NeuroLogica, Danvers, Mass.)

1.25-mm, 2.5-mm, 5.0-mm, and 10-mm slice thickness; and 512 × 512 image resolution with a maximum scan length of 2 m. In addition, this portable body CT scanner is fully integrated with DICOM 3.1, the Hospital Information System, and the Radiology Information System and performs within the Integrating the Healthcare Enterprise.

The characteristics of the workstation are shown in Table 12-3. Several examples of clinical images are shown in Figure 12-28.

| TABLE 12-3 Characteristics of the Workstation of the BodyTom Portable Body CT Scanner |
|---|
| • Slim cart design<br>• Genuine Windows 7 Professional 64 bit<br>• Integrates with PACS<br>• Processor: Intel Quad Core Xeon Processor 2.67 GHz<br>• Memory: 4 GB<br>• Operating system hard drive: 80 GB<br>• Data storage: 1 TB secondary<br>• Advanced visualization software package<br>• 2D/3D MPR viewing<br>• DVD/CD burner<br>• 27″ LCD Monitor Resolution: 2560 × 1440<br>• Dose check<br>• Battery powered<br>• MP3 dock with surround-sound system |

Courtesy NeuroLogica, Danvers, Mass.

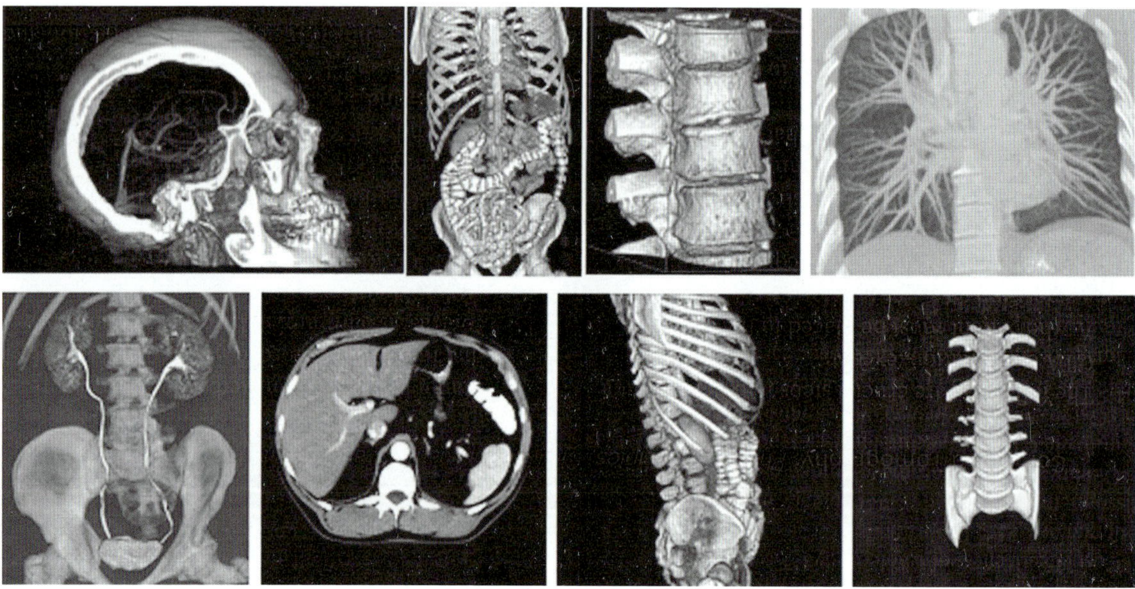

**FIGURE 12-28** Several examples of clinical images produced by the BodyTom portable MSCT scanner. (Courtesy NeuroLogica, Danvers, Mass.)

## REVIEW QUESTIONS

Answer the following questions to check your understanding of the materials studied.

1. One of the major challenges for imaging a rapidly beating heart is that the imaging modality:
   A. must ensure good contrast resolution.
   B. must use two x-ray tubes.
   C. must provide high temporal resolution.
   D. must be capable of high kVp switching.
2. Which of the following influences the spatial resolution in cardiac CT imaging?
   A. detector size
   B. reconstruction interval
   C. pitch
   D. all of the above
3. Which of the following is defined as a CT image of blood vessels opacified by contrast media?
   A. CTA
   B. MRA
   C. CT endoscopy
   D. virtual endoscopy

4. The following are crucial steps in carrying out a CTA examination, except:
   A. the patient must be placed in the supine position.
   B. patient preparation and acquisition parameters.
   C. contrast medium administration.
   D. image postprocessing techniques.
5. The technical requirements that make CT fluoroscopy possible include:
   1. fast data acquisition as in multislice volume CT.
   2. dedicated algorithm for image reconstruction.
   3. continuous image display.
   4. specially activated fluoroscopy exposure switch.

   A. 1 only
   B. 1 and 2
   C. 1, 2, and 3
   D. 1, 2, 3, and 4
6. In which of the following is the dataset for every 60° acquisition added while the dataset for the previous image is discarded as new 60° data sets are processed?
   A. fast continuous scanning
   B. fast imaging reconstruction
   C. continuous image display
   D. interactive cine
7. Manufacturers' automated systems to ensure that images are recorded when —flow-in of contrast is optimum in blood vessels are:
   1. SmartPrep.
   2. CARE Bolus.
   3. SureStart.
   4. OptiEuc.

   A. 1 only
   B. 1 and 2
   C. 1, 2, and 3
   D. 1, 2, 3, and 4
8. In medical image fusion, feature extraction and feature processing belong to:
   A. Fuzi Logic.
   B. image fusion.
   C. image registration.
   D. all of the above.
9. The modality based on the use of pendant geometry cone-beam CT imaging system is:
   A. flat detector CT.
   B. quantitative CT.
   C. CT screening.
   D. breast CT.
10. The most sensitive of all x-ray imaging modalities for the measurement of the mineral content of trabecular bone in osteoporosis is:
    A. film-screen radiography.
    B. quantitative CT.
    C. fluoroscopy.
    D. digital radiography.

## REFERENCES


Ahn, P. H., & Garg, M. K. (2008). Positron emission tomography/computed tomography for target delineation in head and neck cancers. *Seminars in Nuclear Medicine*, *38*, 141–148.

Bai, M., Liu, B., Mu, H., Liu, X., & Jiang, Y. (2012). The comparison of radiation dose between C-arm flat-detector CT (DynaCT) and multi-slice CT (MSCT): a phantom study. *European Journal of Radiology*, *81*(11), 3577–3580.

Beinfield, M. T., Wittenberg, E., & Gazelle, G. S. (2005). Cost effectiveness of whole-body CT screening. *Radiology*, *234*, 415–422.

Bissonnette, J. P., Balter, P. A., Dong, L., et al. (2012). Quality assurance for image-guided radiation therapy utilizing CT-based technologies: a report of the AAPM TG-179. *Medical Physics*, *39*(4), 1946–1963.

Blobel, J., et al. (2008). Heart rate adaptive multisegment image reconstruction in diagnostic cardiac computed tomography. *Visions*, *12*, 12–16.

Boone, J. M., Nelson, T. R., Lindfors, K. K., & Seibert, J. A. (2001). Dedicated breast CT: radiation dose and image quality evaluation. *Radiology*, *221*, 657–667.

Boone, J. M., Shah, N., & Nelson, T. R. (2004). A comprehensive analysis of DgN(CT) coefficients for pendant-geometry cone-beam breast computed tomography. *Medical Physics*, *31*, 226–235.

Bourne, R. (2010). *Fundamentals of digital imaging in medicine*. London: Springer.

Brant-Zawadzki, M. N. (2002). Screening CT: rationale. *Radiographia*, *22*(6), 1536–1539, discussion 1532–1536.

Brenner, D. J. (2006). Radiation risks in diagnostic radiology. In W. Huda (Ed.), *RSNA categorical course in diagnostic radiology physics: from invisible to visible—the science and practice of x-ray imaging and radiation dose optimization* (pp. 41–50). Oak Brook, IL: Radiological Society of North America.

Brunetti, J., Caggiano, A., Rosenbluth, B., & Bialotti, C. (2008). Technical aspects of positron emission tomography/computed tomography fusion planning. *Seminars in Nuclear Medicine*, *38*, 129–136.

Bushong, S. (2012). In *Radiologic science for technologists: physics, biology, and protection* (10th ed.). St. Louis, MO: Mosby.

Carlson, S. K., Bender, C. E., Classic, K. L., Zink, F. E., et al. (2001). Benefits and safety of CT fluoroscopy in interventional radiologic procedures. *Radiology, 219*, 515–520.

Carlson, S. K., Felmlee, J. P., Bender, C. E., Ehman, R. L., et al. (2005). CT fluoroscopy-guided biopsy of the lung or upper abdomen with a breath-hold monitoring and feedback system: a prospective randomized controlled clinical trial. *Radiology, 237*, 701–708.

Chang, C. H., Sibala, J. L., Fritz, S. L., Dwyer, S. J., 3rd., & Templeton, A. W. (1979). Specific value of computed tomography breast scanner (CT/M) in diagnosis of breast diseases. *Radiology, 132*, 647–652.

Chen, B., & Ning, R. (2002). Cone-beam volume CT breast imaging: feasibility study. *Medical Physics, 29*, 755–770.

Dalrymple, N. C., et al. (2005). Introduction to the language of three-dimensional imaging with multidetector CT. *Radiographies, 25*, 1409–1428.

Daly, B., & Templeton, P. A. (1999). Real-time CT fluoroscopy: evolution of an interventional tool. *Radiology, 211*, 309–315.

Dougherty, G. (2009). *Digital image processing for medical applications*. Cambridge, UK: Cambridge University Press.

Ebert, D. S., Heath, D. G., Kuszyk, B. S., et al. (1998). Evaluating the potential and problems of three-dimensional computed tomography measurements of arterial stenosis. *Journal of Digital Imaging, 11*, 1–8.

Fahrig, R., Dizon, R., Payne, T., et al. (2006). Dose and image quality for a cone-beam C-arm CT system. *Medical Physics, 33*, 4541–4550.

Froelich, J. J., et al. (1997). Guidance of non-vascular interventional procedures with real-time CT-fluoroscopy. *Electromedica, 66*, 50–55.

Furlow, B. (2014). CT image visualization: a conceptual introduction. *Radiologic Technology, 86*(2), 187–204.

Furtado, C. D., Aguirre, D. A., Dirlin, C. B., et al. (2005). Whole-body CT screening: spectrum of findings and recommendations in 1192 patients. *Radiology, 237*, 385–394.

Gisvold, J. J., Reese, D. F., & Karsell, P. R. (1979). Computed tomographic mammography (CT/M). *American Journal of Roentgenology, 133*, 1143–1149.

Glick, S. J., Thacker, S., Gong, X., & Liu, B. (2007). Evaluating die impact of x-ray spectral shape on image quality in flat-panel CT breast imaging. *Medical Physics, 34*, 5–9.

Goodnight, N., Wang, R., & Humphreys, G. (2005). Computation on programmable graphics hardware. *IEEE Computer Graphics and Applications, 25*(5), 12–15.

Gupta, R., Jones, S. E., Moovaart, E. A., & Pomerantz, S. R. (2006). Computed tomography angiography in stroke imaging: fundamental principles, pathologic findings, and common pitfalls. *Seminars in Ultrasound, CT, and MRI, 27*, 221–242.

Haghighat, M. B. A., Aghagolzadeh, A., & Seyerdarabi, H. (2011a). Multi-focus image fusion for visual sensor networks in DCT domain. *Computers and Electrical Engineering, 37*(5), 789–797.

Haghighat, M. B. A., Aghagolzadeh, A., & Seyerdarabi, H. (2011b). A non-reference image fusion metric based on mutual information of image features. *Computers and Electrical Engineering, 37*(5), 744–756.

Hohl, C., Suess, C., Wildberger, J. E., et al. (2008). Dose reduction during CT fluoroscopy: phantom study of angular beam modulation. *Radiology, 246*, 525–530.

Horton, K. M., et al. (2004). CT screening: principles and controversies. In E. K. Fishman, & B. Jeffrey (Eds.), *Multidetector CT: principles, techniques, and clinical applications* (pp. 549–559). Philadelphia, PA: Lippincott Williams & Wilkins.

Hsieh, J., Londt, J., Vass, M., Li, J., Tang, X., & Okerlund, D. (2006). Step-and-shoot data acquisition and reconstruction for cardiac x-ray computed tomography. *Medical Physics, 33*, 4236–4248.

Inoue, D., Gobara, H., Hiraki, T., Mimura, H., et al. (2012). CT fluoroscopy-guided cutting needle biopsy of focal pure ground-glass opacity lung lesions: diagnostic yield in 83 lesions. *European Journal of Radiology, 81*(2), 354–359.

James, A. P., & Dasarathy, B. V. (2014). Medical image fusion: a survey of the state of the art. *Information Fusion, 19*, 4–19.

Joe, B. N., & Sickles, E. A. (2014). The evolution of breast imaging: past to present. *Radiology, 273*, S23–S44.

Johnson, P. T., Fishman, E. K., Duckwall, J. R., Calhoun, P. S., & Heath, D. G. (1998). Interactive three-dimensional volume rendering of spiral CT data, current applications in the thorax. *Radiographics, 18*, 165–1987.

Kalender, W. (2005). *Computed tomography: fundamentals, system technology, image quality, applications*. Erlangen, Germany: Publicis Corporation Publishing.

Kalender, W. A., & Kryiakou, Y. (2007). Flat-detector computed tomography (FD-CT). *European Radiology, 17*, 2767–2779.

Katada, K. (1995). Further innovations in CT technology: CT fluoroscopy and real-time helical scan CT. *Medical Review, 53*, 1–11.

Katada, K., Kato, R., Anno, H., et al. (1996). Guidance with real-time CT fluoroscopy: early clinical experience. *Radiology, 200*, 851–856.

Kataoka, M. L., Raptopoulos, V. D., Lin, P. J., et al. (2006). Multiple-image in-room imaging guidance for interventional procedures. *Radiology, 239*, 863–868.

Kato, R., Katada, K., Anno, H., et al. (1996). Radiation dosimetry at CT fluoroscopy: physician's hand dose and development of needle holders. *Radiology, 201*, 576–578.

Keat, N. (2001). Real-time CT and CT fluoroscopy. *British Journal of Radiology, 74*, 1088–1090.

Kessler, M. L. (2006). Image registration and data fusion in radiation therapy. *British Journal of Radiology, 79*, S99–S108.

Kloeckner, R., dos Santos, D. P., Schneider, J., et al. (2013). Radiation exposure in CT-guided interventions. *European Journal of Radiology, 82*(12), 2253–2257.

Kyriakou, Y., & Kalender, W. (2007). Efficiency of antiscatter grids for flat-detector CT. *Physics in Medicine and Biology, 52*, 6275.

Kuszyk, B. S., & Fishman, E. K. (1998). Technical aspects of CT angiography. *Seminars in Ultrasound, CT, and MRI, 19*, 383–393.

Kuszyk, B. S., Beauchamp, N. J., Jr., & Fishman, E. K. (1998). Neurovascular applications of CT angiography. *Seminars in Ultrasound, CT, and MRI, 19*(5), 394–404.

Kwan, A. L. C., Boone, J. M., Yang, K., & Huang, S. Y. (2007). Evaluation of the spatial resolution characteristics of a cone-beam breast CT scanner. *Medical Physics, 34*, 275–281.

Lell, M. M., Anders, K., Uder, M., et al. (2006). New techniques in CT angiography. *Radiographics, 26*, S45–S62.

Machida, H., Yuhara, T., Mori, T., Ueno, E., et al. (2010). Optimizing parameters for flat-panel detector digital tomosynthesis. *Radiographics, 30*, 549–562.

Mah, D., & Chen, C. C. (2008). Image guidance in radiation oncology treatment planning: the role of imaging technologies on the planning process. *Seminars in Nuclear Medicine, 38*, 114–118.

Mahesh, M., & Cody, D. D. (2007). Physics of cardiac imaging with multiple-row detector CT. *Radiographics, 27*, 1495–1509.

Matsuoka, S., Yamashiro, T., Washko, G. R., et al. (2010). Quantitative CT assessment of chronic obstructive pulmonary disease. *Radiographics, 30*(1), 345–350.

McDermott, P., & Orton, C. (2010). *The physics and technology of radiation therapy*. Madison, WI: Medical Physics Publishing.

Meyer, M., Kalender, W. A., & Kyriakou, Y. (2010). A fast and pragmatic approach for scatter correction in flat-detector CT using elliptic modeling and iterative optimization. *Physics in Medicine and Biology, 55*, 99.

Mutic, S., et al. (2003). Quality assurance for CT simulators and computed tomography simulation process. Report to the AAPM Radiation Therapy Committee. Task Group No 66. *Med Phys, 30*, 2762–2792.

Nagel, W., et al. (1987). Recent clinical results on the use of QCT in diagnosis of osteoporosis. *Electromedica, 55*, 104–110.

Nair, A., Godoy, M. C., Holden, E. L., et al. (2012). Multidetector CT and postprocessing in planning and assisting in minimally invasive bronchoscopic airway interventions. *Radiographics, 32*(5), E201–E232.

National Lung Screening Trial Research Team. (2011). Reduced lung-cancer mortality with low-dose computed tomographic screening. *New England Journal of Medicine, 365*, 395–409.

Nawfel, R. D., et al. (2000). Patient and personnel exposure during CT fluoroscopy-guided interventional procedures. *Radiology, 216*, 180–184.

Ozaki, M. (1995). development of a real-time reconstruction system for CT fluoroscopy. *Med Rev, 53*, 12–17.

Paulson, E. K., et al. (2001). CT Fluoroscopy-guided interventional procedures—techniques and radiation dose to radiologists. *Radiology, 220*, 161–167.

Pomerantz, S. R., et al: Computed tomography angiography and computed tomography perfusion in ischemic stroke: s step-by-step approach to image acquisition and three-dimensional post processing, *Semin Untrasound* CT MRI, 29: 243–270, 206

Prat-Gonzalez, S., et al. (2008). Cardiac CT: indications and limitations. *J Nucl Med Technol, 36*, 18–24.

Pratx, G., & Xing, L. (2011). GPU computing in medical physics: a review. *Medical Physics, 38*(5), 2685–2697.

Prosch, H., Stadler, A., Schilling, M., et al. (2012). CT fluoroscopy-guided vs. multislice CT biopsy mode-guided lung biopsies: accuracy, complications and radiation dose. *European Journal of Radiology, 81*(5), 1029–1033.

RadiologyInfo.org (http://www.radiologyinfo.org/en/news/newdetarget.cfm?ID=5), a website produced by the Radiological Society of North America (RSNA) and the American College of Radiology (ACR). Accessed April 28, 2015.

Roth, R. G., Maidment, A. D., Weinstein, S. P., et al. (2014). Digital breast tomosynthesis: lessons learned from early clinical implementation. *Radiographics, 34*, E89–E102.

Sarti, M., Brehmer, W. P., & Gay, S. B. (2012). Low-dose techniques in CT-guided interventions. *Radiographics, 32*(1), 1109–1119.

Schlegel, W., et al. (Eds.). (2006). In *New Technologies in Radiation Oncology*. New York: Springer.

Schoepf, U. J., et al. (2007). Coronary CT angiography. *Radiology, 244*, 448–463.

Shaw, C. C., et al. (2005). Cone-beam CT with flat-panel detector: simulation, implementation and demonstration. In *Proceedings of the IEEE, Engineering in Medicine and Biology 27 Annual Conference*, pp. 4461–4464. Hong Kong, China.

Stoeckelhuber, B. M., Leibecke, T., Schulz, E., et al. (2005). Radiation dose to the radiologist's hand during continuous CT fluoroscopy-guided interventions. *Cardiovascular Interventional Radiology, 28*(5), 589–594.

Struffert, T., Deuerling-Zhen, Y., Kloska, S., et al. (2010). Flat detector CT in the evaluation of brain parenchyma, intracranial vasculature, and cerebral blood volume: a pilot study in patients with acute symptoms of cerebral ischemia. *American Journal of Neuroradiology, 31*, 1462–1469.

Tanenbaum, L. N. (2006). MDCT angiography: tips and techniques. *Applied Radiology, 4*, 3–10.

Udupa, J. K., & Herman, G. T. (Eds.). (2000). *3D imaging in medicine*, 2nd ed. Boca Raton, FL.: CRC Press.

Wagner, L. K. (2000). CT fluoroscopy: another advancement with additional challenges in radiation management. *Radiology, 216*, 9–10.

Webb, S. (2003). The physical basis of IMRT and inverse planning. *British Journal of Radiology, 76*, 678–689.

Yamao, Y., et al. (2010). Optimal scan parameters for CT fluoroscopy in lung interventional radiologic procedures: relationship between radiation dose and image quality. *Radiology, 255*(1), 233–241.

Zhang., et al. (2011). Volume visualization: a technical overview with a focus on medical applications. *Journal of Digital Imaging, 24*(4), 640–664.

# 13

# Three-Dimensional Computed Tomography: Basic Concepts

## OUTLINE



## LEARNING OBJECTIVES

On completion of this chapter, you should be able to:

1. explain each of the following with respect to three-dimensional concepts:
   - four coordinates used in 3D imaging
   - sequence in transforming 3D space or scene space
   - modeling
   - shading
   - lighting
   - rendering.
2. explain what is meant by each of the following:
   - slice imaging
   - projective imaging
   - volume imaging.
3. identify four major components of a typical 3D imaging system.
4. describe briefly each of the four major steps in creating 3D images.
5. describe briefly each of the following 3D rendering techniques:
   - surface rendering
   - volume rendering
   - intensity projection renderings.
6. compare each of the rendering techniques used in 3D imaging.
7. outline the characteristic features of stand-alone workstations for 3D imaging.

## LEARNING OBJECTIVES—cont'd

8. identify the role of the graphics processing unit in 3D imaging.
9. identify several clinical applications of 3D imaging.
10. state the meaning of virtual reality imaging (VRI).
11. describe the four technical aspects of VRI.
12. outline the clinical applications, advantages, and limitations of VRI.
13. identify several software tools for VRI.
14. explain briefly the features of flight path planning.
15. identify the role of the technologist in 3D imaging.

## KEY TERMS TO WATCH FOR AND REMEMBER

The following key terms/concepts are important to your understanding of this Chapter

**Average Intensity Projection (AIP)**
**flight path**
**Maximum Intensity Projection (MIP)**
**Minimum Intensity Projection (MinIP)**
**modeling**
**object delineation**
**qualitative information**
**quantitative information**
**ray tracing**
**rendering**
**segmentation**
**shaded surface display (SSD)**
**thresholding**
**virtual reality (VR) imaging**
**volume rendering**

Three-dimensional imaging in medicine is a method by which a set of data is collected from a 3D object such as the patient, processed by a computer, and displayed on a 2D computer screen to give the illusion of depth. Depth perception causes the image to appear in three dimensions.

In the past, 3D imaging created virtual endoscopy, a technique that allows the viewer to "fly through" the body in an effort to examine structures such as the brain, tracheobronchial tree, vessels, sinuses, and colon (Rubin et al., 1996; Vining, 1996). Additionally, 3D medical reconstruction movie clips are now available on the Internet. Viewers can now fly through the colon, skull, brain, lung, torso, and arteries of the heart. Additionally, 3D imaging unearthed a whole new dimension in examining contrast-filled vessels from volumetric spiral/helical computed tomography (CT) data and **CT angiography** (CTA), respectively. In radiology, 3D imaging has found applications in radiation therapy, craniofacial imaging for surgical planning, orthopedics, neurosurgery, cardiovascular surgery, angiography, and magnetic resonance imaging (MRI; Calhoun et al., 1999; Udupa, 1999; Wu et al., 1999). Another use of 3D imaging has been in the visualization of ancient Egyptian mummies without destroying the plaster or bandages (Yasuda et al., 1992). CTA is described further in Chapter 11. The advances in spiral/helical CT, such as the introduction of the new multislice CT scanners and MRI technologies, have resulted in an increasing use of 3D display of sectional anatomy. As a result, 3D imaging has become commonplace in most large-scale radiology departments, and researchers continue to explore the potential of 3D applications. For example, as early as 2002, Hoffman et al. (2002) used 3D and virtual fly-through techniques as a "noninvasive research tool" to evaluate Egyptian mummies. Pickhardt (2004) presented research findings on the use of 3D images for polyp detection in CT colonography, and Macari and Bini (2005) reviewed the current and future role of CT colonography. Recently, Dalrymple et al. (2005) described the technical aspects of 3D CT with multislice CT scanners and in particular reviewed the basics of intensity **projection** techniques (described later in this chapter). In addition, Lawler et al. (2005) described the use of 3D postprocessing, available with multislice CT scanners, in the study of adult ureteropelvic junction obstruction, and Fayad et al. (2005) discussed the use of 3D techniques to study musculoskeletal diseases of children. Furthermore, Beigelman-Aubry et al. (2005) discussed the use of 3D to assess diffuse lung diseases.

Later, several workers such as Fatterpekar et al. (2006), Lell et al. (2006), and Silva et al. (2006) reported the results of their 3D studies for evaluation of the temporal bone in CTA and virtual dissection at CT colonography, respectively. Additionally, Barnes (2006) reviewed the advancement of medical **image processing** including 3D techniques in a series of three articles. He quoted Dr. Richard Robb, PhD, from the Mayo Clinic in

Rochester, Minnesota, who stated that "we're in a very exciting **generation** in medical imaging. We've got very exciting opportunities to contribute to the well-being of humans around the world because of the advances in medical imaging we have available to us."

3D imaging has now evolved into what is now commonly referred to as 3D **volume visualization** using advanced visualization (AV) techniques to improve the visualization of diagnostic images in an effort to enhance the observers' interpretation of the large image datasets typical of CT and MR examination (Zhang et al., 2011). More recently, Bolan (1993) stated that "in fact, the quantitative attributes of AV technology have reached a new level of sophistication, prompting a paradigm shift in the delivery of patient information, in which 3D imaging may lead to better patient care."

Volumetric image **visualization tools** include three **volume-rendering algorithms** such as **multiplanar reconstruction (MPR),** surface **rendering** (SR) and volume rendering (VR), especially in CT (Dalrymple et al., 2005; Fatterpekar et al., 2006; Furlow, 2014; Udupa & Herman, 2000).

This chapter describes the fundamental concepts of 3D imaging in CT to provide technologists with the tools needed to enhance their scope and interaction with 3D **imaging systems** that are becoming more commonplace in imaging and therapy departments in hospitals. Furthermore, the basics of virtual reality imaging are introduced.

## RATIONALE

The purpose of 3D imaging is to use the vast amounts of data collected from the patient by **volume CT scanning** (and other imaging modalities such as MRI, for example) to provide both qualitative and **quantitative information** in a wide range of clinical applications. **Qualitative information** is used to compare how observers perform on a specific task to demonstrate the diagnostic value of 3D imaging. Quantitative information is used to assess three elements of the technique: precision (reliability), accuracy (true detection), and **efficiency** (feasibility) of the 3D imaging procedure (Furlow, 2014; Pierce et al., 2009; Russ, 2006; Udupa & Herman, 2000).

## HISTORY

In 1970 Greenleaf et al. produced a motion display of the ventricles by using biplane angiography. Soon after, the commercial introduction of CT renewed interest in medical 3D images because it was clearly apparent that a stack of contiguous CT sectional images could generate 3D information. This idea resulted in the development of specialized **hardware** and **software** for the production of 3D images and the development of algorithms for 3D imaging.

Technologic developments in 3D imaging continued at a steady pace throughout the 1970s, and by the early 1980s many CT scanners featured 3D software as an optional package. In the early 1980s, 3D imaging was discovered to be useful for clinical applications when several researchers began using the technology in craniofacial surgery, orthopedics, radiation treatment planning, and cardiovascular imaging. The box at the bottom of the page summarizes the major developments in the evolution of 3D imaging to the year 1991. Today, 3D imaging has evolved as a discipline on its own, demanding an understanding of various image-processing concepts such as preprocessing, visualization, manipulation, and analysis operations (Furlow, 2014; Russ, 2006; Udupa & Herman, 2000).

### BOX 13-1 Early History of Three-Dimensional Medical Imaging

- 1969—Hounsfield and Cormack develop the CT scanner.
- 1970—Greenleaf and colleagues report first biomedical 3D display: computer-generated oscilloscope images relating to pulmonary blood flow.
- 1972—First commercial CT scanner introduced.
- 1975—Ledley and colleagues report first 3D rendering of anatomic structures from CT scans.
- 1977—Herman and Liu publish 3D reconstructions of heart and lung of a dead frog.
- 1979—Herman develops technique to render bone surface in CT datasets; collaborates with Hemmy to image spine disorders.
- 1980—A CT scanner manufactured by General Electric features optional 3D imaging software.
- 1980-1981—Researchers begin investigating 3D imaging of craniofacial deformities.
- 1983—Commercial CT scanners begin featuring built-in 3D imaging software packages.
- 1986—Simulation software developed for craniofacial surgery.
- 1987—First international conference on 3D imaging in medicine organized in Philadelphia, Pennsylvania.
- 1990-1991—First textbooks on 3D imaging in medicine published; atlas of craniofacial deformities illustrated by 3D CT images published.

Adapted from Schwartz, B. (1994). *Medical Devices Research Reports, 1*, 8-10.

# FUNDAMENTAL THREE-DIMENSIONAL CONCEPTS

## Coordinates and Terminology

To understand how 3D images are generated in medical imaging, it is necessary first to identify and outline four coordinate systems that relate to the CT scanner, the display device, the object, and the scene. These coordinate systems are illustrated in Figure 13-1 and include the scanner coordinate system, *abc*; the display coordinate system, *rst*; the object coordinate system, *uvw*; and the scene coordinate system, *xyz*. Each of these is defined in Table 13-1.

The most familiar system is the *xyz*, the scene or Cartesian coordinate system, as it is commonly called. In this system, the *x*-, *y*-, and *z*-axes are positioned at right angles (orthogonal) to one another. The width of an object is described by the *x*-axis, whereas the height is described by the *y*-axis. The **z-axis,** on the other hand, describes the dimension of depth and adds perspective realism to the image.

Use of the coordinate system allows description of an object by measuring distances from the point of intersection, or zero point. Distances can be positive or negative from the zero point, and images can be manipulated to rotate about the three axes. This rotation occurs in what is referred to as *3D space*, and computer software helps the observer to **view** 3D space by displaying the front, back, top, and bottom of the object, providing a perspective from the observer's vantage point. The technique is known as *computer-aided visualization* or *3D visualization*, and the application of 3D visualization in medicine is called *3D medical imaging*.

In medicine, 3D imaging uses a right-handed *x*, *y*, and *z* coordinate system (Russ, 2006; Udupa & Herman, 2000) because images are displayed on a computer screen. The *x*, *y*, and *z* coordinates define a space in which multidimensional data (a set of slices) are represented. This space is called the *3D space* or *scene space*. The coordinate system helps to define the voxels (volume elements) in 3D space and allows use of the voxel information such as **CT numbers** or signal intensities in MRI to reconstruct 3D images.

## Transforming Three-Dimensional Space

Generally, 3D space can be subjected to a series of common 3D transformations (Fig. 13-2). The radiologic technologist can manipulate scene, structure, geometric, and projective transformations and control image processing and image analysis. The technologist may transform 3D space in four ways (Table 13-2).

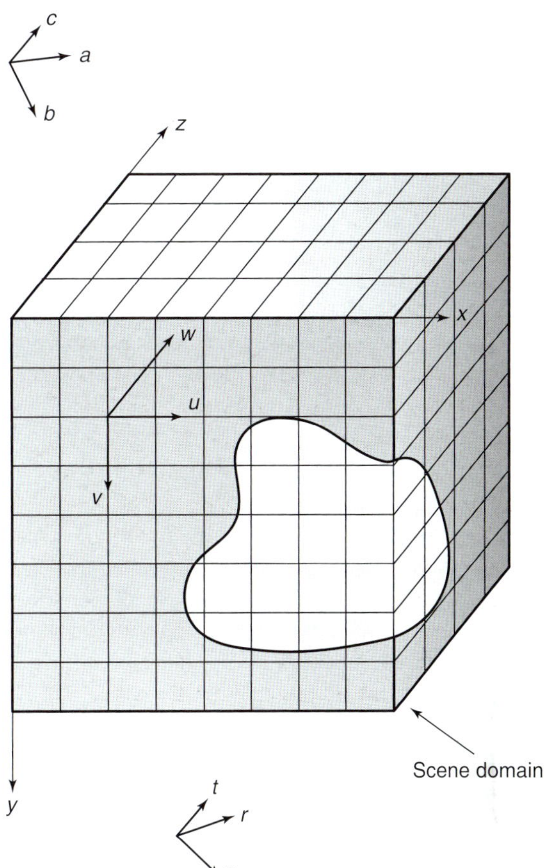


**FIGURE 13-1** Drawing provides graphic representation of the four coordinates used in 3D imaging: *abc*, scanner coordinate system; *rst*, display coordinate system; *uvw*, object coordinate system; *xyz*, scene coordinate system.

## Modeling

The generation of a 3D object using computer software is called ***modeling***. Modeling uses mathematics to describe physical properties of an object. According to one definition, modeling is "a computer simulation of a physical object in which length, width, and depth are real attributes. A model, with *x*-, *y*-, and *z*-axes can be rotated for viewing from different angles" (Microsoft Press, 2002).

Several modeling techniques are used. In extrusion, one of the most common techniques, computer software is used to transform a 2D profile into a 3D object. In Figure 13-3, for example, a square is changed into a box. Extrusion can also generate a wireframe model from a 2D profile. The wireframe is made up of triangles or polygons often referred to as *polygonal mesh*. Wireframes were common during the early development of 3D display in medicine, and they are still used in other applications.

**TABLE 13-1 Frequently Used Terms in Three-Dimensional Medical Imaging**

| Term | Definition |
|---|---|
| Scene | Multidimensional image; rectangular array of voxels with assigned values |
| Scene domain | Anatomical region represented by the scene |
| Scene intensity | Values assigned to the voxels in a scene |
| Pixel size | Length of a side of the square cross section of a voxel |
| Scanner coordinate system | Origin and orthogonal axis systems affixed to the imaging device |
| Scene coordinate system | Origin and orthogonal axis systems affixed to the scene (origin usually assumed to be upper left corner to first section of scene, axes are edges of scene domain that converge at the origin) |
| Object coordinate system | Origin and orthogonal axis systems affixed to the object or object system |
| Display coordinate system | Origin and orthogonal axis systems affixed to the display device |
| Rendition | 2D image depicting the object information captured in a scene or object system |

From Udupa, J. (1999). *Radiographics, 19*, 783-806.

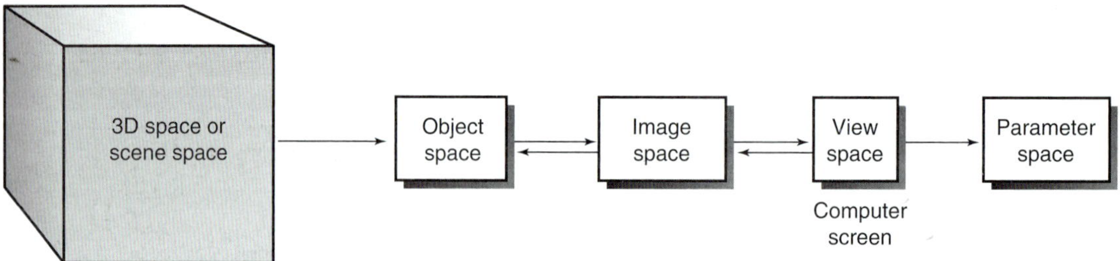


**FIGURE 13-2** Sequence of transformations characteristic of 3D imaging.

**TABLE 13-2 Transforming Three-Dimensional Space**

| Space Desired | Task Required |
|---|---|
| Image space | Translate, rotate, or scale scenes, objects, or surfaces |
| Object space | Extract structural information about the object from the 3D space |
| Parameter space | Take measurements from the image's view space on the computer screen |
| View space | View the 2D screen of the computer monitor |

During the next step of modeling, a surface is added to the object by placing a layer of pixels (image mapping) and patterns (procedural textures) on top of the wireframes. The radiologic technologist can control various attributes of the surface, such as its texture.

## Shading and Lighting

Shading and lighting also add realism to the 3D object. There are several shading algorithms, including wireframe shading, flat shading, Gouraud shading, and Phong shading. Each technique has its own set of advantages and disadvantages; however, a full discussion of shading algorithms is outside the scope of this chapter. The interested reader should refer to Russ (2006) for detailed descriptions of these algorithms.

Although shading determines the final appearance of surfaces of the 3D object, lighting helps us to see the shape and texture of the object (Fig. 13-4). Various lighting techniques are available to enhance the appearance of the 3D image; one of the most common is called **ray tracing,** which is described later in this chapter.

## Rendering

Rendering is the final step in the process of generating a 3D object. It involves the creation of the simulated 3D image from data collected from the object space. More specifically, *rendering* is a computer program that converts the anatomic data collected from the patient into the 3D image seen on the computer screen. With most 3D software, the object must be rendered before the effects of lighting and other attributes can be observed. Rendering therefore adds lighting, texture, and color to the final 3D image.

Two types of 3D rendering algorithms are used in radiology: surface rendering and volume rendering. Surface rendering uses only contour data from the set of slices in 3D space, whereas volume rendering makes use of the entire dataset in 3D space. Because it uses more information, volume rendering produces a better image than surface rendering, but it takes longer and requires a more powerful computer. Rendering is described subsequently.

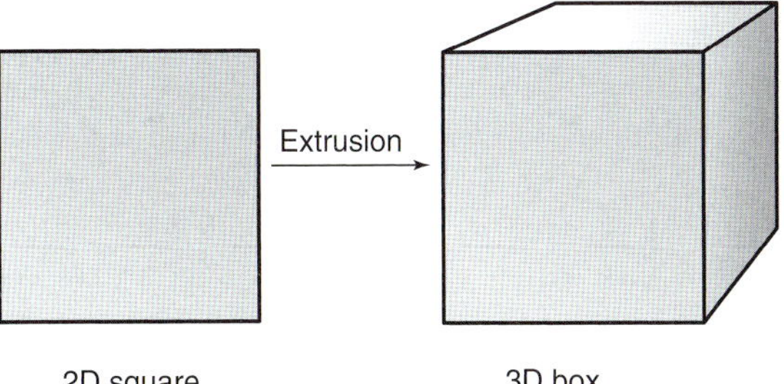


**FIGURE 13-3** Extrusion is a modeling technique that generates a 3D object from a 2D profile on a computer screen.

## CLASSIFICATION OF THREE-DIMENSIONAL IMAGING APPROACHES

Udupa and Herman (2000) identified three classes of 3D imaging approaches: slice imaging, projective imaging, and volume imaging.

### Slice Imaging

Slice imaging is the simplest method of 3D imaging. In 1975 CT operators generated and displayed coronal and sagittal images from the CT axial dataset. This technique is known as *multiplanar reconstruction* (MPR). In the past, other researchers such as Herman and Liu (1977), Marvilla (1978), and Rhodes et al. (1980) also used slice imaging to produce coronal, sagittal, and paraxial images from the transaxial scans. Today, MPR is available on all CT and MRI scanners. However, MPR does not produce true 3D

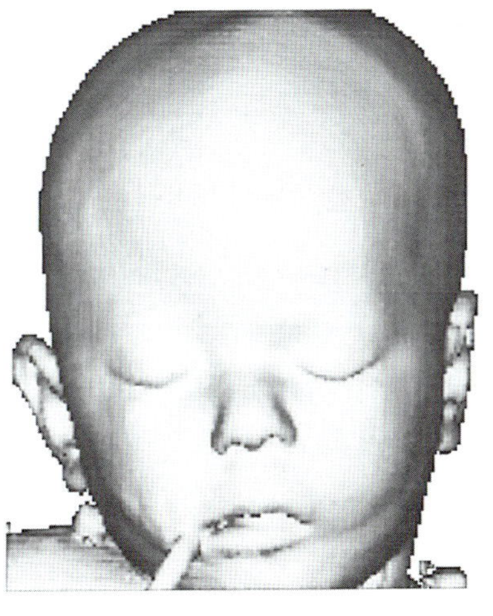
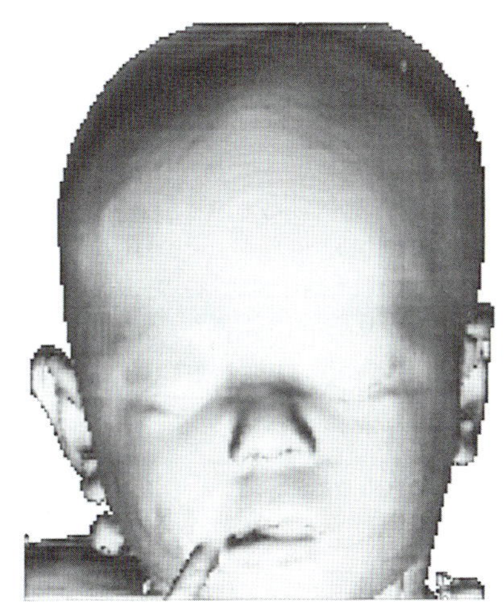
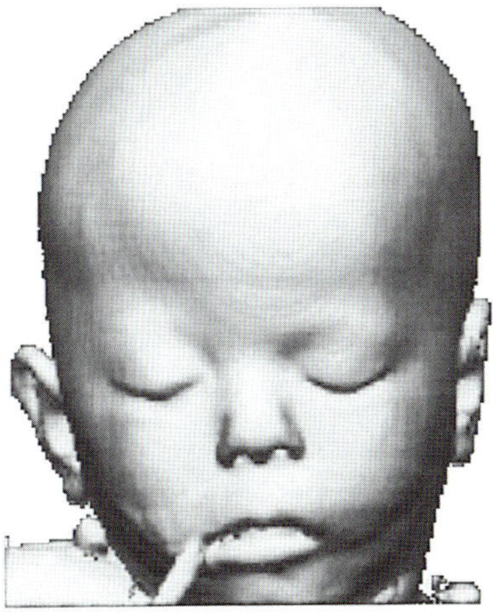
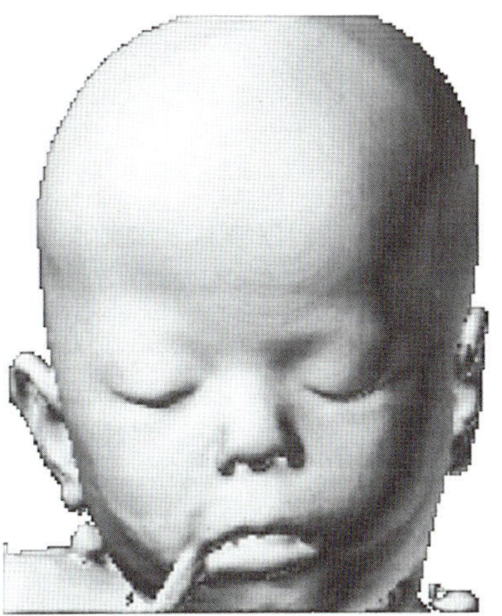

**FIGURE 13-4** The effects of lighting in a surface-rendered 3D image. As the light source is moved to different locations, various features of the image become clearly apparent.

images; rather it produces 2D images displayed on a flat computer screen (Dalrymple et al., 2005).

### Projective Imaging

Projective imaging is the most popular 3D imaging approach. However, it still does not offer a true 3D mode; it produces a "2.5D" mode of visualization, an effect somewhere between 2D and 3D. As Udupa and Herman (2000) explained:

> Projective imaging deals with techniques for extracting multidimensional information from the given image data and for depicting such information in the 2D view space by a process of projection. Surface rendering and volume rendering are two major classes of approaches available under projective imaging.

The technique of projection is illustrated in Figure 13-5. The contiguous axial sections represent the volume image data. Information from this volume image data is projected at various angles into the 2D view space.

### Volume Imaging

Volume imaging must not be confused with volume rendering. Volume rendering belongs to the class of projective imaging, whereas volume imaging produces a true 3D visualization mode. Volume imaging methods include holography, stereoscopic displays, anaglyphic methods, varifocal mirrors, synthalyzers, and rotating multidiode arrays (Jan, 2005). These methods are beyond the scope of this book.

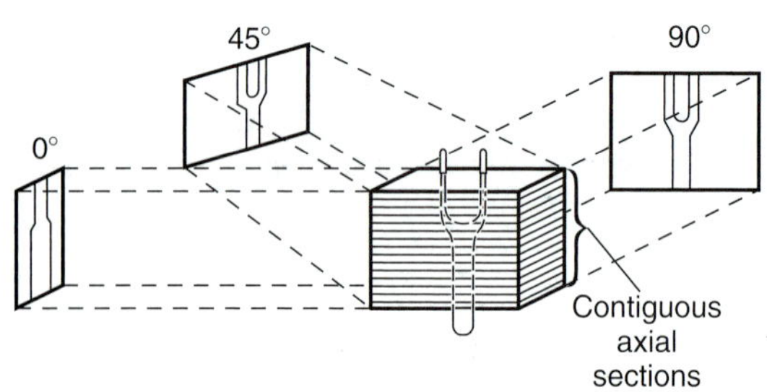


**FIGURE 13-5** The technique of projection used in 3D imaging. This is a major characteristic of projective imaging (one class of 3D imaging techniques).

## GENERIC THREE-DIMENSIONAL IMAGING SYSTEM

In a recent article describing the current perspective of 3D imaging, Udupa and Herman (2000) provided a framework for a typical 3D imaging system (Fig. 13-6). Four major elements are noted: **input,** workstation, **output,** and the user. *Input* refers to devices that acquire data. Imaging input devices, for example, would include CT and MRI scanners. The acquired data are sent to the workstation, which is the heart of the system. This powerful computer can handle various 3D imaging operations. These operations include preprocessing, visualization, manipulation, and analysis. Once processing is completed, the results are displayed for viewing and recording onto output devices. Finally, the user can interact with each of the three components—input, workstation, and output—to optimize use of the system.

The goals of each of the four major 3D imaging operations and the commonly used processing techniques are summarized in Table 13-3.

## TECHNICAL ASPECTS OF THREE-DIMENSIONAL IMAGING IN RADIOLOGY

### Definition of Three-Dimensional Medical Imaging

Dr. Gabor Herman of the Medical Image Processing Group at the University of Pennsylvania defines 3D medical imaging as "the process that starts with a stack of sectional slices collected by some medical imaging device and results in computer-synthesized displays that facilitate the visualization of underlying spatial relationships" (Herman, 1993). Additionally, Udupa and Herman (2000) emphasized that the term

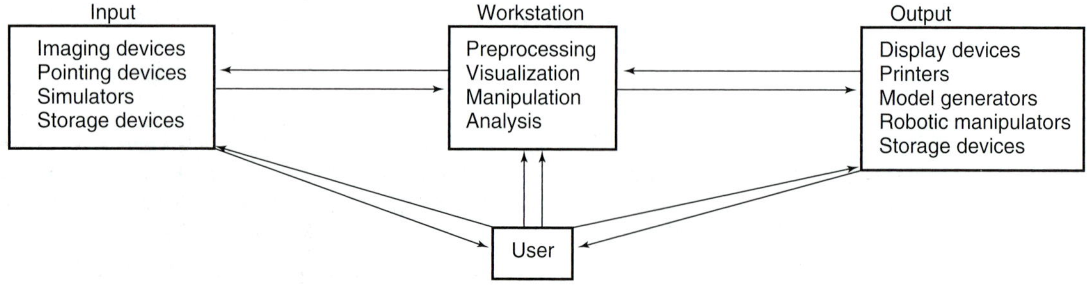


**FIGURE 13-6** A typical 3D imaging system consists of four major components: input, workstation, output, and the user.

**TABLE 13-3 Goals of Various Operations for Three-Dimensional Medical Imaging**

| Classes of 3D Operations | Goals | Commonly Used Operations | Goals |
|---|---|---|---|
| Preprocessing | To take a set of scenes and output computer object models or another set of scenes from the given set, which facilitates the creation of computer object models | Volume of interest | To reduce the amount of data by specifying a region of interest and a range of intensities of interest |
| | | Filtering | To enhance wanted (object) information and suppress unwanted (noise) background, other object information in the output scene |
| | | Interpolation | To change the level of discretization (sampling) of the input scene |
| | | Registration | Takes two scenes or objects as input and outputs a transformation that when applied to the second scene or object matches it as closely as possible to the first |
| | | Segmentation | To identify and delineate objects |
| Visualization | To create renditions from a given set of scenes or objects that facilitate the visual perception of object information | Scene-based visualization<br>• Section mode<br>• Volume mode | To create renditions from scenes |
| | | Object-based visualization<br>• Surface rendering<br>• Volume rendering | To create renditions from defined objects |
| Manipulation | To create a second object system from a given object system by changing objects or their relationships | Rigid manipulation | Operations to cut, separate, add, subtract, move, or mirror objects and their components |
| | | Deformable manipulation | Operations to stretch, compress, bend, and so on |
| Analysis | To generate a quantitative description of the morphology, architecture, and function of the object system from a given set of scenes or object system | Scene-based analysis | Quantitative descriptions obtained from scenes to provide ROI statistics and measurements of density, activity, perfusion, and flow |
| | | Object-based analysis | Quantitative descriptions obtained from objects on the basis of morphology, architecture, change over time, relationships with other objects in the system, and changes in these relationships |

Modified from Udupa, J. (1999). *Radiographics, 19*, 783-806.

*3D imaging* can also refer to the four categories of 3D operations: preprocessing, visualization, manipulation, and analysis.

Four steps are needed to create 3D images (Fig. 13-6):

1. **Data acquisition.** Slices, or sectional images, of the patient's anatomy are produced. Methods of data acquisition in radiology include CT, MRI, ultrasound, **positron emission tomography (PET),** single photon emission tomography, and digital radiography and fluoroscopy.
2. *Creation of 3D space or scene space.* The voxel information from the sectional images is stored in the computer.

3. *Processing for 3D image display.* This is a function of the workstation and includes the four operations listed previously.
4. *3D image display.* The simulated 3D image is displayed on the 2D computer screen.

These four steps vary slightly depending on which imaging modality is used to acquire the data. Each of the four steps is described in detail, using CT as the method of data acquisition.

## Data Acquisition

In CT, data are collected from the patient by x-rays and special electronic detectors. Data can be acquired slice by slice with a conventional CT scanner or in a volume with a spiral/helical CT scanner. During *slice-by-slice acquisition*, the **x-ray tube** and detectors rotate to collect data from the first slice of the anatomic area of interest; then the data are sent to the computer for **image reconstruction.** After the first slice is scanned, the tube and detectors stop, the patient is moved into **position** for the second slice, and scanning continues. The data from the second slice are transferred to the computer for image reconstruction. This "stop-and-go" technique continues until the last slice has been scanned.

One of the fundamental problems of slice-by-slice CT scanning is that certain portions of the anatomy may be missed because motion caused by the patient's respiration can interfere with scanning or be inconsistent from scan to scan. This problem can lead to inaccurate generation of 3D and multiplanar images. The final 3D image can have the appearance of steplike contours known as the *stairstep* **artifact.**

In **volume data acquisition,** a volume of tissue rather than a slice is scanned during a single breath-hold. This means that more data are sent to the computer for image reconstruction. **Volume scanning** is achieved because the x-ray tube rotates continuously as the patient moves through the **gantry.** One advantage of this technique is that more data are available for 3D processing, improving the quality of the resultant 3D image.

## Creation of Three-Dimensional Space or Scene Space

All information collected from the voxels that compose each of the scanned slices goes to the computer for image reconstruction. The voxel information is a CT number calculated from tissue **attenuation** within the voxel. In MRI the voxel information is the signal intensity from the tissue within the voxel. The result of image reconstruction is the creation of 3D space, where all image data are stored (Fig. 13-7).

Data in 3D space are systematically organized so that each point in 3D space has a specific address. Each point in 3D space represents the information (CT number or MRI signal intensity) of the voxels within the slice.

## Processing for Three-Dimensional Image Display

Processing, which is a major step in the creation of simulated 3D images for display on a 2D computer screen, is accomplished on the workstation. Although it is not within the scope of this chapter to address these operations in detail, it is important that technologists have an understanding of how sectional images are transformed into 3D images as illustrated in Figure 13-7.

In 1990, Mankovich et al. (1990) identified two classes of processing to explain 3D image display: voxel-based processing and object-based processing. *Voxel-based processing* "makes determinations about each voxel and decides to what degree each should contribute to the final 3D display," whereas *object-based processing* "uses voxel information to transform the images into a collection of objects with subsequent processing concentrating on the display of the objects."

Voxel-based processing was used as early as 1975 as a means of generating coronal, sagittal, and oblique images from the stack of contiguous transverse axial set of images—the technique of MPR. Although MPR is not a true 3D display technique, it does provide additional information to enhance our understanding of 3D anatomy (Beigelman-Aubry et al., 2005; Lell et al., 2006). In MPR, the computer scans the 3D space and locates all voxels in a particular plane to produce that particular image (Fig. 13-8).

Object-based processing involves several processing methods to produce a model (called an *object model* or *object representation*) from the 3D space and transforms it into a 3D image displayed on a computer screen. According to Russ (2006) and others (Dalrymple et al., 2005; Lell et al., 2006; Udupa & Herman, 2000), the processing of an object model into a simulated 3D image involves steps such as the following:

1. **Segmentation** is a processing technique used to identify the structure of interest in a given scene. It determines which voxels are a part of the object and should be displayed and which are not and should be discarded. **Thresholding** is a method of classifying the types of tissues, such as bone, soft tissue, or fat, represented by each of the voxels. The CT number is used for assigning thresholds to tissues.

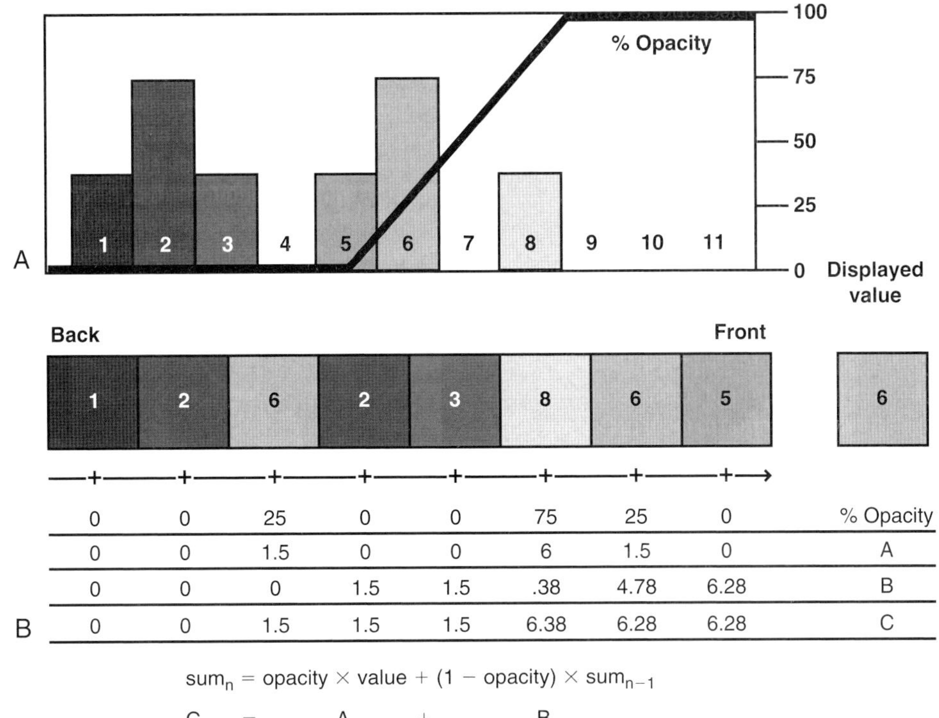


| | | | | | | | | |
|---|---|---|---|---|---|---|---|---|
| 0 | 0 | 25 | 0 | 0 | 75 | 25 | 0 | % Opacity |
| 0 | 0 | 1.5 | 0 | 0 | 6 | 1.5 | 0 | A |
| 0 | 0 | 0 | 1.5 | 1.5 | .38 | 4.78 | 6.28 | B |
| 0 | 0 | 1.5 | 1.5 | 1.5 | 6.38 | 6.28 | 6.28 | C |

$$sum_n = opacity \times value + (1 - opacity) \times sum_{n-1}$$

$$C = A + B$$

**FIGURE 13-14** Diagram illustrates volume-rendering technique. A histogram of the voxel values **(A)** in the data "ray" **(B)**.

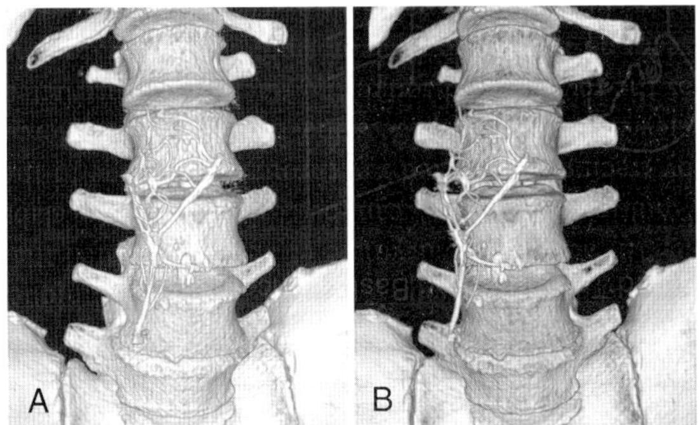


**FIGURE 13-15** SSD and volume-rendered images of an inferior vena cava filter overlying the spine. **A,** SSD creates an effective 3D model for looking at osseous structures in a more anatomic perspective than is achieved with axial images alone. It was used in this case to evaluate pelvic fractures not included on this image. **B,** Volume rendering achieves a similar 3D appearance to allow inspection of the bone surfaces in a relatively natural anatomic perspective. In addition, the color assignment tissue classification that is possible with volume rendering allows improved differentiation of the inferior vena cava filter from the adjacent spine. (From Dalrymple, N. C., Prasad, S. R., Freckleton, M. W., & Chintapalli, K. N. (2005). *Radiographics, 25,* 1409-1428. Figure and legend reproduced by permission of the Radiological Society of North America and the authors.)

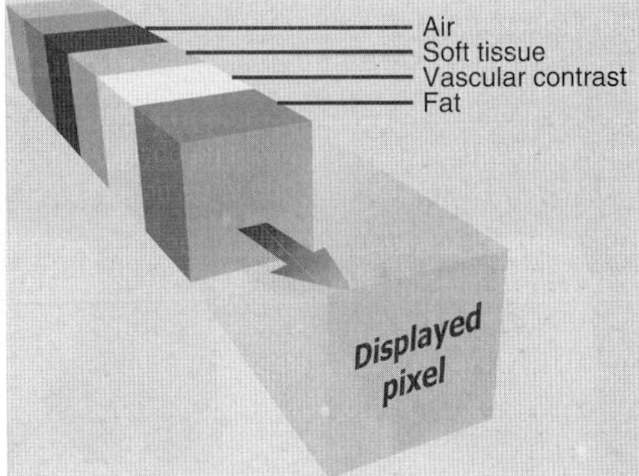


**FIGURE 13-16** Row of data encountered along a ray of projection. These data consist of attenuation information calculated in Hounsfield units. The value of the displayed 2D pixel is determined by the amount of data included in the calculation (slab thickness) and the processing algorithm (MIP, MinIP, or AIP, or ray sum). (From Dalrymple, N. C., Prasad, S. R., Freckleton, M. W., & Chintapalli, K. N. (2005). *Radiographics, 25,* 1409-1428. Figure and legend reproduced by permission of the Radiological Society of North America and the authors.)

The algorithms for sliding thin slabs (STS; or thickening of MPR images) include **average intensity projection (AIP), maximum intensity projection (MIP),** and **minimum intensity projection (MinIP).**

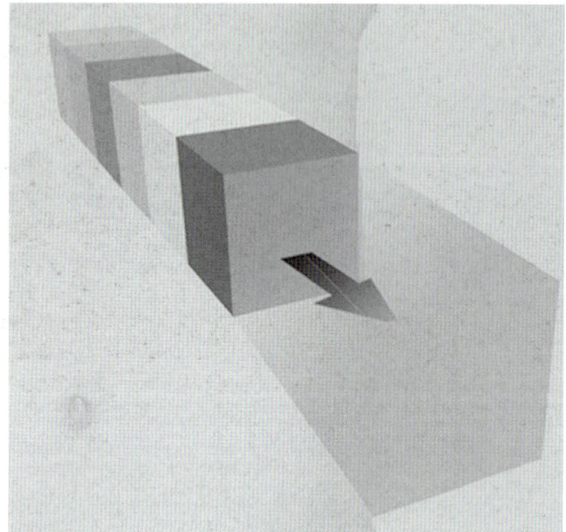

**FIGURE 13-17** AIP of data encountered by a ray traced through the object of interest to the viewer. The included data contain attenuation information ranging from that of air (black) to that of contrast media and bone (white). AIP uses the mean attenuation of the data to calculate the projected value. (From Dalrymple, N. C., Prasad, S. R., Freckleton, M. W., & Chintapalli, K. N. (2005). *Radiographics, 25,* 1409-1428. Figure and legend reproduced by permission of the Radiological Society of North America and the authors.)

## Average Intensity Projection

The AIP technique is an algorithm intended to create a thick MPR image by using the average of the attenuation through the tissues of interest to calculate the pixel viewed on the computer, as is clearly illustrated in Figure 13-17. The effects of the AIP algorithm on an image are shown in Figure 13-18.

## Maximum Intensity Projection

MIP is a volume-rendering 3D technique that originated in magnetic resonance angiography (MRA) and is now used frequently in CTA. In MIP, the algorithm is such that only the tissues with the greatest attenuation will be displayed for viewing by an observer, as is illustrated in Figure 13-19.

MIP does not require sophisticated computer hardware because, like surface rendering, it makes use of less than 10% of the data in 3D space. Figure 13-20 details the underlying concept of MIP. Essentially, the MIP computer program renders a 2D image on a computer screen from a 3D dataset (slices) as follows:

1. A mathematical ray (similar to the one in ray tracing) is projected from the viewer's eye through the 3D space (dataset).
2. This ray passes through a set of voxels in its path.
3. The MIP program allows only the voxel with the maximum intensity (brightest value) to be selected.

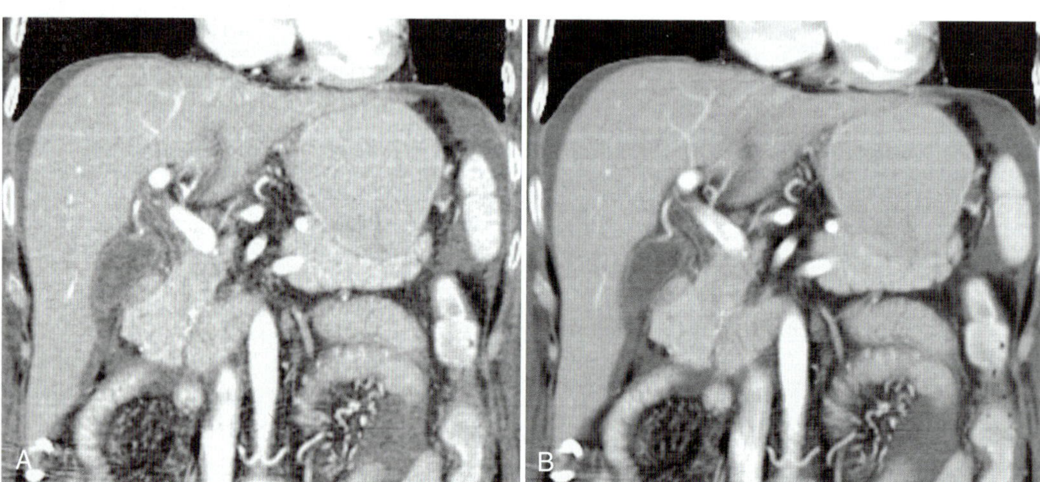


**FIGURE 13-18** Effects of AIP on an image of the liver. **A,** Coronal reformatted image created with a default thickness of 1 pixel (approximately 0.8 mm). **B,** Increasing the slab thickness to 4 mm by using AIP results in a smoother image with less noise and improved contrast resolution. The image quality is similar to that used in axial evaluation of the abdomen. (From Dalrymple, N. C., Prasad, S. R., Freckleton, M. W., & Chintapalli, K. N. (2005). *Radiographics, 25,* 1409-1428. Figure and legend reproduced by permission of the Radiological Society of North America and the authors.)

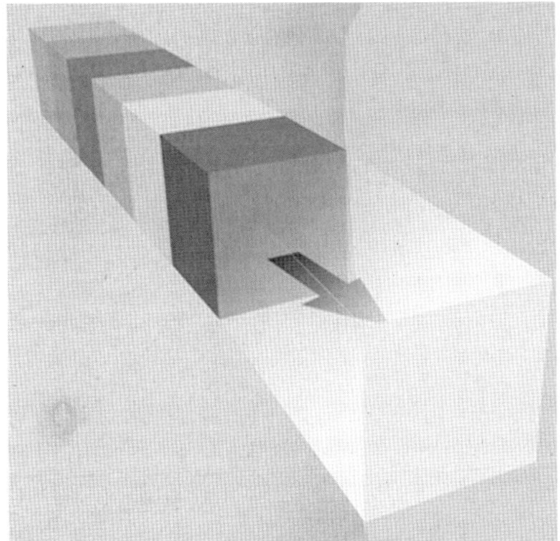

**FIGURE 13-19** MIP of data encountered by a ray traced through the object of interest to the viewer. The included data contain attenuation information ranging from that of air (black) to that of contrast media and bone (white). MIP projects only the highest value encountered. (From Dalrymple, N. C., Prasad, S. R., Freckleton, M. W., & Chintapalli, K. N. (2005). *Radiographics*, *25*, 1409-1428. Figure and legend reproduced by permission of the Radiological Society of North America and the authors.)

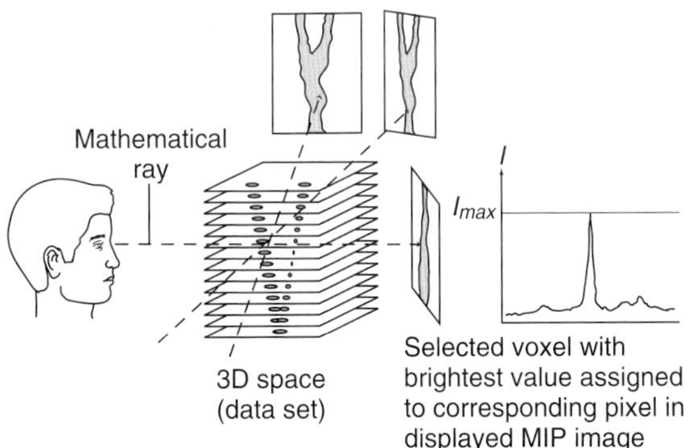


**FIGURE 13-20** MIP. The intensity, *I*, is plotted as a function of slice number.

4. The selected voxel intensity is then assigned to the corresponding pixel in the displayed MIP image.
5. The MIP image is displayed for viewing (Fig. 13-21).

A numerical illustration the MIP technique is clearly shown in Figure 13-22.

MIP images can also be displayed in rapid sequence to allow the observer to view an image that can be rotated continuously back and forth to enhance 3D visualization of complex structures with postprocessing techniques. Figure 13-23 shows multiple projections that vary only slightly in degree increments.

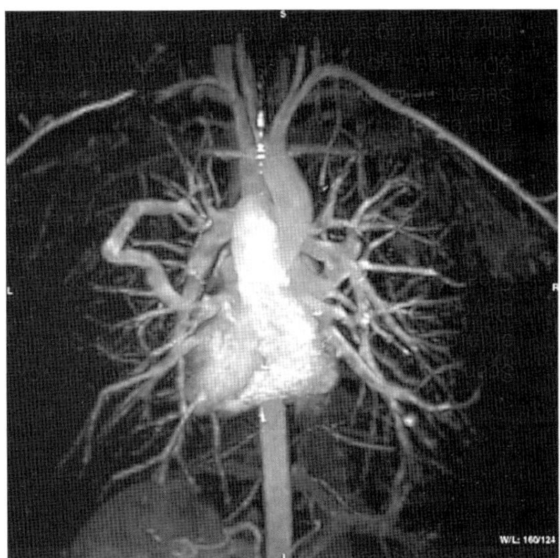


**FIGURE 13-21** Example of an MIP image. (Courtesy Vital Images, Minneapolis, Minn.)

In the past, one of the basic problems with the MIP technique is that "images are three-dimensionally ambiguous unless depth cues are provided" (Heath et al., 1995). To solve this problem, a depth-weighted MIP can be used to deal with the intensity of the brightest voxel, depending on its **distance** from the viewer. Other limitations include the inability of the MIP program to show superimposed structures because only one voxel (the one with the maximum intensity) in the set of voxels traversed by a ray is used in the MIP image display. Additionally, MIP generates a "string of beads" artifact because of volume averaging problems with tissues that have lower intensity values (Heath et al., 1995) and artifacts arising from pulsating vessels and respiratory motion.

A significant advantage of the MIP algorithm is that it has become the most popular rendering technique in CTA (Dalrymple et al., 2005; Fishman et al., 2006; Lell et al., 2006) and MRA (Dalrymple et al., 2005) because vessels containing contrast medium are clearly seen. Additionally, because MIP uses less than 10% of the volume data in 3D space, it takes less time to produce 3D-simulated images than to produce volume-rendering algorithms.

## Minimum Intensity Projection

The MinIP algorithm ensures that only the tissues with the minimum or lowest attenuation will be displayed for viewing by an observer. This is illustrated in Figure 13-24. Of the three intensity projection techniques, the MinIP is the least used; however, MinIP images may be useful in providing a "valuable

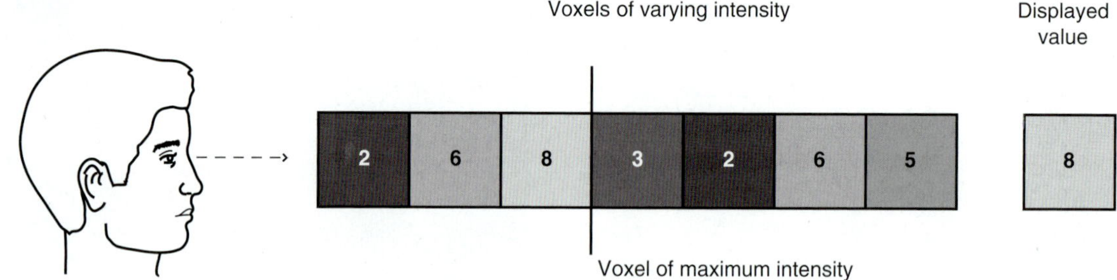


**FIGURE 13-22** Numerical representation of the MIP rendering technique.

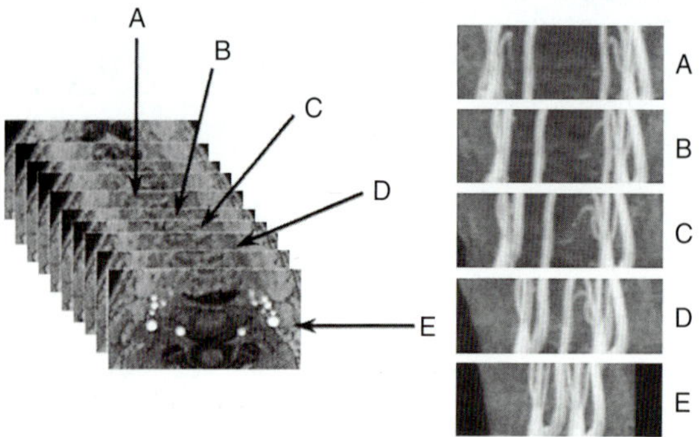


**FIGURE 13-23** A complete projection image at different viewing angles. Postprocessing of the 3D dataset can generate different views to allow the observers to rotate the image back and forth to enhance the perception of 3D relationships in the vessels. (From Laub, G., et al. (1998). *Electromedica, 66*, 68-75.)

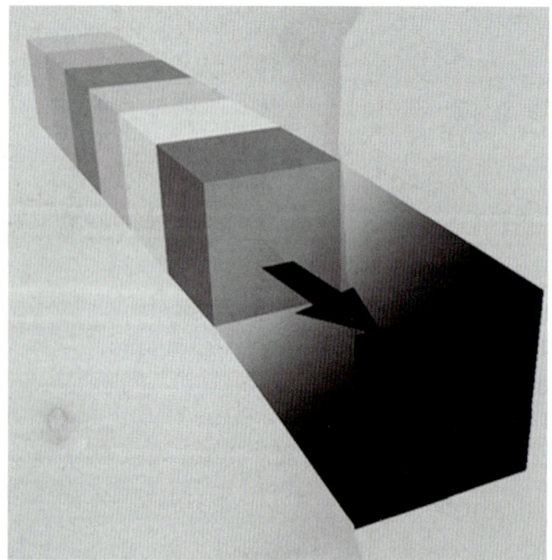

**FIGURE 13-24** MinIP of data encountered by a ray traced through the object of interest to the viewer. The included data contain attenuation information ranging from that of air (black) to that of contrast media and bone (white). MinIP projects only the lowest value encountered. (From Dalrymple, N. C., Prasad, S. R., Freckleton, M. W., & Chintapalli, K. N. (2005). *Radiographics, 25*, 1409-1428. Figure and legend reproduced by permission of the Radiological Society of North America and the authors.)

perspective in defining lesions for surgical planning or detecting subtle small airway diseases" (Dalrymple et al., 2005).

## Comparison of Three-Dimensional Rendering Techniques

One early comprehensive comparison of surface- and volume-rendering techniques was performed in 1991 by Udupa and Herman. They concluded that the surface method had a minor advantage over the volume methods with respect to display ability, clarity of the display, smoothness of ridges and silhouettes, computational time, and storage requirements. It had a significant advantage with its time and storage requirements.

Later in 1995, Heath et al. (1995) compared surface rendering, volume rendering, and MIP with spiral/helical CT during arterial portography. They compared the techniques with respect to seven parameters: depiction of 3D relationships, edge delineation, demonstration of overlapping structures, depiction of vessel lumen, percentage of data used, artifacts, and computational cost. Their results are summarized in Table 13-4. It is clearly apparent that volume rendering is superior in all parameters compared; however, it has the highest computational cost.

One of the characteristic features of the MIP technique is that it removes discarded data that have low values. The SSD technique removes all data with the exception of the data that are associated with the surface and, as mentioned in Table 13-4, typically uses less than 10% of the data. The effect of this data limitation is illustrated in Figure 13-25.

Although volume-rendered images may look similar to images generated by the SSD technique, the use of 100% of the acquired dataset and "assigning a full spectrum of opacity values and separation of the tissue classification and shading processes provide a much more robust and versatile dataset than the binary system offered by SSD" (Dalrymple et al., 2005). This is clearly shown in Figure 13-26.

In the past, 3D volume rendering has been shown to be useful in a wide range of clinical applications (Calhoun et al., 1999), including the thoracic aorta

**TABLE 13-4 Comparison of Three-Dimensional Rendering Techniques in Medical Imaging**

| | Surface Rendering | MIP | Volume Rendering |
|---|---|---|---|
| Depiction of 3D relationships | Good | Fair | Good |
| Edge delineation | Good | Good | Fair |
| Demonstration of overlapping structures | No | No | Yes |
| Depiction of vessel lumen | No | Depicts section that is 1 pixel thick | Yes |
| Percentage of data used | Typically <10% | Typically <10% | Up to 100% |
| Artifacts present in medical images | Many false surfaces | MIP artifact and background enhancement | Few if properly segmented |
| Computational cost | Low | Low | High |

From Heath, D. G., et al. (1995). *Radiographics*, 15, 1001-1011.

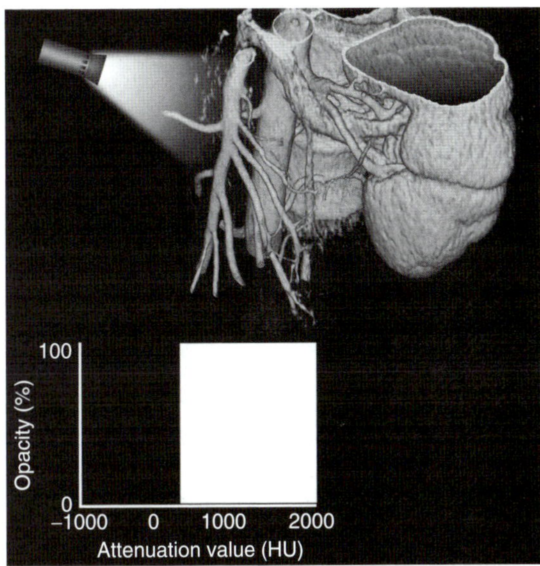


**FIGURE 13-25** Data limitations of SSD. Surface data are segmented from other data by means of manual selection or an attenuation threshold. The graph in the lower part of the figure represents an attenuation threshold selected to include the brightly contrast-enhanced renal cortex and renal vessels during CTA. The "virtual spotlight" in the upper left corner represents the grayscale shading process, which in reality is derived by means of a series of calculations. To illustrate the "hollow" dataset that results from discarding all but the surface-rendering data, the illustration was actually created by using a volume-rendered image of the kidney with a cut plane transecting the renal parenchyma. Subsequent editing was required to remove the internal features of the object while preserving the surface features of the original image. *HU*, Hounsfield units. (From Dalrymple, N. C., Prasad, S. R., Freckleton, M. W., & Chintapalli, K. N. (2005). *Radiographics, 25*, 1409-1428. Figure and legend reproduced by permission of the Radiological Society of North America and the authors.)

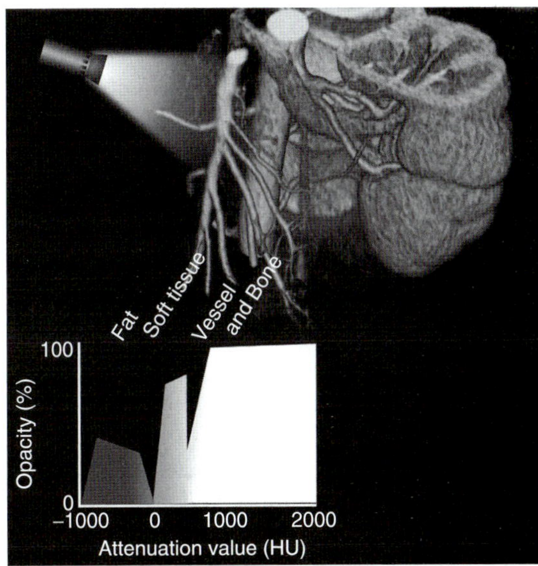


**FIGURE 13-26** Data-rich nature of volume rendering. The graph in the lower part of the figure shows how attenuation data are used to assign values to a histogram-based tissue classification consisting of deformable regions for each type of tissue included. In this case, only fat, soft tissue, vessels, and bone are assigned values, but additional classifications can be added as needed. Opacity and color assignment may vary within a given region, and the shape of the region can be manipulated to achieve different image effects. Because there is often overlap in attenuation values between different tissues, the classification regions may overlap. Thus, accurate tissue and border classification may require additional mathematical calculations that take into consideration the characteristics of neighboring data. *HU*, Hounsfield units. (From Dalrymple, N. C., Prasad, S. R., Freckleton, M. W., & Chintapalli, K. N. (2005). *Radiographics, 25*, 1409-1428. Figure and legend reproduced by permission of the Radiological Society of North America and the authors.)

(Wu et al., 1999) and in evaluating carotid artery stenosis (Leclerc et al., 1999).

More recent discussions of the use of 3D rendering techniques for clinical imaging using the data obtained from multislice CT scanners have been reported by several authors, including Kalender (2005), Dalrymple et al. (2005), Silva et al. (2006), Lell et al. (2006), and Fishman et al. (2006), and the interested student should refer to these original reports for more information.

When these 3D imaging techniques are used, these considerations are noted by several authors:

- "Appreciation of the strengths and weaknesses of rendering techniques is essential to appropriate clinical application and is likely to become increasingly important as networked 3D capability can be used to integrate real-time rendering into routine image interpretation" (Dalrymple et al., 2005).
- "My own expectation is that volume rendering with user friendly, preset evaluation protocols and intelligent editing tools will prevail as the method of choice in 3D display forms. However, they will only supplant and augment, but not replace 2D displays" (Kalender, 2005).
- "Generating 'boneless' 3D images became possible with modern postprocessing techniques, but one should keep in mind the potential pitfalls of these techniques and always double-check the final results with source or MPR images" (Lell et al., 2006).
- "Although different systems have unique capabilities and functionality, all provide the options of volume rendering and maximum intensity projection for image display and analysis. These two post processing techniques have different advantages and disadvantages when used in clinical practice, and it is important that radiologists understand when and how each technique should be used" (Fishman et al., 2006).
- "To avoid potential pitfalls in image interpretation, the radiologist must be familiar with the unique appearance of the normal anatomy and of various pathologic findings when using virtual dissection with two-dimensional axial and 3D endoluminal CT colonographic image datasets" (Silva et al., 2006).

## EDITING THE VOLUME DATASET

The purpose of editing the volume dataset is for clarity of 3D image display. This is well described by Fishman et al. (2006), and the interested reader should refer to the article for a detailed account of the procedure. In summary, Fishman et al. (2006) noted the following:

1. The volume-rendered 3D technique is much better than the MIP technique for a clear display of the anatomy of interest in the volume dataset. The MIP cannot display the 3D anatomic relationships, only because it is 2D.
2. For better clarity of anatomic details, the volume dataset must be edited by using thinner slabs compared with the entire volume dataset.
3. Several editing tools are available to change the appearance of the images. These include **windowing** (window width and window length manipulation), color and shading tools, and tools that allow the operator to change the opacity or the transparency of the image display (Fishman et al., 2006) and segmentation (Dalrymple, 2005; Lell et al., 2006).

## EQUIPMENT

Equipment for 3D image processing falls into two categories: the CT or MRI scanner console and stand-alone computer workstations. Both types of equipment use software designed to perform several image-processing operations, such as interactive visualization, multi-image display, analysis and measurement, intensity projection renderings, and 3D rendering. Most postprocessing for 3D imaging is done on stand-alone dedicated workstations that are becoming more popular as their costs decrease.

### Stand-Alone Workstations

A number of popular CT equipment manufacturers provide 3D packages for their CT and MRI scanners, and many are offering both 3D hardware and software packages for use in radiology (Furlow, 2014). Although the technical specifications of each workstation vary depending on the manufacturer, typical 3D processing techniques include software to perform the following:

- MPR
- Surface and volume rendering
- Slice plane mapping. This technique allows two tissue types to be viewed at the same time.
- Slice cube cuts. This is a processing technique that allows the operator to slice through any plane to demonstrate internal anatomy.
- Transparency visualization. This processing technique allows the operator to view both surface and internal structures at the same time.
- MIP, AIP, MinIP
- 4D angiography. This technique shows bone, soft tissue, and blood vessels at the same time and allows the viewer to see tortuous vessels with respect to bone.
- Disarticulation. This SSD technique allows the viewer to enhance the visualization of certain structures by removing others.

- Virtual reality imaging. Some workstations are also capable of virtual endoscopy, a processing technique that allows the viewer to look into the lumen of the bronchus and colon, for example. It is also possible for the viewer to "fly through" the 3D dataset. Virtual CT endoscopy is described later in this chapter.

### The Graphics Processing Unit

In Chapter 7, the **graphics processing unit (GPU)** was introduced as an innovative piece of computer hardware for use in medical physics and medical imaging. GPUs offer powerful computing performance in computer graphics and visualization (Goodnight et al., 2005). The basic architecture of the GPU can be found in a paper by Lefohn et al. (2006) for those readers who are interested in the hardware configuration. As reviewed by Pratx and Xing (2011), the GPU is now used in the following image reconstruction, image processing, dose calculation, and treatment plan optimization, as well as in other applications

## CLINICAL APPLICATIONS OF THREE-DIMENSIONAL IMAGING

One of the major motivating factors for the development and application of 3D imaging in medicine is to improve the communication gap between the radiologist and the surgeon. 3D imaging can help radiologists locate the condition and identify the best way to demonstrate it. Interestingly, craniofacial surgery was one of the first clinical applications of 3D medical imaging. Today, 3D medical imaging is used for applications ranging from orthopedics (bone fractures) to cardiovascular and pulmonary assessment to radiation therapy (Furlow, 2014; Calhoun et al., 1999; Dalrymple et al., 2005; Kalender, 2005; Lell et al., 2006; Silva et al., 2006; Udupa & Herman, 1991; Zonneveld & Fukuta, 1994).

The applications of 3D imaging in CT, MRI, nuclear medicine, and ultrasonography continue to evolve at a rapid rate, with most of the work done in CT and MRI. For example, 3D imaging has provided the basis for endoscopic imaging, where the viewer can fly through CT and MRI datasets with the goal of performing "virtual endoscopy." The most recent clinical application of 3D imaging is virtual dissection, "an innovative technique whereby the three-dimensional (3D) model of the colon is virtually unrolled, sliced open, and displayed as a flat 3D rendering of the mucosal surface, similar to a gross pathologic specimen" (Silva et al., 2006).

To date, clinical applications of 3D imaging in CT have been in the craniomaxillofacial complex, musculoskeletal system, central nervous system, cardiovascular system, pulmonary system, gastrointestinal system, and genitourinary system and in radiation treatment planning for therapy. In the craniomaxillofacial complex, for example, 3D imaging has been used to evaluate congenital and developmental deformities (shape of the deformed skull and the extent of suture ossification) and to assess trauma (bone fragment displacement and fractures).

3D imaging can demonstrate complex musculoskeletal anatomy and is used to study acetabular and calcaneal trauma, muscle atrophy, spinal conditions, and trauma of the spine, knee, carpal bones, and shoulder.

The development of CTA opened up additional avenues for the use of 3D imaging in the evaluation of cerebral aneurysms and arteriovenous malformations. It has been applied in CT of the gastrointestinal system, primarily imaging the liver, and genitourinary systems, primarily in kidney and bladder assessment. 3D volume rendering provides accurate evaluation of the thoracic aorta and internal carotid artery stenosis.

In radiation therapy, 3D imaging is especially used to superimpose isodose curves on sectional anatomy for the purpose of providing a clear picture of tissues and organs that receive various degrees of radiation dose. This is essential to demonstrate that the tumor receives maximum dose with minimum dose to the surrounding healthy tissues.

The student should refer to the reports by Beigelman-Aubry et al. (2005), Dalrymple et al. (2005), Fatterpekar et al. (2006), Fayad et al. (2005), Fishman et al. (2006), Furlow (2014), Lawler et al. (2005), Lell et al. (2006), Pickhardt (2004), and Silva et al. (2006) for more recent applications of 3D imaging in clinical practice.

## FUTURE OF THREE-DIMENSIONAL IMAGING

The first two decades of 3D imaging have generated a new and vast knowledge base on the technology of 3D imaging and on its clinical role in medicine. It has provided additional information that has helped in the diagnostic interpretation of images and enhanced communication among radiologists and surgeons and other physicians. Zhang et al. (2011) stated that "more recently, further efficiencies have been attained by designing and implementing volume rendering algorithms on graphics processing units (GPUs)."

Software developments will include improvements in segmentation techniques, for example. Also the cost of dedicated computer hardware and software will decrease, and personal computer-based workstations will become available. 3D rendering is now possible on the Internet.

As the technology for 3D imaging becomes increasingly sophisticated and better refined, clinical applications will expand and 3D imaging will be applied to other areas of the body. Applications in CT, MRI, and other imaging modalities will expand with the goal of providing additional information to support and validate diagnostic interpretation. Finally as noted by Furlow (2014):

> Increasing automation is also a common theme in registration, segmentation, ... of potential pathologies in CT datasets. This trend will continue, but it is unlikely to ever become error free. It will remain crucially important to visually inspect postprocessed images carefully, rather than relying entirely on the algorithms that produce them

## VIRTUAL REALITY IMAGING: TECHNICAL CONSIDERATIONS

The perception of 3D anatomy from 2D images often is difficult for some individuals because of the complexity of the structures in terms of their geometrical shapes. One solution is a 3D image-processing technique referred to as **virtual reality (VR) imaging.**

VR is a branch of computer science that immerses users in a computer-generated environment and allows them to interact with 3D scenes. The use of VR concepts to the creation of inner views of tubular structures is called *virtual endoscopy* (Vining, 1996). As explained by Higgins et al. (1998):

1. A virtual endoscope is a graphics-based software system used for simulating endoscopic exploration inside a 3D image. In virtual endoscopy, a 3D image acts as a "copy" or virtual environment, representing the scanned anatomy. With the use of computer-based rendering tools, a virtual endoscope produces endoluminal surface views inside the virtual environment similar to those from a real endoscope. A virtual endoscope permits essentially unrestricted exploration because it cannot traumatize the virtual environment.
2. A real endoscope uses optical video-assisted technology to help physicians interactively examine the inside of tubular anatomic structures. Because of the nature of the physical device, the patient may feel some discomfort, and other risks may also exist.

The topic of VR imaging received significant attention at the 2006 Computer Assisted Radiology and Surgery conference held in Osaka, Japan, where researchers presented their work on VR imaging applications. At the conference, Dr. Naoki Suzuki described a number of projects at Japan's Institute of Medical Imaging at the Jikei University School of Medicine in Tokyo and made an important comment that "our vision is to utilize VR techniques to improve medical simulation and navigation" (Barnes, 2006). VR applications in medicine, surgery, and 4D imaging range from diagnosis using 3D and 4D image datasets, **image fusion,** and virtual surgery to treatment simulation, human body dynamics, and medical education in virtual space (Barnes, 2006).

Several technical requirements must be taken into account when CT virtual endoscopy is considered. The four fundamental requirements are data acquisition, image preprocessing, 3D rendering, and image display and analysis (Fig. 13-27). Each of these techniques is currently being researched in an effort to improve the performance of virtual CT colonoscopy, although some controversy still exists among gastroenterologists and radiologists (Macari & Bini, 2005).

### Data Acquisition

The first step in virtual endoscopy imaging is careful selection of the **scan parameters** to be used for creating the dataset. These parameters, which optimize image display while reducing the radiation dose to the patient, include **slice thickness,** spiral/helical **pitch,** slice reconstruction overlap, and the scanning **exposure** technique (i.e., peak kilovolts [kVp], milliamperes [mA]/revolution, and scan time/revolution). In addition, the reconstruction parameters with respect to the type of **interpolation** algorithm and reconstruction kernel are also vital to the optimization of the procedure (Jolesz et al., 2007).

The selection of these parameters has been discussed in the literature for several virtual endoscopic examinations. For CT bronchoscopy, for example, Hopper (1999) reported that a 2-mm slice thickness, a pitch of 1, and a 75% slice reconstruction overlap produce significantly better virtual images than do a slice thickness of 4 to 8 mm, a pitch of 1.5 to 2, and a 25% to 50% slice overlap. In addition, Jolesz et al. (2007) recommended the use of parameters such as 120 kVp, 70 mA to 165 mA, 20 seconds' to 40 seconds' exposure time; 3-mm to 5-mm **collimation;** 5-mm to 6-mm table feed with a pitch of 1 or 2, 512 × 512 **matrix** size, and 180 degrees of linear interpolation

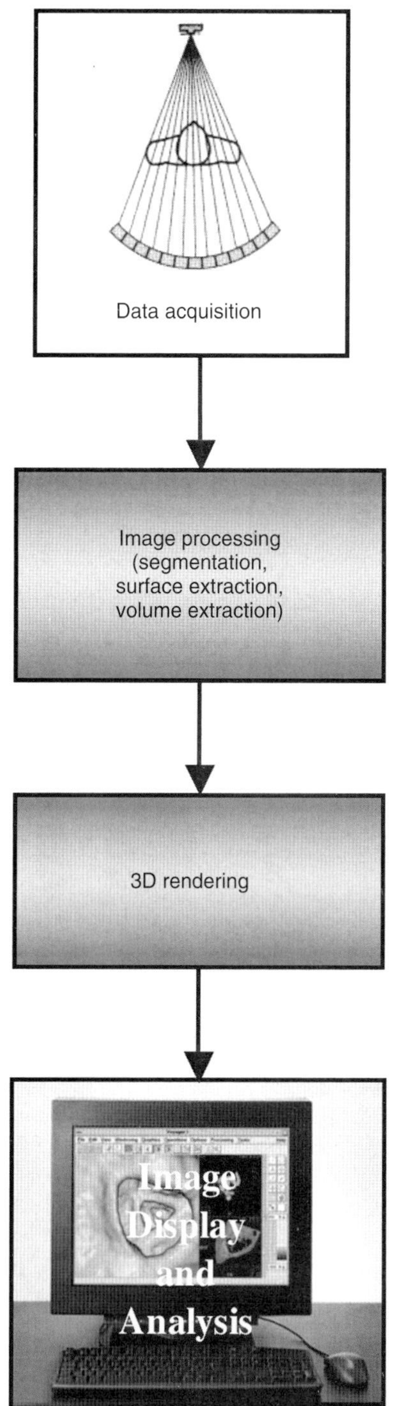


**FIGURE 13-27** Technical requirements for CT virtual endoscopy.

algorithm with a standard reconstruction algorithm; and 3-mm table incrementation. In addition, for virtual colonoscopy, proper patient **preparation** is an essential element of the success of the examination.

The imaging parameters represent a trade-off between radiation dose and image quality. The effect of slice thickness, for example, on image quality is demonstrated in Figure 13-28. Techniques for virtual studies in bronchoscopy, colonoscopy, and angioscopy also require consideration of several parameters such as kilovolts, mA/revolution, scan time/revolution, pitch, slice thickness, and so forth. The choice of the actual values for each will depend on the clinical facility and radiologists. For example, typical values for a virtual bronchoscopy may include 120 kV, 150 mA/30 revolutions, 1 s/revolution, and a pitch of 1, a slice thickness of, say, 5 mm, and an image index of 1 mm.

## Image Preprocessing

Preprocessing of image data is the next step after data acquisition (Fig. 13-27), and it is intended to optimize the images before they are subject to further processing and analysis. Preprocessing involves the use of various noise-filtering algorithms; image segmentation; defining paths through tubular structures; and other tools, such as classification, "cropping," and "cutting."

Image segmentation is an important step in the creation of VR images in CT. Segmentation can be performed by the operator (semiautomatic), or it can be done automatically. In the semiautomatic mode, the user selects objects to include in the dataset through the use of windowing. These objects are then prepared for rendering. For bronchoscopy the result of this procedure defines a 3D image mask that, as Higgins et al. (1998) explained, "excludes voxels not belonging to the lungs or major airways. All **mediastinal** structures, bones, and other extraneous structures are removed."

Another preprocessing tool is volume extraction, a technique where 3D surfaces are extracted from a volume (Doi et al., 2002; Takanashi et al., 1997). Another approach to volume extraction is one discussed by Lakarc and Kaufman (2003), a technique where voxels (rather than 3D surfaces) are extracted from a volume into another 3D segmented region. These techniques are beyond the scope of this book.

## Three-Dimensional Rendering

Two rendering techniques used in virtual CT endoscopy are surface rendering and volume rendering. Both have been used in various virtual CT examinations, but most experts agree that surface rendering is not best suited for use in CT VR imaging (Fleiter et al., 1997; Higgins et al., 1998) because of problems such as the production of **partial volume-averaging** artifacts.

Volume rendering provides the best results because it produces optimum visualization of the anatomy

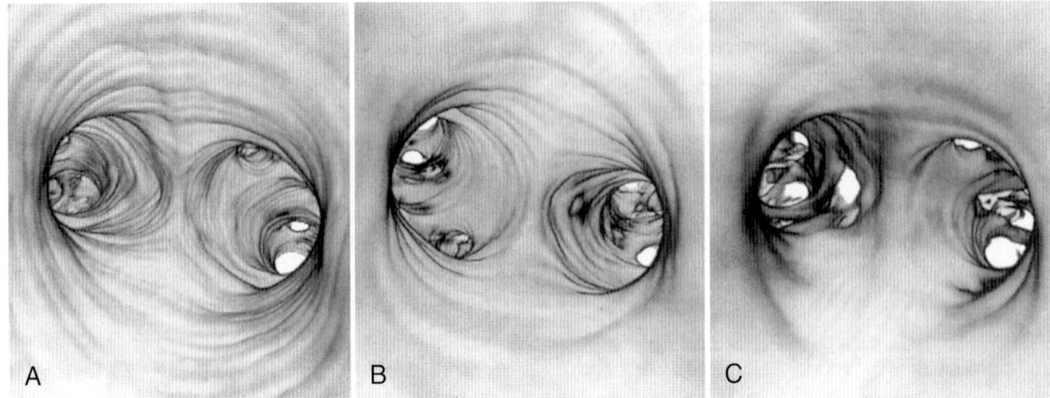


**FIGURE 13-28** The effect of slice thickness on image quality in CT virtual endoscopy. Thin (2-mm) slices produce sharper images **(A)** compared with 4-mm-thick **(B)** and 8-mm-thick **(C)** slices. These images were obtained with 50% reconstruction overlap using a pitch of 1. (From Hopper, K. D. (1999). *Seminars in Ultrasound, CT, and MRI, 20,* 10-15.)

(e.g., mucosal patterns and lesions), minimizes partial volume averaging artifacts, and adds life-like reality to images (Hopper, 1999, 2000; Tomandl et al., 2000; Vining, 1996). Hybrid rendering, or techniques that combine features of both surface- and volume-rendering algorithms, are under investigation (Vining, 1999).

## Image Display and Analysis

Because of the nature of the visualizations and interactivity needed for optimum viewing and evaluation of images, image display and analysis in CT VR imaging require powerful computer workstations (Fig. 13-29) to handle both data acquisition and advanced visualization processing operations.

As an alternative, some CT consoles may also facilitate virtual endoscopy. Virtual CT endoscopy includes image analysis techniques that allow the user to assess images interactively with a wide range of software tools. These tools will allow the user to perform a wide range of operations such as the following:

- Pan through a stack of 2D images (axial CT display mode)
- Fly through the 3D-rendered anatomic models (virtual endoscopic mode)
- Navigate the 3D anatomic models by using automated **flight path** programs
- Split or unfold anatomic models
- Identify pathologic conditions through computer-aided detection
- Depict topography of inner colonic surfaces as flattened structures (panoramic endoscopic display mode)

In an early study conducted by Beaulieu et al. (1999), the researchers found that panoramic endoscopy is more sensitive than virtual endoscopy for detection of polyps. This has been supported more recently by Silva et al. (2006).

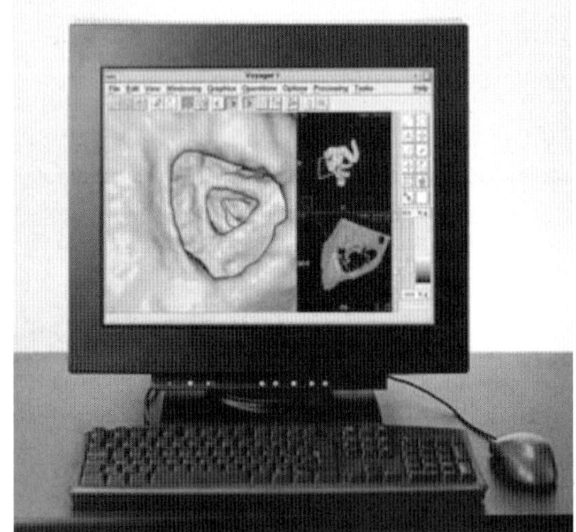

**FIGURE 13-29** A workstation for CT virtual reality image display and analysis. (Courtesy Phillips Medical Systems.)

## APPLICATIONS OF VIRTUAL ENDOSCOPY

Virtual endoscopy is evolving into a clinical tool with a wide range of applications. It has been used to evaluate the colon (virtual colonoscopy; Vining, 1999), airways (virtual bronchoscopy; Hopper, 1999), paranasal sinuses, bladder, spinal canal, and, more recently, the pancreatic and common bile ducts (virtual cholangiopancreatoscopy; Prassopoulos et al., 1998) and the inner ear (virtual labyrinthoscopy;

Tomandl et al., 2000). Figure 13-28 shows an example of images from CT virtual endoscopy of the bronchus. Of these applications, virtual colonoscopy, or CT colonoscopy as it is popularly referred to, has received much attention in the literature (Macari & Bini, 2005; Pickhardt, 2004; Silva et al., 2006).

## CT Colonoscopy: A Brief Overview

The developments in multislice CT scanners have provided the motivation for a number of improvements in CT colonoscopy. Furthermore, CT colonoscopy has become an integral tool for the evaluation of colorectal polyp detection, and it may be used routinely in the future for colorectal **screening** (Furlow, 2013; Macari & Bini, 2005; Silva et al., 2006; Taylor et al., 2006). In a special review of CT colonography, Macari and Bini (2005) pointed out that there are two schools of thought regarding the clinical use of CT colonography. Although some individuals are excited about the noninvasiveness of the technique, others believe that much more work needs to be done to not only demonstrate the **sensitivity** of CT colonography but also to emphasize that a certain degree of expertise in radiology is required for diagnostic interpretation of the images. Furthermore, the study by Taylor et al. (2006) concluded that "for polyps smaller than 1 cm, measurement differences of up to 2.5 mm are within the expected limits of inter- and intraobserver agreement for all measurement techniques. Automated and manual 3D polyp measurements are more accurate than manual 2D measurements."

### Display Tools

A typical CT colonoscopy imaging examination may generate a thousand plus images; therefore, it is important that radiologists have the necessary display tools to expedite the viewing of such a large image dataset. In this respect, CT manufacturers have provided various software tools for display, viewing, and interpretation. For example, Figure 13-30 shows one manufacturer's workstation display tools for CT virtual colonoscopy, and Figure 13-31 presents another display structure showing several views displayed simultaneously. For a detailed discussion of CT colonoscopy, the interested reader should refer to the paper by Furlow (2013).

### Virtual Dissection

A recent report by Silva et al. (2006) identified the work of various researchers who have used display tools such as 2D axial images, 2D MPR images,

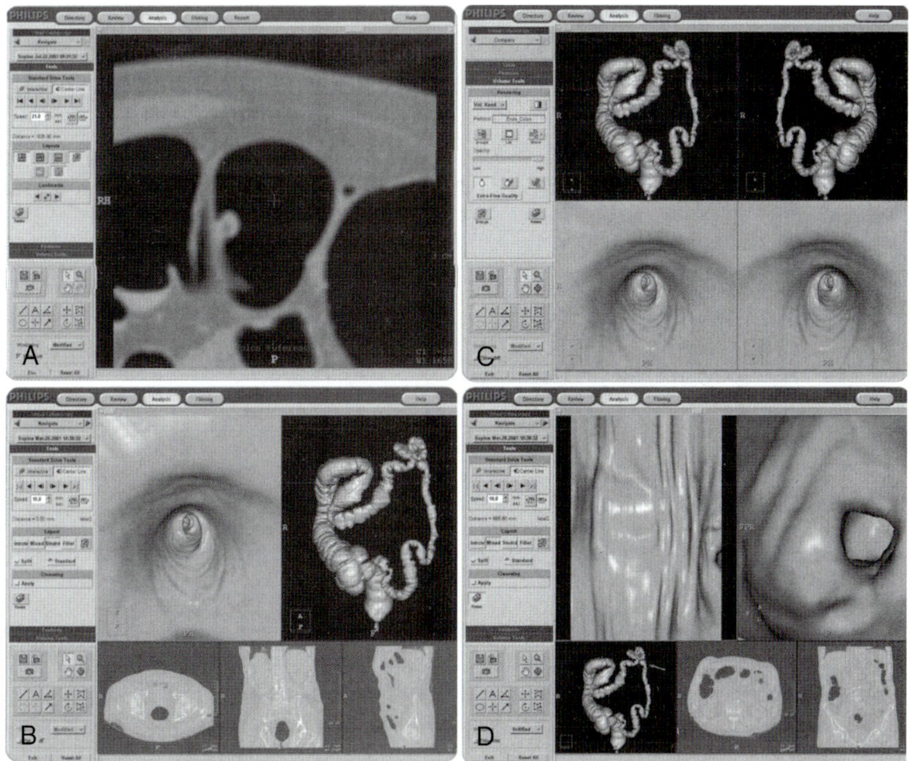

**FIGURE 13-30** Examples of various display tools for CT colonoscopy. **A,** 2D/3D mode for primary inspection. **B,** Forward/reverse mode. **C,** Compare mode. **D,** Layout mode with Forward Filet view, 2D, and other reference views. (Courtesy Philips Medical Systems.)

3D images, CAD images, and virtual dissection images. They note that virtual dissection

> is an innovative technique whereby the three dimensional (3D) model of the colon is virtually unrolled, sliced open, and displayed as a flat 3D rendering of the mucosal surface, similar to a gross pathologic specimen. This technique has the potential to reduce evaluation time by providing a more rapid 3D image assessment than is possible with an antegrade and retrograde 3D endoluminal fly-through. It may also ultimately improve accuracy by reducing blind spots present with endoluminal displays and by reducing reader fatigue (Silva et al., 2006).

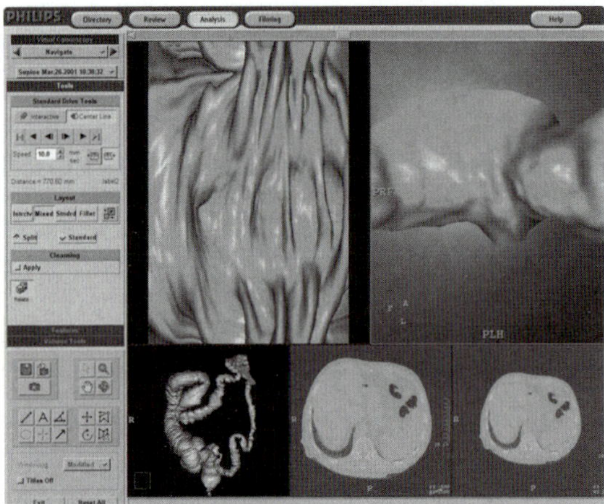


**FIGURE 13-31** Simultaneous display of Filet View and split view and the location on the volume-rendered reference view offers optimum flexibility in viewing images obtained in a CT colonoscopy examination. (Courtesy Philips Medical Systems.)

Figure 13-32 illustrates the technique of virtual dissection, whereas Figures 13-33 and 13-34 show the 3D volume-rendered image of the colon and the associated virtual dissection image of the same colon, respectively.

## ADVANTAGES AND LIMITATIONS

The various features of virtual endoscopy and real endoscopy have been described in the literature (Blezek & Robb, 1997; Higgins et al., 1998; Hopper, 1999; Vining, 1999). Early results indicate that virtual endoscopy offers unique features and advantages for gathering both endoluminal and extraluminal information. (Table 13-5 presents a comparison of the features of virtual and real bronchoscopy.) Virtual endoscopy can also reduce complications (e.g., infection and perforation) that could arise from real endoscopy.

More recently, and as pointed out by Macari and Bini (2005), although CT colonography is a useful tool for the evaluation of colorectal neoplasia, "substantial controversy" still exists as to its clinical efficacy. Silva et al. (2006), on the other hand, explained that the technique of virtual dissection can provide radiologists with more information to ensure accurate diagnosis compared with 3D endoluminal image displays.

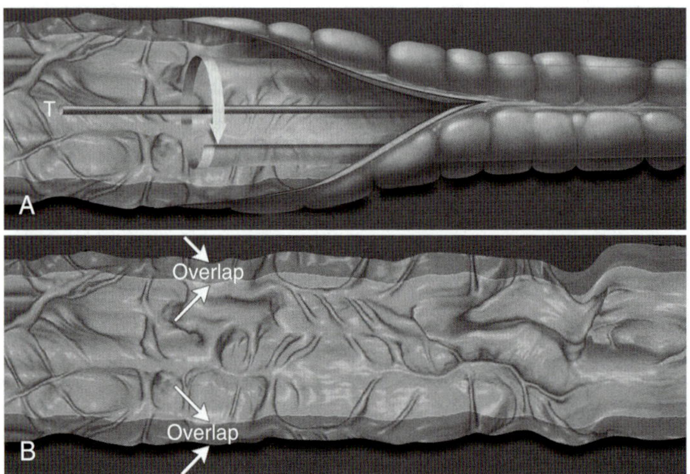


**FIGURE 13-32** Virtual dissection schema. **A,** The virtual dissection software slices the colon open and unfolds it longitudinally by reconstructing the axial CT source image data from the perspective of a virtual camera with an orientation perpendicular to the midline of the colonic tract. **B,** A 360-degree view of the inner colonic surface is presented as a flattened 3D panel with a few degrees of overlap at the edges (*arrows*). (From Silva, A. C., Wellnitz, C. V., & Hara, A. K. (2006). *Radiographics, 26*, 1669-1686. Figure and legend reproduced by permission of the Radiological Society of North America and the authors.)

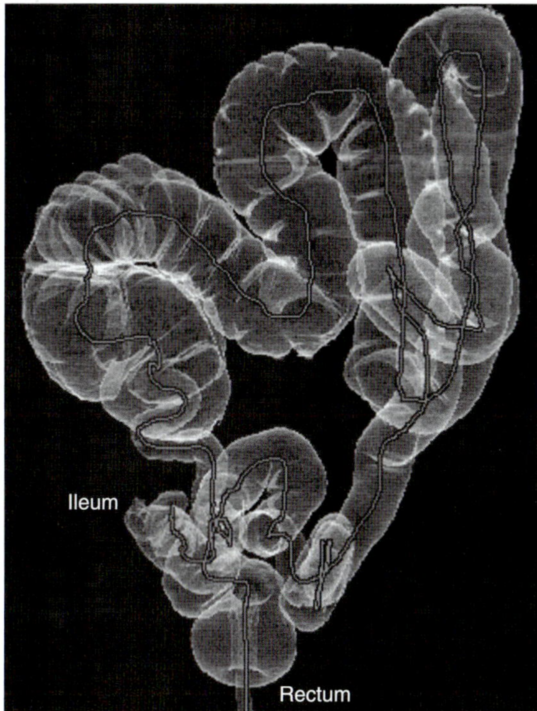


**FIGURE 13-33** Normal anatomy and common features in a complete CT colonographic examination. Volume-rendered image of the colon from the rectum to the distal ileum. (From Silva, A. C., Wellnitz, C. V., & Hara, A. K. (2006). *Radiographics, 26*, 1669-1686. Figure and legend reproduced by permission of the Radiological Society of North America and the authors.)

## SOFTWARE FOR INTERACTIVE IMAGE ASSESSMENT

A wide range of software tools for interactive image assessment is available, and CT vendors offer various categories of packages that feature a variety of visual and quantitative tools specifically for use in virtual endoscopy imaging.

### CT Endoscopy Tool

The CT virtual endoscopy tool is an advanced visualization package that can provide real-time fly through within and around tubular anatomy in the same manner that a real endoscope is used. The tool features an intuitive user interface that provides considerable flexibility in interactive image assessment. For example, mouse technology is used to guide the user through the anatomy. In addition, this tool can provide movie loop presentations, which can be recorded on videotape and used for remote **communications.**

A unique feature of the CT endoscopy tool is compositing (a volumetric imaging technique that displays bone, soft tissues, and vessels at the same time), also called *4D angiography*, which provides 3D images with a fourth dimension, opacity. There are other features as well, but they are beyond the scope of this chapter. For example, this tool makes use of an exclusive technology referred to as the

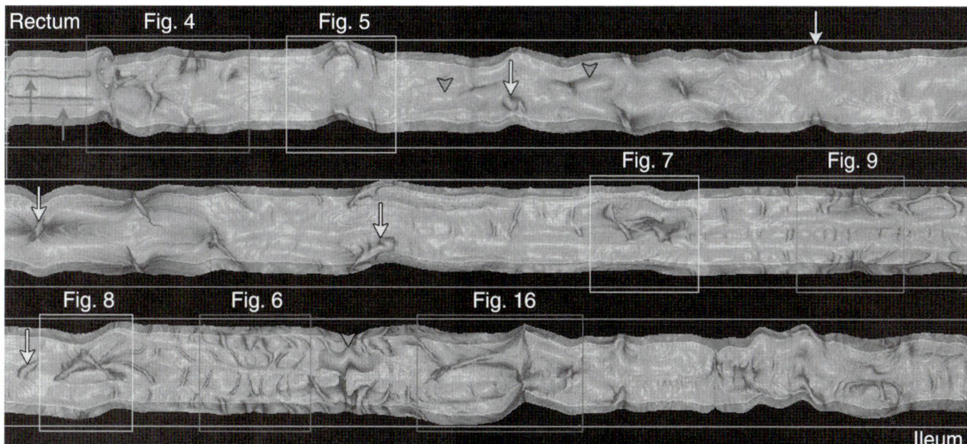


**FIGURE 13-34** Virtual dissection image of the same colon shows the rectal tube as an elongated horizontal structure that parallels the midline of the tract (*red arrows*). The adjacent section outlined in red (*Fig. 6* in image) shows the normal appearance of haustral folds in a straight colonic segment. Sections outlined in yellow (*Fig. 5, Fig. 7,* and *Fig. 8* in image) and yellow arrows indicate haustral distortions related to the degree of colonic curvature and the relative position of the haustral folds on the virtual dissection image. The section outlined in green (*Fig. 9* in image) and the green arrowheads indicate areas of the colon that contain residual fluid. (From Silva, A. C., Wellnitz, C. V., & Hara, A. K. (2006). *Radiographics*, 26, 1669-1686. Figure and legend reproduced by permission of the Radiological Society of North America and the authors. Please visit http://evolve.elsevier.com/Seeram/ to view a color image.)

*Filet View*, which is intended to display all details of the structure in a single view. Figure 13-35 shows Filet Views (Fig. 13-35, *B* and *C*) compared with the typical straight-on colonoscopy view (Fig. 13-35, *A*).

The tool can be used in a wide range of clinical applications, including pre-endoscopic evaluation of lesion screening and planning of endoscopic or surgical procedures. It also can be used to explore hollow anatomic structures such as the bronchus,

**TABLE 13-5 Comparison of Features of Virtual and Real Bronchoscopy**

| Virtual Bronchoscopy | Real Bronchoscopy |
|---|---|
| Imaging environment is a virtual environment as captured in a 3D CT image | Imaging environment is illuminated in in vivo endoluminal regions |
| Awareness is enhanced by the many display tools | Video is the only display tool |
| Many quantitative measurements can be taken | Quantitation is limited |
| Viewing direction is unrestricted | Only frontal views are possible |
| Views inside and outside solid structures are possible | Only endoluminal views are possible |
| Viewing geometry is controllable | Perspective is fixed |
| User can track 3D position during navigation | User must remember position of scope |
| Multiple simultaneous views are possible | User can see only one view at a time |
| Cine sequences can be recorded | High-quality video can be recorded |
| No information on the mucosal surface can be obtained | Detailed information on the mucosal surface can be obtained |
| Performance of interventional procedures with views is not possible without linkage to a real bronchoscope | Real intervention is possible |
| View quality is limited by image resolution | High-resolution video is used. |

From Hopper, K. D. (1999). *Seminars in Ultrasound, CT, and MRI. 20*, 10-15.

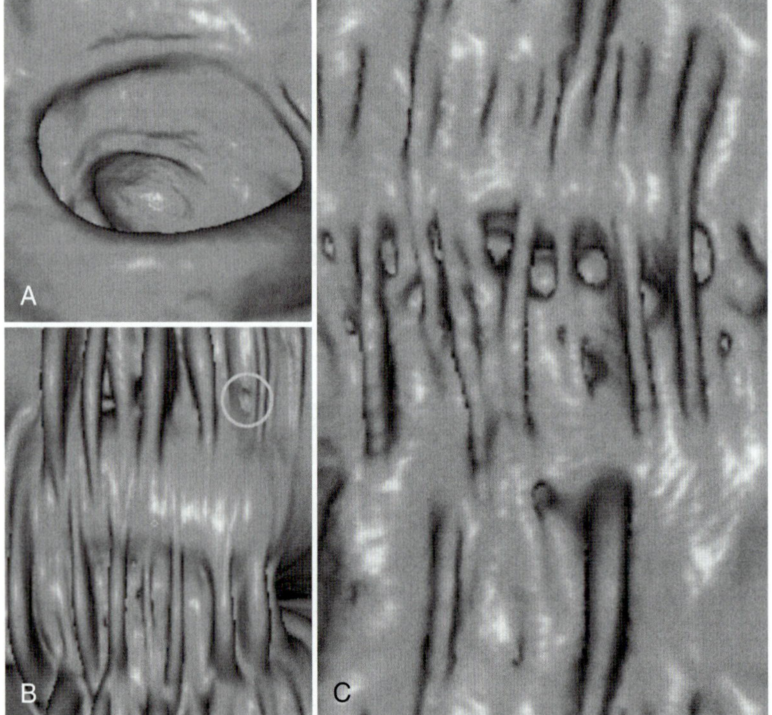


**FIGURE 13-35** The effect of the Filet view in demonstrating pathologies of interest compared with the typical straight-on view in CT colonoscopy. Although the straight-on view **(A)** does not show the polyp, the Filet View **(B)** shows not only the polyp (*circle*) but also the entire lumen of the colon on a single view as well as a polyp (*circle*). **C,** The diverticulosis and the haustral folds are demonstrated. (Courtesy Philips Medical Systems.)

colon, stomach, blood vessels, upper respiratory tract and larynx, paranasal sinuses, bladder, and spinal canal.

It is important to note that other interactive image assessment tools are currently available. These tools allow the user to perform several tasks, including:

- Showing the inside of hollow structures
- Correlating 3D endoscopic and MPR images, and a number of fly modes
- Provide image visualization of the colon for masses, cancers, polyps, and other lesions
- Perform 3D measurements, translucent rendering, automated 2D flights, real-time volume rendering, automatic and interactive navigation, and automatic segmentation, to mention only a few

### Three-Dimensional Navigator

The Navigator advanced visualization software provides a single icon-driven interface for ease of use and interaction with virtual endoscopic images. For example, it allows real-time navigation of structures, unique fly through of tubular structures, enhanced visualization capabilities for viewing inside cavities, smooth or edge detail viewing, and endoluminal viewing of 3D surface-rendered abnormalities of tubular structures (e.g., polyps, tumors, clots, vascular strictures or aneurysms, and blockages). The Navigator also allows the user to fly around the outside of the anatomy, such as in the circle of Willis.

It is important to note that other interactive image assessment tools are currently available. These tools allow the user to perform several tasks, including showing the inside of hollow structures, correlating 3D endoscopic and MPR images, and a number of fly modes, for example, to enhance diagnostic interpretation. Other tools can be used to provide image visualization of the colon for masses, cancers, polyps, and other lesions and allows the user to perform 3D measurements, translucent rendering, automated 2D flights, real-time volume rendering, automatic and interactive navigation, and automatic segmentation.

### Functional and Molecular Imaging Tools

The introduction of image fusion techniques for hybrid imaging such as PET/CT, which combines functional or molecular data with anatomic images produced by CT and MRI alone, will require new tools to assist radiologists to navigate and interpret multidimensional multimodality images. One such tool, called Osirix, was introduced and described by Rosset et al. (2006). This tool is also compliant with Digital Imaging and Communication in Medicine (DICOM) software that can be used to navigate through the huge image datasets generated by PET/CT scanners, multislice CT scanners that produce dynamic cardiac images, and MRI scanners that produce functional cardiac images.

## FLIGHT PATH PLANNING

Figure 13-36 shows the difference between surface-rendered and volume-rendered images in CT virtual

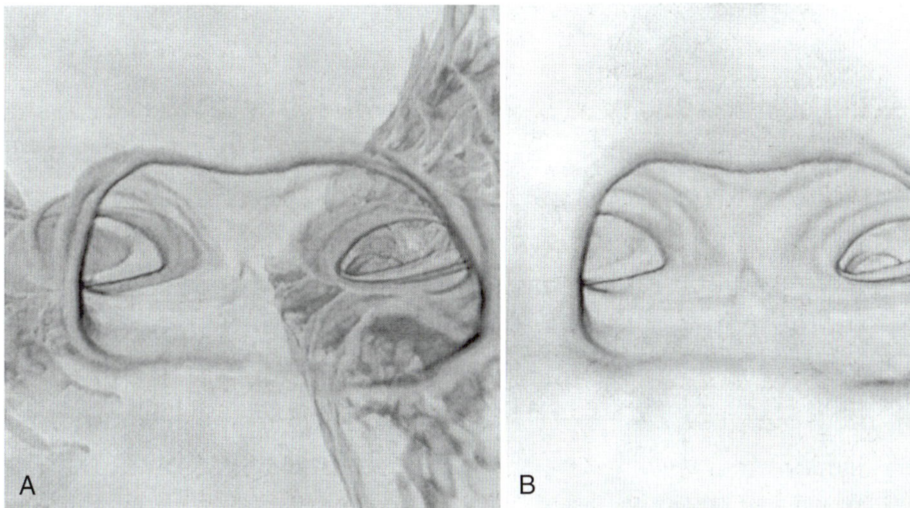


**FIGURE 13-36** Visual comparison of a surface-rendered image **(A)** and a volume-rendered image **(B)** in CT virtual endoscopy. Volume rendering not only improves image quality but also reduces artifacts caused by partial volume averaging. (From Hopper, K. D. (1999). *Seminars in Ultrasound, CT, and MRI, 20*, 10-15.)

endoscopy. Figure 13-37 shows the use of the navigation tool, one of the visualization tools of the CT endoscopy tool. Three orthogonal projections are created from the image dataset sent to the computer workstation to assist the user in navigating through the anatomy. First, the navigation path is outlined by placing markers along the anatomy to be examined. This is followed by a fly through of the path. The active virtual image is shown in the middle of the screen.

## Navigation

Successful navigation within the hollow anatomic region is essential so that structures of interest can be located and examined; such navigation depends on flight path algorithms. Because manual planning of flight paths can be time-consuming, algorithms have been developed that plan the flight paths automatically.

An early algorithm, described by Paik et al. (1998), uses a virtual "camera" to fly through the anatomy. First, the camera's position and orientation (straight pointing and angled pointing) are defined. Then a sequence of views along a path can be rendered as a sequence of frames to make a virtual endoscopic movie. Figure 13-38 presents an example of flight path planning. It shows a portion of a hollow anatomic structure in which a path has been defined. The path has three segments: start voxel ($V_{start}$) to $S_1$ segment, a segment from $S_1$ to $S_2$, and a segment from $S_2$ to an end voxel ($V_{end}$). The authors of the algorithm, Paik et al. (1998), explain this initial path selection as follows:

> Our algorithm determines the voxel on the surface that is closest to the start voxel, $S_1$, and the voxel closest to the end voxel, $S_2$. With a goal voxel of $V_{start}$, the algorithm computes a Euclidean distance map for the union of the surface and the voxels in the $V_{start}$ to $S_1$ line segment and the $S_2$ to $V_{end}$ line segment. This distance map is computed by assigning the goal voxel a distance of zero and iteratively assigning neighbor voxels the minimum Euclidean distance along a voxel path back to the goal voxel in a breadth first traversal until all voxels are reached. The algorithm follows the shallowest descent to find a path connecting $V_{end}$ to $V_{start}$.

## FUTURE OF CT VIRTUAL ENDOSCOPY

CT virtual endoscopy is an evolving diagnostic imaging tool. Investigators involved in research and practical applications of virtual endoscopy have noted that its future is promising. It has great potential as a diagnostic tool for providing better visualization of various anatomic structures such as the colon, airways, and other tubular structures, from both outside and inside perspectives. A special review of CT colonoscopy (Macari & Bini, 2005) indicates that it is a "viable alternative imaging tool for colorectal polyp detection" and that a good deal of education in CT colonoscopy techniques will be necessary if it is to have an impact on screening the colon for cancer.

Developments in the technology for virtual endoscopy, such as digital image-processing and computer visualization tools and automated techniques, can

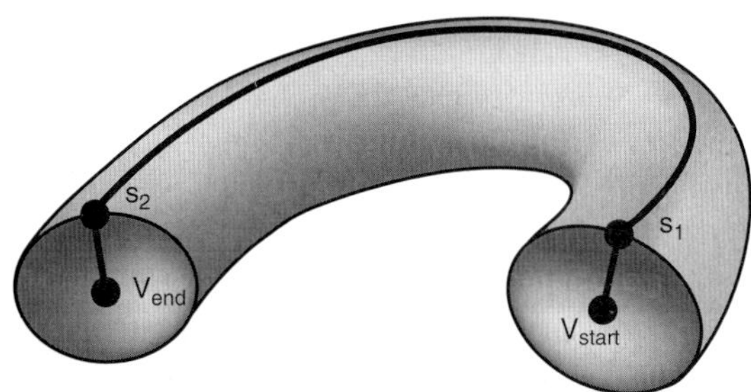


**FIGURE 13-38** An example of planning a flight path in virtual endoscopy. (From Paik, D. S., Beaulieu, C. F., Jeffrey, R. B., et al. (1998). *Medical Physics, 25,* 629-637.)

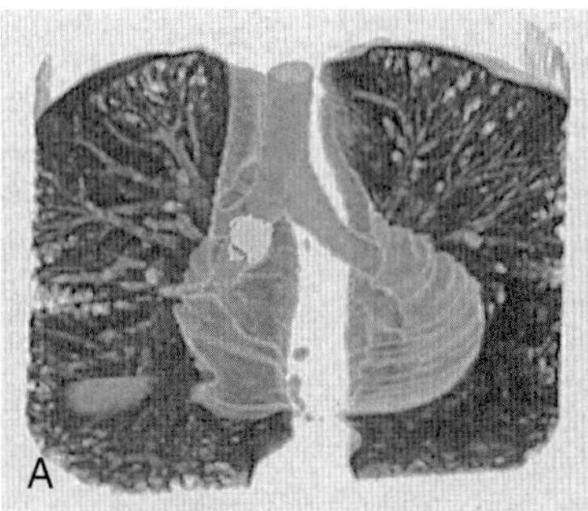

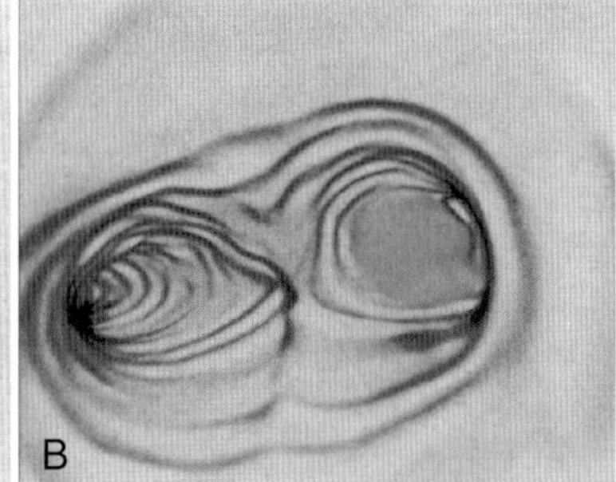

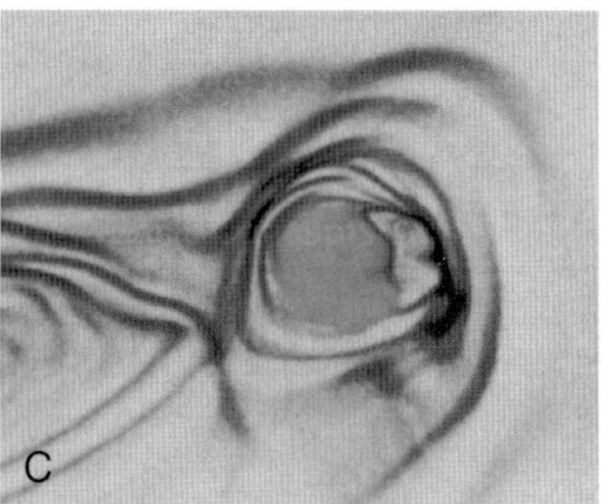


**FIGURE 13-37** The appearance of CT virtual endoscopy images of the bronchus. **A,** Holographic projection helps the observer to localize the exact position and shows the "flow in flight path." **B** and **C,** Virtual endoscopic images. (Courtesy Picker International, Cleveland, Ohio.)

only lead to improvement of virtual endoscopy as a clinically useful tool. Multislice CT technology will have a significant impact on the accuracy of virtual endoscopy. The vast amount of datasets collected from a multislice CT scanner will generate much better virtual endoscopic images than those obtained with single-slice datasets (Kopecky, 1999). A more recent study indicates that the use of computer software for making 3D measurements and manual 3D measurements provide more accurate results than 2D manual measurements (Taylor et al., 2006).

Already, studies are under way to validate the clinical usefulness of CT virtual endoscopy in a wide range of applications, including colonoscopy and bronchoscopy, which have received more attention in the literature because of the prevalence of colorectal and bronchogenic carcinoma (Higgins et al., 1998; Hopper, 1999; Vining, 1999). Some of these studies have shown that, compared with real endoscopy, virtual endoscopy is much cheaper and risk free and causes the patient less discomfort.

As noted by Vining (1999) and others such as Macari and Bini (2005), Silva et al. (2006), and Taylor et al. (2006), other factors must be considered before the use of virtual endoscopy becomes commonplace, such as the following:

- It must be better than real endoscopy in detecting various anatomic structures and pathologic conditions.
- Radiologists must be well versed in interpreting normal and abnormal features of the anatomy under investigation to make an accurate diagnosis.
- It should be easy to perform on patients and easy for technologists and radiologists to use.
- It should be available on all multislice CT scanners and MRI scanners.
- The use of computer software to make measurements provides more accuracy than manual measurements.
- It must be accepted by primary care physicians and insurance companies.
- It must be accepted by the public.

Finally, Brenner (2006) reported that currently, virtual colonoscopy is undergoing clinical trials in the United States and in other countries and will ultimately provide definitive results as to its efficacy as a screening tool for lesions in the colon. Later in this regard, the American College of Radiology (ACR) has made available a practice parameter and technical standard that represent a policy statement of the ACR (2014) entitled "ACR–SAR–SCBT-MR Practice Parameter for the Performance of **Computed Tomography (CT)** Colonography in Adults." This document provides guidance on the performance of CT colonography in the CT clinical environment. It includes topics such as indications and contraindications, qualifications and responsibilities of personnel, specifications of the examination, documentation and communication of the results, equipment specifications, radiation safety, quality control and improvement, safety, infection control, and patient education.

## ROLE OF THE RADIOLOGIC TECHNOLOGIST

As 3D and VR imaging technologies expand and become commonplace in medical imaging and radiation therapy, it is likely that radiologic technologists will play an increasing role in image-processing and analysis techniques. Radiologic technologists may need to expand their knowledge base to include a basic understanding of 3D imaging concepts. Educational programs in radiologic technology may need to offer courses that prepare students to perform 3D imaging and various types of **image postprocessing** for digital images in medical imaging.

In a study conducted by Pierce et al. (2009) the researchers sought to "reveal the frequency and type of postprocessing tasks being performed by computed tomography (CT) technologists by discussing the longitudinal results of the American Registry of Radiologic Technologists (ARRT) CT practice analysis surveys from 1993 to 2007." Having conducted a randomized survey of 3000 CT technologists, and selecting a sample of 1475 technologists who worked in CT performing a number of tasks including 3D CT imaging, they found that "the proportion of respondents responsible for 3-D imaging increased from 47% in 1993 to 74% in 2001 and to 82% in 2007 ($P < 0.001$). This increase occurred in all employment settings ($P < 0.001$) and department sizes ($P < 0.001$), including small departments. Daily frequency of occurrence grew from 4% in 1993 to 11% in 2001 and 53% in 2007 ($P < 0.001$)" and concluded that "routine 3-D postprocessing has become typical practice in radiology CT departments across all employment settings."

The ASRT (2015) developed an Educational Framework for 3-D Image Postprocessing to assist program planners "with a detailed listing of the knowledge and skill items required of individuals tasked with performing 3-D and other postprocessing reformations." In particular, the framework includes topics such as 2D (planar) and 3D (volumetric) anatomy, image postprocessing, pathology correlation in 3D postprocessing, procedures for 3D image postprocessing, and quality assurance in 3D image postprocessing.

To perform quality 3D medical imaging, including VR imaging, the technologist and the radiologist must work as a team. Technical ability in performing CT or MRI examinations and an understanding of the 3D imaging process and other postprocessing digital techniques are equally important. In addition, effective communication between the technologist and radiologist is vital in performing 3D medical imaging and will become even more important as the technology expands to provide new clinical applications.

## REVIEW QUESTIONS

Answer the following questions to check your understanding of the materials studied.

1. In 3D imaging, the space defined by *x, y,* and *z* coordinates that houses data from a set of slices acquired by multi-slice volume CT scanning is referred to as:
   A. 3D space or scene space.
   B. image space.
   C. parameter space.
   D. view space.
2. The final step in processing for 3D image display is:
   A. preprocessing.
   B. rendering.
   C. data filtering.
   D. object delineation.
3. In which of the following are pixels farthest away from the viewer darker, while those pixels closer to the viewer are lighter?
   A. volume rendering
   B. maximum intensity projection
   C. shaded surface display
   D. minimum intensity projection
4. Which of the following uses the entire data set in 3D space to produce good quality images but requires more computing power?
   A. shaded surface display
   B. surface shading
   C. maximum intensity projection
   D. volume rendering
5. Which of the following allows for the creation of inner views of tubular structures for the purpose of enhancing diagnosis?
   A. CTA
   B. surface shading
   C. virtual reality imaging
   D. CT fluoroscopy
6. Which of the following is a branch of computer science that allows users to interact with 3D scenes, in a computer-generated environment?
   A. artificial intelligence
   B. expert systems
   C. virtual reality
   D. programming
7. In transforming 3D space, which is the desired space for taking measurements from the image view space is a function of:
   A. image space.
   B. object space.
   C. parameter space.
   D. view space.
8. Which of the following 3D operations is intended to identify and delineate objects?
   A. segmentation
   B. filtering
   C. registration
   D. interpolation
9. The percentage of data from 3D image space used by MIP rendered 3D algorithms is typically:
   A. 100%.
   B. 10%.
   C. 25%.
   D. 50%.
10. Volume rendering algorithms typically use ____ of the data in 3D space:
    A. 100%
    B. 50%
    C. 25%
    D. 10%

## REFERENCES

ASRT. (2015). *Educational Framework for 3-D Image Postprocessing.* http://www.asrt.org/docs/default-source/educators/ed_frmwrk_3dimagepostprocessingfinal_011411.pdf?sfvrsn=2. Accessed Jan 2015.

Barnes, E. (2006). *Medical image processing has room to grow: parts 1, 2, and 3.* AuntMinni.com. Accessed December 2006.

Beaulieu, C. F., Jeffrey, R. B., Jr., Karadi, C., Paik, D. S., & Napel, S. (1999). Display modes for CT colonography. *Radiology, 212,* 203–212.

Beigelman-Aubry, C., Hill, C., Guibal, A., Savatovsky, J., & Grenier, P. A. (2005). Multi-detector row CT and postprocessing techniques in the assessment of diffuse lung disease. *Radiographics, 25,* 1639–1652.

Blezek, D. J., & Robb, R. A. (1997). Evaluating virtual endoscopy for clinical use. *Journal of Digital Imaging, 10*, 51–55.

Brenner, D. J. (2006). Radiation risks in diagnostic radiology. In *RSNA categorical course in diagnostic radiology: from invisible to visible—the science and practice of x-ray imaging and radiation dose optimization* (pp. 41–50). Oak Brook, IL: Radiological Society of North America.

Bolan, C. (1993). Routine 3D imaging becomes a reality. *Applied Radiology*, 27-31.

Calhoun, P. S., Kuszyk, B. S., Heath, D. G., Carley, J. C., & Fishman, E. K. (1999). Three-dimensional volume rendering of spiral CT data: theory and method. *Radiographics, 19*, 745–764.

Dalrymple, N. C., Prasad, S. R., Freckleton, M. W., & Chintapalli, K. N. (2005). Introduction to the language of three-dimensional imaging with multidetector CT. *Radiographics, 25*, 1409–1428.

Doi, A., et al. (2002). 3D volume extraction and mesh generation using energy minimization techniques. In *Proceedings of the 1st international symposium on 3D data processing visualization and transmission*. New York: IEEE.

Fatterpekar, G. M., et al. (2006). Role of 3D CT in the evaluation of the temporal bone. *Radiographics, 26*, S117–S132.

Fayad, L. M., Johnson, P., & Fishman, E. K. (2005). Multidetector CT of the musculoskeletal disease in the pediatric patient: principles, techniques, and clinical applications. *Radiographics, 25*, 603–618.

Fleiter, T., Merkle, E. M., & Aschoff, A. J. (1997). Comparison of real-time virtual and fiberoptic bronchoscopy in patients with bronchial carcinoma: opportunities and limitations. *American Journal of Roentgenology, 169*, 1591–1595.

Fishman, E. K., Ney, D. R., Heath, D. G., et al. (2006). Volume rendering versus maximum intensity projection in CT angiography: what works best, when, and why. *Radiographics, 26*, 905–922.

Furlow, B. (2013). Computed tomography colonoscopy. *Radiologic Technology, 84*(5), 493–511.

Furlow, B. (2014). CT image visualization: a conceptual introduction. *Radiologic Technology, 86*(2), 187–204.

Goodnight, N., Wang, R., & Humphreys, G. (2005). Computation on programmable graphics hardware. *IEEE Computer Graphics and Applications, 25*(5), 12–15.

Greenleaf, J. F., et al. (1970). Computer-generated three dimensional oscilloscopic images and associated techniques for display and study of spatial distribution of pulmonary blood flow. *IEEE Transaction on Nuclear Science-NS, 17*, 353–359.

Heath, D. G., Soyer, P. A., Kuszyk, B. S., et al. (1995). Three-dimensional spiral CT during arterial portography: comparison of three rendering techniques. *Radiographics, 15*, 1001–1011.

Herman, G. T. (1993). 3D display: a survey from theory to applications. *Computerized Medical Imaging and Graphics, 17*, 131–142.

Herman, G. T., & Liu, H. K. (1977). Display of three-dimensional information in computed tomography. *Journal of Computer Assisted Tomography, 1*, 155–160.

Higgins, W. E., Ramaswamy, K., Swift, R. D., McLennan, G., & Hoffman, E. A. (1998). Virtual bronchoscopy for three dimensional pulmonary image assessment: state of the art and future needs. *Radiographics, 18*, 761–778.

Hoffman, H., Torres, W. E., & Ernst, R. D. (2002). Paleoradiology: advanced CT in the evaluation of Egyptian mummies. *Radiographics, 22*, 377–385.

Hopper, K. D. (1999). CT bronchoscopy. *Seminars in Ultrasound, CT, and MRI, 20*, 10–15.

Hopper, K. D, Iyriboz, A. T., Wise, S. W., Neuman, J. D., Mauger, D. T., & Kasales, C. J. (2000). Mucosal detail at CT virtual reality: surface versus volume rendering. *Radiology, 214*, 517–522.

Jan, J. (2005). *Medical image processing, reconstruction and restoration (signal processing and communications)*. Boca Raton, FL: CRC Press.

Jolesz, F. A., et al. (2007). Interactive virtual endoscopy. *American Journal of Roentgenology, 169*, 1229–1235.

Kalender, W. (2005). *Computed tomography: fundamentals, system technology, image quality, applications*. Munich, Germany: Publicis.

Kopecky, K. K. (1999). Multislice CT spirals past single-slice CT in diagnostic efficiency. *Diagnostic Imaging, 21*, 36–42.

Laub, G., et al. (1998). Magnetic resonance angiography techniques. *Electromedica, 66*, 68–75.

Lawler, L. P., Jarret, T. W., Corl, F. M., & Fishman, E. K. (2005). Adult ureteropelvic junction obstruction: insights with three-dimensional multi-detector row CT. *Radiographics, 25*, 121–134.

Leclerc, X., Godefroy, O., Lucas, C., et al. (1999). Internal carotid artery stenosis: CT angiography with volume rendering. *Radiology, 210*, 673–682.

Lefohn, A. E., Kniss, J., Strzodka, R., & Sengupta, S. (2006). Glift: generic, efficient, random-access GPU data structures. *ACM Transactions on Graphics, 25*(1), 60–99.

Lell, M. M., Anders, K., Uder, M., et al. (2006). New techniques in CT angiography. *Radiographics, 26*, S45–S62.

Macari, M., & Bini, E. J. (2005). CT colonography: where have we been and where are we going? *Radiology, 237*, 819–833.

Mankovich, N. J., Robertson, D. R., & Cheeseman, A. M. (1990). Three-dimensional image display in medicine. *Journal of Digital Imaging, 3*, 69–80.

Marvilla, K. R. (1978). Computer reconstructed sagittal and coronal computed tromography head scans: clinical applications. *J Comput Assist Tomogr, 2*, 12–123.

Microsoft Press. (2002). *Computer dictionary* (5th ed.). Redmond, WA: Microsoft Press.

Neri, E., et al. (Eds.) (2007). *Image processing in radiology*. New York: Springer.

Paik, D. S., Beaulieu, C. F., Jeffrey, R. B., et al. (1998). Automated flight path planning for virtual endoscopy. *Medical Physics, 25*, 629–637.

Pickhardt, P. J. (2004). Differential diagnosis of polypoid lesions seen at CT colonoscopy (virtual colonoscopy). *Radiographics, 24*, 1535–1559.

Pierce, L., Rosenberg, J., & Neustel, S. (2009). Trends in CT 3D postprocessing. *Radiologic Technology, 81*(1), 24–31.

Prassopoulos, P., Raptopoulos, V., Chuttani, et al. (1998). Development of virtual CT cholangiopancreatoscopy. *Radiology, 209*, 570–574.

Pratx, G., & Xing, L. (2011). GPU computing in medical physics: a review. *Med Phys, 38*(5), 2685–2687.

Rhodes, M. L., Glenn, W. V., & Azaawi, Y. M. (1980). Extracting oblique planes from serial CT sections. *Journal of Computer Assisted Tomography, 4*, 649–657.

Rosset, A., Spadola, L., Pysher, L., & Ratib, O. (2006). Navigating the fifth dimension: innovative interface for multidimensional multimodality image navigation. *Radiographics, 26*, 299–308.

Rubin, G. D., Beaulieu, C. F., Argiro, V., et al. (1996). Perspective volume rendering of CT and MR images: applications for endoscopie imaging. *Radiology, 199*, 321–330.

Russ, J. C. (2006). *The image processing handbook* (5th ed.). Boca Raton, FL: CRC Press.

Schwartz, B. (1994). 3D computerized medical imaging. *Medical Device Research Reports, 1*, 8–10.

Silva, A. C., Wellnitz, C. V., & Hara, A. K. (2006). Three-dimensional virtual dissection at CT colonography: unraveling the colon to search for lesions. *Radiographics, 26*, 1669–1686.

Takanashi, I., et al. (1997). 3D active net-3D volume extraction. *Journal of Institute of Image Information and Television Engineers, 51*, 2097–2106.

Taylor, S. A., Slater, A., Halligan, S., et al. (2006). CT colonoscopy: automated measurement of colonie polyps compared with manual techniques—human in vitro study. *Radiology, 242*, 120–128.

Tomandl, B. E., Hastreiter, P., Eberhard, K. E., et al. (2000). Virtual labyrinthoscopy: visualization of the inner ear with interactive direct volume rendering. *Radiographics, 20*, 547–558.

Udupa, J. K. (1999). Three-dimensional visualization and analysis methodologies: a current perspective. *Radiographics, 19*, 783–803.

Udupa, J., & Herman, G. (1991). *3D imaging in medicine.* Boca Raton, FL: CRC Press.

Udupa, J. K., & Herman, G. T. (Eds.). (2000). *3D imaging in medicine* (2nd ed.) Boca Raton, FL: CRC Press.

Vining, D. J. (1996). Virtual endoscopy flies viewer through the body. *Diagnostic Imaging, 3*, 127–129.

Vining, D. J. (1999). Virtual colonoscopy. *Seminars in Ultrasound, CT, and MRI, 20*(1), 56–60.

Wu, C. M., Urban, B. A., & Fishman, E. K. (1999). Spiral CT of the thoracic aorta with 3D volume rendering: a pictorial review of current applications. *Cardiovascular Interventional Radiology, 22*, 159–167.

Yasuda, T., et al. (1992). 3D visualization of an ancient Egyptian mummy. *IEEE Computer Graphics and Applications, 2*, 13–17.

Zhang, Q., Eagleson, R., & Peters, T. M. (2011). Volume visualization: a technical overview with a focus on medical applications. *Journal of Digit Imaging, 24*(4), 640–664.

Zonneveld, F. W., & Fukuta, K. (1994). A decade of clinical three-dimensional imaging: a review, 2: clinical applications. *Investigative Radiology, 29*, 574–589.

14

# Positron Emission Tomography/CT (PET/CT) and Single-Photon Emission Computed Tomography/CT (SPECT/CT) Hybrid Scanners

*Frederic H. Fahey, D.Sc., Matthew R. Palmer, Ph.D.*

## OUTLINE



## LEARNING OBJECTIVES

On completion of this chapter, you should be able to:

1. outline basic principles of radionuclide imaging, single-photon emission computed tomography (SPECT) and positron emission tomography (PET).
2. define the fundamentals of annihilation coincidence detection as it is applied to PET.
3. describe the concepts behind time-of-flight (TOF) PET.
4. outline the basic steps of SPECT data acquisition.
5. describe three components of a rotating gamma camera SPECT device.
6. list four differences between PET and SPECT.
7. discuss two approaches to attenuation correction for PET or SPECT.
8. discuss three ways that CT can be used in the context of hybrid imaging.
9. list three clinical applications where PET/CT has been shown to be of substantial value. Do the same for SPECT/CT.

## KEY TERMS TO WATCH FOR AND REMEMBER

The following key terms/concepts are important to your understanding of this chapter:

**attenuation correction**
**coincidence detection**
**fluorine-18 ($^{18}F$; FDG)**
**gallium-68 ($^{68}Ga$)**
**gamma camera**
**gamma ray**
**lymphoscintigraphy**
**myocardial perfusion SPECT**
**positron**
**positron emission tomography (PET)**
**radioactive radionuclide**
**radiopharmaceutical**
**random coincidences**
**rubidium-82 ($^{82}Rb$)**
**scattered coincidence**
**single-photon emission computed tomography (SPECT)**
**technetium-99m ($^{99m}Tc$) sestamibi**
**time-of-flight PET**
**true coincidence**

**Computed tomography (CT)** of the patient can provide exquisite anatomic detail that is often invaluable for diagnosis, whereas **positron emission tomography (PET)** and single-photon emission computed tomography (SPECT) provide functional information regarding the patient. For example, malignant tumors tend to be more highly metabolic than surrounding normal tissues with a higher rate of glycolysis. Therefore a radioactive pharmaceutical that distributes throughout the body according to glucose metabolic rate, such as fluorine-18 ($^{18}$F)-labeled 2-fluoro-2-deoxy-D-glucose (FDG), can yield additional diagnostic information to that provided by the CT scan. Likewise, the anatomic information provided by CT can be invaluable in trying to localize the uptake of **technetium-99m ($^{99m}$Tc) sestamibi** in the evaluation of parathyroid adenomas. PET and SPECT lack anatomic detail; thus, it is often difficult to accurately localize features with high uptake. For these reasons, it is extremely useful, if not essential, to correlate the functional information provided by PET and SPECT with the anatomy shown on CT. In many cases, separately viewing the PET or SPECT scans alongside CT studies is adequate to make a diagnosis, but in a number of cases it is very helpful to register the two datasets such that they are displayed as a single fused image. E-Figure 14-1 shows two slices of a PET/CT scan from a patient with lung cancer. The CT images are shown on the right and the PET images in the middle. On the left are the fused color images with the PET results overlaid on top of the CT images. The registration and fusion of the PET or SPECT with the CT data can be performed either by using **software** approaches that determine the transformation that will best match the datasets or by using hybrid PET/CT or SPECT/CT scanners that combine both modalities into a single **gantry.** The example in e-Figure 14-1 was acquired on a hybrid PET/CT scanner. Currently PET is only marketed in the context of hybrid PET/CT scanners, but SPECT as well as hybrid SPECT/CT scanners are still marketed. This chapter briefly describes the basics behind PET and SPECT imaging (collectively referred to as *emission tomography*), basic approaches to instrumentation, imaging considerations, and a review of some of the clinical applications for both PET/CT and SPECT/CT.

## PRINCIPLES OF PET IMAGING

The atomic nucleus contains a number of protons and neutrons. There may be too many of one or the other or they may be configured in such a way that the nucleus is unstable. Such atoms are said to be "radioactive." In these cases, the nucleus may seek to become more stable by undergoing a nuclear transformation with the emission of a particle such as a gamma ray or an alpha or beta particle. If the nucleus contains too many protons, the nucleus may transform by emitting a positive beta particle, also known as a "positron," or by capturing an orbital electron. A positron is a positively charged beta particle. It has the same mass as an electron but has a positive rather than a negative charge (Cherry et al., 2012; Evans, 1982). One of the advantages of PET compared with other nuclear imaging is that many of the radioactive isotopes of elements of biological interest, such as carbon, oxygen, and nitrogen, are positron emitters; therefore, pharmaceuticals incorporating these radioisotopes can be imaged using a PET scanner. In addition, radioactive fluorine can also be very useful as it can often be chemically substituted for a hydrogen atom or a hydroxyl (OH) group Therefore, radiopharmaceuticals such as $^{15}$O-labeled water, $^{13}$N-labeled ammonia, $^{11}$C-labeled methionine, $^{11}$C-raclopride, or FDG can be produced. Other radionuclides of current interest include **rubidium-82 ($^{82}$Rb)** used for cardiac imaging and **gallium-68 ($^{68}$Ga)** for oncologic imaging. After these are administered to a patient, the in vivo distribution can be imaged using a PET scanner. Such studies can provide quantitative, in vivo images of blood flow, protein synthesis, neuroreceptor site density, or glucose metabolic rate.

Consider that an $^{18}$F-labeled **radiopharmaceutical** has been administered to a patient and one of the $^{18}$F atoms has been incorporated into the cell of a tumor. As shown in Figure 14-1, after some time the $^{18}$F atom will transform to an $^{18}$O atom by emitting a positron. The positron will travel several millimeters in the tissue until it loses most of its kinetic energy, at which point it will combine with a neighboring electron to form an entity known as "positronium." After a very short time (~$10^{-10}$ seconds) the positron–electron pair will "annihilate," converting its mass into two photons that are emitted back to back, almost exactly in opposite directions. The energy of the two photons is determined using Einstein's equation

$$E = mc^2$$

where $m$ is the mass of the electron (or positron) and $c$ is the speed of light. Therefore, the two photons each have energy of 511 kiloelectron volts (keV).

If each of these photons interacts with detectors on opposite sides of the PET scanner and are detected within a short time window (5 to 15 nanoseconds [ns], i.e., 5-15 × $10^{-9}$ seconds), a "coincidence" detection occurs, and the annihilation event can be assumed to have occurred along the line that connects the two detectors, referred to as the "line of response" (LOR). More accurately, the event can be localized to within the envelope defined by the two detectors and shown as the dotted lines in Figure 14-1. Thus, to a first approximation, the **spatial resolution** of a PET scanner is determined by the size of the radiation detectors used in the scanner. Therefore, if the scanner uses 4-millimeter (mm) detectors, as most modern clinical PET scanners do, the spatial resolution can be assumed to be approximately 4 mm or, perhaps, slightly more. Even if one could localize the annihilation event exactly, this is really not the locus of interest. It is more important to know from where the positron was emitted, that is, the location of the $^{18}F$ atom within the tissue. Since the positron traveled several millimeters prior to annihilation (referred to as the positron range), the radiopharmaceutical distribution cannot be localized exactly. In addition, the two photons may not be emitted at exactly 180 degrees to each other. If the positron–electron pair was not completely at rest when annihilation occurred, conservation of momentum would dictate that they would be emitted at an angle slightly different from 180 degrees. These two factors, the positron range and the slight noncolinearity of the two photons, lead to the best possible spatial resolution, even in a perfect PET scanner, of about 3 mm for a whole-body PET scanner and 1 mm for a small-bore, animal PET scanner (Levin & Hoffman, 1999; Palmer et al., 2005).

Two small detectors on either side of the patient would not collect very many photons; thus, the placement of a large number of small detectors about the patient is necessary to acquire high-resolution PET data in a reasonable amount of time. In Figure 14-2, a single detector on one side of the patient is not only in coincidence with one detector on the opposite side but with several hundred detectors. Each detector maps out a fan beam with the detectors on the opposite side with which they are in coincidence. In a single ring, there may be as many as 500 to 700 small detectors. To acquire PET data simultaneously from a number of imaging planes, several detector rings can be placed back to back, making a single detector module a rectangular mosaic of small detectors (Casey & Nutt, 1986). Figure 14-3 shows a detector block from a PET scanner that is a 6 × 6 array of small, scintillating detectors with two dual-channel photomultiplier tubes behind it. Each scintillating detector measures 4 × 8 mm so the entire 6 × 6 array is 24 × 48 mm. By taking the weighted sum of the signal from the photomultiplier tubes, the system determines within

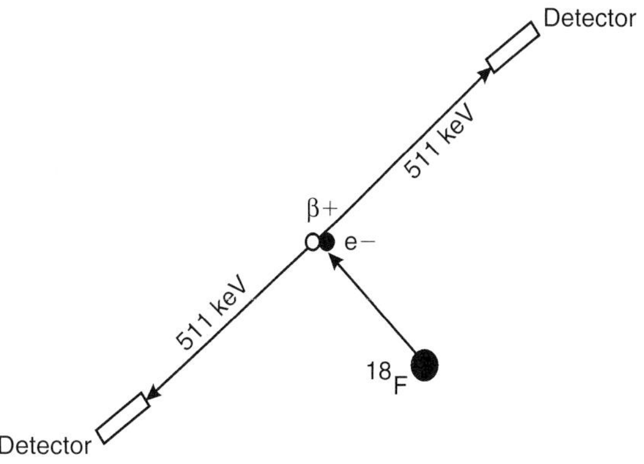


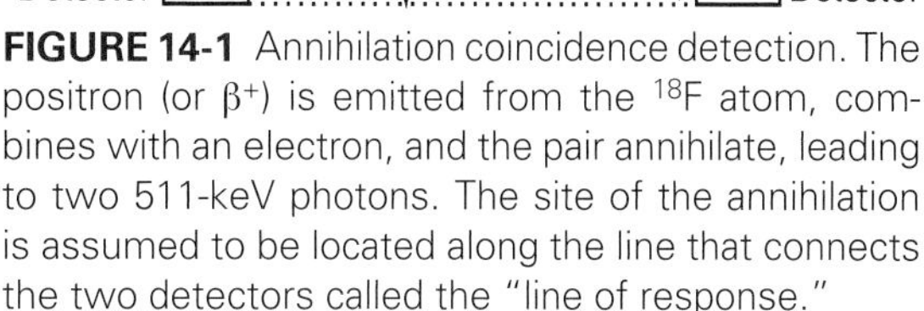


**FIGURE 14-1** Annihilation coincidence detection. The positron (or $\beta^+$) is emitted from the $^{18}F$ atom, combines with an electron, and the pair annihilate, leading to two 511-keV photons. The site of the annihilation is assumed to be located along the line that connects the two detectors called the "line of response."

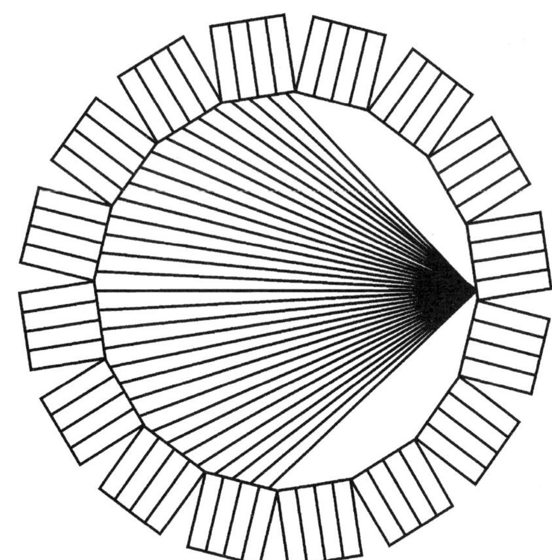

**FIGURE 14-2** Ring of detectors. In a modern PET scanner, the object is surrounded by a ring of detectors. A single detector is allowed to be in coincidence with many detectors on the opposite side of the scanner.

which of the 36 detectors the interaction occurred. A modern PET scanner may have several hundred such blocks of detectors with a total of tens of thousands of small, scintillating detectors.

Not all **coincidence detection** events are of the same quality as shown in Figure 14-4. When both annihilation photons exit the patient without

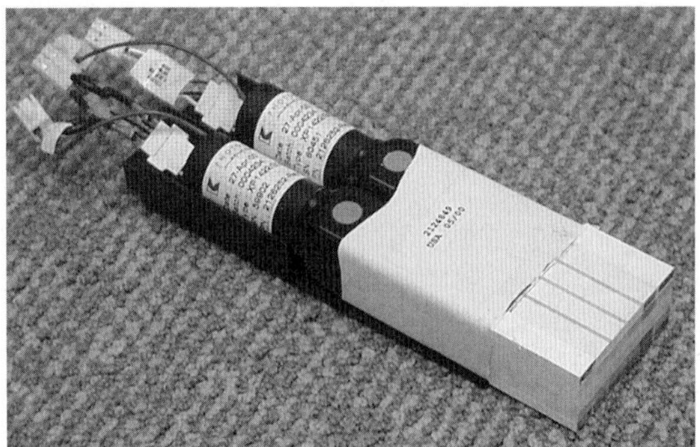

**FIGURE 14-3** Block detector module from a PET scanner. A single detector module from a PET scanner consisting of a rectangular array of small detector elements and a photomultiplier tube array.

**TABLE 14-1 Potential PET Scanner Scintillating Materials**

| Scintillator | NaI | BGO | LSO | GSO |
|---|---|---|---|---|
| Density (g/cc) | 3.67 | 7.13 | 7.40 | 6.71 |
| Photoelectric lin atten ($cm^{-1}$) | 0.06 | 0.39 | 0.23 | 0.18 |
| Compton lin atten ($cm^{-1}$) | 0.28 | 0.52 | 0.56 | 0.46 |
| Relative light yield | 100 | 15 | 75 | 40 |
| Decay constant (ns) | 230 | 300 | 40 | 50 |
| Peak wavelength (nm) | 410 | 480 | 420 | 440 |
| Effective *Z* | 51 | 75 | 66 | 59 |
| Index of refraction | 1.85 | 2.15 | 1.82 | 1.85 |
| Hygroscopic? | Yes | No | No | No |

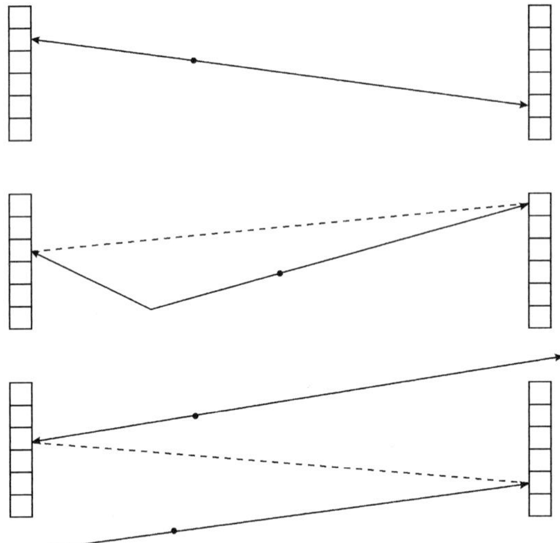

**FIGURE 14-4** True, scatter, and random coincidence events. If an annihilation event occurs and the two 511-keV annihilation photons are detected without incident, this is referred to as a "true" coincidence event (*top*). If one of the photons scatters prior to detection, this is referred to as a "scatter" coincidence event (*middle*). If two unrelated events are detected at the same time, this is referred to as a "random" coincidence event (*bottom*).

incident and are detected in coincidence, it is referred to as a "true" coincidence detection. This is shown at the top of Figure 14-4. However, there is a possibility that one of the photons will undergo Compton scattering prior to exiting the patient, as shown in the middle of Figure 14-4. The LOR associated with this coincidence detection may not pass through the annihilation event; therefore, it does not accurately localize the event. This is referred to as a "scatter" coincidence detection. Last, there is a possibility at higher count rates that two independent events occur simultaneously and that two photons are randomly detected in coincidence, as shown at the bottom of Figure 14-4. The resulting LOR does not accurately localize either annihilation event. This is referred to as a "random" or "accidental" coincident detection and, without compensation, leads to background activity that reduces image contrast. The random coincidence rate can be reduced by either reducing the detector count rates or by reducing the coincidence timing window (Fahey, 2001, 2003; Hoffman & Phelps, 1986).

The crystals used in the construction of PET scanner detectors are called scintillators. Photons interact in the crystal, resulting in the emission of light, which is collected by an array of photomultiplier tubes. Table 14-1 lists some common scintillating materials that have been used for PET detectors. Sodium iodide (NaI), the material used in **gamma cameras,** emits the most light per photon, yielding the best energy resolution. However, the lower density and lower effective *Z* number (the average number of protons per atom) leads to lower detection **efficiency**—a smaller fraction of the photons that strike the detector will be detected. Bismuth germanate (BGO) has both a higher density and effective *Z* number so it has a higher detection efficiency. However, both NaI and BGO emit their scintillation light rather slowly, requiring a 12-ns coincidence timing window. Lutetium oxyorthosilicate (LSO) and gadolinium oxyorthosilicate (GSO) have reasonably high detection efficiency (densities and effective *Z* numbers almost as high as BGO) and emit their light much more quickly (Daghighian et al., 1993; Surti et al., 2000). Lutetium yttrium oxyorthosilicate, used by some manufacturers, has detection properties very similar to LSO. This allows the coincidence timing window to be reduced by at least a factor of two (from 12 to 5 ns or 6 ns). Since the random coincidence rate is proportional to the coincidence timing window, this results in a corresponding reduction in random coincidence rate.

The ring diameter of most clinical PET scanners is 70 to 100 centimeters (cm). Thus it takes about 3 ns for an annihilation photon to traverse the scanner. If the scanner's **temporal resolution** is fast enough, one might be able to determine the time difference between the detections of the two annihilation photons and discern where along the LOR the event occurred. This approach is referred to as "time-of-flight" (TOF) PET. Such localization data can be used by the reconstruction **algorithm** and lead to a more accurate reconstruction of the PET data (Lewellen, 1998; Surti, 2015).

Consider an annihilation event that occurs along a specific LOR as shown in Figure 14-5. The photon moving toward the left will travel a **distance** $x_1$ before it hits the detector, and the other photon will travel a distance $x_2$ before it is detected. The time difference between the two detections, $t_{diff}$, is given by the following:

$$t_{diff} = (x_2 - x_2)/c$$

where $c$ is the speed of light. The question is whether the temporal resolution of the scanner is fast enough to resolve this very short time difference. Alternatively, if the scanner's temporal resolution is given by $\Delta t$, then the shortest distance that could be determined is given by the following:

$$\Delta x = c\Delta t/2$$

Modern **time-of-flight PET** scanners using LSO have temporal resolutions of approximately 0.6 ns ($0.6 \times 10^{-9}$ seconds), and light travels about 30 cm in 1 ns. This indicates that the annihilation event can be localized to within about 7 cm. Although 7 cm does not sound very impressive, it means that the resulting detection event needs to be back-projected only along 7 cm rather than across the entire patient's width during the reconstruction process. Since the detection events are more accurately placed, this leads to less **noise** as if it were acquired with more counts. For example, if the patient is 30 cm wide along the LOR of interest, the study will appear as if it was acquired with more than twice as many counts leading to a reduction in image noise and a subsequent improvement in image quality. Since this improvement depends on the patient size, time of flight should have a greater positive impact in larger patients rather than smaller ones such as children. All of the major vendors that market PET/CT scanners provide time of flight as an option.

Some older scanners provided interplane septa that allowed for the acquisition of PET data in 2D mode, which substantially reduces the amount of

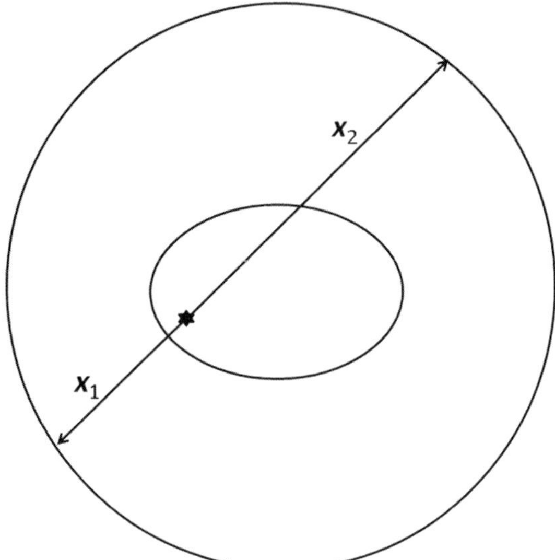


**FIGURE 14-5** Time-of-flight PET. In this figure, the photon moving to the left travels $x_1$ distance while the other photon travels $x_2$. Thus the time difference between the two detections is $(x_2 - x_1)/c$, where $c$ is the speed of light. If the temporal resolution is sufficient, the scanner can localize this detection along the line of response to within a certain distance. Current scanners with time-of-flight capability can localize the detection to within about 7 cm, which leads to notable improvement in image quality, particularly in large patients.

interplane scatter and **random coincidences** from activity outside the axial field of **view.** Alternatively, 3D mode leads to an increase by a factor of 4 or 5 in **sensitivity.** These interplane septa were retractable, which provided the option of acquiring data in either the 2D or 3D mode. Modern PET scanners do not provide this capability and acquire in 3D mode only.

At this point in time, all commercial, whole-body PET scanners are hybrid scanners, the vast majority of which are PET/CT scanners, but a few PET/MR scanners are currently marketed as well. The CT portion of hybrid PET/CT systems uses multidetector CT technology. Modern scanners may incorporate CT with 32 or more slices. Figure 14-6 shows two views of a PET/CT system. Figure 14-6, *A* shows the CT component of the system, and Figure 14-6, *B* shows the PET component. In reality, PET/CT scanners are two separate machines in close proximity with a single bed that moves the patient between the two. The PET and CT data are acquired sequentially. The CT scout scan is initially acquired to define the field of view. The CT image is then acquired followed by the PET acquisition. A typically whole-body (i.e., from the base of the skull to mid-thigh) PET/CT acquisition may take 20 to 30 minutes to complete.

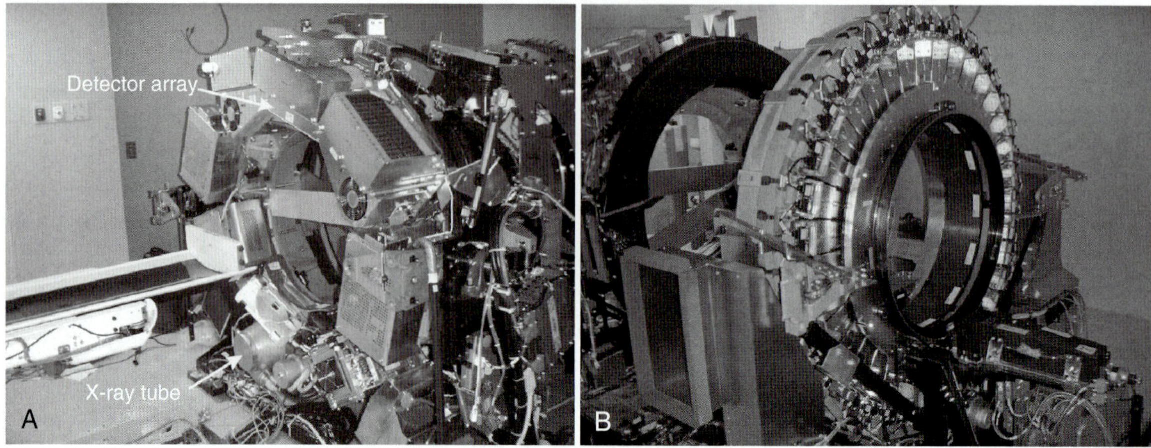


**FIGURE 14-6** PET/CT scanner. **A,** CT portion of a modern PET/CT scanner with the covers removed. The detector array and the x-ray tube are noted. **B,** PET component of the PET/CT scanner. Note the ring of block detector modules with photomultiplier tubes.

## PRINCIPLES OF SPECT IMAGING

In conventional nuclear medicine imaging, the patient is administered a radiopharmaceutical and imaged with a device referred to as a gamma camera. The gamma camera is a large area (typically 300 × 500 cm) radiation detector that can localize each detection of a **gamma ray** incident upon it. The radiation detector material is most commonly a thallium-drifted NaI scintillating crystal. The gamma camera is fitted with a collimator that defines the directionality of the detected photon. In most cases, a parallel-hole collimator is used that restricts the detected photons to those that basically strike the detector at right angles to its surface. This is quite restrictive; only about 1 in 10,000 gamma rays emitted within the patient are actually detected by the scintillating crystal. A variety of different parallel-hole collimators can be used with a particular gamma camera, depending on the energy of the gamma rays to be detected (there are low-, medium-, and high-energy collimators) and other desired imaging parameters. For example, the collimator may consist of smaller holes, and it is referred to as a "high-resolution" collimator. Alternatively, a collimator with larger holes can be used when the image task requires higher sensitivity where sensitivity can be defined as the number of counts per minute per a certain quantity of radioactivity. This would be considered a "high-sensitivity" collimator. In general, there is a trade-off between spatial resolution and sensitivity. Last, the thickness of the septa between holes is varied depending on the energy of the photon of interest. In the context of nuclear medicine, photons in the 80- to 200-keV range (such as $^{133}$Xe, $^{201}$Tl, and $^{99m}$Tc) are considered "low energy"; 200 to 300 keV (such as $^{111}$In) is medium energy; and >300 keV (e.g., $^{131}$I) is high energy. Depending on the imaging task at hand and the radiopharmaceutical to be used, a low-energy high-resolution collimator or a medium-energy all-purpose collimator can be considered.

If a tomographic representation of the in vivo radiopharmaceutical distribution is to be performed, then gamma camera images or **"projections"** at a number of angles about the patient (Fig. 14-7) can be acquired. Typically these projection images are acquired about every 3 degrees such that a complete set for 360 degrees would consist of approximately 120 projections. Assuming parallel-hole **collimation** is used, a detection at a particular location on the crystal can be assumed to have come from the **ray** intersecting the detection crystal at that point at a right angle and extending back through the patient. Thus the acquired data can be back-projected through the patient at each projection angle, and a reconstruction of the object can be generated just as in CT or PET using filtered **back-projection** or iterative approaches. This technique is referred to as "single-photon emission computed tomography," or SPECT, to distinguish it from PET, which requires two photons to back-project a detection event.

Compared with PET, the advantage of SPECT is that it does not require the radiopharmaceutical to be a positron emitter so all of the radiopharmaceuticals routinely imaged in conventional nuclear medicine can potentially be imaged tomographically with SPECT. These include radiopharmaceuticals labeled with $^{99m}$Tc, $^{201}$Tl, $^{123}$I, $^{111}$In, $^{131}$I, and so on. Thus SPECT has been routinely used to image the heart, the brain, the skeleton, and the kidneys and has also been used for tumor imaging. Some clinical examples

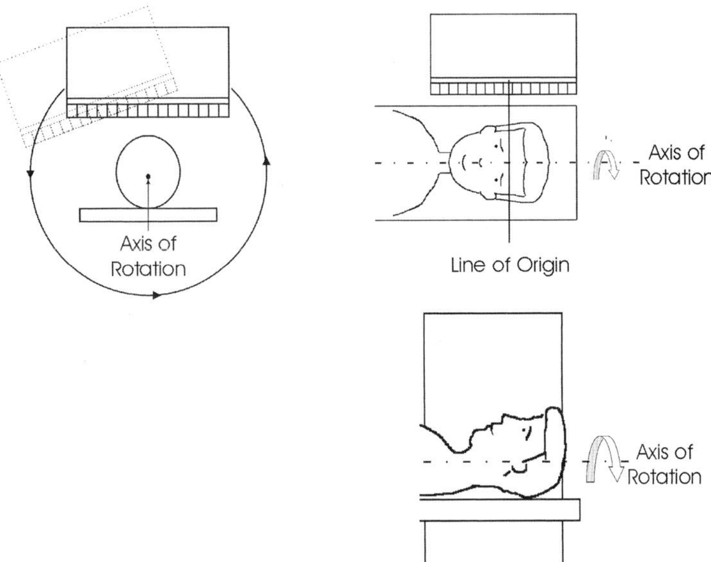


**FIGURE 14-7** SPECT acquisition. The patient is placed on the imaging table and the gamma camera rotates, acquiring a projection image at set angular intervals, typically every 3 degrees. The gamma camera also moves radially to stay as close to the patient as possible to maintain the highest spatial resolution. Assuming the use of a parallel hole collimator, a gamma ray detected at a particular location is assumed to have been emitted someplace along the line of origin (*upper right*).

will be shown later in this chapter. The disadvantage is its relatively low sensitivity compared with PET because it needs to use absorptive collimation. As a result, SPECT is typically more than 100 times less sensitive (in terms of the detected count rate per unit activity) compared with PET.

In a typical SPECT acquisition, the patient is administered the radiopharmaceutical, most typically by intravenous injection, although in certain cases, other routes of administration might be used. After an appropriate uptake period that may be as short as several minutes and as long as several days, the patient is placed on the imaging table and moved in place for imaging. Once the patient is in place, a large number of projection images (from tens to hundreds) are acquired, which are subsequently reconstructed into a tomographic dataset consisting of a series of transverse slices through the patient in a manner very similar to that used in PET or CT. Because of the extended acquisition times, dynamic studies (i.e., a time sequences of scans) are not commonly acquired in SPECT; however, gating the acquisition on the electrocardiogram (ECG) is very common and found to be quite useful for cardiac SPECT. In these instances, the acquisition of each projection is gated to the ECG, and the complete, acquired dataset is reconstructed to provide a tomographic dataset at various points in the cardiac cycle.

The most common instrumentation used for SPECT is the rotating gamma camera. Most current SPECT gamma camera systems consist of two rectangular, large field of view (30 × 50 cm) camera heads mounted opposite each other on a rotating gantry. In addition, the camera heads can be placed in a 90-degree configuration such that a complete set of projections over 180 degrees can be acquired with a 90-degree rotation of the gantry. The gamma camera gantry rotates about the patient, typically acquiring 60 to 120 projection images that are subsequently reconstructed. The camera heads can also move radially as close to the patient as possible to maintain high spatial resolution. Figure 14-8 shows a SPECT/CT scanner. The two gamma camera heads are seen in the front with the CT component in the rear, which is typical of hybrid SPECT/CT scanners. This configuration is different from PET/CT, where the CT component is typically in the front.

In the past decade, systems that can only acquire SPECT have been introduced to the clinic. These dedicated devices typically are designed for a specific clinical application, such as cardiac SPECT with higher sensitivity and a smaller footprint to more easily fit within the limited space often available in an outpatient clinic (Slomka et al., 2014). The higher sensitivity of these devices allows for much faster **data acquisition** or a substantial reduction in the amount of administered activity necessary to perform the exam. Reducing the amount of

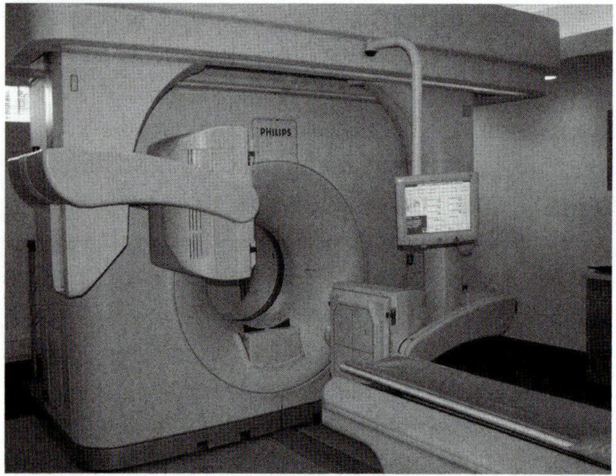


**FIGURE 14-8** SPECT/CT scanner. In this figure, the two gamma camera heads of the SPECT component are seen in the front with the CT component in the rear. This configuration is typical of hybrid SPECT/CT scanners.

administered activity leads directly to a lower radiation dose to the patient. An alternative to the use of a dedicated SPECT scanner is the use of specially designed focused collimators. The use of such special collimators provides higher sensitivity for cardiac imaging while allowing the camera to be used for other types of imaging and even conventional planar nuclear medicine imaging, when the device is not being used for cardiac SPECT.

## Attenuation Correction

The probability of detecting a photon emitted from the center of an object is less than that for an event on the periphery due to the fact that the photon is more likely to be absorbed or scattered if it has to travel through more material. If there are two features, each with exactly the same amount of activity, the one on the periphery will have a higher signal than the one at the center. To achieve uniform quantitative accuracy the spatial variation in **attenuation** must be corrected (Cherry et al., 2012).

Consider two PET detectors in coincidence and the intersection of the LOR and an object of uniform attenuating material, where $L$ is the length of the LOR within the object. Also consider an annihilation event that occurs at a point within the object along this LOR (Fig. 14-9, *A*). If the distance from this point to the edge of the object in one direction is $x$ and in the other direction it is $(L - x)$, the probability of one of the annihilation photons escaping the object without being attenuated is $e^{-\mu x}$ and in the other direction it is $e^{-\mu(L-x)}$, where $\mu$ is the **linear attenuation coefficient** for material and $e$ is equal to ~2.718 and is the base of the natural logarithm. Thus the probability of both photons escaping without being attenuated is the product of these two probabilities:

$$P = (e^{-\mu x}) \times \left(e^{-\mu(L-x)}\right) = e^{-\mu L}$$

Therefore, the total probability that both photons escape without attenuation does not depend on where along the LOR the event occurs. It only depends on the thickness of the object along LOR, $L$. If $x$ is small, photons traveling in the $x$ direction are less likely to be attenuated, but those moving in the other direction are more likely and the total probability remains the same. To know how many annihilation events would have been detected along this LOR if there were no photon attenuation, divide the number of detected events by $e^{-\mu L}$ or, alternatively, multiply the number of detected events by $e^{\mu L}$. If the attenuating material is uniform and the object outline can be defined, then the value of $L$ for each LOR can be determined and the above formula can be used to apply corrections to each LOR prior to reconstruction. The resultant reconstructed data would be free of the attenuation **artifact.** This process is referred to as "calculated **attenuation correction.**"

In SPECT, only one photon is emitted. As shown in Figure 14-9, *B*, the probability of the photon being detected is given by the following:

$$P = e^{-\mu x}$$

where $x$ is the distance from the point of emission to the edge of the patient. Note that there is no opposing photon in SPECT as there is in PET. Therefore, the probability of detecting a photon emitted from the center of a patient is actually higher for SPECT than it is for PET, even though the photon energies used in SPECT are typically considerably lower than 511 keV. For example, the probabilities of detecting photons from the center of a 30-cm-thick patient are 5.8% and 10.5% for PET and SPECT (with $^{99m}$Tc), respectively. In the case of uniform attenuation as in the abdomen, one calculated approach for SPECT attenuation correction is to estimate the distance, $x_i$, from each point of emission to the edge of the body along a number of rays distributed at equal angular intervals about the body, as shown in Figure 14-9, *C*. For this purpose, the patient's body outline must be estimated. The average attenuation effect can be estimated by taking the average attenuation probability along these rays. By dividing the counts, $C$, at that location (or pixel), one could estimate the attenuation corrected counts, $Ccor$:

$$Ccor = C / \left( \sum_i e^{-\mu x_i} \right)$$

This correction, known as the first-order Chang correction, needs to be applied at every **pixel** for every

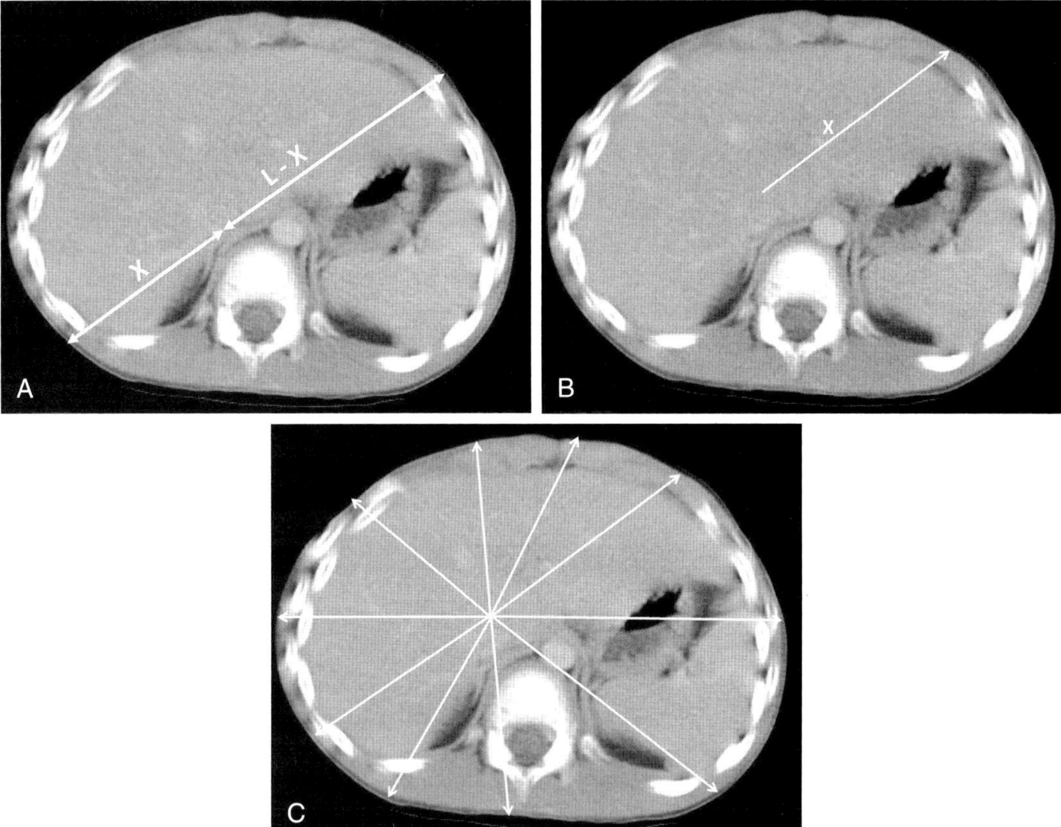


**FIGURE 14-9** Photon attenuation. **A,** This figure illustrates a positron-electron annihilation event in the abdomen of a patient. The photon going in one direction must traverse a distance of $x$, whereas the photon going in the opposite direction must traverse $L - x$. The total probability that both photons will escape the body is given by $e^{-\mu L}$, which depends only on the total thickness of the patient along the LOR and not on the location of the event along the LOR. **B,** In SPECT, only one photon (gamma ray) is emitted. Thus the attenuation compensation must also estimate the depth of the emission. **C,** For the first-order Chang attenuation correction, the length of a number of rays that are evenly spaced angularly is determined and the average attenuation at that pixel estimated assuming uniform attenuation.

slice within the SPECT study (Chang, 1978). For thoracic and cardiac SPECT, the assumption of uniform attenuation is not adequate since the region contains both lungs and soft tissue. To do an adequate job of attenuation correction in the thorax, transmission data must also be available. Some scanners provide external radioactive sources that allow for the acquisition of transmission data, which can later be used to apply the nonuniform attenuation correction.

## CT-Based Attenuation Correction

A very effective approach to attenuation correction for PET or SPECT is to use the data from a registered CT scan; that is, it is the same size and in the same orientation and sliced along the same planes as the PET or SPECT scan (Kinahan et al., 2003; Seo et al., 2005). Such registration can be achieved by acquiring both datasets with a hybrid scanner or by applying a software registration algorithm to the emission and CT data that were acquired on separate machines.

CT inherently provides images of the attenuation properties of the object being imaged. The pixel values are recorded in CT or Hounsfield units (HU):

$$HU = \frac{\mu - \mu_{water}}{\mu_{water}}$$

where $\mu$ and $\mu_{water}$ are the linear attenuation coefficients, at the CT x-ray energy, of the material within the pixel and water, respectively. HU for water is zero, for air is −1000, for soft tissue is −100 to 100, and for bone is ~1000. Therefore, if CT data are available, it is reasonable to use these data for attenuation correction. However, there are several major differences between the attenuation data available from CT and that necessary for attenuation correction. First, photons used in CT have substantially lower energy than the photons from

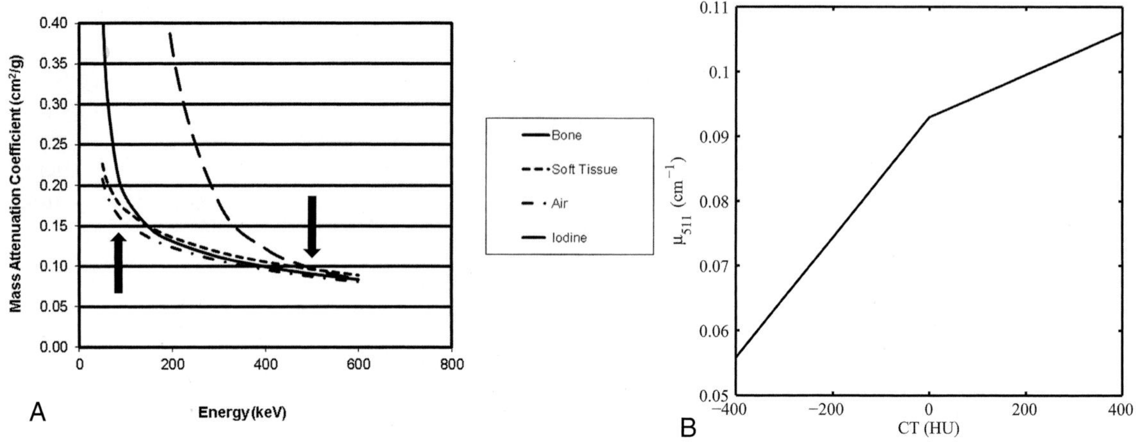


**FIGURE 14-10** CT-based attenuation correction for PET. **A,** The mass attenuation coefficients (that is, the linear attenuation coefficient per unit mass) for bone, soft tissue, air, and iodine as a function of photon energy. The arrow on the left denotes the mean energy range for CT, whereas the arrow on the right indicates 511 keV. **B,** Multilinear transformation from CT HUs to the linear attenuation coefficient for 511 keV for PET attenuation correction.

PET or SPECT. The tube voltages typically used in CT are between 80 and 140 kVp, leading to mean energies in the 35- to 50-keV range compared with the 511-keV photons used in PET or SPECT photons with energies between 80 and 360 keV. In Figure 14-10, *A*, the linear attenuation coefficients for soft tissue, air, bone, and iodine are plotted as a function of energy, and there is a substantial difference between those in the CT energy range (35 to 140 keV) and those at 511 keV. Even for 140-kVp x-rays, the mean x-ray energy is about half that of the 140-keV photons for $^{99m}$Tc. Thus, a transformation must be applied between CT HU values and the linear attenuation coefficient suitable for the PET or SPECT photons. Such a transformation is shown for PET in Figure 14-10, *B*. The shape of the graph would be very similar for SPECT, although the specific linear attenuation coefficient values on the vertical axis would be different. The linear attenuation coefficients for soft tissue at 140 and 511 keV are 0.093 and 0.15 $cm^{-1}$, which corresponds to the value of the transformation at HU equals 0. For HU values between −1000 and 0, the material is assumed to be a mixture of air and soft tissue, which on a per density basis has very similar attenuation properties, thus there is a single linear slope in this region. For HU values >0, the material is assumed to be a mixture of soft tissue and bone so the linear transformation has a different slope (Lonn, 2003).

There is also a substantial difference in the spatial resolution between CT (on the order of 1.0 mm) and PET (6 to 8 mm) or SPECT (typically 10 to 15 mm). Applying a very sharp CT correction to these smoother image data can lead to artifacts at the edge of structures within the object. To compensate for this, the transformed CT data are smoothed to a more appropriate spatial resolution. The resultant transformed, smoothed CT data are subsequently reprojected into an array of attenuation correction factors that can be applied during PET or SPECT reconstruction. Compared with traditional measured-attenuation correction, the CT data have substantially less noise; the application of CT-based attenuation correction adds very little additional noise to the reconstructed image. Also, the CT data are acquired in a very short amount of time (<1 minute) compared with the SPECT transmission data.

## Clinical PET/CT Data Acquisition

The following describes a typical workflow of a clinical PET procedure. The patient arrives in the PET center, is taken to a preparatory/injection room, and is injected with the PET radiopharmaceutical. The patient may wait in this room while the radiopharmaceutical distributes within the body. The amount of waiting time depends on the biokinetics associated with the particular tracer. The patient is then escorted to the scanner room and placed on the imaging table. The CT scout view can be used to **position** the study anatomically. The CT scan is typically acquired just prior to the PET emission acquisition.

As discussed previously, one of the advantages of PET is that many of the elements considered biologically pertinent (e.g., carbon, nitrogen, and oxygen) have isotopes that are positron emitters. Additionally, $^{18}$F can often be substituted for a hydrogen or a hydroxyl group. However, the disadvantage of these isotopes is their relatively short half-lives—2, 10, 20, and 110 minutes for $^{15}$O, $^{13}$N, $^{11}$C, and $^{18}$F, respectively. Although $^{18}$F has a sufficiently long half-life so that its radiopharmaceuticals can be produced in regional radiopharmacies and delivered to clinical PET centers, the other three radioisotopes must be produced on-site with the use of a medical cyclotron. These cyclotrons typically can generate accelerated charge particle beams in excess of 10 MeV and can be used for the routine production of $^{11}C$, $^{13}N$, $^{15}O$, and $^{18}F$.

In some cases, a radiopharmaceutical generator system, similar to the $^{99}Mo$-$^{99m}Tc$ generator routinely used in conventional nuclear medicine, can be used to deliver PET radioisotopes. For example, the strontium-82/rubidium-82 ($^{82}Sr$-$^{82}Rb$) generator can be used to provide $^{82}Rb$ to the PET clinic. $^{82}Sr$ (25-day half-life) decays to $^{82}Rb$ (75-second half-life). The $^{82}Sr$ is chemically bound to a ceramic column. Some of the $^{82}Sr$ will decay to $^{82}Rb$, which has different chemistry and, thereby, will no longer be bound to the column. The column is eluted with saline, and $^{82}Rb$ is washed away into a vial where it is available to be administered to the patient. $^{82}Rb$ distributes to the myocardium in a manner similar to $^{201}Tl$, providing a PET alternative to measuring myocardial perfusion and viability. Its use has been shown to be of significant clinical value, particularly in larger patients. The PET clinic can purchase a generator every 4 to 6 weeks and have $^{82}Rb$ available every day without relying on a regional radiopharmacy. More recently, germanium-68/gallium-68 ($^{68}Ge$-$^{68}Ga$) generators have been introduced. In particular, $^{68}Ga$ DOTATOC has been used as a somatostatin receptor agent in patients with neuroendocrine tumors (Sharma et al., 2013).

By far, the most commonly used radiopharmaceutical for PET imaging is FDG, which is a radioactive analog of glucose that distributes in tissues that are actively metabolizing glucose. This makes FDG a useful radiopharmaceutical for a number of very different clinical applications, including neurology, cardiology, and, most important, oncology. Although some PET clinics have their own medical cyclotrons, most receive delivery of their FDG in unit doses from a regional radiopharmacy. They contact the radiopharmacy the previous day and inform them of the types of studies to be performed and how much activity they need for each exam. On the day of the exam, the clinic receives a shipment of the syringes needed for that day. Prior to injection, the syringe is assayed in the dose calibrator to ensure that the appropriate amount of activity is in the syringe for that study.

As an example, let us consider a whole-body FDG scan. Once the patient arrives at the clinic and is registered, he or she is taken to the preparatory/injection room. The patient is injected with the FDG and then must wait for the radiopharmaceutical to distribute within his body. This uptake waiting period is typically 40 to 60 minutes and 45 to 90 minutes for brain and whole-body imaging, respectively. Since most of the time the patient will be sitting in this room with radioactivity on-board, the room should be sufficiently removed from the PET scanner and other gamma counting or imaging equipment or appropriately shielded. After the uptake period, the patient is moved to the imaging room and placed on the imaging table. Since the imaging session will take at least 20 minutes, it may be helpful to secure the patient with Velcro wraps or tape.

Most modern PET scanners have an axial field of view of at least 15-cm. If the portion of the patient to be scanned is larger than that, multiple scans are acquired at different axial offsets by moving the couch in precisely controlled steps. The resultant reconstructed images will be formatted such that they can be reviewed as one continuous study. The time to acquire the emission scan at each position typically ranges from 3 to 5 minutes, depending on the equipment used and the diagnostic task at hand. A whole-body PET scan typically incorporates data from the patient's thighs up to their eyes and thus, on a machine with a 15-cm axial field of view, would be comprised of as many as six or seven bed positions. For PET/CT with 3 minutes per bed position, the CT acquisition takes less than a minute to acquire, and the imaging could be completed in about 20 minutes.

One major consideration of hybrid PET/CT is the higher radiation dose delivered to the patient. The radiation dose delivered by CT depends on a number of factors including tube voltage, tube current, and **exposure** time. In addition, the **effective dose** to the patient would depend on the region of the body scanned. Typical effective doses for helical CT of the chest and abdomen/pelvis are in the 7- to 10-millisieverts (mSv; Cohnen et al., 2003; Pantos et al., 2011) range. Since the CT portion of a PET/CT is acquired over an extended part of the body, it is reasonable to assume that the effective dose for this may be slightly higher for a CT scan of diagnostic quality. This can be compared with the typical effective dose for an FDG PET study involving a 370-MBq injection of 7 mSv (ICRP, 2008). Therefore, the effective dose to the patient arising from the CT portion of the study can be double that from the PET portion, particularly if the CT scan is acquired of diagnostic quality (Fahey, 2009). In these cases, the CT scan might be acquired with the administration of contrast and an adequate dosage level to clearly delineate the patient's anatomy. However, the patient's arms may be down by his or her side, and the data may be acquired with the patient breathing lightly to minimize misregistration with the subsequent PET scan, given the fact that the PET scan may need 20 to 30 minutes to acquire.

In some instances, it may be necessary to acquire a separate diagnostic-quality CT scan. Alternatively, an anatomic localization scan could be acquired that provides enough anatomy to localize the features on the PET scan but not considered to be of diagnostic quality. This scan may be acquired with a substantial reduction in radiation dose, perhaps by a factor of 2 or 3, compared with the diagnostic-quality CT scan. Last, the CT scan may be acquired only for attenuation correction. In some cases, a diagnostic CT scan may not be indicated for this type of study (e.g., for brain imaging, where magnetic resonance [MR] is the anatomic imaging modality of choice) so the CT scan is only used for attenuation correction. Even if CT is indicated, a diagnostic CT scan may be acquired separately from the PET/CT scan as described previously. In these cases, the acquisition of a CT scan with a much lower radiation dose may be appropriate. A CT scan adequate for attenuation correction can be obtained with a much reduced tube current (10 milliamperes [mA] instead of 200 mA or more), and in the case of smaller patients, lower tube voltages (as low as a peak kV [kVp] of 80) could be used. Lowering the tube current from 200 to 10 mA reduces the radiation dose by a factor of 20, and reducing the tube voltage from 120 to 80 kVp can lead to a further reduction by at least a factor of 3 (Fahey, 2009; Fahey et al., 2007). Although such reduction in tube current and voltage would still lead to an adequate attenuation correction, the utility of the resultant CT images for anatomic correlation would be limited due to the excessive quantum noise.

In some cases, the use of CT-based attenuation correction can lead to artifacts in the reconstructed PET data. There are two assumptions associated with CT-based attenuation correction, and if either one of these is not met, notable artifacts can occur that can affect the ability to interpret the study. The first assumption is that the patient is in exactly the same position and state during the acquisition of both the CT and PET scans. The second assumption is that the transformation used to convert CT HU values to the linear attenuation coefficient at 511 keV is appropriate for all materials within the field of view. Typically, the CT scan is acquired first, starting at the head and moving toward the feet. As previously noted, this acquisition can take less than 1 minute. The PET scan is then acquired starting below the bladder and moving toward the head. This acquisition can take 20 to 30 minutes to acquire. Thus, for the head and neck in a whole-body PET scan, there can be 20 to 30 minutes between the time the CT scan was acquired and when the PET scan was acquired. It is possible that the patient could move in this time such that the CT and PET scans are no longer registered. This can lead to an artifact in the reconstructed PET data. For example, if the CT scan is shifted laterally relative to the PET scan, then one side of the patient will be undercorrected and the other side will be overcorrected. The asymmetry introduced could be interpreted as due to pathology; therefore, it is crucial to keep the patient immobilized from the beginning of the CT scan until the end of the PET scan. In addition, the final reconstructed data should be visually evaluated for the presence of this artifact. If this artifact is suspected, one can reconstruct the PET data without attenuation correction and see if the asymmetry exists in the underlying emission data. If this artifact is noted and the patient is still on the imaging table, it might be possible to acquire a low-dose CT scan for attenuation correction of this part of the body, or a calculated attenuation correction could be applied.

Even if the patient is kept very still, the motion of internal organs from breathing can also lead to artifacts in the reconstructed PET data. It is routine practice in conventional CT of the chest to have a patient hold his or her breath during the acquisition of the helical CT scan. However, since it takes 20 to 30 minutes to acquire the PET emission scan, it is impossible to have patients hold their breath for that period of time, so they are typically instructed to breathe quietly during the PET scan. The attenuation in the area of the diaphragm during the PET study will be an average over the entire breathing cycle and over many cycles. Applying attenuation correction from the CT data acquired during a particular instant over the liver and diaphragm can lead to substantial overcorrections in regions of the lung, resulting in regions of apparent high uptake in the lungs that could either be confused for tumor or obscure actual pathology.

Several approaches have been used to better control breathing during the data acquisition to help minimize these artifacts (Goerres et al., 2003). One approach is to allow the patient to breathe during the acquisition of the CT scan. Patients can also be instructed to hold their breath at mid- rather than at end inspiration. This probably leads to the diaphragm being in about the same position in the two studies. A more complicated, technical approach is to gate the CT and PET acquisitions on the respiratory cycle and use these data to better register the two datasets. In these studies, an apparatus is used to monitor the breathing cycle during the data acquisition. This leads to a number of scans acquired at different parts of the respiratory cycle. The resultant data can be averaged over the breathing cycle prior to attenuation correction so that it more closely matches the PET data. In addition to providing better registration between the CT and the PET data for artifact-free attenuation correction, respiratory gating can also improve the quantification of lung tumors by reducing the blurring from breathing motion.

The use of contrast material in CT can also lead to artifacts in the reconstructed PET data. Barium contained in oral **contrast media** and iodine contained in IV contrast media are high atomic number elements (*Z* of 56 and 53, respectively). At CT photon energies (<140 keV), on a per unit mass basis, barium and iodine attenuate x-ray photons to a much greater degree than does tissue. This is precisely why they are used as contrast materials in diagnostic CT. At 511 keV, however, attenuation per unit mass of barium, iodine, and all the tissue components is virtually the same. The attenuation map obtained by transforming HUs from a CT image containing contrast material is therefore inaccurate. The transformed attenuation coefficient for 511-keV photons will be too high because of the presence of contrast material leading to an overcorrection of the PET emission image. This can be either focal hot-spots that might be misinterpreted as pathology or larger regions or structures that may be recorded with higher uptake values in quantitative analyses.

Increased activity in PET images from contrast material being present in high concentrations in the CT images used for attenuation correction are typically on the order of 10% to 20%. The advantages of using contrast materials and the improvement in diagnostic quality probably outweigh the problems associated with these errors. For this reason, the routine use of oral and IV contrast materials in conjunction with PET/CT is common. One method to reduce these errors is to use alternative transformation curves that compensate for the presence of contrast media. This option is available on commercial PET/CT scanners. It must be understood, however, that this solution is a compromise since the revised curve must assume some typical mix of water, bone, and now iodine to explain higher density pixels. Another method is to have available routinely the uncorrected emission images and use them to rule out false-positive findings that might appear in areas where contrast material pools. One advantage of this latter method is that it can also be used to rule out a number of artifacts introduced by attenuation correction errors such as motion between CT and PET acquisitions and the presence of metallic prostheses (Antoch, et al., 2002).

## Clinical Examples of PET/CT

### Oncology: Lung

PET with FDG is a powerful imaging modality for use in the initial diagnosis, staging, and follow-up of lung cancer. Most lung cancer nodules are FDG avid and are generally surrounded by tissue with relatively low FDG uptake. E-Figure 14-1 illustrates a case of lung cancer in a 66-year-old male. Panels *A* through *C* contain transaxial CT, PET, and PET/CT fusion images, respectively, through the primary lung tumor mass (labeled p on the PET image). A collapsed portion of the lung adjacent to the mass is also clearly visible on the CT scan. Panels *D* through *F* contain transaxial sections inferior to the previous set and illustrate a metastasis in the adrenal gland (a). High activity seen in the kidney (k), however, is a normal finding.

### Oncology: Lymphoma

Another disease where PET is invaluable is lymphoma. Figure 14-11 contains FDG PET images of a 17-year-old male patient with Hodgkin's lymphoma acquired for initial staging and follow-up about 7 weeks later at mid-treatment. Coronal CT and PET sections through the primary site of involvement pretreatment are shown in panels *A* and *B*, respectively. Follow-up images are shown in panels *C* and *D*. The CT images show a slight reduction in tumor volume, but the corresponding PET images document a dramatic reduction in FDG avidity from initial scan to follow-up. The whole-body **maximum intensity projection (MIP)** images also show other areas of normal high FDG uptake in the heart and bladder (marked H and B, respectively).

### Cardiac: FDG

Although the clinical mainstay of PET with FDG is in oncology, there is growing interest in cardiac applications. The myocardium is normally quite variable in its affinity for FDG, but it can be made to be FDG avid to assess myocardial viability. In an FDG myocardial viability study, the patient is first given a drink high in glucose followed by a series of insulin injections. When blood glucose has returned to normal, the FDG is injected. E-Figure 14-2 shows coronal reconstructions through the chest of a 72-year-old male who was administered 500 MBq (14 mCi) of FDG 45 minutes prior to image acquisition. The PET images clearly show little or no uptake in the inferior myocardial wall, which indicates the lack of viable tissue there. Often this study would be performed and interpreted in conjunction with a **myocardial perfusion SPECT** study.

### Epilepsy: FDG

FDG PET has also been shown to be useful in the localization of epileptic seizures (Ollenberger et al., 2005). Seizure foci tend to be hypometabolic on the interictal PET scan, that is, a scan acquired when the patient is not having a seizure. Figure 14-12 shows a

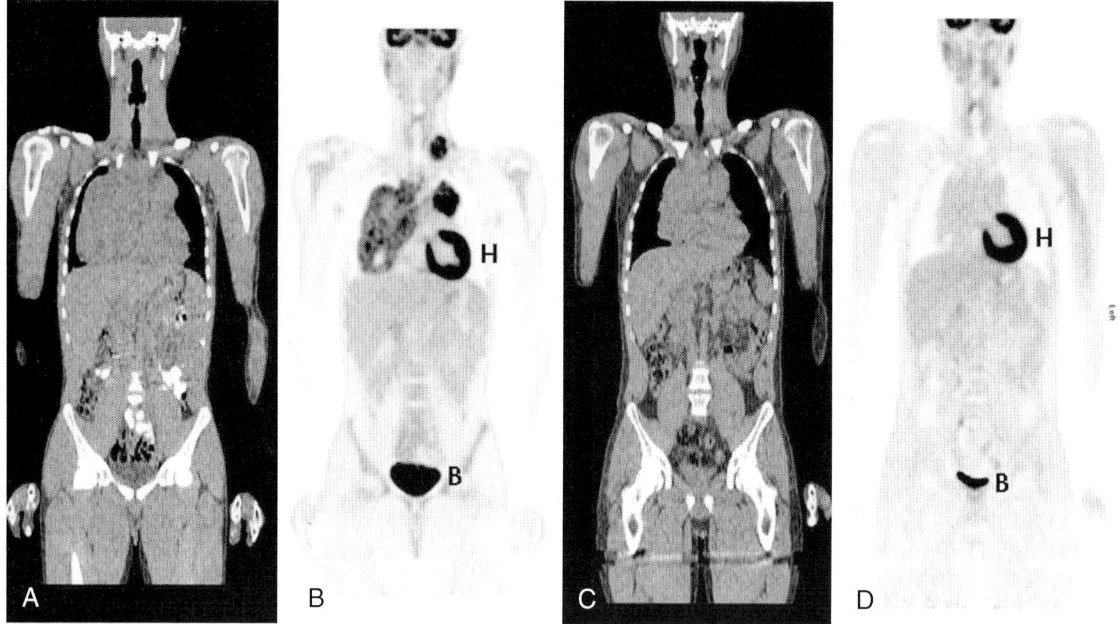


**FIGURE 14-11** FDG PET/CT scan in a patient with Hodgkin's lymphoma. FDG PET/CT images of a 17-year-old male patient with Hodgkin's lymphoma acquired for initial staging and follow-up about 7 weeks later at mid-treatment. **A,** Pretreatment coronal CT section. **B,** Pretreatment FDG-PET section. **C,** Follow-up coronal CT section. **D,** Follow-up FDG-PET section. The CT images show a slight reduction in tumor volume, but the corresponding PET images document a dramatic reduction in FDG avidity from initial scan to follow-up. The whole-body MIP images also show areas of normal high FDG uptake in the heart and bladder (marked *H* and *B*, respectively).

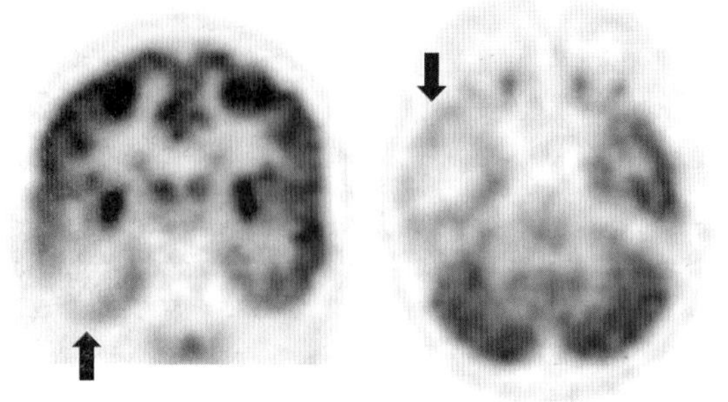

**FIGURE 14-12** FDG PET in patient with temporal lobe epilepsy. Transverse (*right*) and coronal (*left*) slices through an interictal FDG PET scan of a patient with temporal lobe epilepsy. The seizure focus in the patient's right (viewer's left noted with arrows) temporal lobe is hypometabolic.

transverse (right) and coronal (left) slice through the FDG PET scan of a patient with right-sided intractable temporal lobe epilepsy. It is clearly shown that the patient's right temporal lobe (arrow on the left) has substantially reduced signal on the FDG PET compared with the left temporal lobe. This information can be invaluable to the neurosurgeon treating this patient. For example, this scan indicates that this patient has unilateral disease limited to the right temporal lobe, indicating that this is an appropriate candidate for surgical intervention.

## Clinical SPECT/CT Data Acquisition

In many cases, the decision to use SPECT/CT is determined on a case-by-case basis and, in some cases, in addition to the initial case to assist in anatomic localization. In this way, the acquisition of SPECT/CT can be fundamentally different from PET/CT where the PET is always acquired in conjunction with CT. In addition, SPECT/CT is acquired with a wide variety of radiopharmaceuticals whereas PET/CT is almost always acquired with $^{18}$F FDG. As a result, the clinical workflow associated with a SPECT/CT study can be highly variable depending on the specific exam performed and radiopharmaceutical used.

The basic procedure that may be followed for a SPECT/CT scan will be described, but certain aspects may vary from patient to patient. First, the patient comes to nuclear medicine to be imaged. Depending on the particular procedure to be performed, the radiopharmaceutical might be injected, inhaled, or ingested in advance of the imaging session or, in some cases, after acquisition has been initiated. The time between the

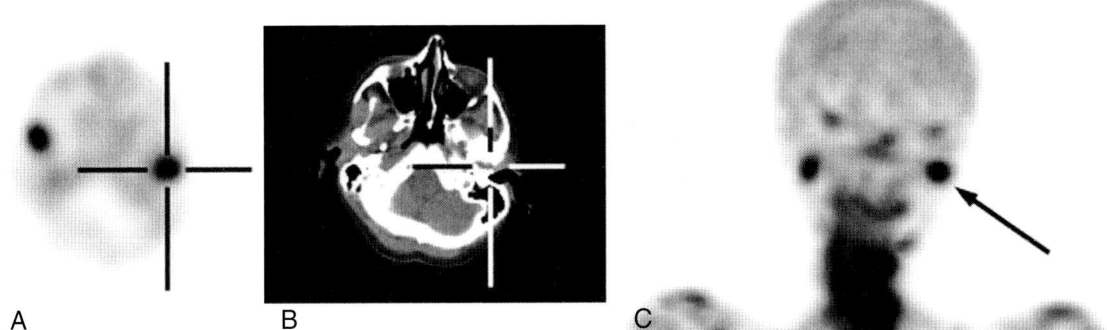


**FIGURE 14-13** $^{99m}$Tc-MDP bone SPECT/CT. Transaxial SPECT **(A)** and CT **(B)** images from a $^{99m}$Tc-MDP bone scan. **C,** Frontal MIP showing focal uptake of the tracer in the skull and uptake in the vertebral bodies of the cervical spine. The arrow **(C)** corresponds to the focus delineated on the SPECT and CT images.

administration of the radiopharmaceutical and the imaging could vary from seconds to days. The choice of how and when to introduce the tracer depends on tracer dynamics and the clinical objectives of the study.

There are some imaging procedures where SPECT/CT is routinely performed and others where its use is decided during an ongoing study as discussed earlier. For example, SPECT/CT may be used routinely for parathyroid or cardiac imaging whereas it might be determined that anatomic localization may be of particular value in certain skeletal or tumor imaging cases. In either case, once the decision has been made that SPECT/CT is clinically indicated, the patient is placed on the imaging table after waiting appropriately for uptake of the radiopharmaceutical. Similar to PET/CT, a CT scout study is acquired and, based on this, the field of view is determined for the study. The CT study is acquired followed by the SPECT study. The CT and SPECT studies are reconstructed and registered to provide the fused image set for review by the nuclear medicine physician and radiologist. The SPECT/CT acquisition typically takes ~20 minutes to acquire. Based on the size of a typical gamma camera used for SPECT/CT, this provides a 30-cm field of view in the axial direction. In a large majority of cases a 30-cm field of view is considered adequate, but multiple bed positions can be acquired similar to the PET/CT if necessary. Although the dynamics of time sequence acquisitions is common in conventional nuclear medicine, such acquisitions are not practical for SPECT/CT because of the time necessary to acquire a complete set of projection data. However, the SPECT acquisition may be acquired in conjunction with a physiologic gate (such as the ECG) as previously described. This is also true for SPECT/CT.

The artifacts that may be encountered with SPECT/CT are similar to those in PET/CT, that is, misregistration between the SPECT and CT scans and inadequate compensation for contrast material. As with PET/CT, the time difference between the CT and SPECT studies can be 10 seconds to minutes, so there can be movement between the two studies leading to misregistration in the data. Respiratory motion can also provide artifacts in the region near the diaphragm. Last, the use of CT contrast can potentially lead to artifacts in the SPECT study if not properly processed.

## Clinical Examples of SPECT/CT

### Musculoskeletal Image

Bone scintigraphy is a common imaging procedure used to diagnose and monitor certain bone pathologies. The radiopharmaceutical most often used as a bone-scanning agent is methylene diphosphonate (MDP) labeled with $^{99m}$Tc. The patient is typically injected with ~20 mCi of $^{99m}$Tc-MDP, which concentrates in bone tissue according to the rate of turnover. Patients are scanned ~3 hours after administration.

The SPECT/CT study shown in Figure 14-13 is of a middle-aged woman with a history of cancer who presented with pain in her jaw. The study was performed to look for the possibility of metastatic disease. The scan shows areas of focal uptake in the skull corresponding to the temporomandibular joint and uptake in the neck is in the vertebral bodies of the cervical spine.

### Parathyroid Imaging

The diagnosis of hyperparathyroidism is made primarily on the basis of laboratory testing. Surgery for the removal of parathyroid adenomas or excision

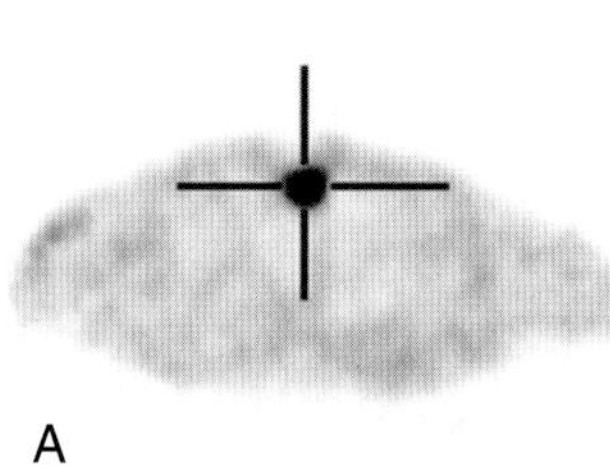


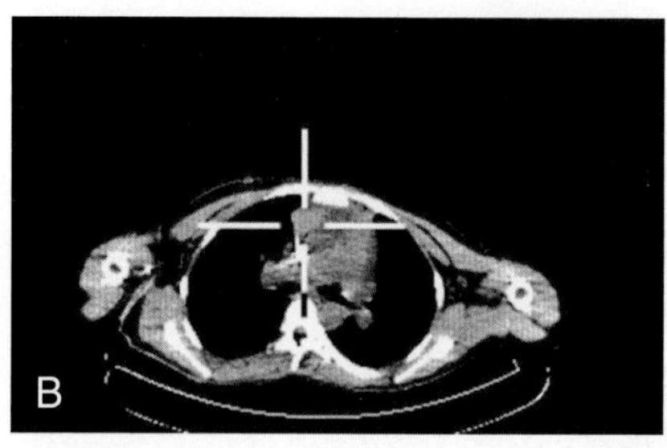


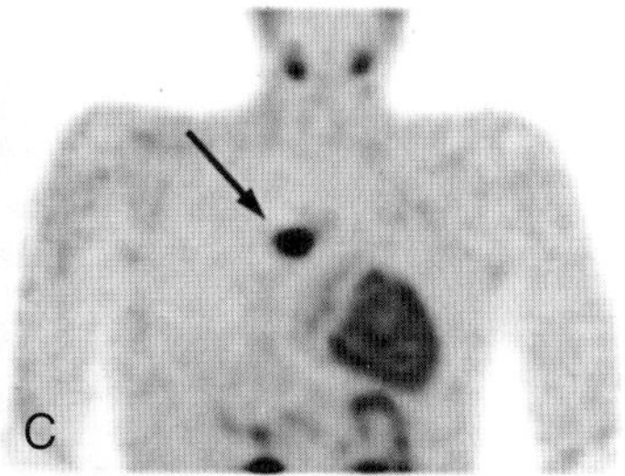


**FIGURE 14-14** $^{99m}$Tc sestamibi SPECT/CT in patient with parathyroid tumor. Transaxial section through SPECT **(A)** and CT **(B)** images from a woman being investigated for a parathyroid tumor. The tumor is seen in the chest in the area of the mediastinum. **C,** A frontal MIP that shows the tumor (*arrow*) as well as normal uptake in the myocardium, neck, and gut.

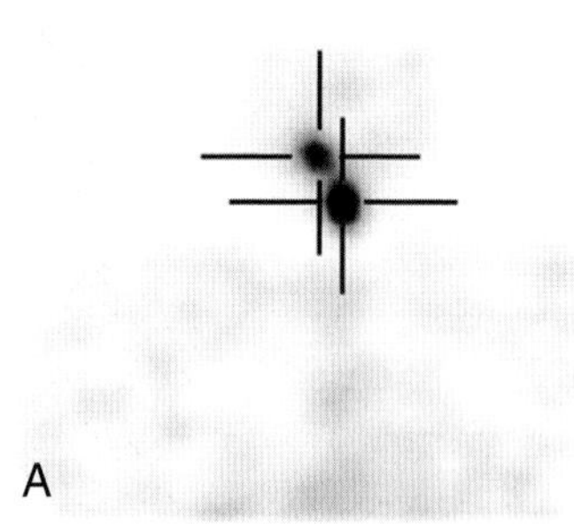


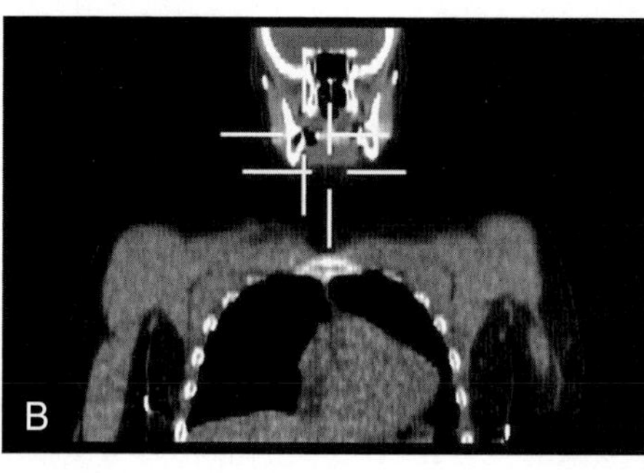


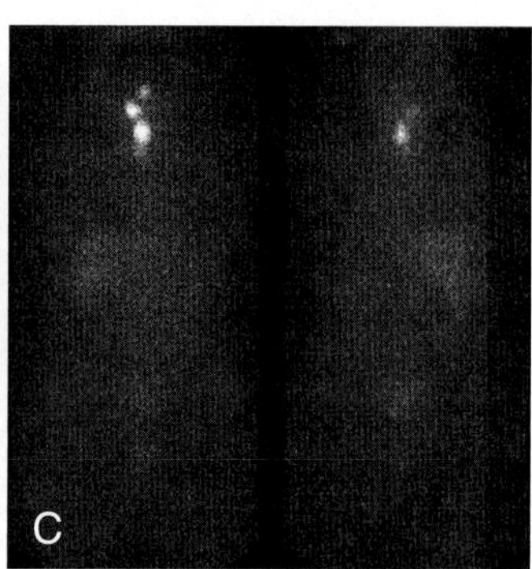


**FIGURE 14-15** $^{131}$I SPECT/CT in patient treated for thyroid cancer. Coronal sections through SPECT **(A)** and CT **(B)** images obtained 7 days after administration of a therapeutic dose of $^{131}$I for the treatment of thyroid cancer. **C,** Shows the anterior and posterior whole-body images that were obtained on the SPECT camera setup to acquire planar images. The whole-body images demonstrate the absence of distance sites. SPECT/CT was performed to further evaluate the foci in the head and neck.

of hyperfunctioning parathyroid glands is the standard treatment for symptomatic disease. SPECT/CT imaging can be a valuable tool for tumor localization and surgical planning.

In a typical parathyroid-imaging protocol, the study is initiated with the injection of ~20 mCi of $^{99m}$Tc sestamibi. The neck is imaged at 20 minutes and 2 hours. A pinhole collimator is used to obtain a magnified image in the area of the thyroid gland, followed by a SPECT acquisition of the thorax.

Images in Figure 14-14 are of the neck and chest of a young woman with elevated parathyroid hormone. SPECT images show focal uptake, which is clearly located on the CT as being in the mediastinum. The focal uptake in the neck, myocardium, and gut are all normal.

## Thyroid Imaging

Iodine concentrates in thyroid tissue, and imaging and therapy with radioiodine have been central to the practice of nuclear medicine since its inception. The two radioisotopes used most frequently in the clinic are $^{123}$I, which has a half-life of 13 hours, and $^{131}$I, which has a half-life of 8 days. Images obtained with a SPECT camera following the uptake of radioiodine have very high contrast since most organs and tissues in the body do not concentrate iodine. This property of iodine makes radioiodine very useful, but it also frames the challenge of nuclear image with a near-ideal imaging agent. Foci of uptake cannot easily be located anatomically since few landmarks can be visualized, making anatomic correlation with CT particularly valuable.

The images of Figure 14-15 are of a middle-aged woman with thyroid cancer. Images were obtained 7 days after the therapeutic administration of 150 mCi of $^{131}$I. The whole-body images (Fig. 14-15, *C*) show several foci in the area of the neck and head. The coronal image formed from the SPECT data intersects two of those foci, which can be localized by CT to the mouth and the thyroid bed. The intense uptake in the thyroid is the intended consequence of the therapy. Uptake in the mouth is most likely normal due to salivary excretion.

## Somatostatin Receptor Imaging

Octreotide is a pharmaceutical that mimics somatostatin and can be labeled with a number of radiotracers to image the distribution of somatostatin receptors in the body. A common radiolabel used in clinical imaging is $^{111}$In, which has a half-life of almost 3 days. As such $^{111}$In-octreotide is a potent marker for neuronal and endocrine tumors that express high concentrations of somatostatin receptors. The long half-life of $^{111}$In allows time for the unbound tracer to clear from the body, resulting in a high target-to-background ratio that yields a highly sensitive test for diseased tissue. In a typical study, an adult patient is injected with ~6 mCi of $^{111}$In-labled octreotide and imaged at 4 and 24 hours post injection.

E-Figure 14-3 shows images from an elderly man who was suspected of having a neuroendocrine tumor. Two abnormal foci are evident in the coronal section of the SPECT image—one in the dome of the liver and the other in the lower abdomen.

## Myocardial Perfusion Imaging

Myocardial perfusion SPECT using $^{99m}$Tc sestamibi is the most commonly performed nuclear medicine study and accounts for ~50% of radiopharmaceutical imaging procedures. These studies provide a method to directly assess the blood flow or perfusion to the myocardium. Often the procedure is performed twice, once with the patient administered $^{99m}$Tc sestamibi (typically ~8 mCi) during rest and again with the patient undergoing stress (typically ~30 mCi), either through exercise or the use of vasodilating drugs. Comparing the two studies can help the clinician determine whether the myocardium is normal, ischemic, or infarcted.

These studies can be subject to photon attenuation artifacts, and uniform attenuation correction is not possible when imaging the thorax. Thus the use of SPECT/CT can assist in alleviating these attenuation artifacts and lead to more accurate interpretation of the images. E-Figure 14-4 shows a SPECT/CT of a patient with normal myocardial perfusion.

## Brain Imaging

Two common $^{99m}$Tc-lableled radiopharmaceuticals are used for imaging brain perfusion with SPECT. Exametazime (commonly referred to as HMPAO) and ethyl cysteinate dimer (ECD) are two agents that cross the blood-brain barrier and distribute in proportion to perfusion in the brain. Since function is coupled to perfusion, the brain scan images acquired after the tracer clears from the blood represent a crude map of brain function. Clinically, SPECT brain imaging is used for a number of indications such as evaluating dementia, localizing epileptic foci, or evaluating brain injury following head trauma.

A typical brain scan protocol involves the injection of ~20 mCi of the radiopharmaceutical and imaging 1 to 2 hours post injection. During the injection and uptake the patient should be made comfortable in a quiet, dimly lit room and should not engage in any activity including reading or speaking as these activities can elevate perfusion in the corresponding areas of the brain and affect the tracer distribution seen in the SPECT images.

The images in Figure 14-16 show a single transaxial section through the brain of a young man. The radiotracer was $^{99m}$Tc-labled ECD. The distribution was judged to be normal.

## Lymphoscintigraphy

**Lymphoscintigraphy** is a technique that involves the injection of tiny amounts of radioactivity (<1 mCi) intradermally. The objective is to mark the sentinel lymph nodes (i.e., the first node to receive lymph drainage from a tumor). If the tumor has metastasized to the lymphatic system, the sentinel lymph node is highly likely to be positive for disease. Lymphoscintigraphy is typically done prior to a surgical procedure, which is very often performed soon after the imaging study so that the radioactive lymph node can be located using an intraoperative probe or **imaging system.** SPECT/CT is an extremely powerful tool for surgical planning. The very high contrast of the SPECT images makes it very difficult to visualize the surrounding anatomy. The registered CT allows the surgeon to localize the target node and to make measurements of location in three dimensions.

Many radiotracer formulations have been tried for lymphoscintigraphy. One of the common formulations is sulfur colloid, a suspension of particles labeled with $^{99m}$Tc. The particles are drained through the lymphatic system and, if the particle size is controlled carefully, the collection in a sentinel node is rapid enough to be well visualized in the nuclear medicine clinic but persists long enough in the sentinel node to be detected during subsequent surgery.

Figure 14-17 shows a sentinel node studied with SPECT/CT. Several intradermal injections were made near a melanoma lesion in the patient's calf. The SPECT images show an inguinal focus clearly located when overlaid on the CT images.

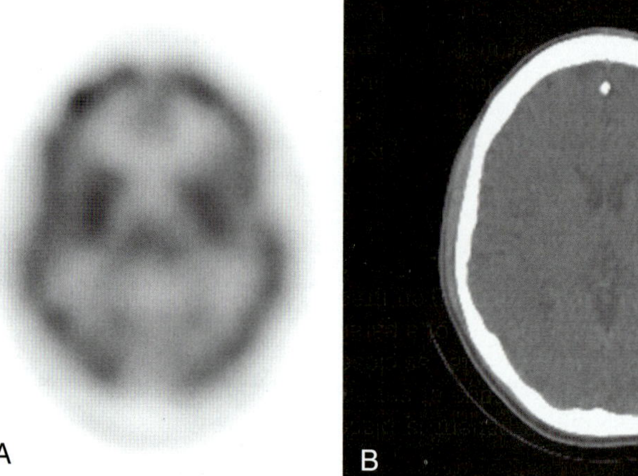


**FIGURE 14-16** $^{99m}$Tc ECD brain SPECT/CT. Transaxial SPECT **(A)** and CT **(B)** images obtained 1 hour after administration of $^{99m}$T-lableled ECD. The images show a normal pattern of perfusion in the brain with the tracer concentrating in the gray matter structures of the cortex and the basal ganglia.

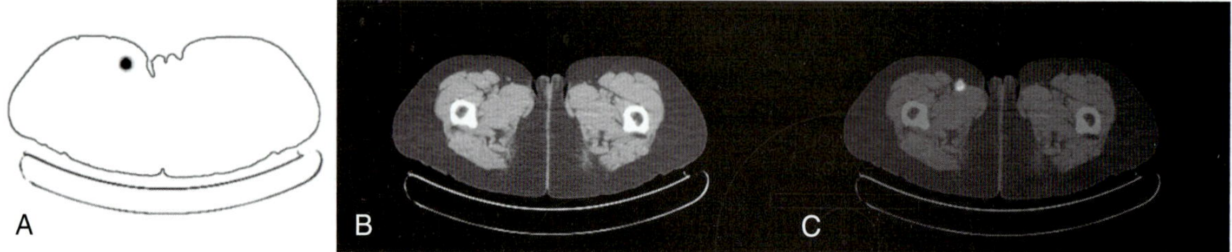


**FIGURE 14-17** Lymphoscintigraphy using $^{99m}$Tc-lableled sulfur colloid. Transaxial SPECT **(A)**, CT **(B)**, and fused **(C)** images at the level of the groin of a patient with melanoma. An inguinal lymph node is clearly identified by the SPECT images. The radiotracer was $^{99m}$Tc-lableled sulfur colloid injected intradermally near the tumor in the calf. The outline seen on the SPECT image was drawn using the CT scan as a guide and then transferred to the SPECT image to better visualize the anatomic location.

## SUMMARY

In the past 30 years PET and SPECT have become invaluable clinical tools providing images of function, physiology, and molecular processes. Emission tomography can provide outstanding images of function and metabolism, which augments the anatomic information provided by CT and MR. For these reasons, it is very useful to register the functional and anatomic data of emission tomography to CT to provide a more complete view of the patient. Thus, in the past 10 years, hybrid PET/CT and SPECT/CT scanners have been developed that can provide both anatomic and functional imaging in a single setting. Although there are many advantages to this hybrid approach, there are also some limitations of which one needs to be cognizant to more optimally use these devices and to better interpret their data. Recent advancements in the imaging technology along with the development of novel radiopharmaceuticals will continue the rapid growth of hybrid emission tomography in the new era of molecular medicine.

## REVIEW QUESTIONS

Answer the following questions to check your understanding of the materials studied.

1. A positron-emitting, radioactive atom, upon transformation, may emit a _________.
   A. alpha particle
   B. positive beta particle
   C. infrared photon
   D. neutron

2. The process by which a positron and an electron combine and are converted to energy is referred to as ______.
   A. Compton scattering
   B. filtered backprojection
   C. internal conversion
   D. annihilation

3. In time-of-flight PET, ________.
   A. the difference in detection time is used to improve reconstruction
   B. the PET study is acquired as a dynamic time sequence of images
   C. the time for the gamma camera to rotate about the patient is measured
   D. the radioactive half-life of the radiopharmaceutical is estimated
4. The device most commonly used to acquire SPECT data is the _______.
   A. high-energy collimator
   B. hybrid PET scanner
   C. photomultiplier tube
   D. rotating gamma camera
5. SPECT data acquisition ___________.
   A. requires a positron-emitting radiopharmaceutical
   B. uses annihilation coincidence detection
   C. can be acquired using an electrocardiogram gate.
   D. does not typically require the use of a collimator
6. Attenuation correction __________.
   A. can be performed using the CT portion of the hybrid scan
   B. is not necessary for PET
   C. compensates for two photons detected at the same time.
   D. requires the acquisition of an emission image
7. An advantage of the incorporation of CT into a hybrid imaging study is it can ______.
   A. lead to faster iterative reconstruction
   B. reduce the radiation dose to the patient
   C. provide anatomic correlation for PET or SPECT
   D. enhance the study with excellent functional imaging
8. Which of the following statements is NOT true about PET/CT?
   A. Practically all current PET devices are PET/CT hybrid scanners.
   B. The PET provides higher spatial resolution than the CT.
   C. The CT study is generally acquired before the PET study.
   D. Both the PET and CT studies deliver radiation dose to the patient.
9. Which of the following statements is NOT true about SPECT/CT?
   A. Practically all current SPECT devices are SPECT/CT hybrid scanners.
   B. CT can be used for attenuation correction in SPECT.
   C. The anatomic information from CT can be very helpful in reading SPECT.
   D. SPECT/CT can be used for cardiac, thyroid, or skeletal imaging.
10. An advantage of SPECT over PET is the ability to image _____________.
    A. with higher sensitivity.
    B. isotopes of carbon, oxygen, and nitrogen.
    C. with better quantitative accuracy.
    D. radiopharmaceuticals used in planar nuclear medicine.

## REFERENCES


Antoch, G., Freudenberg, L. S., Egelhof, T., Stattaus, J., Jentzen, W., Debatin, J. F., et al. (2002). Focal tracer uptake: a potential artifact in contrast-enhanced dual-modality PET/CT scans. *Journal of Nuclear Medicine, 43*, 1339–1342.

Casey, M. E., & Nutt, R. (1986). A multicrystal 2-dimensional BGO detector system for positron emission tomography. *IEEE Transactions on Nuclear Science, 33*, 460–463.

Chang, L. T. (1978). A method for attenuation correction in radionuclide tomography. *IEEE Transactions on Nuclear Science, 25*, 638.

Cherry, S. R., Sorenson, J. A., & Phelps, M. E. (2012). *Physics in nuclear medicine* (4th ed.). Philadelphia, PA: Saunders. 356–360.

Cohnen, M., Poll, L. W., Puettmann, C., Ewen, K., Saleh, A., & Modder, U. (2003). Effective doses in standard protocols for multi-slice CT scanning. *European Radiology, 13*, 1148–1153.

Daghighian, F., Shenderov, P., Pentlow, K. S., Graham, M. C., Eshaghian, B., Melcher, C. L., et al. (1993). Evaluation of cerium doped lutetium oxyorthosilicate (LSO) scintillation crystal for PET. *IEEE Transactions on Nuclear Science, 40*, 1045–1047.

Evans, R. D. (1982). *The atomic nucleus*. New York: Krieger.

Fahey, F. H. (2001). Positron emission tomography instrumentation. *Radiologic Clinics of North America, 39*, 919–929.

Fahey, F. H. (2003). Instrumentation in positron emission tomography. *Neuroimaging Clinics of North America, 13*, 659–669.

Fahey, F. H. (2009). Dosimetry of pediatric PET/CT. *Journal of Nuclear Medicine, 50*, 1483–1491.

Fahey, F. H., Palmer, M. R., Strauss, K. J., Zimmerman, R. E., Badawi, R. D., & Treves, S. T. (2007). Dosimetry and adequacy of CT-based attenuation correction for pediatric PET. *Radiology, 243*, 96–104.

Goerres, G. W., Burger, C., Kamel, E., Seifert, B., Kaim, A. H., Buck, A., et al. (2003). Respiration-induced attenuation artifact at PET/CT: Technical considerations. *Radiology, 226*, 906–910.

Hoffman, E. J., & Phelps, M. E. (1986). Positron emission tomography: principles and quantitation. In M. E. Phelps, J. C. Mazziotta, & H. R. Schelbert (Eds.), *Positron emission tomography and autoradiography: principles and applications for the brain and heart.* New York: Raven.

International Commission on Radiation Protection (ICRP). (2008). *ICRP Report 106, Radiation dose to patients from radiopharmaceuticals* (pp. 85–87).

Kinahan, P. E., Hasegawa, B. H., & Beyer, T. (2003). X-ray-based attenuation correction for positron emission tomography/computed tomography scanners. *Seminars in Nuclear Medicine, 33*, 166–179.

Levin, C. S., & Hoffman, E. J. (1999). Calculation of positron range and its effect on the fundamental limit of positron emission tomography system resolution. *Physics in Medicine and Biology, 44*, 781–799.

Lewellen, T. K. (1998). Time-of-flight PET. *Seminars in Nuclear Medicine, 28*, 268–275.

Lonn, A. (2003). *Evaluation of method to minimize the effect of x-ray contrast in PET-CT attenuation correction.* IEEE Medical Imaging Conference, *M6*, 146.

Ollenberger, G. P., Byrne, A. J., Berlangieri, S. U., Rowe, C. C., Pathmaraj, K., Reutens, D. C., et al. (2005). Assessment of the role of FDG PET in the diagnosis and management of children with refractory epilepsy. *European Journal of Nuclear Medicine and Molecular Imaging, 32*, 1311–1316.

Palmer, M. R., Zhu, X., & Parker, J. A. (2005). Modeling and simulation of positron range effects for high resolution PET imaging. *IEEE Transactions on Nuclear Science, 52*, 1392–1395.

Pantos, I., Thalassinou, S., Argentos, S., Kelekis, N. L., Panayiotakis, G., & Efstathopoulos, E. P. (2011). Adult patient radiation doses from non-cardiac CT examinations: a review of published results. *British Journal of Radiology, 84*, 293–303.

Seo, Y., Wong, K. H., Sun, M., Franc, B. L., Hawkins, R. A., & Hasegawa, B. H. (2005). Correction of photon attenuation and collimator response for a body-contouring SPECT/CT imaging system. *Journal of Nuclear Medicine, 46*, 868–877.

Sharma, P., Mukherjee, A., Bal, C., Malhotra, A., & Kumar, R. (2013). Somatostatin receptor-based PET/CT of intracranial tumors: a potential area of application for 68 Ga-DOTA peptides? *American Journal of Roentgenology, 201*, 1340–1347.

Slomka, P. J., Berman, D. S., & Germano, G. (2014). New cardiac cameras: single-photon emission CT and PET. *Seminars in Nuclear Medicine, 44*, 232–251.

Surti, S. (2015). Update on time-of-flight PET imaging. *Journal of Nuclear Medicine, 56*, 98–105.

Surti, S., Karp, J. S., Freifelder, R., & Liu, F. (2000). Optimizing the performance of a PET detector using discrete GSO crystals on a continuous lightguide. *IEEE Transactions on Nuclear Science, 47*, 1030–1036.

# 15

# Computed Tomography of the Head, Cerebral Vessels, Neck, and Spine*

*Jocelyne S. Lapointe*

## OUTLINE



## LEARNING OBJECTIVES

On completion of this chapter, you should be able to:

1. discuss the indications for CT of the head and face, cerebral blood vessels, neck, and spine.
2. compare the role of CT with other imaging modalities.
3. identify various anatomic structures for CT of the head, neck, and spine.
4. identify relevant patient preparation details that will minimize artifacts, ensure patient safety and comfort, and produce a study of optimal diagnostic quality when performing CT of the head, neck, and spine.
5. identify various positioning considerations when performing CT of the head, neck, and spine.
6. describe briefly scanning protocols used for CT of the head, neck, spine, and cerebral blood vessels.
7. discuss the elements of radiographic techniques, including the influence of slice thickness, matrix size, and reconstruction algorithms used in CT of the head, neck, and spine.
8. outline the use of contrast media in CT of the head, cerebral blood vessels, neck, and spine.

## KEY TERMS TO WATCH FOR AND REMEMBER

The following key terms/concepts are important to your understanding of this chapter

**contrast media**
**magnetic resonance imaging (MRI)**
**position**
**preparation**

*The assistance of CT technologists Donna Lopez and Ron Chitsaz in the preparation of the manuscript is very much appreciated.

Beginning in 1972, **computed tomography (CT)** has provided anatomic information about the body in ways that have greatly increased the diagnosis of pathological conditions in a noninvasive fashion. Neuroradiology is the subspecialty of radiology that deals with the central nervous system and conditions affecting the head and neck. It was revolutionized by CT scanning. It became possible to see inside the brain (i.e., inspect the gray and white matter without the need for a brain biopsy) and to see inside the spinal canal and evaluate disks.

With the advent of multidetector CT scanners at the beginning of the twenty-first century, visualizing the entire vascular tree in a few seconds after an intravenous contrast injection has become feasible. More uses will follow, with further technical developments.

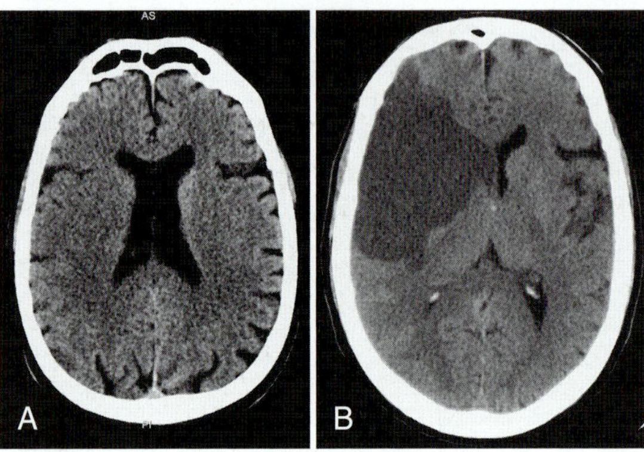


**FIGURE 15-1** **A,** Early subtle infarction. **B,** Late well-defined cerebral infarction. Subtle loss of the distinction between the gray and the white matter is present on the early CT, in the right middle cerebral artery territory, with good delineation of the affected area on the later CT.

## INDICATIONS

### Head and Face

CT is valuable for assessing intracranial pathological conditions, especially in the acute stage. It is performed to guide further investigations and therapy. It is fast and causes no security concerns, in contrast to **magnetic resonance imaging (MRI).** (Patients must be screened before being positioned in the MRI machine, which causes delays.) Motion can cause **artifacts,** but it is less of an issue than with MRI. (Terminology commonly found on imaging requests is written in *italics*, to help the student identify conditions. Not all the conditions mentioned later are illustrated.)

A common indication for CT scanning is acute neurological dysfunction, often presenting as paralysis (*stroke*) or transient ischemic attack (*TIA*). The neurological deficit can be caused by a cerebral infarction from blockage of a blood vessel in the neck or head, by a spontaneous brain hemorrhage caused by hypertension or an underlying blood vessel abnormality such as an aneurysm, by an infection (*viral encephalitis* or *bacterial abscess*), or by a *primary or metastatic tumor*.

*Cerebral infarction* is the result of loss of adequate blood supply to a portion of the brain. In the early stages, it may be difficult to see the location of the infarcted tissue on CT. Early edema (as seen in Fig. 15-1, *A*) causes loss of gray-white matter differentiation, which is the earliest CT sign of infarction. As the infarct matures, it becomes more obvious and better defined. Because of the increased water content of the infarcted tissue, the density is decreased (i.e., dark; Fig. 15-1, *B*).

*Hemorrhage* in the brain substance (Fig. 15-2, *A*) can occur spontaneously, either because of an underlying vascular anomaly, such as a tumor or an *arteriovenous malformation* (*AVM*) or because the patient's hypertension has weakened the walls of the capillary vessels. Hemorrhage can also occur in the subarachnoid space (Fig. 15-2, *B*), resulting in bloody cerebrospinal fluid (CSF; from a leaking aneurysm) or between the brain and its meninges (epidural and subdural spaces). Acutely extravasated blood is of increased density (i.e., white). The degree of mass effect caused by the hematoma is reflected in the amount of brainstem compression from the shift of the midline structures. This affects the patient's level of consciousness, which is measured by the *Glasgow Coma Scale* (range 3 to 15). A normal score is 15 and the lowest score is 3. Delay in **scanning** any patient with a score less than 13 or 14 after a head injury should be avoided because this score can change in less than 5 minutes in the presence of an expanding intracranial hematoma. The technologist should always advise the medical personnel immediately if

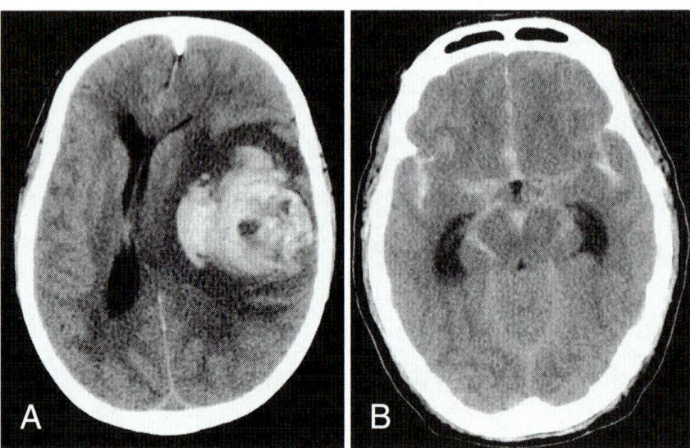


**FIGURE 15-2** **A,** Large left parenchymal hematoma causing a marked midline shift to the right. **B,** Severe *subarachnoid hemorrhage* outlining all the cisterns of the skull base.

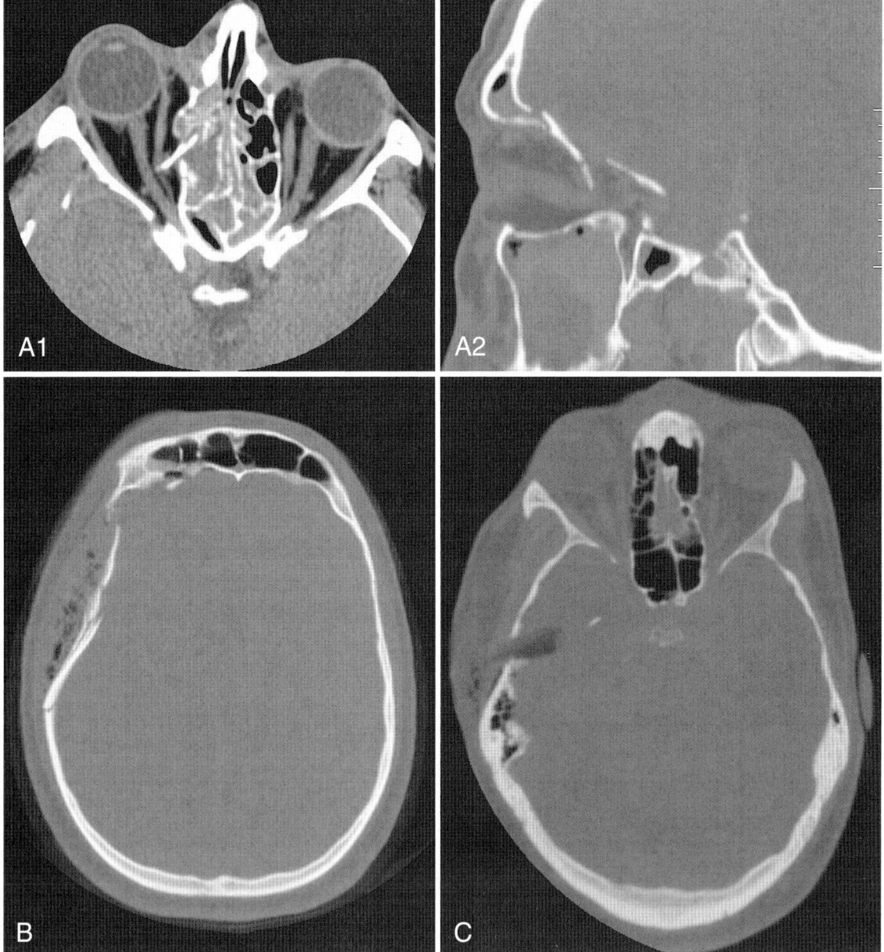


**FIGURE 15-3** **A,** Orbital roof fractures. The transverse image on orbit settings shows the bone fragment spearing the right medial rectus muscle and the sagittal image on bone windows shows the rotation of this fragment. **B,** Comminuted depressed skull fracture with *subcutaneous emphysema* and fluid in the right frontal sinus. **C,** Wooden stick piercing the right temporal bone and lobe, displacing a fragment of bone into the brain, better appreciated on wide windows (it mimics air on routine brain windows, not shown).

a dramatic change in level of consciousness is seen while the patient is in the scanner. (This is one type of patient who should not be left unsupervised, while waiting for transport, for example.)

Hematomas evolve in density over time, becoming less and less dense and finally approaching CSF in density. The clot will be jellylike in the acute phase and will eventually liquefy and shrink. *Chronic subdural hematoma* is the most common condition followed up by repeated CT scanning to document its complete disappearance. Re-accumulation of a chronic subdural hematoma is also common, requiring repeated drainage.

When a traumatic brain or facial injury is suspected, CT provides rapid information about *contusions* (brain bruise) and *hematomas* (blood clot) in the brain and in the spaces between skull and brain (*epidural* and *subdural hematomas*). Facial and skull *fractures* are easily seen (Fig. 15-3, *A*), except linear cranial vault fractures coursing in the plane of section. The depth of depressed bone fragments can be measured (Fig. 15-3, *B*). The results of corrective surgery and the location of metallic **hardware** in the face, as well as the degree of healing callus, are easily appreciated on follow-up examinations.

The most common brain tumor is a *metastasis*; which are often multiple (metastases; Fig. 15-4, *A*). Common primary brain tumors are *meningioma* and *glioblastoma multiforme* (GBM; Fig. 15-4, *B*). Their location and pattern of enhancement is used to predict their histological grade preoperatively.

Stereotaxic procedures by various methods are commonplace in neurosurgery. They are used to accurately localize the lesion before biopsy or resection.

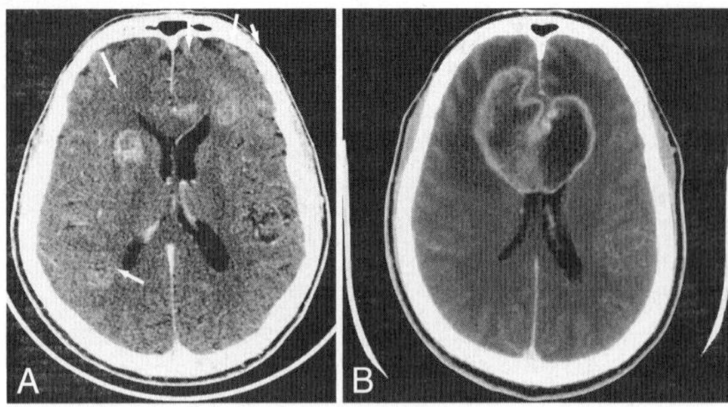


**FIGURE 15-4 A,** Multiple ring enhancing metastases in both frontal lobes. **B,** Enhancing bifrontal (butterfly) GBM; it is surrounded by edema, causing mass effect on the frontal horns.

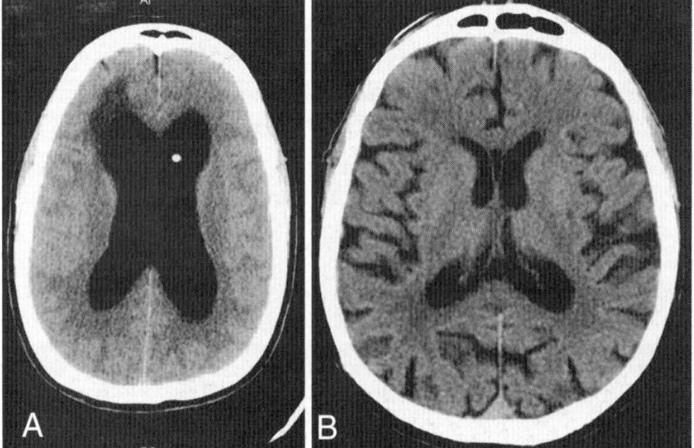


**FIGURE 15-5 A,** Shunted *hydrocephalus* (enlarged ventricles caused by obstruction to CSF flow) can fail, requiring shunt revision. **B,** Brain *atrophy* can also result in large ventricles, without CSF obstruction.

The preoperative studies can be obtained with fiducial markers applied to the scalp or with the head in a stereotaxic frame. Different systems are available, with some frames attaching to the CT table, in place of the head holder. Newer systems are frameless, using a combination of computer programs to superimpose the images and correlate them to the patient's anatomy.

In the case of *meningitis* or *encephalitis*, it is useful to analyze the CSF for the presence of cells and various compounds, such as glucose, proteins, antibodies, and bacteria and viruses. A lumbar puncture (LP) can only be safely performed if the possibility of an intracranial mass (hydrocephalus [Fig. 15-5, *A*], tumor or abscess) has been ruled out. Many physicians prefer the certainty of CT before proceeding with the LP because signs of an intracranial mass are not always present. Brain atrophy can also result in large ventricles and must be distinguished from hydrocephalus (Fig. 15-5, *B*).

Many *congenital brain abnormalities* are diagnosed in childhood, whereas others are only recognized in adulthood. Some types of *seizure* disorders are caused by localized arrested brain development (for example, *cortical dysplasia*). Surgery may alleviate the seizures. Some brain anomalies remain asymptomatic and are an imaging curiosity (for example, cavum of the septum pellucidum, cisterna magna).

Apart from the brain, conditions affecting other components of the head, such as the sinuses, temporal bones, and orbits, are commonly evaluated by CT scanning.

Sinus disease (*sinusitis*, tumor) is readily seen with CT (Fig. 15-6, *A*). Sinus anatomy shows many variations important to the ear, nose, and throat surgeon. To avoid complications such as entering the brain or orbit inadvertently, sinus surgery is often performed with direct correlation with the CT images, a procedure known as functional endoscopic sinus surgery.

The mandible, being a curved bone, is not optimally assessed for pathological conditions with plain films; it is easily evaluated with CT by using two-dimensional (2D) and three-dimensional (3D) reformatted images; a 3D reformatted mandible is shown in Figure 15-6, *B*.

Orbital CT scan images should always be available in at least two planes (transverse and coronal) because of the pyramidal shape of the bony orbit. The intraorbital fat delineates the optic nerve, extraocular muscles, and superior ophthalmic veins. For example, CT accurately localizes radiopaque *foreign bodies* for the surgeon. Wood is not radiopaque and may mimic air, so bone windows should be available (shown in Fig. 15-3, *C*). Although orbital ultrasonography is used widely to study the ocular globe, CT is better at characterizing orbital mass lesions and identifying the cause of *proptosis* (displacement of the globe).

Other uses of CT include looking for pituitary *microadenoma* in the pituitary gland situated in the sella turcica (cause of many endocrine problems) and masses in the middle ear (*cholesteatoma*) and internal auditory canal (*acoustic neuroma*) as causes for hearing loss (Fig. 15-7).

## Cerebral Blood Vessels

Helical scanning makes it possible to image structures during the continued intravenous (IV) injection of a bolus of iodinated contrast medium. Multislice CT scanners extend the length of the vascular tree that can be imaged with one contrast injection. Because of the speed of image acquisition, a pump is used to inject the contrast. A greater scan length (i.e., length of travel of the tabletop) is possible with a greater number of simultaneous slices. At this time, the artifacts caused over the carotid arteries by metal in the

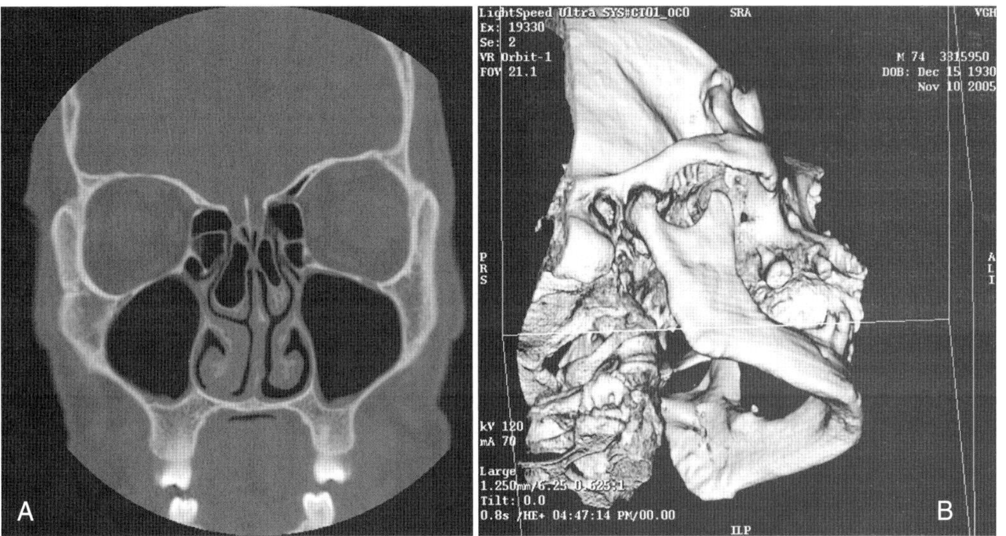


**FIGURE 15-6 A,** Paranasal sinuses obtained prone to better see the drainage pathways of the maxillary sinuses (known as the ostia). **B,** Reformatted 3D image of the mandible. The image can be rotated on the computer to evaluate all the margins of this curved bone.

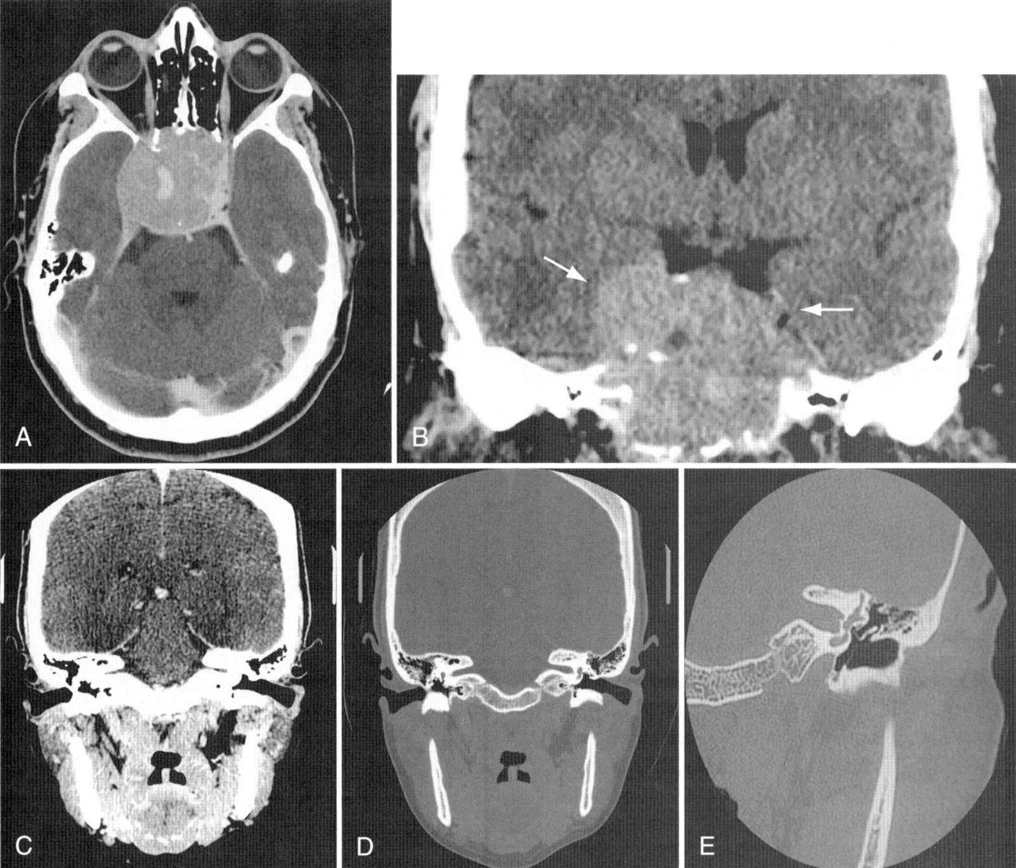


**FIGURE 15-7 A** and **B,** Very large pituitary adenoma, filling the sphenoid sinus but not abutting on the optic chiasm, imaged in transverse plane and reformatted in coronal plane. **C** and **D,** Direct (i.e., with neck extension) coronal images of the internal auditory canals, on soft tissue **(C)** and bone **(D)** algorithms. **E,** Left petrous bone, acquired in direct coronal plane, showing the ossicles in the middle ear, surrounded by air.

mouth (dental fillings, caps, and braces) cannot be completely eliminated. Magnetic resonance angiography (MRA) or catheter angiography may be necessary to rule out or confirm a vascular abnormality suggested by **CT angiography** (CTA).

CTA can outline the cerebral blood vessels from their origin on the aortic arch to their various intracranial branches, as shown in Figure 15-8. Because of the ease and convenience of CTA, the number of patients investigated for vascular conditions has multiplied. The vessels supplying the brain originate from the aortic arch (the innominate or brachiocephalic trunk, left common and left subclavian arteries). The subclavian and the vertebral arteries, the common carotid artery bifurcations (site of most *stenoses*), the internal carotid arteries, the intracranial arteries (anterior, middle, posterior cerebral, basilar, and cerebellar, which are aneurysm sites) are readily visible (Fig. 15-9).

A delay of a few seconds between injection and acquisition of images of the entire brain increases the visualization of the jugular veins and dural sinuses (sagittal and transverse sinuses), which are sites of possible *thrombosis*. This is known as a CT venogram (CTV; not shown).

An important use of CTA is in suspected acute cerebral infarction because rapid intervention may result in lessening the extent of brain damage. After a noncontrast CT of the brain to rule out hemorrhage, CT perfusion (CTP) at the level of the suspected

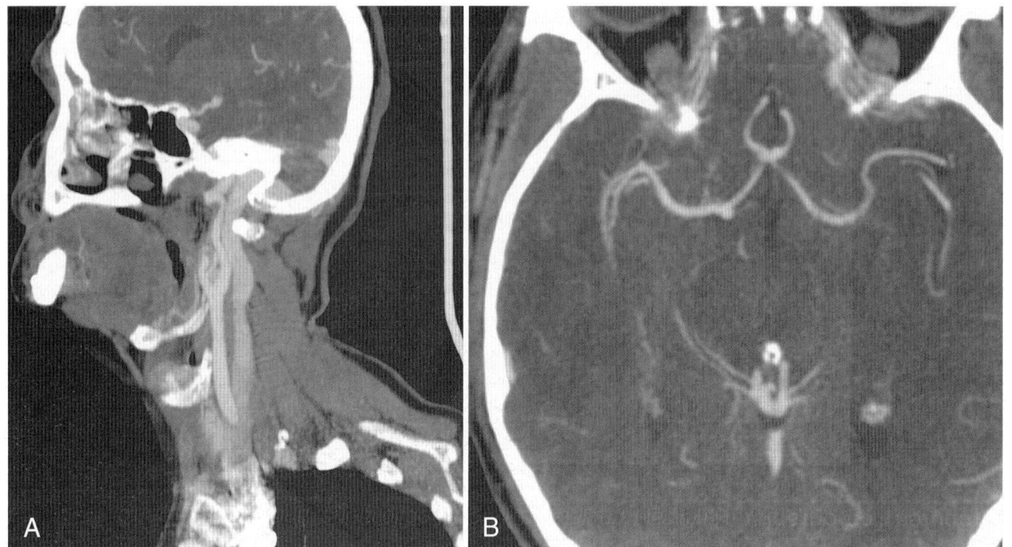


**FIGURE 15-8 A,** Normal CTA of the common carotid bifurcation, showing the Y-shaped arteries and the large jugular vein posterior to it. **B,** Normal CTA of the circle of Willis, showing the anterior communicating artery and both middle cerebral arteries.

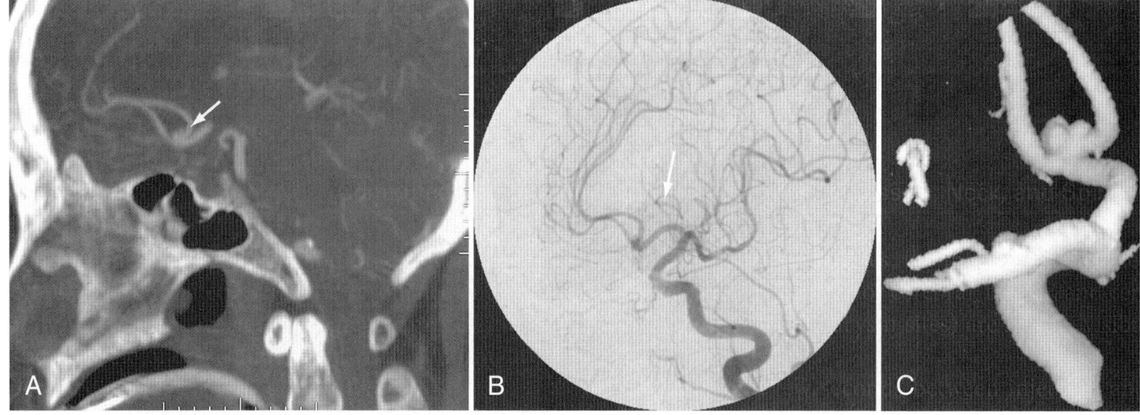


**FIGURE 15-9 A** to **C,** The same *anterior communicating artery aneurysm* is shown on the CTA, the cerebral angiogram, and the 3D model constructed from this angiogram.

infarct is obtained (in some centers) to delineate the amount of brain at risk for permanent damage; CTA of the cerebral vessels follows to identify the presence of clot in a major intracranial artery (usually the middle cerebral or the basilar artery) before a "clot-busting" drug, known as a thrombolytic agent (such as thrombin plasminogen activator) is administered.

Patients with a hemorrhage caused by a suspected aneurysm or an AVM can undergo a CTA to confirm the diagnosis before being transferred to a more specialized treatment center. This is particularly useful in smaller or more remote localities where a neurosurgeon or neurologist is not available.

## Spine and Neck

In many centers CT has replaced plain films of the cervical spine in cases of trauma because it shows injuries not detectable otherwise (see examples of fractures in Fig. 15-10). A certain amount of "pathology" overlap is seen in the cervical region because conditions affecting the vessels, the bones, and the soft tissues are often found when one type of cervical examination is performed. This is most evident when the study is a CTA covering the neck. In addition to bone and vessels, abnormalities of the thyroid gland, the salivary glands, lymph nodes, and neck muscles can be appreciated.

As a result of trauma the carotid or vertebral arteries may be injured (resulting in a *dissection* or *occlusion*) during the violent neck motion that caused a spinal fracture or *dislocation*. Patients with *carotid stenosis* caused by arteriosclerosis are usually older. The cervical spine often shows *disk herniation* or osteophytes causing nerve root compression or *spinal stenosis*. The converse is also true. Studies looking for cervical disk herniation may also show carotid bifurcation calcification, a possible cause of symptomatic carotid artery disease and a potential cause of stroke or TIA.

Masses can occur along the chains of lymph nodes in the neck (for example, *lymphoma*, *Hodgkin's disease*), along nerves (such as vagus nerve *schwannoma*), or adjacent to the vessels (*carotid body tumor*; Fig. 15-11, *A*). Tumors occurring in the salivary glands, nasopharynx, tongue, and floor of the mouth can metastasize to the neck nodes, changing the tumor grade and treatment protocol and the survival rate (Fig. 15-11, *B*).

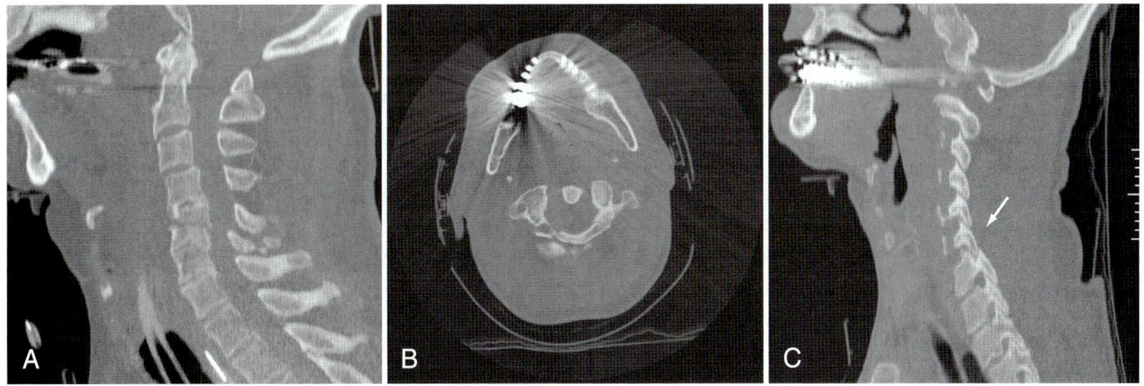


**FIGURE 15-10** **A,** Reformatted image of the cervical spine showing fractures of C2 and C5. Multiple *spinal fractures* are not uncommon. **B,** Metal causes streak artifacts but still demonstrates the C1 fracture. **C,** Alignment is a critical component of spinal assessment. A *facet lock* is present.

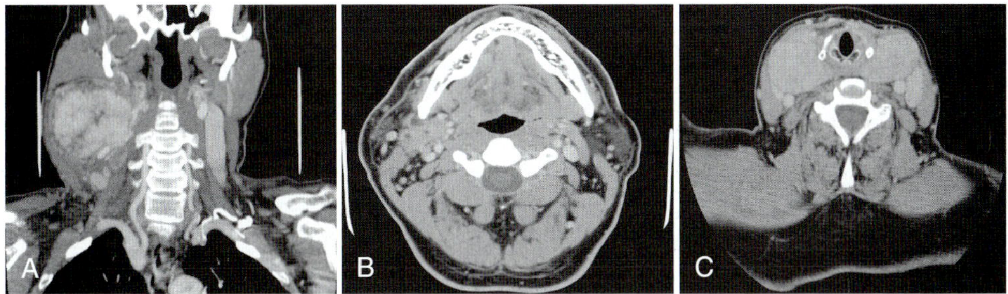


**FIGURE 15-11** **A,** Large vascular mass (carotid body tumor) shown on CTA. **B,** Metastatic ring enhancing necrotic lymph nodes, abutting on the right submandibular gland. **C,** Large thyroid goiter encircling the trachea.

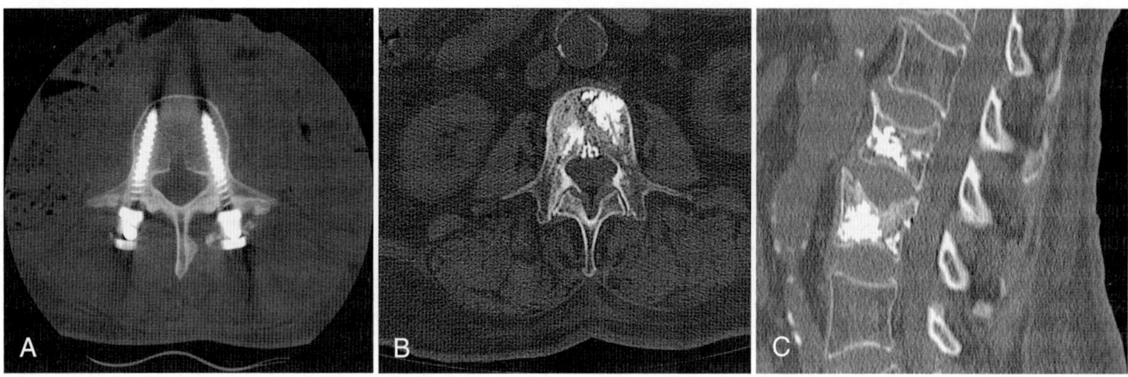


**FIGURE 15-12 A,** Pedicle screws in the lumbar spine, with bone graft material around the head of the left screw. **B** and **C,** Vertebroplasty: radiopaque cement is injected through the pedicles into the vertebral body: transverse and sagittal images.

Preservation of the voice can be achieved in localized laryngeal cancers when treatment consists of a partial laryngectomy. This emphasizes the need for accurate delineation of tumor.

Enlargement of the thyroid gland as the result of a *goiter* is a frequent incidental finding when the neck is imaged for any reason (Fig. 15-11, *C*). When large, a goiter can plunge into the superior mediastinum and cause airway obstruction. Thyroid hormone production can be abnormal, resulting in various symptoms.

Many infections start in the disk space (*diskitis, osteomyelitis*) at any level of the spine. They can spread to the epidural space (*epidural abscess*), resulting in spinal cord compression and paralysis. Other infections extend into the prevertebral or paraspinal tissues. In the neck, they can obstruct the airway or cause difficulty swallowing and drooling. An acutely swollen neck can be life threatening because of the potential for obstruction of the airway, particularly in children.

Tumors affecting the spine or spinal cord can originate as primary tumors or metastasize from other sites to bone or soft tissue, affecting the vertebral bodies, the pedicles, laminae, and facet joints. Their treatment often requires removal of a great deal of bone, resulting in possible instability of the spine. Bone grafts and metallic instrumentation are frequently inserted to preserve patient mobility. Metallic instrumentation may fail, requiring frequent follow-up by imaging (plain films/CT) and occasionally surgical revision.

Instrumentation of the spine is also used in treating atlantoaxial (C1-2) instability in *rheumatoid arthritis* and in treating *scoliosis*, spine fractures, *spinal stenosis*, and *spondylolisthesis*. It requires accurate placement of pedicle screws, hooks, wires, and plates. CT accurately depicts the **position** of the instrumentation. In some cases, screws may traverse a foramen and impinge on a nerve root or a vertebral artery; a neurological deficit or pain can ensue (Fig. 15-12, *A*).

Another type of spinal procedure is vertebroplasty. Radiopaque cement (methylmethacrylate) is injected under fluoroscopic control into spinal compression fractures to reduce pain and in some cases to decrease the kyphosis.

Postprocedure CT scans of the many types of spinal interventions described previously are common to assess the results (Fig. 15-12, *B* and *C*).

## ROLE OF CT COMPARED WITH OTHER IMAGING MODALITIES

The recent advent of multislice CT scanners with the capacity to image multiple organ systems at one sitting without having to move the patient has revolutionized the evaluation of a number of acute conditions. Multiple trauma patients in particular are assessed from head to toe by CT scan, in many cases replacing plain radiographs and catheter angiography. The sequencing of these examinations is important to increase diagnostic accuracy while minimizing the radiation dose and the volume of IV contrast. Ideally, the sequence should evaluate the patient for the most life-threatening conditions first on the basis of the initial assessment.

The noncontrast head CT (using thin slices for later reformatted images if facial fractures are readily apparent) should be followed by CTA of the thoracic aorta (to rule out a dissection) and CT of the chest, abdomen, and pelvis (to look for solid and hollow organ injury). CTA of the neck vessels can be obtained last.

Reformatted images of the entire spine on bone **algorithm** in three planes, obtained from the previous series, are used to rule out spine fractures and evaluate alignment. Reformatted facial bone and mandible images, also on bone algorithm, are produced if required.

More subtle fractures can be diagnosed with CT than with plain films. Nursing practices (for example, turning the patient in the intensive care unit to avoid bed sores) can be influenced by the presence of spine fractures not visible on plain films.

Such multiple studies can easily result in 2000 to 2500 images in total. Better quality images are obtained if the patient's arms can be moved (down for the head and neck CTA and up for the chest-abdomen; i.e., if the patient has no clavicle, scapula, or humeral fractures). Some trauma cases also require other orthopedic scans (e.g., pelvis, hips) or a CT cystogram.

CTA can complement duplex ultrasonography. It is not hampered by calcification, unlike ultrasonography. Also unlike ultrasonography, it cannot determine direction or velocity of blood flow. The CTA can image the cervical blood vessels over a longer segment than can duplex ultrasonography.

Transcranial Doppler imaging (another form of ultrasonography) can be used to evaluate flow in intracranial vessels, but it is not widely available. The CTA images are more "user friendly" than ultrasonography for most clinicians. MRA currently does not provide the same rapid answers as CTA in acute stroke in most institutions.

Enlarged thyroid glands can indicate an increased or decreased production of thyroid hormone, resulting in symptoms affecting various organ systems. Initial evaluation of a thyroid goiter by ultrasonography allows for fine-needle aspiration. Gadolinium-enhanced MRI of the neck does not affect thyroid iodine metabolism. It can be used as a substitute for CT when iodine therapy of a thyroid nodule is planned.

Although MRI is the preferred imaging technique for the spinal cord and the intervertebral disks, CT scanning continues to provide valuable information about calcification and the bones. Similar to brain CT, spine lesions such as tumor and infection will enhance with IV contrast. CT can thus be used when MRI is dangerous, as in the presence of a cardiac pacemaker or the older types of cerebral aneurysm clips.

In the absence of trauma, CT (or MRI) can be used when acute spinal cord compression is diagnosed by the sudden loss of sensation, motor function, or bowel or bladder function. Common causes include *epidural abscesses* in IV drug users and *spinal metastasis*. (Symptoms caused by metastasis to the brain or spine are often the presenting complaint in individuals with no known primary cancer; up to half of new cases of cancer are discovered because of their metastases.)

CT-guided procedures such as nerve root blocks, facet blocks, and spine biopsies require scanning the same levels repeatedly. Some CT scanners have a "fluoroscopy" option to assist in these procedures. These procedures are also performed on the usual fluoroscopic units.

Patients with spinal instrumentation sometimes need re-evaluation of the contents of their spinal canal. Metallic artifacts can impede CT and MRI diagnosis because the spinal canal is obscured or distorted by the artifact. Some newer CT scanners can reduce this metallic spray artifact by extending the Hounsfield units thanks to a special metal artifact-reduction **software** program.

Another way around this problem is a myelogram followed by a CT scan: water-soluble contrast medium specific for subarachnoid use is injected under fluoroscopy by LP or C1-2 puncture into the subarachnoid space by the radiologist. After suitable fluoroscopic images are obtained, CT images are acquired on bone algorithm (kernel) and reformatted in the appropriate planes. Adhesions of spinal cord or nerve roots (*arachnoiditis*), spinal cord cavities (*syrinx*), and other conditions obscured by the metallic artifacts can be diagnosed and treated appropriately (Fig. 15-13).

## SECTIONAL ANATOMY: A REVIEW

**R. A. Nugent, revised by J. S. Lapointe**

Image acquisition is obtained in the transverse (axial) plane with the patient in a (usually) supine position or (occasionally) in a prone or decubitus position. Knowledge of sectional anatomy is mandatory. A readily available reference text is an invaluable tool.

Because the acquisition of images with most CT scanners now in use is multiplanar (i.e., 4 to 64 slices), the review of coronal and sagittal reformatted images is now commonplace. These planes, by presenting the anatomy in a more traditional fashion, illustrate variations in the expected anatomy and the spread of disease. The student gains a better understanding of sectional anatomy by correlating transverse images with reformatted images in the other two planes. The angle of an oblique structure, such as the lateral wall of the orbit, is subsequently easier to appreciate.

As with plain radiographs, such as a chest x ray, transverse (axial) images and coronal reformatted

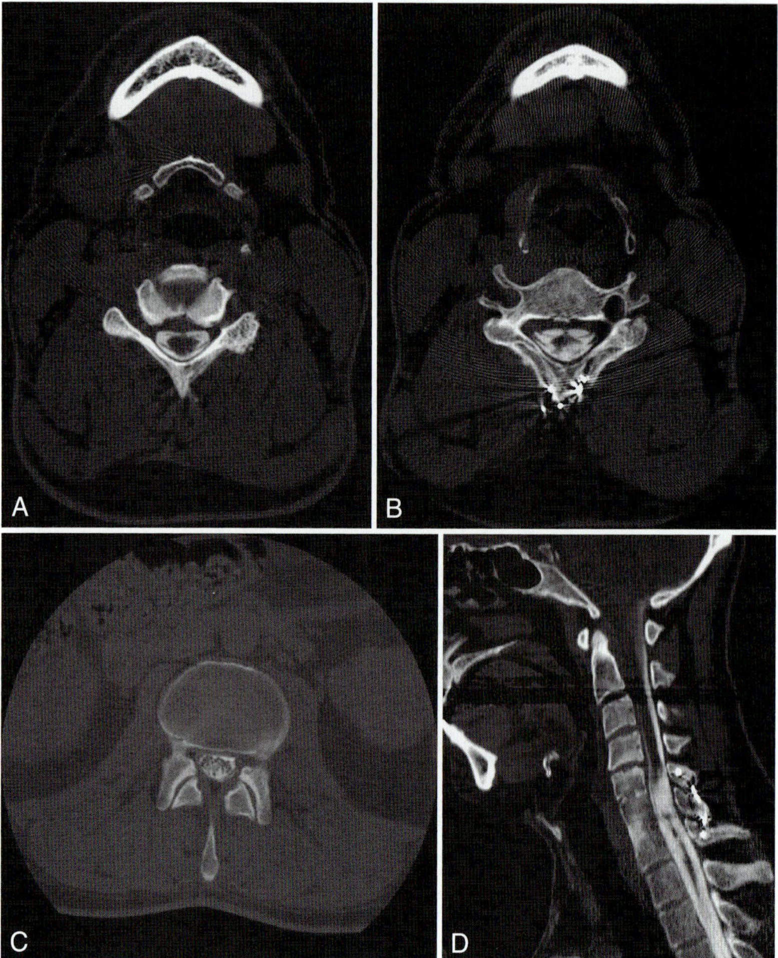


**FIGURE 15-13 A,** CT myelogram delineates a normal cervical spinal cord and nerve roots. **B,** The cervical spinal cord (outlined by contrast) is distorted by injury. **C,** The normal lumbar nerve roots are outlined by the intrathecal contrast. **D,** A sagittal reformatted image shows how using the bone algorithm (or equivalent) minimizes the artifact caused by the posterior metallic wiring of the spine.

images are viewed with the patient's right side on the viewer's left (i.e., as if facing the individual). Local preference (usually the radiologist) dictates whether the transverse (axial) images are viewed from top to bottom or vice versa and if the sagittal images are viewed from right to left or left to right. Labeled scout (topogram, scanogram) images must be available to decrease uncertainty about slice location and for accurate reporting.

## Head

### Transverse Sections

The anatomic structures of the normal appearance of the brain by use of a standard algorithm are shown in Figure 15-14. Slices through the skull base (Fig. 15-15) give exquisite detail of the foramina, facial structures, pituitary fossa, and temporal bones. CSF in the basal cisterns and ventricles helps define the anatomy, as does calcium in normal structures such as the choroid plexus, pineal gland, and falx cerebri. Differentiation of white and gray matter allows for definition of the basal ganglia, thalamus, and external and internal capsules.

### Coronal Sections

Coronal images (Figs. 15-16 through 15-19) are particularly useful for assessing bone when the plane of the bone runs parallel to the axial slice. Coronal images therefore are valuable for scans of the floor and roof of the orbit, the skull base, and the top of the cranial vault. The pituitary gland is well defined as a fairly rectangular structure within the sella turcica, which is intersected in the midline, slightly posteriorly, by the pituitary stalk. The cranial nerves in the

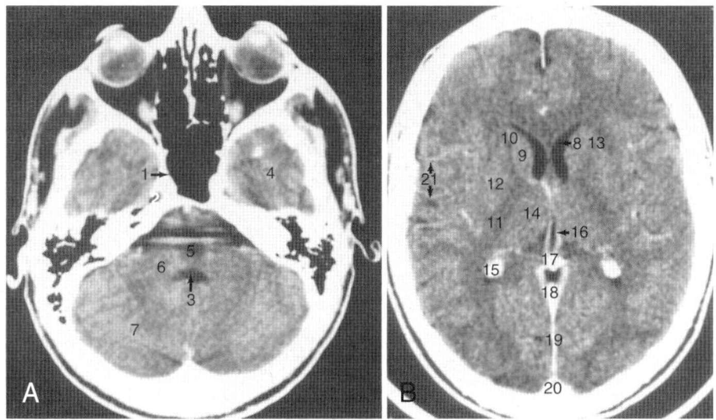


**FIGURE 15-14** **A** and **B,** Brain. The normal appearance of the brain using a standard algorithm and 5-mm-thick images, obtained with IV contrast enhancement. *1,* Sphenoid sinus; *2,* trigeminal ganglion; *3,* fourth ventricle; *4,* temporal lobe; *5,* pons (partly obscured by streak artifact); *6,* middle cerebellar peduncle; *7,* cerebellar hemisphere; *8,* frontal horn of the lateral ventricle; *9,* head of the caudate nucleus; *10,* anterior limb of the internal capsule; *11,* posterior limb of the internal capsule; *12,* lentiform nucleus; *13,* external capsule; *14,* thalamus; *15,* calcified choroid plexus; *16,* internal cerebral vein; *17,* pineal calcification; *18,* straight sinus; *19,* falx cerebri; *20,* superior sagittal sinus; *21,* branches of the middle cerebral artery. The use of a standard algorithm with a relatively narrow window (80 units) results in good contrast between white and gray matter.

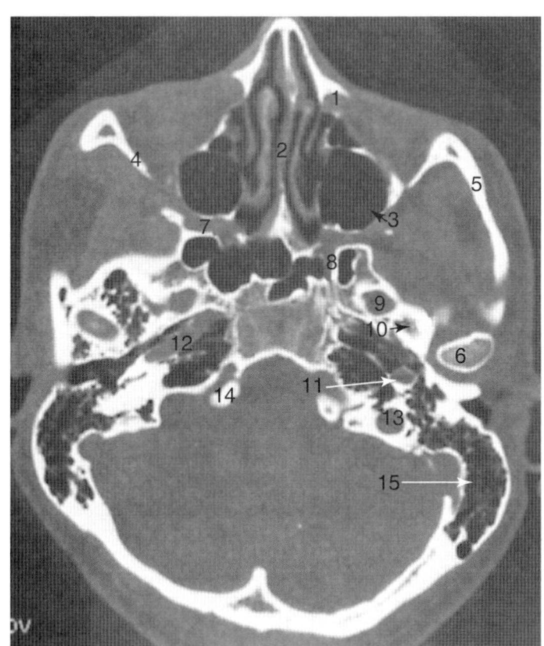


**FIGURE 15-15** A 1.5-mm-thick axial slice through the base of the skull using the bone algorithm shows excellent spatial resolution. *1,* Opening of the nasolacrimal duct; *2,* nasal septum; *3,* maxillary sinus; *4,* lateral orbital wall; *5,* zygomatic arch; *6,* mandibular condyle; *7,* pterygopalatine fossa; *8,* vidian (pterygoid) canal; *9,* foramen ovale; *10,* foramen spinosum; *11,* ascending carotid canal; *12,* horizontal carotid canal; *13,* jugular fossa; *14,* jugular tubercle; *15,* mastoid air cells.

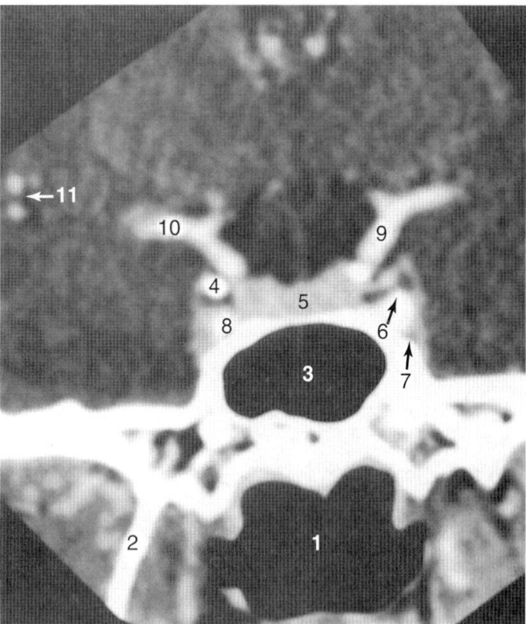


**FIGURE 15-16** Sella turcica. A 1.5-mm-thick coronal slice through the sella turcica, obtained with IV contrast enhancement, demonstrates these structures: *1,* oropharynx; *2,* lateral pterygoid plate; *3,* sphenoid sinus; *4,* anterior clinoid; *5,* pituitary gland; *6,* cranial nerve III; *7,* cranial nerve VI; *8,* cavernous portion of the internal carotid artery; *9,* supraclinoid portion of the internal carotid artery; *10,* middle cerebral artery; *11,* branches of the middle cerebral artery.

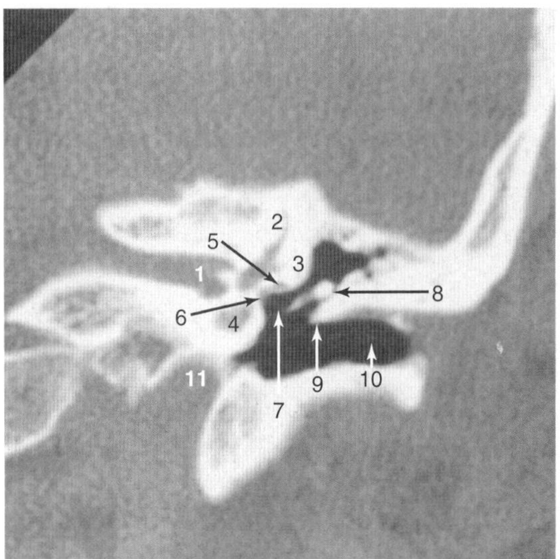


**FIGURE 15-17** Temporal bone. A 1-mm coronal image through the left temporal bone using the high-resolution bone algorithm is demonstrated. The thinness of the slice, as well as the smaller FOV, helps maximize the spatial resolution. *1*, Internal auditory canal; *2*, superior semicircular canal; *3*, lateral semicircular canal; *4*, cochlea; *5*, horizontal portion of the facial canal; *6*, oval window; *7*, stapes; *8*, malleus; *9*, Chausse spur; *10*, external auditory canal; *11*, carotid canal.

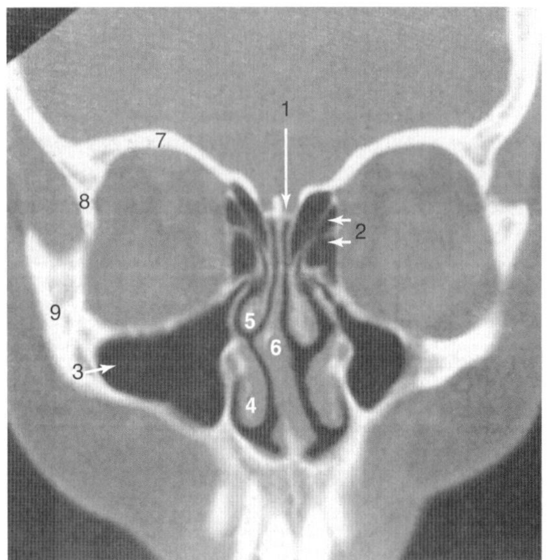


**FIGURE 15-18** Paranasal sinuses and facial bones. A 3-mm-thick coronal image using the bone algorithm demonstrates the air-containing paranasal sinuses and nasal airway. *1*, Cribriform plate; *2*, ethmoid sinuses; *3*, maxillary sinus; *4*, inferior turbinate; *5*, middle turbinate; *6*, nasal septum; *7*, roof of the orbit; *8*, lateral orbital wall; *9*, zygoma.

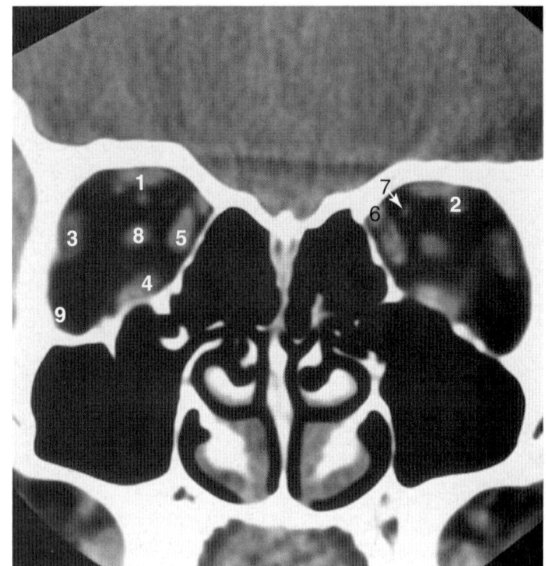


**FIGURE 15-19** Orbits. A 3-mm-thick coronal view of the orbits, obtained without IV contrast enhancement, demonstrates that orbital fat produces excellent contrast, resulting in good definition of the extraocular muscles and optic nerve. *1*, Superior rectus muscle; *2*, superior ophthalmic vein; *3*, lateral rectus muscle; *4*, inferior rectus muscle; *5*, medial rectus muscle; *6*, superior oblique muscle; *7*, ophthalmic artery; *8*, optic nerve.

cavernous sinus can be identified on either side of the pituitary gland.

Coronal images of the temporal bone can highlight the relationships of the ossicles and structures along the medial wall of the middle ear, including the facial canal, oval window, and lateral semicircular canal. Coronal images intersect the tentorium and demonstrate its tentlike appearance. They help define whether a lesion is supratentorial or infratentorial, which aids in surgical planning.

A tumor that abuts a ventricle can be assessed in the coronal plane to determine whether it arises from or is extrinsic to the ventricle.

### Sagittal Sections

Sagittal sections are not used routinely in most institutions, but are now easier to obtain with multislice scanners. They are particularly helpful in evaluating the midline structures.

## Neck

When an IV contrast medium is used to enhance images, major vascular structures such as the carotid arteries and jugular veins can be identified. Both the superficial mucosa and the submandibular glands enhance. The parotid gland, with its high fat content,

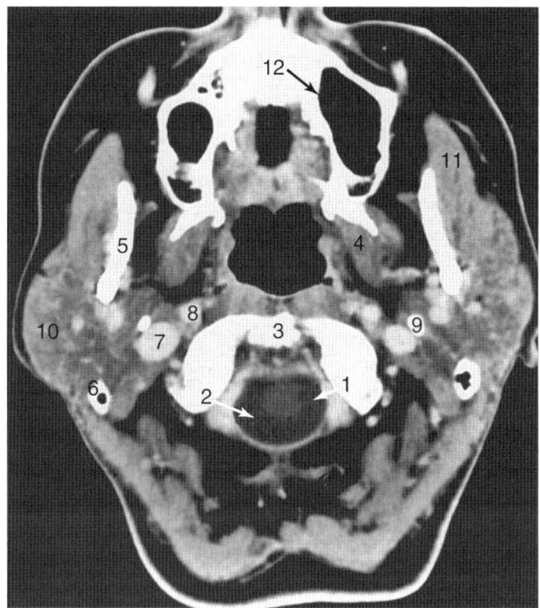


**FIGURE 15-20** Neck. This 3-mm-thick axial slice through the upper neck was obtained with IV contrast enhancement. *1*, Spinal cord; *2*, cerebrospinal fluid; *3*, top of the odontoid; *4*, pterygoid muscles; *5*, mandible; *6*, tip of the mastoid; *7*, internal jugular vein; *8*, internal carotid artery; *9*, styloid process; *10*, parotid gland; *11*, masseter muscle; *12*, maxillary sinus.

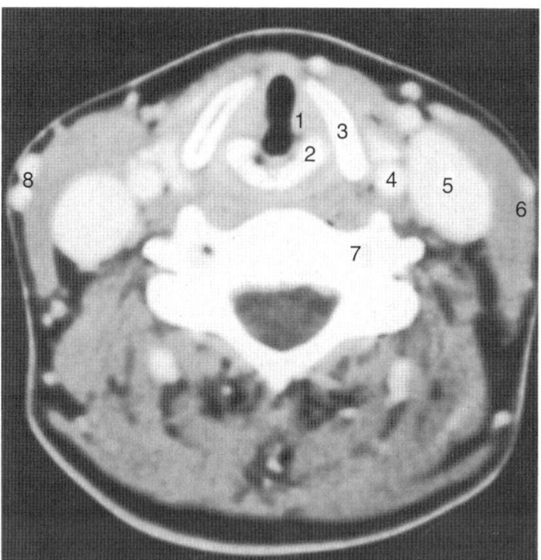


**FIGURE 15-21** Larynx. A 3-mm-thick axial slice through the larynx obtained at the level of the vocal cords demonstrates prominent enhancement of the vascular structures. The laryngeal cartilages are better defined on the bone setting, which is not included here. *1*, True vocal cord; *2*, arytenoid cartilage; *3*, thyroid cartilage; *4*, common carotid artery; *5*, internal jugular vein; *6*, sternocleidomastoid muscle; *7*, vertebral artery; *8*, superficial veins.

demonstrates an intermediate density between those of fat and muscle (Fig. 15-20).

Thin sections of the larynx show the relationship of the cartilages to the adjacent soft tissue. The level of the true vocal cords is defined by the position of the arytenoid cartilages (Fig. 15-21).

## Spine

The sectional anatomy of the lumbar and cervical spines is illustrated in Figures 15-22 and 15-23, respectively. Spine images are acquired in the transverse plane, either helically or by varying the **gantry** tilt. Coronal or sagittal images can now be obtained easily with multiplanar CT scanners. CT differentiates the disk from the adjacent ligamentum flavum, thecal sac, intraspinal fat, and bone. The nerve roots are easily identified as they exit through the intervertebral foramina. Epidural veins can be seen, particularly in the lumbar spine, but are better visualized with contrast medium enhancement.

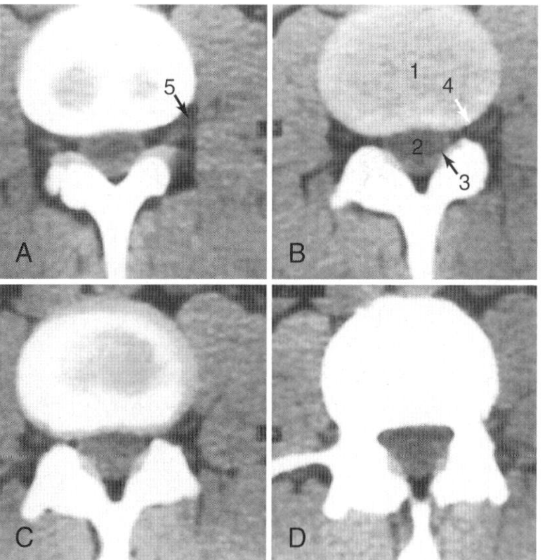


**FIGURE 15-22** Lumbar spine. Four sections **(A-D)** through the L3-4 disk space were obtained every 4 mm using a slice thickness of 5 mm. The disk (*1*) is slightly higher in density than the adjacent paravertebral muscle and the thecal sac (*2*). The ligamentum flavum (*3*) is also slightly denser than the thecal sac. Fat in the spinal canal and intervertebral foramen (*4*) helps define the root sleeve (*5*).

# PATIENT PREPARATION

Little **preparation** is needed in most cases. Attention to the following details will minimize artifacts,

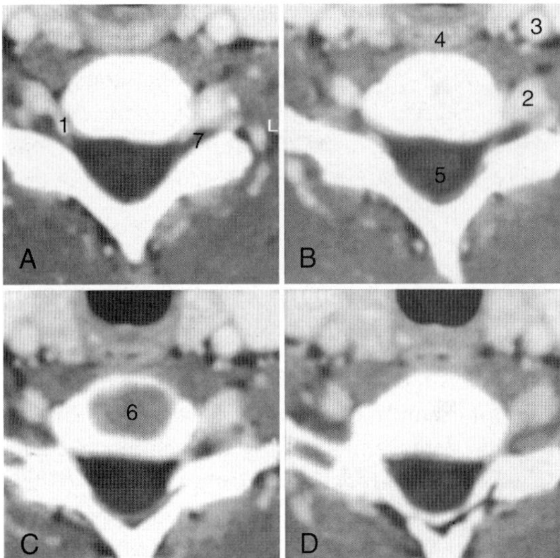


**FIGURE 15-23** Cervical spine. Sequential 3-mm-thick images **(A-D)** obtained every 2 mm through the C6-7 disk space demonstrate prominent enhancement of the epidural veins (*1*), vertebral artery (*2*), and carotid artery (*3*), as well as the esophagus (*4*), spinal cord (*5*), and disk (*6*). The dorsal root ganglion (*7*) is outlined by the epidural veins.

ensure patient safety and comfort, and produce a study of optimal diagnostic quality.

- *Metallic objects*: The area to be scanned should be free of all jewelry, hairpins, metal gown snaps, wires attached to the patient, and other devices. They can be moved out of the field when they are noted on the scout (scanogram, topogram) images, without having to repeat the scout in most cases. Glasses are removed but contact lenses remain in place for brain scanning.
- *Fasting* is not required. However, if IV contrast is being used, a large meal immediately before the CT scan is discouraged in case the contrast causes nausea or vomiting.
- An *empty bladder* is important, especially if the time in the CT scan may be prolonged, as for a CT-guided biopsy or nerve root block.
- *Patient anxiety* may be eased by the technologist's calm demeanor. After confirming the patient's identity, the technologist introduces himself, gives a short explanation of the procedure and the reason for using contrast, and describes expected sensations (heat, **noise,** table movement, and need for staying still).
- *Contrast injection* requires a review of known drug/contrast allergies and of the renal function to minimize contrast reactions and kidney impairment resulting from contrast-induced nephropathy. (This step may be done before the study is scheduled, but the technologist should be aware of this information before contrast is administered.) The appropriate needle size and injection site for the requested study can then be chosen.
- *Cardiac medications* may indicate poor cardiac function. This is relevant information for CTA.
- A *comfortable position* on the scanning table, with holding straps and warm blankets or cushions under the knees and elbows, may result in less motion, reducing image repetition and radiation dose.
- The *eyes* should be closed when the laser positioning light is used near the eyes.

The following may be helpful when the technologist is faced with challenging patients:

- *Combative or uncooperative patients* (for example, because of head injury, psychiatric problems, dementia, and alcohol) require special precautions. More restraints than usual may be needed to obtain a diagnostic study. Use of rapid helical scanning (for example, 800 milliseconds [ms], instead of the usual 1000 to 2000 ms) reduces the resolution between gray and white matter, but the study will be of sufficient quality to demonstrate life-threatening lesions, such as an intracerebral hematoma and the degree of midline shift it has caused, necessitating urgent surgical intervention. The technologist must be very vigilant to avoid personal injury.
- *Body fluid protection* should always be observed (the minimum is gloves when dealing with a trauma patient). When appropriate, the patient or the technologist will need to wear a mask and gown (when working with carriers of antibiotic-resistant bacteria, for example, methicillin-resistant *Staphylococcus aureus* or vancomycin-resistant *Escherichia coli*).

## POSITIONING

Image acquisition is obtained with the patient in a supine position. Occasionally, the prone position is required, as for paranasal sinuses, sella turcica, and some CT-guided procedures such as biopsies or nerve root or facet blocks.

A decubitus position, which is seldom used, is reserved for patients who cannot tolerate the supine position. The images can be rotated to a correct position on the reporting console. However, proper annotation of the images, as to side, is necessary for accurate reporting.

Patients with ankylosing spondylitis may present a special positioning challenge because of their severe kyphosis. Stabilizing the patient with cushions or folded blankets minimizes motion. If tilting the gantry to the desired plane is not feasible, helical images reformatted in the usual plane are often diagnostic. Severe scoliosis can be assessed in a similar fashion.

The technologist must center the area to be scanned in the center of the gantry, both horizontally and vertically. Choosing the correct **field of view (FOV)** to encompass the anatomy in question ensures a quality study. The reference detectors must not receive interference from equipment or coverings, such as restraints or blankets, to produce accurate **CT numbers.**

## SCANNING PROTOCOLS

CT scanners are equipped with preset protocols/techniques and a variety of slice thicknesses, which may vary depending on the model and the manufacturer. Adjustments to radiation dose can be made on the basis of patient size. Locally developed protocols can also be used. This usually consists of choosing a **slice thickness** and a plane of section for the organ or structure in question, as well as determining the route of contrast administration and dose.

Standardized departmental protocols, developed in collaboration with the radiologists, help to ensure image quality and facilitate patient throughput. Technological changes/updates will require protocol adjustments from time to time.

The following information is based on current usage at a single institution, which has four different types of helical CT scanners (single-slice, 8-slice, 16-slice, and 64-slice scanners). Protocols are adjusted to approximate results from each of the four scanners for the sake of uniformity. Some studies are only carried out on certain scanners to optimize the images (for example, temporal [petrous] bone).

Circumstances such as excessive motion may require changing the technique (milliamperage and time). Image quality will be decreased when a shorter scanning time is used, but the study should be adequate to rule out a surgical emergency.

### Head and Its Contents

Two transverse scanning planes are widely used in brain imaging. In adults, the orbitomeatal baseline (OM line, also called Reid's baseline or RBL) joining the infraorbital rim to the superior border of the external auditory meatus is favored because it results in better images of the orbits, sella turcica, posterior fossa, and brainstem. Some centers use the canthomeatal line (CM line), which joins the lateral canthus of the eye to the center of the external auditory canal. The angle measured between these two lines is 10 degrees.

In children, a steeply angled plane, commonly 20 to 25 degrees to the OM or CM line is used to scan the brain to avoid radiating the ocular lens leading to early cataracts (Fig. 15-26, *A*, later in this section).

The transverse plane is still the most used plane for image interpretation of the skull and its contents. If reformatted images are required, it is better to acquire thin slices initially and to reformat the images. This technique is useful when scanning the orbits; for example, the lenses of the eyes are scanned only once, dental amalgam artifact is eliminated, and images in true coronal plane (perpendicular to the hard palate) are generated. Patient comfort is also increased compared with direct coronal imaging, when the neck must be hyperextended to achieve a near coronal position and the gantry tilted appropriately. Coronal sections are particularly useful when structures that run parallel to the transverse plane are assessed, such as the floor and roof of the orbits, the sella turcica and adjoining cavernous sinuses, and the skull base and vertex.

Exceptions to this approach exist. Direct coronal images of the temporal petrous bones/internal auditory canals and sella turcica are preferred because the resolution of the 0.6 to 1.25 millimeter (mm) slices is greater than with reformatted images and the orbits are avoided. Prone direct coronal images are also preferred in some centers for the study of paranasal sinuses because air-fluid levels tend to pool away from the path of drainage, known as the ostia, resulting in a better study than the supine transverse or hyperextended (supine coronal) positions. Thin transverse images with sagittal and coronal reformatted images are used when extension of the neck is not possible.

Sagittal images have not been used routinely in the past but are gaining in popularity. They are particularly useful when assessing midline structures and midline abnormalities of the brain and spine.

The algorithm (or kernel) chosen will affect the resolution of the images. In some cases, it may be possible to acquire diagnostic images using low milliamperage, as with paranasal sinuses or facial bones. Fractures, *sinusitis*, and *nasal polyps* can easily be assessed this way, using only a bone algorithm or equivalent kernel. Temporal (petrous) bones, on the other hand, need higher milliamperage to get accurate detail of the densest bone in the body and its small structures, such as the cochlea, semicircular canals, and ossicles.

Contrast enhancement is not visible on bone algorithm or bone windows. When contrast is used, images on soft tissue algorithms (standard or equivalent) are also required to see the enhancing tissue, such as with sinus tumors and chronic sinus infections.

## Neck, Spine, and Cerebral Blood Vessels

Traditionally, the transverse plane was the preferred plane for interpretation. However, multiplanar reconstructions in coronal, sagittal, and oblique planes greatly enhance the radiologist's ability to diagnose conditions affecting these areas, which contain bony curves (cervical lordosis and mandible), soft tissue curves (carotid bifurcation and cervical disk), and many overlapping organ systems (salivary glands, airway, and lymph nodes).

To avoid artifacts on soft tissue algorithm caused by dental amalgam and capped teeth, when possible, transverse angled images on either side of the teeth can be obtained by tilting the gantry. The artifacts are not as distracting if only a bone algorithm (kernel) is needed, for example, to study only the bones; in that case, a single set of images may be acquired. Newer computer software allows reformation of images scanned with a different gantry tilt. This software may be on the scanner workstation or on the picture archiving **communications** systems unit used for reporting.

### The Neck

The face and neck contain salivary glands, chains of lymph nodes, and blood vessels. Fat delineates many compartments in the neck. Neck studies usually include images from the nasopharynx to the manubrium/jugular notch. IV contrast is used to help distinguish blood vessels from lymph nodes and muscles because *metastatic lymph nodes* are common in head and neck cancer.

Patients with neck masses may have difficulty breathing in the supine position. This presents a special challenge in positioning the patient. Some patients require a tracheostomy to lie supine, often resulting in the presence of subcutaneous emphysema marring some images.

Transverse images acquired in the same plane as the cervical disks are preferred because they are in the same plane as the true vocal cords, which are situated at the level of the small bilateral arytenoid cartilages. Sequential, rather than helical, acquisition is used because it improves resolution.

Special phonation techniques are occasionally used to assess the mobility of the vocal cords. After the routine image acquisition, the level of the true vocal cords is determined. A limited number of slices are then acquired while the patient vocalizes E-E-E-E-E (in expiration) or a reversed E-E-E-E (in inspiration).

The larynx is surrounded by a number of cartilages (Fig. 15-24). They can be fractured or dislocated with a blow to the front of the neck, affecting the airway and the voice. This is why bone algorithm of the cartilages of the neck is sometimes requested. The thyroid cartilage is larger and more calcified in men than in women. Reformatted sagittal and coronal images depict the cartilaginous abnormality to best advantage before repair.

The salivary glands include the parotid glands, the submandibular glands, the sublingual glands, and minor salivary glands scattered throughout the mouth. Benign and malignant tumors arise in them (Fig. 15-25). *Calculi* can obstruct salivary gland ducts.

### The Spine

Spine imaging is acquired either perpendicular to the tabletop or by tilting the gantry to align the plane of

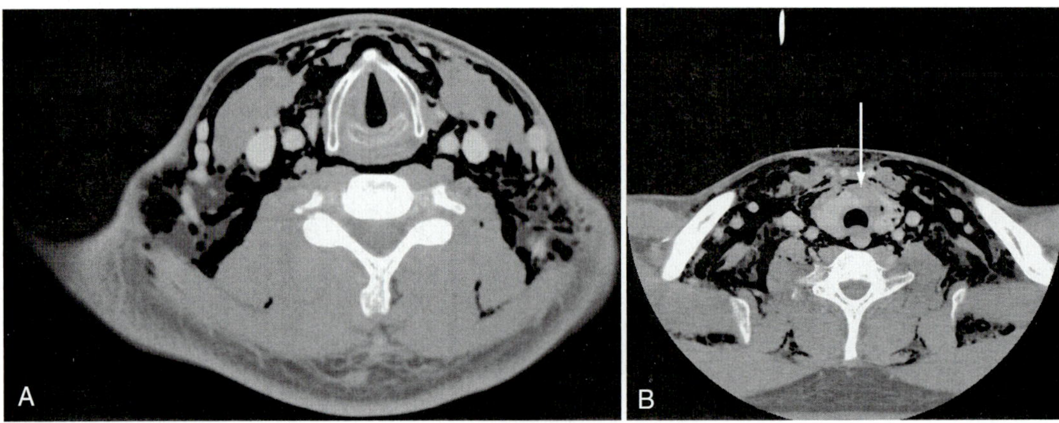


**FIGURE 15-24 A,** Extensive *subcutaneous emphysema* outlines a normal thyroid cartilage. **B,** The thyroid gland is lacerated in the same patient.

section with the vertebral body end plate, as seen on the lateral scout image (Fig. 15-26, *B*).

The use of sequential versus helical scanning depends on the type of equipment available as well as the need for reformatted images. The equipment may or may not allow a gantry tilt with helical scanning. Depending on the indication for spine imaging, bone algorithm (kernel), with or without soft tissue algorithm, is obtained.

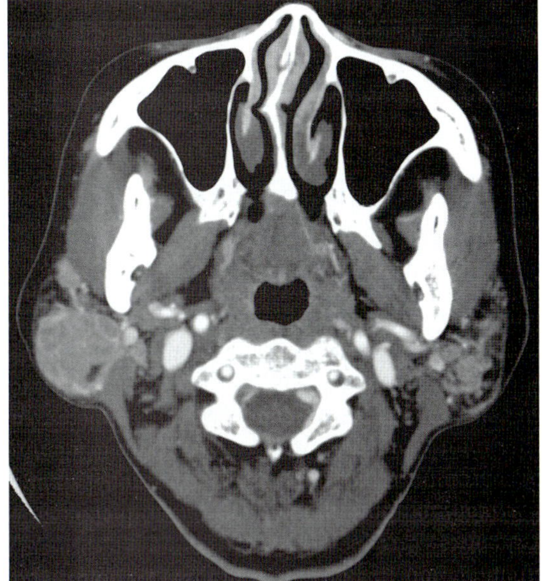

**FIGURE 15-25** Bilateral parotid tumors.

Disk disease, spinal stenosis, and trauma do not require IV contrast. The disk, as shown in Figure 15-27, *A*, can be differentiated from the dural sac (filled with spinal cord, nerves, and CSF), intraspinal fat, ligaments (ligamentum flavum, posterior longitudinal ligament), and bones.

Reformatted sagittal and coronal images help in the assessment of the alignment and the evaluation of *scoliosis* and *spondylolisthesis*. They show the nerves in the intervertebral foramina, and they help to determine whether the nerves are compromised by *disk herniation* or osteophytes. Quality coronal images are produced when the curves (*kyphosis* and *lordosis*) seen on the sagittal images are taken into account.

Because of its curved outline and smaller size, a cervical disk herniation is more difficult to diagnose than a lumbar disk herniation. Because IV contrast highlights the epidural veins and a herniated disk will displace these veins, it is used frequently (but not by everyone) to better outline a cervical disk herniation (Fig. 15-27, *B*). A continuous drip infusion or preferably a pump injection will highlight these veins.

## Cerebral Blood Vessels

CTP is one form of CTA used in suspected acute brain infarction to determine the amount of brain tissue at risk of permanent damage. The perfusion study is usually followed immediately by the CTA study. The CTP and CTA each require injection of a bolus

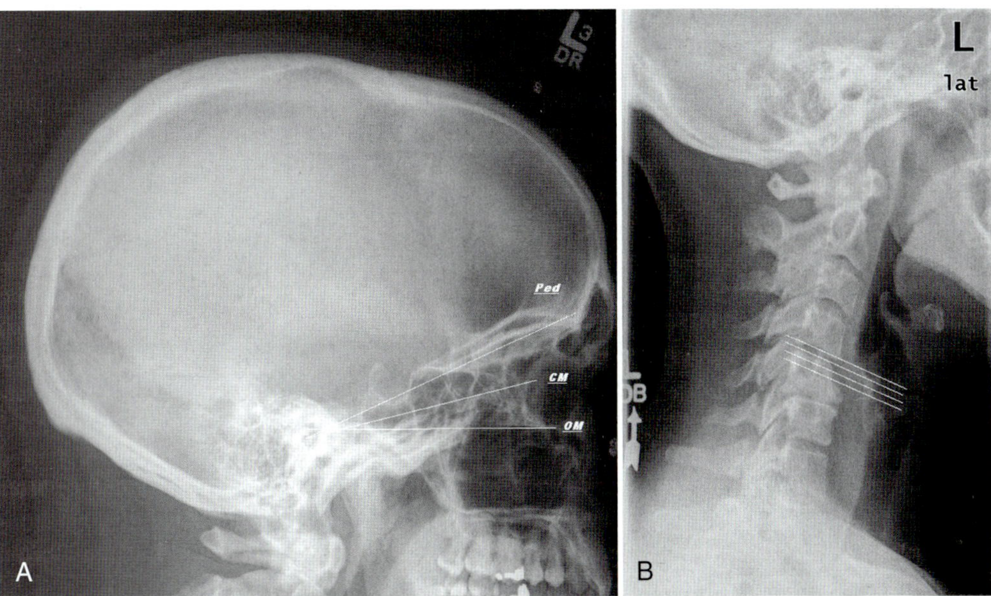


**FIGURE 15-26** **A,** Lateral scout of skull with a selection of scanning planes: orbitomeatal (*OM*), canthomeatal (*CM*), and steeper "pediatric" angle to avoid the lens. **B,** Lateral scout of the cervical spine shows the optimum plane of section for imaging the cervical disks and larynx/vocal cords.

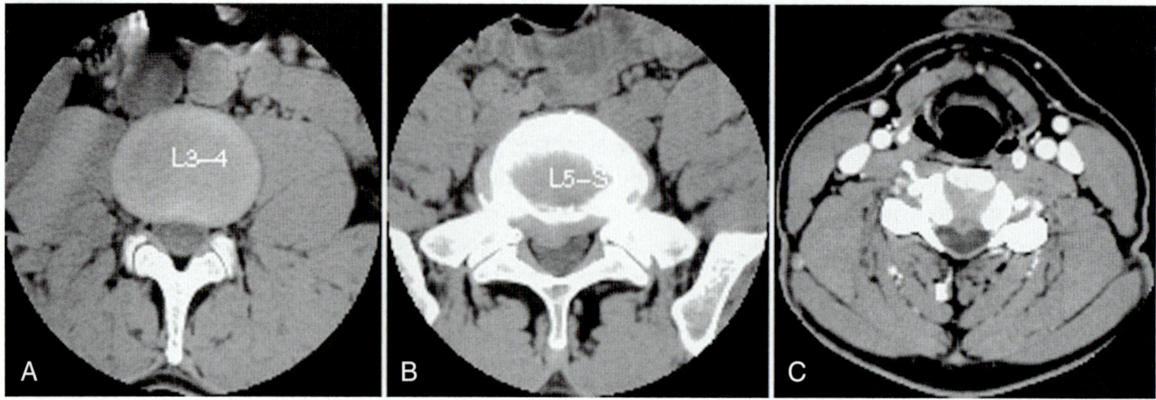


**FIGURE 15-27** **A,** Normal lumbar disk (no contrast used). Lumbar **(B)** and cervical disk **(C)** herniations: the herniation of the smaller cervical disk is better seen when IV contrast is used.

of contrast. The amount of contrast is adjusted to limit the total amount used in this instance. Our current practice is to use 50 milliliters (ml) of contrast for the CTP and 100 ml for the CTA. A CTA without CTP receives 100 to 150 ml of contrast, our limit for a single dose study (see later section, **Contrast Media** Usage).

A limited area of brain is repeatedly scanned (two to four locations currently) during the first contrast bolus for the CTP. These levels are determined by the radiologist or neurologist from the findings on the unenhanced CT and from the presumed area of infarction on the basis of the neurological examination.

Bolus tracking is used for the CTA to time the image acquisition to the peak of contrast in the cervical vessels by **sampling** the carotid just below the skull base. This is immediately followed by the second bolus (if a CTP preceded the CTA) and acquisition of images from the aortic arch to the circle of Willis.

The technologist can produce maximum intensity **projection** reformatted images or 3D surface-shaded images while the radiologist evaluates the CTP study on an independent workstation using a CTP software program provided by the manufacturer. Values of cerebral blood flow, blood volume, and mean transit time are determined by the radiologist to further evaluate the brain infarction and the amount of potentially salvageable brain.

A CTV images the head from the skull base to the vertex to look for thrombus in the dural (sagittal and transverse) sinuses and in the cortical veins. An 8- to 10-second delay is added to the CTA protocol before images are acquired. Sagittal and coronal reformatted images delineate the patency of these channels.

## RADIOGRAPHIC TECHNIQUE

### Milliamperage, Kilovoltage, Helical Pitch, and Rotation Time

The preset techniques and protocols supplied by manufacturers are helpful. However, the technologist must be able to manipulate milliamperage, kilovoltage, helical **pitch,** scan time, and slice thickness to suit the circumstances.

Increasing the milliamperage and the kilovoltage will improve the signal-to-noise ratio. Sufficiently high technique is necessary for contrast resolution of soft tissue in the brain (gray-white matter differentiation). Similarly, spine imaging in large patients can be improved by increasing the technique (by using the maximum kilovoltage and increasing the scan time).

Increasing the scan rotation time will result in better resolution because each image is generated from more projections.

Increasing the helical pitch results in a shorter scan time but reduces the overall image quality because of more **interpolation** in the scan data and vice versa.

Longer scan times can result in longer tube cooling and the possibility of patient motion (often a result of back pain).

### Slice Thickness

Slice thickness should be adapted to the area of interest. Studies requiring reformatted images are acquired helically, with thin slices. Sequential image acquisition is preferred for brain, petrous bones, and neck masses, for better resolution.

Thin transverse sections show the base of the skull well, giving excellent definition of the temporal bones, pituitary fossa, facial bones, and foramina. Thicker slices increase the definition of gray and white matter in the brain.

The low density of various brain tissues, such as fat (in the myelin of white matter) and CSF, outlines components of the brain such as frontal and temporal lobes, basal ganglia, and ventricles. The high density of calcium is found in many normal structures inside the skull (pineal gland and choroid plexus) and must be differentiated from pathological calcium (tumor and AVM).

**Spatial resolution** is improved with thinner slices, at the cost of a decreased signal-to-noise ratio. Increasing the milliamperage and kilovoltage will improve the signal-to-noise ratio but will also increase the radiation dose.

The average slice thickness has decreased over the years, with the old 10-mm slice of the brain now being 2.5 to 5 mm. Our current practice for a routine head scan consists of 2.5- to 3-mm sequential slices in the posterior fossa and 5-mm slices for the rest of the head.

Orbits are studied with 1- to 2-mm helical slices and a small FOV (13 to 15 cm).

Temporal bone images are sequential 0.6 to 1 mm thick with a 10-cm FOV.

CTA image acquisition is 1-mm helical. CTP, on the other hand, uses cine mode and 5- to 10-mm thick slices; the tabletop may toggle back and forth during CTP image acquisition, depending on the scanner.

The cervical spine is imaged with helical 1- to 2-mm slices every 1 to 2 mm when good bone detail is needed. On the other hand, 2.5- to 3-mm sequential slices overlapped every 2 mm are used to look for a disk herniation. Wide shoulders present a challenge. Enlarging the field of view and increasing the technique may not always be successful in preventing over-range artifacts from the humeral heads. A swimmer's position is used in some settings to decrease these artifacts.

Lumbar images consist of 3- to 5-mm sequential slices every 3 to 4 mm. One method uses overlapping thicker slices (for example, 7-mm slices every 4 to 5 mm) to improve visualization of herniated lumbar disks, for example, when scatter radiation is increased because of a large girth.

### Matrix Size and Reconstruction Algorithms

**Matrix** size is predetermined at 512 × 512 on most current equipment. Some systems have a 1024 × 1024 matrix (e.g., Philips).

Many reconstruction algorithms are available. The three basic algorithms used for the brain, neck, and spine are the standard, the bone, and the detail algorithms (General Electric) or the Siemens kernels (31, 70, and 45 seconds).

The standard algorithm (and its equivalents) is chosen for most soft tissue imaging, such as the brain and the intervertebral disk, because it provides good contrast resolution. It is important to distinguish gray from white matter when looking for acute cerebral infarction.

The detail algorithm is useful when studying the soft tissues of the neck. It increases edge definition, especially when good definition of lymph nodes and fat planes is required.

The bone algorithm is used to increase the sharpness of the bony detail. This algorithm optimizes spatial resolution, but contrast resolution is poor. It should not be used in isolation when IV contrast is administered because tissue enhancement is not visible on bone windows or bone settings. However, bone algorithm is the preferred technique when subarachnoid (intrathecal) contrast has been injected by LP. This is true whether the imaging is of the spine (post myelography CT) or of the brain (CT cisternography).

## CONTRAST MEDIA USAGE

Intravenously injected iodinated contrast media have been used since the early days of CT scanning to improve visualization of normal and abnormal structures. In recent years, safer nonionic and iso-osmolar contrast media have become available. Iodinated contrast does not interfere with MRI studies done on the same day.

By further attenuating the x-ray beam, structures containing the iodinated contrast are denser and thus more visible. In the brain, a number of normal structures enhance, including the blood vessels, the choroid plexus, the pineal gland, the pituitary stalk, and the meninges.

In the spine, the enhanced epidural veins, situated along the posterior margin of the vertebral bodies, outline the disk margin along the spinal canal and adjoining nerve roots; the ability to diagnose a small disk herniation by the displacement of these veins is increased. In the neck, the enhanced vessels make the lymph nodes distinct because the nodes run chain-like along the vessels.

Abnormal tissue can enhance, either because the blood-brain barrier has been breached (e.g., malignant tumor or abscess in the brain) or because of an inflammatory response (e.g., scarring in the postoperative spine). The degree of enhancement is related to the method of contrast administration (drip infusion versus pump injection) and the dose and concentration of contrast received, as well as the delay between contrast administration and image acquisition.

In the brain and spine, most studies are performed with the IV drip method. This allows the contrast to "percolate" and enhance lesions such as meningioma and metastasis. At least 3 to 5 minutes is required after most of the contrast has been injected to reach satisfactory enhancement. A delay in image acquisition (up to 1 hour) can result in more pronounced enhancement. Because enhancement persists for hours, at least 6 to 8 hours should elapse after a contrast scan before an unenhanced CT is obtained. This will confirm that the enhancement is real and not the result of calcification or hematoma.

CT angiography (CTA and CTP) requires the opposite method. Images are acquired during rapid contrast injection by a pump to best opacify the cerebral blood vessels.

An antecubital vein and a large-bore needle (18 to 20 gauge) help deliver the contrast efficiently, at a rate of 3 to 5 ml per second. Care to avoid contrast extravasation in the arm is required. The volume injected per second in the vein should take its size in consideration. (Skin necrosis caused by extravasation may require a skin graft.) Specific instructions on what to do in such a case must be available to the technologist.

Use of indwelling catheters, such as percutaneous indwelling central venous catheter lines, is not recommended for pump infusion because their small size cannot handle the rate (volume/second) of injection. Site-specific instructions should be respected.

Pump injection is also used in studying the pituitary gland (sella turcica) for the presence of a microadenoma and the cervical spine for disk disease (to best outline the epidural veins) and neck masses.

Nonionic contrast media have decreased the number of mild and moderate contrast reactions (nausea, vomiting, urticaria, and rigor) but have not altered the risk of anaphylactic reaction and death. Efforts to minimize contrast use and contrast volume are encouraged.

A standard dose of contrast is administered for each type of examination on the basis of patient weight up to a maximum. For example, our adult-only practice uses 3 ml of nonionic contrast per kilogram (kg), to a maximum of 150 ml for both the drip and pump methods. The current contrast concentration is 320 mg/ml of iodine. A single dose of iodine is thus 48 grams (g) of iodine and a double dose is limited to 200 ml of contrast or 68 g of iodine.

Variations do occur. Sella turcica studies use a bolus of 100 ml of contrast (32 g of iodine).

Postoperative lumbar studies looking for epidural fibrosis (scar) use 200 ml of contrast by the drip method (unless the patient weighs <100 pounds/45 kg) because enhancement can be quite subtle with a single dose.

In younger patients with lung carcinoma, a workup for brain metastasis consists of 200 ml of contrast and at least a 30-minute delay to allow the contrast to enhance small (<3 to 5 mm) metastases. Patients older than 75 years of age receive a single dose to protect their renal function.

Great care must always be exercised when iodinated contrast is administered. *Contrast-induced nephropathy* (deteriorated kidney function as a result of iodine-based contrast) has been shown to significantly increase morbidity (and length of stay in hospital) and mortality rates. Patients at risk of having borderline or poor renal function, such as diabetics, heart patients, hypertensives, and the elderly, should have documented laboratory values such as a creatinine and estimated glomerular **filtration** rate (eGFR) before the contrast CT. A creatinine level in the normal range does not mean that the renal function is normal. The eGFR is a better indicator of normal function.

Our current practice is to look for alternative imaging if the creatinine is greater than 120 micromoles (μmol) per liter (normal in our laboratory is 45 to 110 μmol/L) or the eGFR is less than 60 ml/min/1.73 m$^2$ (normal >59).

Exceptions include acute trauma, when life is in danger from bleeding, and acute stroke, when "time is brain."

Contrast media can be used (cautiously) in patients with multiple myeloma and a normal renal function. Re-evaluation of the kidney function in the days after the CT is desirable. Good hydration after the CT may help prevent worsening of kidney function.

All our patients are encouraged to increase their intake of water or juice (but not coffee or cola, which are diuretics) in the hours before and after the examination.

Other types of central nervous system contrast media include air and subarachnoid iodinated contrast. Both are types of intrathecal (subarachnoid) contrast media.

Air was used, by an LP, to outline the internal auditory canal before the advent of MRI to look for an intracanalicular acoustic neuroma as a cause of deafness. When air is found today in the brain or spinal canal, it indicates that a communication exists between the environment and the central nervous system (such as a penetrating injury), raising the possibility of meningitis, or that a recent LP has been performed.

Iodinated subarachnoid contrast is used to look for leakage of CSF from the nose or ear (*rhinorrhea, otorrhea*) or in the spine (*intracranial hypotension*) and to study instrumented spines (postmyelogram). This type of contrast remains visible on CT for hours, even when it is no longer visible on fluoroscopy or plain films, so CT can be used to "rescue" a myelogram. A CT study in the first hour after intrathecal contrast injection is preferable. Occasionally, repeat CT scans after 6-, 12-, or 24-hour delays are used to detect clearance or accumulation of contrast, for example, in a spinal cord syrinx.

A CT of the brain obtained less than 24 hours after a myelogram will have an unusual appearance because of the reabsorption of the contrast by the brain before excretion by the kidneys; it will show greater gray-white matter differentiation than normal. This finding is most puzzling when the history of a myelogram performed at another institution in the prior 24 hours is not provided.

## REVIEW QUESTIONS

Answer the following questions to check your understanding of the materials studied.

1. Indications for CT imaging of the head are:
   1. stroke and cerebral infarction
   2. hemorrhage in the brain substance
   3. chronic subdural hematoma
   4. primary brain tumors are *meningioma* and *glioblastoma multiforme*

   A. 1 and 2
   B. 2 and 3
   C. 3 and 4
   D. 1, 2, 3, and 4
2. Which of the following conditions relates to a loss of adequate blood supply to a portion of the brain?
   A. tumor in the brainstem
   B. hemorrage in the brain substance
   C. cerebral infarction
   D. meningioma
3. CT of the neck would not be performed if the indication written on the request is:
   A. polyps.
   B. mass.
   C. stenosis of the carotid vessels.
   D. goiter.
4. The following are indications for CT of the spine *except*:
   A. herniation of the vertebral disk.
   B. strokes.
   C. osteomyelitis.
   D. spondylolisthesis.
5. When performing a CT examination of the head, images are principally obtained in the following plane:
   A. sagittal plane
   B. oblique plane
   C. coronal plane
   D. transverse axial plane
6. When positioning a patient for a skull CT examination, the image plane that still remains the most popular is the:
   A. sagittal plane.
   B. oblique plane.
   C. coronal plane.
   D. transverse axial plane.
7. When performing CT of the head, neck, and spine, the technologist uses all of the following algorithms except:
   A. bone algorithm.
   B. lung algorithm.
   C. standard algorithm.
   D. detail algorithm.
8. The slices that provide optimum generation of reformatted CT images are:
   A. thick slices.
   B. thin slices.
   C. good quality reformatted images are absolutely dependent on the technologist.
   D. 15-mm slice thickness.
9. Which of the following pitches will result in the greatest dose to the patient having a CT of the head?
   A. 1
   B. 1.5
   C. 2
   D. 3
10. Which of the following pitches will result in the poorest image quality?
    A. 1
    B. 1.5
    C. 2.5
    D. 3.5

## FURTHER READING


Bainbridge, J., Hirwadkar, H., & Hourihan, M. D. (2012). Vomiting–is this a good indication for CT head scans in patients with minor head injury? *The British Journal of Radiology*, *85*, 183–186.

Becker, M., Leuchter, I., Platon, A., Becker, C., Dulguerov, P., & Varoquaux, A. (2014). Imaging of laryngeal trauma. *European Journal of Radiology*, *83*, 142–154.

Birenbaum, D., Bancroft, L. W., & Gelsberg, G. J. (2011). Imaging in acute stroke. *Western Journal of Emergency Medicine*, *12*(1).

*CT anatomy of the brain, head and neck and spine.* (2015). <http://w-radiology.com/index.html> Accessed January 2015.

*Head, cerebral vessels, neck, and spine.* <http://headneckbrainspine.com/Skull-Base-CT.php> (This is a website "intended for those interested in neurology anatomy and learning from neurology"). Accessed January 19, 2015.

Hourani, R., Taslakian, B., Shabb, N. S., Nassar, L., Hourani, M. H., Moukarbel, R., et al. (2015). Fibroblastic and myofibroblastic tumors of the head and neck: comprehensive imaging-based review with pathologic correlation. *European Journal of Radiology*, *84*, 250–260.

Ippolito, D., Besostri, V., Bonaffini, P. A., Rossini, F., Di Lelio, A., & Sironi, S. (2013). Diagnostic value of whole-body low-dose computed tomography (WBLDCT) in bone lesions detection in patients with multiple myeloma (MM). *European Journal of Radiology*, *82*, 2322–2327.

Kritsaneepaiboon, S., Siriwanarangsun, P., Tanaanantarak, P., & Krisanachinda, A. (2014). Can a revised paediatric radiation dose reduction CT protocol be applied and still maintain anatomical delineation, diagnostic confidence and overall imaging quality? *The British Journal of Radiology*, *87*(1041), 23–27.

O'Connor, J. P., Tofts, P. S., Milles, K. A., Parkes, L. M., Thompson, G., & Jackson, A. (2011). Dynamic contrast-enhanced imaging techniques: CT and MRI. *The British Journal of Radiology*, *84*(2011), S112–S120.

O'Laughlin, K. N., Hoffman, J. R., Go, S., Gabayan, G. Z., Iqbal, E., Merchant, G., et al. (2013). Nonconcordance between clinical and head CT findings: the specter of overdiagnosis. *Emergency Medicine International*, *2*, 1–7.

Takeyama, N., Kuroki, K., Hayashi, T., Sai, S., Okabe, N., Kinebuchi, Y., et al. (2012). Cerebral CT angiography using a small volume of concentrated contrast material with a test injection method: optimal scan delay for quantitative and qualitative performance. *The British Journal of Radiology*, *85*, e748–e755.

Thomas, C., Korn, A., Krauss, B., Ketelsen, D., Tsiflikas, I., Reimann, A., et al. (2010). Automatic bone and plaque removal using dual energy CT for head and neck angiography: feasibility and initial performance evaluation. *European Journal of Radiology*, *76*, 61–67.

Yuh, E. L., Cooper, S. R., Ferguson, A. R., & Manley, G. T. (2012). Quantitative CT improves outcome prediction in acute traumatic brain injury. *Journal of Neurotrauma*, *29*, 735–746.

16

# Computed Tomography of the Body

*Borys Flak*

## OUTLINE



## LEARNING OBJECTIVES

On completion of this chapter, you should be able to:

1. list the clinical indications for each of the following:
   - mediastinum
   - lung
   - cardiac
   - spleen
   - bowel
   - pancreas
   - kidneys
   - adrenal glands
   - retroperitoneum
   - pelvis
   - trauma
   - vascular system.
2. identify planning considerations for CT of the body procedures.
3. state the important information that should be provided by the technologist to a patient having CT scans of the body.
4. discuss the use of both oral contrast media and intravenous contrast agents in body CT procedures.
5. outline examples of CT scanning protocols for each of the following:
   - thorax
   - abdomen
   - pelvis
   - musculoskeletal system.

## KEY TERMS TO WATCH FOR AND REMEMBER

The following key terms/concepts are important to your understanding of this chapter

**interventional procedures**
**intravenous (IV) contrast agents**
**lymphadenopathy**
**mediastinal**
**sensitivity**
**specificity**

In the early years of **computed tomography (CT)**, many were skeptical about its usefulness outside the central nervous system (CNS). Earlier scanners were unsuitable for examining the body because of the image degradation that occurred with patient motion and movement of internal organs during the 2 to 5 minutes required for a single slice. Within several decades, however, astonishing technological advances including helical **scanning** techniques, multidetector arrays, subsecond scan times, near real-time reconstruction of images, and advanced viewing workstations have completely revolutionized CT. The latest **generation** of scanners can obtain up to 64 slices simultaneously at 0.5-millimeter (mm) **collimation** with 400 millisecond (ms) scan times. This enables extended ranges of coverage with thinner collimation and increased speed, allowing for large **volume data acquisitions** during single short breath-holds. The resultant 3D and multiplanar reformations (MPRs) are outstanding. Therefore, CT of the body has not only fulfilled but in fact surpassed the expectations of its early supporters and has become an important means of evaluating many pathological conditions. **Magnetic resonance imaging (MRI)** has replaced CT as the primary method of investigation for most diseases of the cranium, spinal cord, and musculoskeletal system; however, CT is still superior to MRI for most clinical indications in the chest and abdomen.

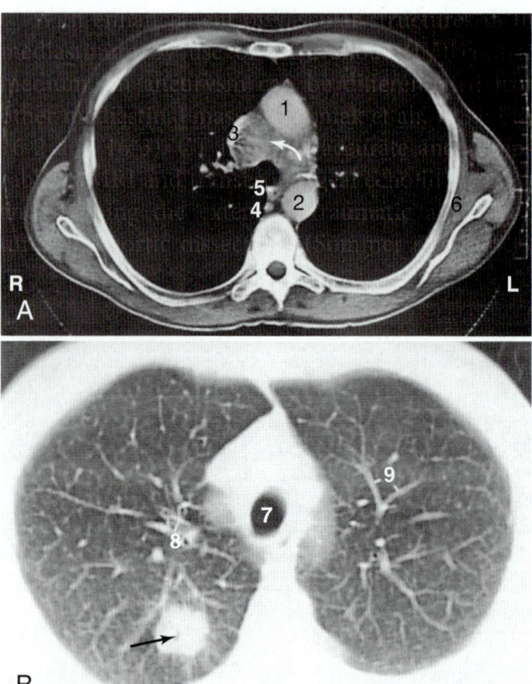


**FIGURE 16-1** Bronchogenic carcinoma (*black arrow*) with pretracheal mediastinal lymphadenopathy (*white arrow*). **A,** *1,* Ascending aorta; *2,* descending aorta; *3,* superior vena cava; *4,* azygos vein; *5,* esophagus; *6,* subscapular muscle. **B,** *7,* trachea; *8,* segmental bronchi; *9,* pulmonary vessels.

## CLINICAL INDICATIONS

In addition to CT, a wide variety of radiologic techniques are available for studying diseases of the body, including plain radiographs, barium studies, angiography, nuclear medicine, ultrasonography, and MRI. Clinicians are faced with the dilemma of which imaging method or methods to use and in what order. Often too many examinations are requested or studies are performed in the wrong sequence before a diagnosis is reached. For these reasons, the use of algorithms or flowcharts has become popular. The suggested approach, however, may not be the most appropriate for the individual institution when the limitations of available equipment and expertise are considered. The radiologist, acting as a consultant, should discuss the clinical problem with the referring physician and choose the most expeditious and cost-effective method or methods for answering the clinician's questions. This chapter presents the major indications for CT of the body.

### Chest and Mediastinum

#### Mediastinum

Almost all **mediastinal** abnormalities detected on chest radiographs (typically suspected masses) or suspected from clinical evidence can be confirmed with CT (Gamsu, 1992). CT is most commonly used to detect **lymphadenopathy** in patients suspected of having bronchogenic carcinoma, lymphoma, or other malignancies (Fig. 16-1). Although highly sensitive, CT and MRI have some limitations; they are less efficient at detecting tumors within normal-size nodes or differentiating between enlarged hyperplastic nodes without a tumor and tumor-containing nodes. CT is useful in patients known to have or suspected of having bronchogenic carcinoma. In these cases, CT is used to determine the extent of invasion of the chest wall, mediastinum, and diaphragm and to detect extrathoracic metastases in the liver and adrenal glands. MRI better demonstrates chest wall invasion and is more accurate in detecting mediastinal invasion and staging apical tumors (Manfredi et al., 1996; Tateishi et al., 2003).

With enhancement of vascular structures in the mediastinum by use of intravenous (IV) contrast medium, an aneurysm can be differentiated from other mediastinal masses (Posniak et al., 1989; Figs. 16-2 and 16-3). CT is highly accurate and comparable to MRI and transesophageal echo in detecting and defining the extent of traumatic aortic ruptures and aortic dissections (Sommer et al., 1996).

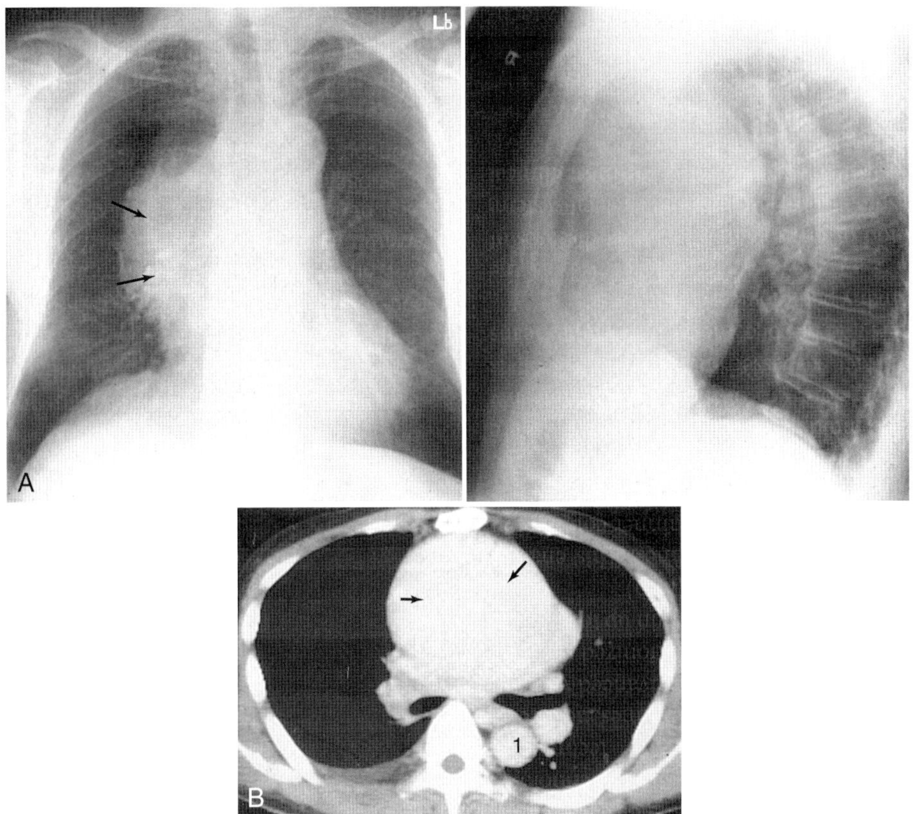


**FIGURE 16-2** Dissecting aneurysm of the ascending aorta (*arrows shown in A and B*). *1*, Descending aorta.

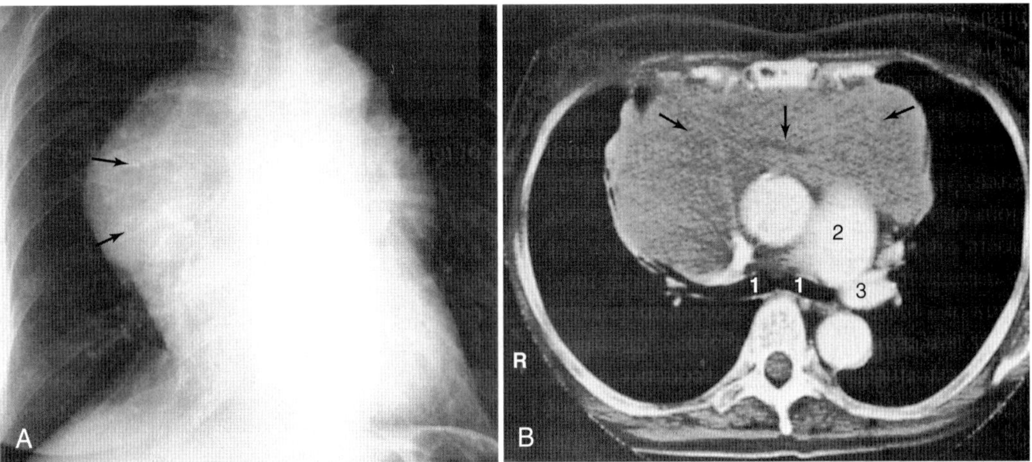


**FIGURE 16-3 A,** Lymphoma seen as an anterior mediastinal mass involving the thymus on helical CT scan (*arrows*). **B,** *1*, Right and left main stem bronchi; *2*, main pulmonary artery; *3*, left pulmonary artery.

Angiography is now rarely used to confirm these diagnoses.

In patients with myasthenia gravis, CT can detect thymic masses not evident on chest radiographs (Fon et al., 1982). Cysts and fatty deposits are distinguished by their characteristic **CT numbers.** A specific diagnosis cannot be made with most other masses, but the relationship of the mass to surrounding structures and its location and extension within the mediastinum can be readily defined and a differential diagnosis suggested.

## Lung

CT is the most sensitive technique for detecting pulmonary metastases (Muhm et al., 1978; Schaner et al., 1978). However, the increased **sensitivity**

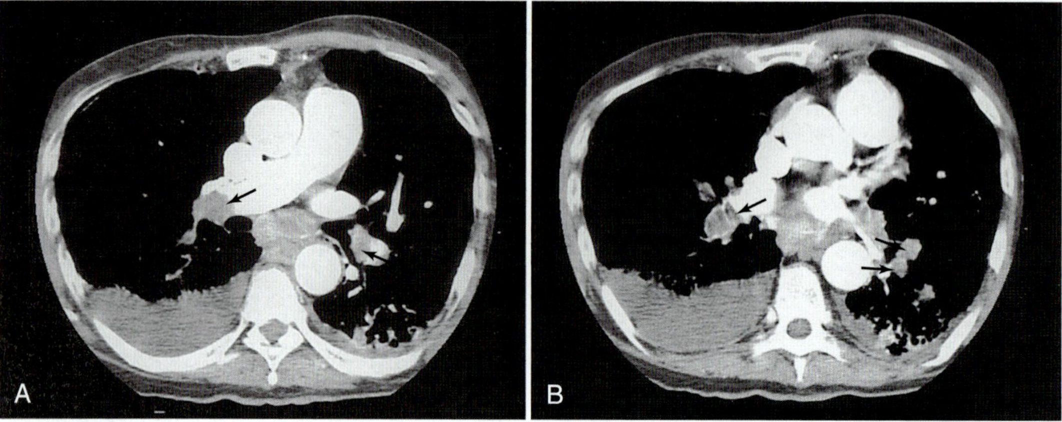


**FIGURE 16-4** Multiple filling defects caused by pulmonary emboli in the pulmonary arteries of both lungs (*arrows shown in A and B*).

is achieved at the price of decreased **specificity**.* Benign lesions such as subpleural lymph nodes and granulomas and a greater number of metastatic lesions can be detected. Therefore, CT is most useful in patients being evaluated for resection of metastatic pulmonary nodules, such as patients with osteogenic sarcoma. In the appropriate clinical setting, high-resolution CT (HRCT) can be diagnostic for lymphangitic carcinomatosis (Munk et al., 1988). CT also can be used to detect occult primary lung tumors in patients who show malignant cells on sputum cytological studies but who have normal chest x-ray films. Some investigators have used nodule densitometry (i.e., the measurement of nodule density with Hounsfield numbers; Zerhouni et al., 1986) or the degree of contrast enhancement (Swensen et al., 1996) on CT to evaluate solitary pulmonary nodules that are indeterminate for malignancy on conventional radiographs.

Helical CT is more sensitive than ventilation/perfusion scans and of equal specificity in detecting pulmonary emboli (Mayo et al., 1997). Emboli are seen as filling defects in the enhanced pulmonary arteries (Fig. 16-4). CT will miss clots in the smaller subsegmental branches, but this may not be clinically significant unless the patient has severe underlying cardiac or pulmonary disease (Stein et al., 1995).

HRCT using thin sections has become the established method for evaluating diffuse lung diseases (Muller, 1991; Fig. 16-5). When the CT findings are analyzed in the context of the clinical history, physical findings, pulmonary function tests, and laboratory data, characteristic HRCT findings may allow a confident diagnosis in conditions such as asbestosis, silicosis, and idiopathic pulmonary fibrosis. In some cases such as allergic alveolitis, HRCT findings may preclude the need for lung biopsy, or it can be used as a guide in selecting the best site for a biopsy. HRCT is more sensitive than chest radiography for detecting emphysema (Fig. 16-6), and it has replaced bronchography as the definitive method for detecting bronchiectasis (Pang et al., 1989).

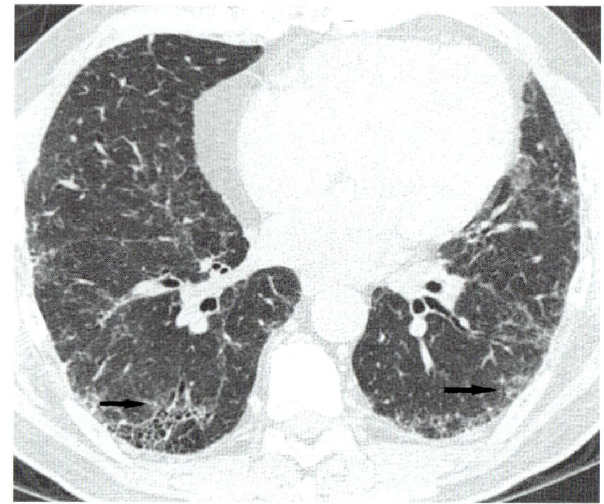

**FIGURE 16-5** Peripheral interstitial changes (*arrows*) in both lungs typical of usual interstitial pneumonia. (Image courtesy Dr. Nestor Muller, Vancouver Hospital.)

Multislice CT is the most effective way to image patients after blunt chest trauma, which is second only to CNS injury as a cause of post-trauma death. A myriad of injuries may result, including

*Sensitivity is defined as the likelihood that a test will be positive in an individual who has disease (i.e., the ability to detect disease). Specificity is defined as the likelihood that a test will be negative in an individual who has no disease (i.e., the ability to detect normalcy).

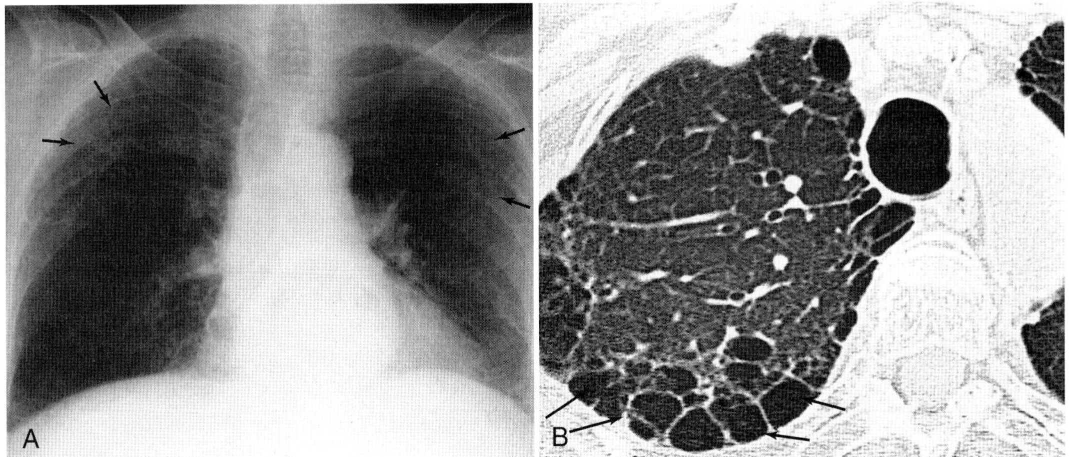


**FIGURE 16-6** Additional interstitial changes (*arrows*) on plain films **(A)** are shown to have occurred as a result of paraseptal emphysema on high-resolution thin sections **(B)**.

pulmonary contusion or laceration, pneumothorax, hemothorax, tracheobronchial laceration, diaphragmatic injury, and chest wall and spinal injuries. Although the chest radiograph is useful in detecting a number of potentially life-threatening conditions (e.g., tension pneumothorax, gross hemothorax), chest radiography is simply not sensitive enough to reliably identify or quantify the extent of most thoracic injuries.

**Screening** CT studies of the lungs to detect nodules has recently become popular, but this remains a highly controversial indication. This is primarily due to the high false-positive rate caused by benign nodules such as granulomas and lymph nodes and current lack of adequate studies to confirm decreased mortality rates from earlier tumor detection (Swensen et al., 2002). **CT screening** is discussed further in Chapter 12.

## Cardiac

The technology of the latest generation of CT scanners combining very rapid scanning with thin collimation, extended range, and electrocardiographic gating now has the ability to help accurately study the coronary arteries noninvasively. It is possible to assess the degree of coronary artery calcification, to obtain angiograms of the coronary arteries, and to display these images in 3D and multiple other projections, and in some cases eliminate the need for more invasive and risky catheter angiography. The same technology also enables the determination of ventricular volume as a function of time from which cardiac **output,** ejection fraction, stroke volume, and so forth can be calculated.

Coronary artery calcium scoring examinations are now widely performed to detect the extent of calcification in the coronary arteries and help clinicians manage patients at risk for a myocardial infarction. "Coronary artery disease is the single most important cause of death in North America, but traditional Framingham risk factor assessment* predicts only 60-65% of acute myocardial infarctions or sudden cardiac deaths. Coronary artery calcification has been shown to be an accurate marker for atherosclerotic disease" (Forster & Isserow, 2005). Typically 45 to 65 images are obtained, areas of calcification in the five major coronary branches are marked, and each plaque is assigned a score on the basis of its area and density. All the scores are added and adjusted for age and sex on the basis of existing data files.

The coronary arteries represent the ultimate challenge for **CT angiography** because of their small size, tortuous course, and pronounced rapid motion. Catheter coronary angiography has been the undisputed gold standard for many years; however, recent studies by Leschka et al. (2005) and Raff et al. (2005) have shown that CT can reliably identify significant coronary stenoses in vessels as small as 1.5 mm with a sensitivity of 94% to 95%, a specificity of 90% to 97%, and, more important, negative predictive values of 93% to 98%.† The latter indicates that multislice CT angiography (CTA) can be reliably used to noninvasively exclude significant coronary artery disease

* Framingham risk factor assessment is a predictive algorithm that estimates the risk for development of angina, myocardial infarction, or coronary disease death over the course of 10 years. The factors considered include age, blood cholesterol levels, blood pressure, cigarette smoking, and diabetes mellitus.

† Negative predictive value is defined as the likelihood that a patient with a negative test truly has no disease.

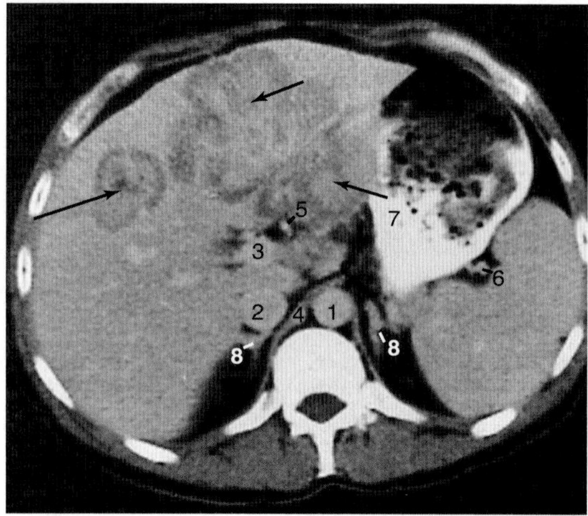


**FIGURE 16-7** Hepatoma (*arrows*) involving the lateral and medial segments of the left lobe of the liver. *1*, Aorta; *2*, inferior vena cava; *3*, portal vein; *4*, crus; *5*, hepatic artery; *6*, splenic artery; *7*, stomach; *8*, adrenals.

in patients with chest pain of uncertain etiology or whose other test results may be inconclusive or conflicting. The image quality is truly impressive.

## Liver

Although CT is more sensitive than ultrasonography in the initial screening of the liver for focal lesions, ultrasonography continues to play a significant role in this regard because of the large volume of patients. CT is always used when ultrasonography results are inconclusive or when more detailed localization and characterization of lesions are required (Fig. 16-7).

Proper use of an IV contrast medium is important for detecting focal masses in the liver. Helical CT used with power injection boluses of contrast medium, with or without the help of bolus-tracking **software,** allows a so-called triphasic examination of the liver. This examination includes one series during the early arterial phase, a second during the venous phase, and a delayed scan. Dynamic CT, which involves multiple repeat scans at the same level or several selected levels, is helpful for demonstrating the characteristic contrast medium-enhancement pattern seen with hemangiomas (Freeny & Marks, 1986; Fig. 16-8). CT hepatic angiography and CT arterial portography are probably still the most sensitive methods available for detecting additional tumor nodules (Hori et al., 1998) and are especially useful for planning hepatic resection. The introduction of multidetector scanners, however, has allowed the use of very thin scans (e.g., 2.5-mm collimation through the entire liver), and a study by Weg et al. (1998) confirmed higher rates of detection and improved conspicuity of small liver lesions (<10 mm) compared with 5- to 10-mm collimation.

With a few exceptions, diffuse liver disease cannot be diagnosed by CT. Hemochromatosis, amiodarone therapy, and some glycogen storage diseases are associated with dense livers on CT (Goldman et al., 1985), whereas fatty infiltration is evidenced by a liver that is less attenuating than the spleen on unenhanced scans (Alpern et al., 1986).

CT and ultrasonography are equally accurate in demonstrating intrahepatic and extrahepatic bile ducts in jaundiced patients (Baron et al., 1982; Fig. 16-9). CT is performed only if the ultrasound technique is unsuccessful. If dilated ducts are demonstrated and the obstructing lesion is not delineated, the next investigation usually is direct cholangiography (transhepatic cholangiography or endoscopic retrograde cholangiopancreatography) or MRI cholangiography.

The liver is the second most common solid abdominal organ to be injured in blunt trauma; however, the majority of injuries can be treated conservatively. Contrast-enhanced CT can identify hematomas that may be subcapsular or parenchymal, lacerations, and evidence of active hemorrhage, which could mean the presence of a more severe vascular injury involving the inferior vena cava, portal veins, or hepatic artery (Shanmuganathan, 2004).

## Spleen

The spleen is the most commonly injured solid organ in the abdomen, and trauma is the most common indication for scanning the spleen. Contrast-enhanced CT can diagnose the principal types of injury, namely, hematoma, laceration, and vascular injury (Fig. 16-10). The latter two more often require surgical intervention (Shanmuganathan 2004). Although focal masses can be seen in the spleen with both CT and ultrasonography, the results of spleen assessment in patients with lymphoma have unfortunately remained poor for both methods (Castellino et al., 1984).

## Bowel

Barium studies and endoscopy traditionally have been the mainstays of alimentary tract investigation. CT is assuming an ever-increasing role because of its ability to delineate not only the lumen but also the bowel wall and adjacent structures. Virtual colonoscopy, or CT colonography, is a new development in gastrointestinal (GI) radiology that is challenging the barium enema and even colonoscopy in the detection of colon polyps (Hara et al., 1997). This technique involves cleansing the colon with a standard bowel **preparation,** insufflating the colon with air or carbon dioxide (or both), performing thin-section

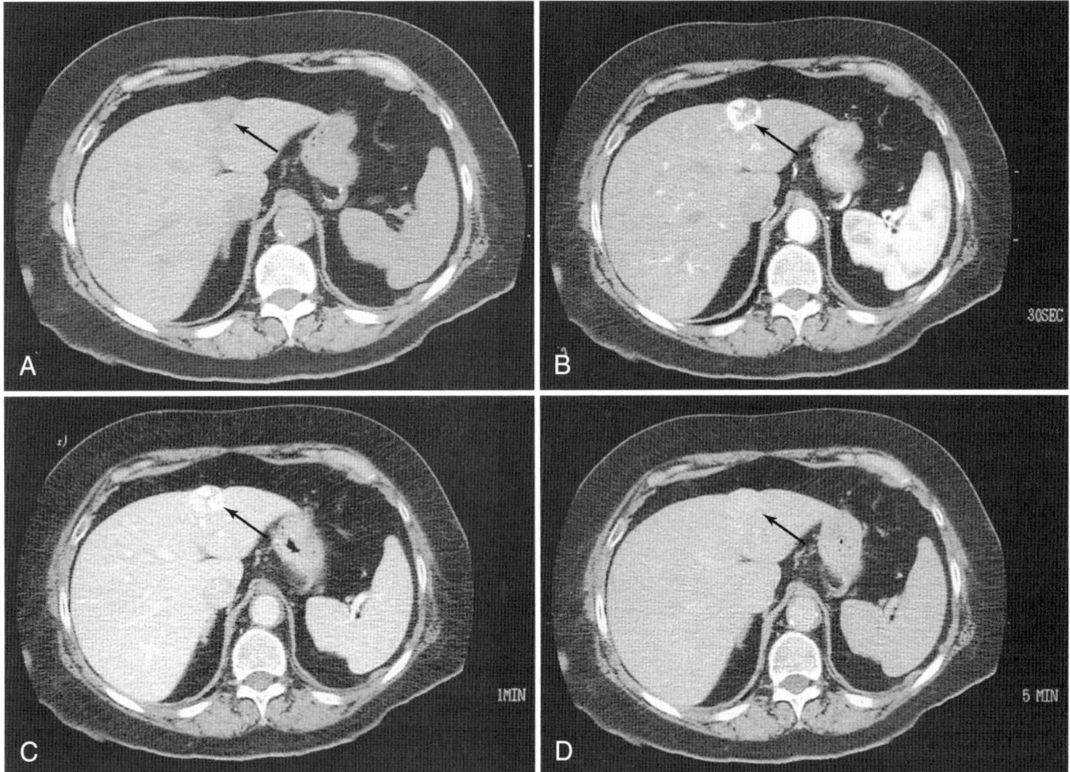


**FIGURE 16-8** Hemangioma of the liver. **A,** Low-density mass in the left lobe (*arrow*). **B,** Arterial phase study demonstrates dense, lobulated peripheral enhancement (*arrow*). **C,** Venous phase study demonstrates that the lesion is filling in with the contrast medium (*arrow*). **D,** Delayed scan demonstrates complete filling in of the lesion, which is nearly isodense (*arrow*).

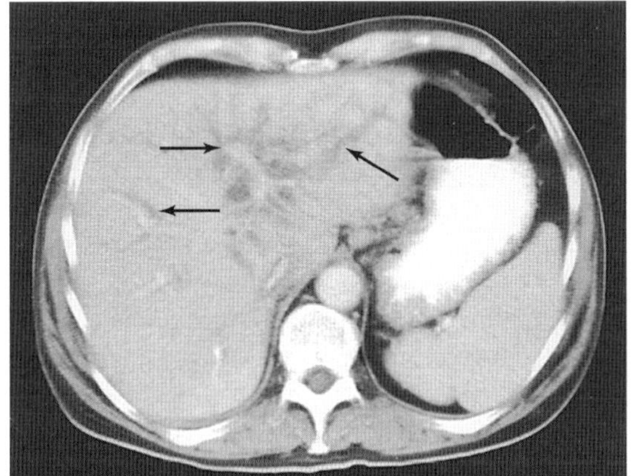

**FIGURE 16-9** Dilated intrahepatic ducts (*arrows*) in a jaundiced patient known to have cholangiocarcinoma.

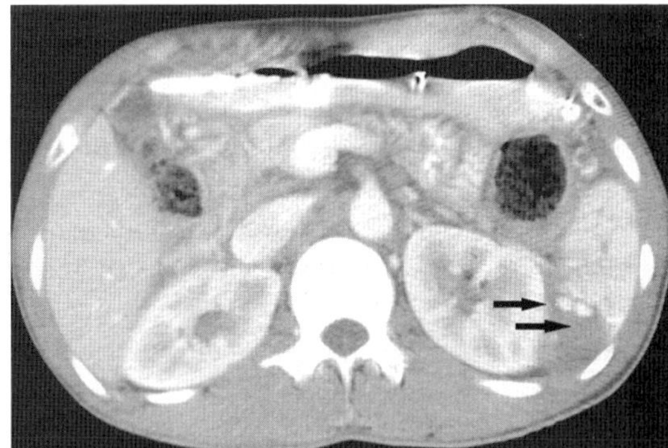

**FIGURE 16-10** Splenic rupture with pseudoaneurysms (*arrows*). (Image courtesy Dr. Luck Louis, Vancouver Hospital.)

helical scans (typically 2 to 3 mm with overlapping reconstruction in both the supine and prone positions), and subsequently reviewing the images in cine or movie mode and performing MPR. The data also can be volume rendered and displayed in a "fly through" navigation mode simulating colonoscopy (Fenlon et al., 1999). The results of preliminary studies have been extremely encouraging, rivaling or surpassing those of conventional methods (Pickhardt et al., 2003).

Although CT has proved not very accurate for staging of GI malignancies, it is still widely used for this purpose, primarily to prevent unnecessary surgery in cases that demonstrate strong evidence of unresectability because of local invasion or distant metastases, such as to the liver (Davies et al., 1997).

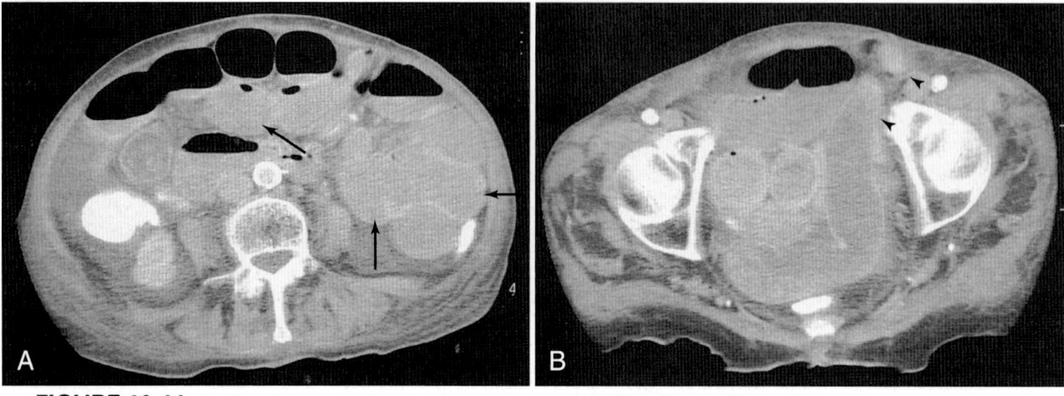

**FIGURE 16-11** **A,** Small bowel obstruction as evidenced by the multiple dilated loops of proximal small bowel (*arrows*). **B,** A herniated loop in the left groin (*arrowheads*).

Plain radiographs are diagnostic in only about 50% to 60% of small bowel obstructions, equivocal in 20% to 30%, and normal or nonspecific in 10% to 20% (Mucha, 1987). CT can confirm an obstruction, determine the level and perhaps the cause, and often indicate whether vascular compromise is present in uncertain cases (Fig. 16-11; Balthazar, 1994).

Barium studies remain the primary procedure for evaluating patients with inflammatory bowel disease, but CT is the key to studying the mural extent and detecting any extraintestinal involvement or complications such as phlegmons, abscesses, sinus tracts, and fistulas (Gore et al., 1996).

In approximately 20% to 33% of patients suspected of having appendicitis, the clinical presentation is atypical (Berry & Malt, 1984), requiring imaging. We prefer to perform graded compression sonography as the initial test; however, a number of studies have demonstrated greater accuracy with CT; therefore, this should be considered an alternative, especially in obese patients or if the sonogram is inconclusive (Lane et al., 1997; Fig. 16-12). Clinically, patients with diverticulitis typically have a fever and a tender mass in the left lower quadrant. CT can accurately determine the severity of involvement and whether a complicating abscess is present (Ambrosetti et al., 1997).

Although bowel injury resulting from blunt trauma is uncommon, CT can be used to differentiate between a full-thickness bowel wall injury that requires surgery and a less serious bowel wall contusion/hematoma or serosal tear.

## Retroperitoneum

### Pancreas

Previously the pancreas was a difficult organ to evaluate, clinically or with routine radiologic studies.

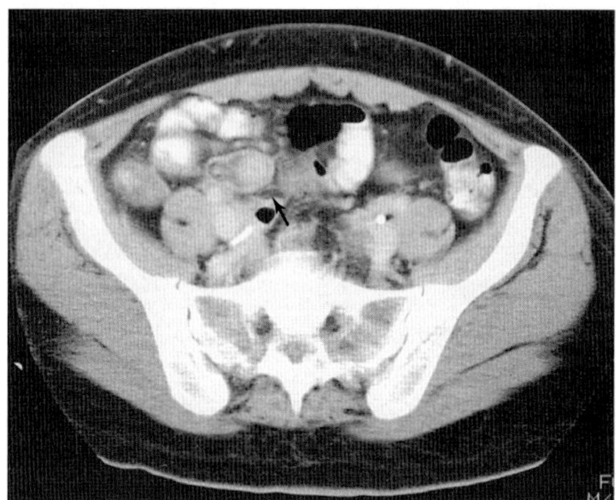

**FIGURE 16-12** Thickened, inflamed appendix (*arrow*) in the right lower quadrant.

Cross-sectional imaging methods such as ultrasonography, CT, and MRI now permit direct demonstration of the pancreas. The role of MRI in the diagnosis of pancreatic disorders is still questionable, and the technique probably offers no significant advantages over CT. When the pancreas is well visualized on a sonogram, the accuracy is comparable to that of CT. In general, the success rate for delineating the entire pancreas is much higher with CT than with ultrasonography because bowel gas often obscures part or all of the pancreas (Hessel et al., 1982; Fig. 16-13).

Acute pancreatitis is a clinical diagnosis, and normally neither CT nor ultrasonography is necessary. Imaging should be performed only when the diagnosis is uncertain, when complications are suspected (Siegelman et al., 1980), or when the clinical course is severe or unexpected. With acute pancreatitis CT is preferred mainly because of the high incidence of associated paralytic ileus, which obscures visualization of the pancreatic region by

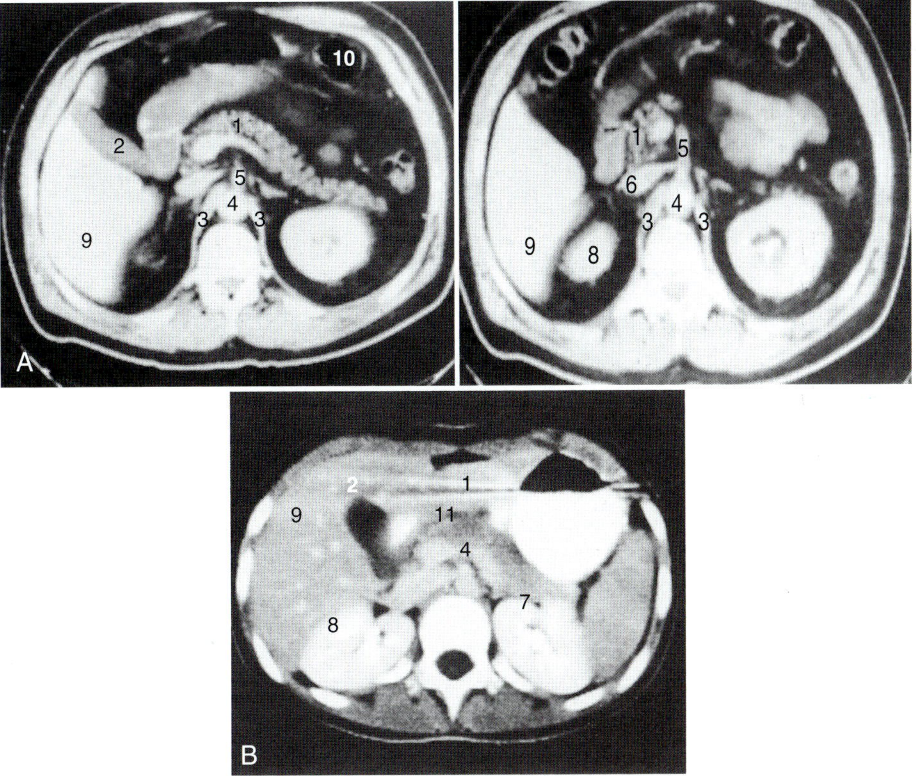


**FIGURE 16-13** Normal pancreas in patient with abundant **(A)** and little **(B)** intra-abdominal fat. *1*, Pancreas; *2*, gallbladder; *3*, crus of the diaphragm; *4*, aorta; *5*, superior mesenteric artery; *6*, inferior vena cava with left renal vein; *7*, left kidney; *8*, right kidney; *9*, liver; *10*, bowel; *11*, splenoportal confluence.

sonogram (Fig. 16-14). Larger pseudocysts can be monitored with ultrasonography, although CT generally provides a more graphic and complete delineation of the extent of involvement, and smaller changes in size and extent can be appreciated. A specific diagnosis of chronic pancreatitis can be made with CT if pancreatic calcification (often not seen on plain films) and pancreatic ductal dilation are noted.

Biphasic or triphasic examinations of the pancreas are helpful when searching for potential solid lesions in the pancreas. The arterial phase study with MPR or 3D reconstruction can delineate the vascular anatomy and help stage lesions by determining whether any vascular invasion is present. The parenchymal phase identifies adenocarcinomas as an area of diminished density because they tend to be hypovascular, whereas islet cell tumors, which are small and often difficult to identify (Rossi et al., 1985), appear as increased in density because of their hypervascularity. Solid pancreatic masses may be caused by a tumor (Fig. 16-15) or by focal inflammation, and differentiation may be difficult unless an ancillary finding such as liver metastases is also present. In most cases percutaneous aspiration or core needle biopsy under CT or ultrasonographic guidance for cytological and histological diagnosis is required (Sundaram et al., 1982; Fig. 16-16).

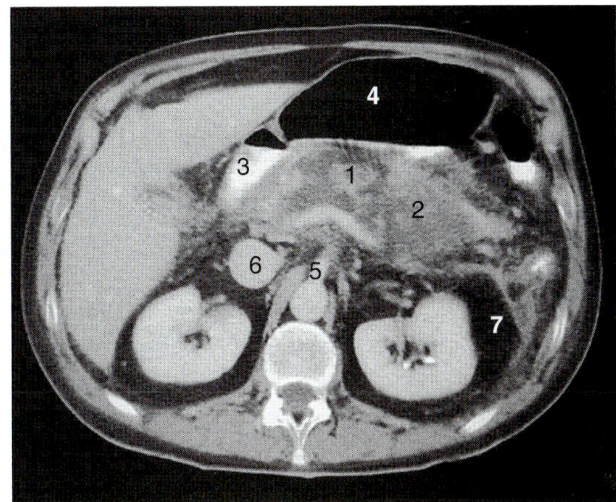


**FIGURE 16-14** Acute pancreatitis. Necrotic pancreas *(1)* surrounded by fluid *(2)*, duodenum *(3)*, air-filled stomach *(4)*, superior mesenteric artery *(5)*, inferior vena cava *(6)*, and perirenal fat *(7)*.

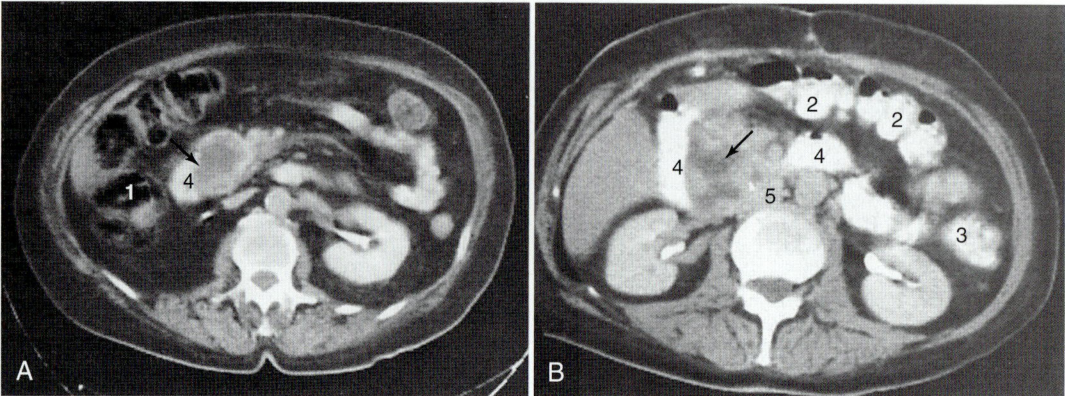


**FIGURE 16-15** Enlargement of the head of the pancreas (*arrows*) caused by carcinoma **(A)** and pancreatitis that has occurred as a result of a perforated ulcer **(B)**. *1,* Ascending colon; *2,* transverse colon; *3,* descending colon; *4,* duodenum; *5,* inferior vena cava.

## Kidneys

Renal ultrasonography and excretory urography (or IV pyelography) traditionally have been the primary means of investigating the kidney, but CT has rapidly gained ground and conventional IV pyelography is now rarely performed. The investigation of renal colic, which was the exclusive domain of the IV pyelogram, now is more effectively and rapidly diagnosed with noncontrast CT (Chen & Zagoria, 1999; Fig. 16-17). CT is more sensitive in detecting stones (Smith et al., 1995), can delineate signs associated with obstruction (Smith et al., 1996), and aids in treatment planning primarily by determining stone size and location (Fielding et al., 1998). Although this study can certainly identify other causes of abdominal pain that may mimic renal colic, it is a limited examination because no contrast is administered and significant pathological conditions such as renal tumors may be missed. Another concern is the radiation dosage, especially if repeated studies might be needed.

In most cases, ultrasonography can distinguish a cystic from a solid mass. When a solid lesion is identified, CT is useful for preoperative staging (Johnson et al., 1987). It is also useful for detecting local recurrence after a nephrectomy. Bowel loops and displaced normal organs make ultrasonographic evaluation difficult. In patients with polycystic kidneys, the demonstration of cysts with higher **attenuation** is consistent with a diagnosis of an infected cyst or bleeding into a cyst (Levine & Grantham, 1985). Angiomyolipomas have a characteristic CT appearance demonstrating areas of fatty attenuation (Totty et al., 1981). Occasionally calculi may appear as filling defects in the renal pelvis, mimicking tumors or blood clots on pyelography. In these cases CT may be useful for differentiating a tumor (Fig. 16-18) from a faintly calcified stone, a distinction that may not be evident on plain film (Pollack et al., 1981). CT IV pyelographic examinations that combine two contrast injections with MPRs of the kidneys and collecting system are used to assess patients for unexplained hematuria, which previously required IV or retrograde pyelography studies.

Preoperative assessment of renal donors with 3D CT CTA studies provides the surgeon with a very graphic road map that demonstrates the number and location of renal arteries.

## Adrenal Glands

CT has made it possible to delineate healthy adrenal glands easily and reliably, except when the patient is extremely thin (Abrams et al., 1982). If clinical and biochemical evidence of hyperfunction is present, CT usually is the only imaging method necessary. Pheochromocytomas and tumors causing Cushing's and Conn's syndromes that are larger than 5 mm are consistently demonstrated on CT. In adrenal hyperplasia, the adrenals may appear normal in size or may be slightly enlarged. Because small aldosteronomas may be missed on CT, adrenal venous **sampling** and venography are still important (Geisinger et al., 1983). Adrenal metastases, most commonly seen with bronchogenic and breast carcinomas, are readily demonstrated on CT and can be confirmed by biopsy.

A common clinical problem is the incidentally discovered, nonfunctioning small adrenal mass. These masses most often are nonfunctioning adenomas with a high lipid content. Recent studies have concluded that if the attenuation coefficient of the mass is low (10 or lower) on a noncontrast scan or if there is >50% washout of enhancement on 10-minute delayed scanning compared with an 80-second

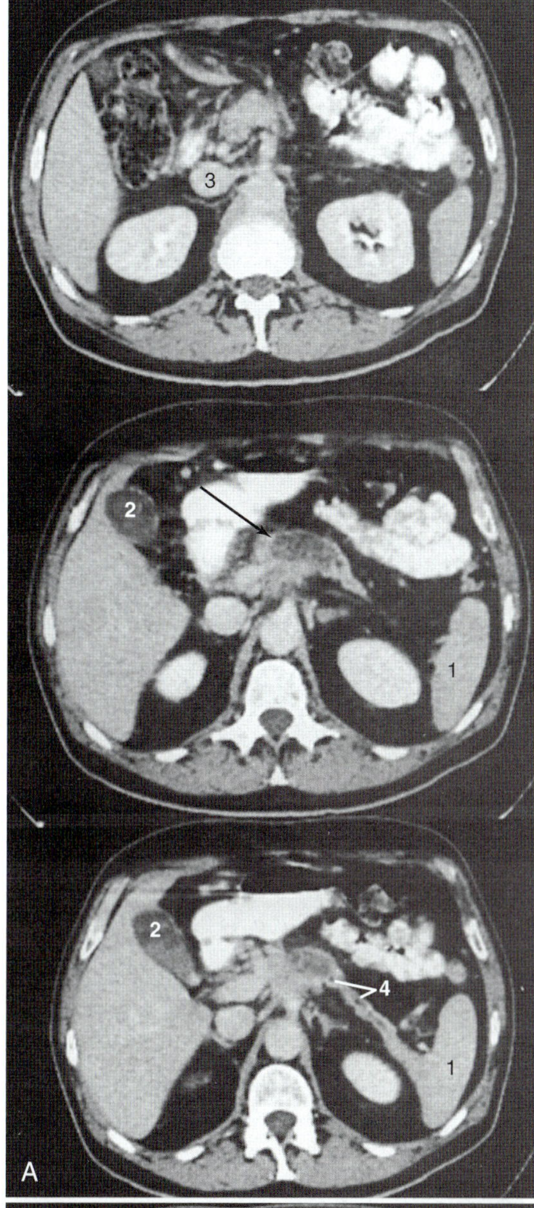


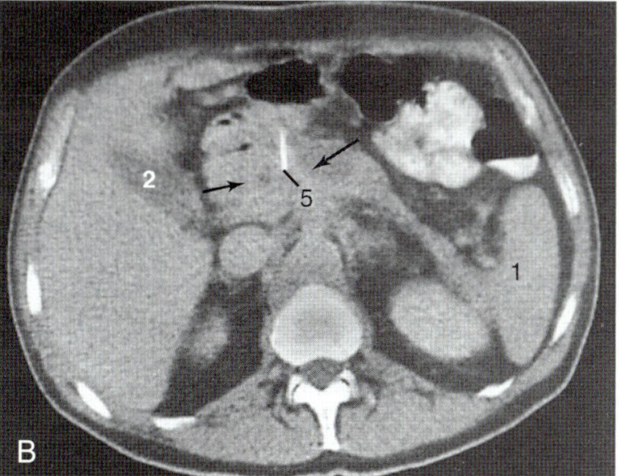


**FIGURE 16-16 A,** Carcinoma of the neck of the pancreas (*arrows*) with associated atrophy and dilation of the pancreatic duct. **B,** Aspiration biopsy of the mass with a 22-gauge needle. *1,* Spleen; *2,* gallbladder; *3,* inferior vena cava with left renal vein; *4,* dilated pancreatic duct with cystic changes; *5,* needle tip.

delayed scan, a confident diagnosis of adenoma can be made (Mayo-Smith et al., 2001; Fig. 16-19).

## Miscellaneous

The other main indications for imaging of the retroperitoneum are detection of lymphomatous or metastatic lymph nodes (Fig. 16-20) and assessment of abdominal aortic aneurysms.

The retroperitoneum often is obscured on a sonogram because of bowel gas, fat, and bony structures. CT therefore is the superior and obvious imaging method of choice. Because the main criterion for abnormality is lymph node enlargement, false-negative CT results may occur when the internal architecture of the lymph node is distorted without any associated enlargement.

Ultrasonography is adequate for sizing and following up on abdominal aortic aneurysms. Preoperative assessment, however, generally requires CT (Siegel & Cohan, 1994) or MRI (Prince et al., 1995) to determine the relationship of the aneurysm to the renal arteries, to precisely size the entire aneurysm, and to assess the iliac arteries, especially if endovascular grafting is considered. CT is also more useful when complications are suspected, such as rupture of an aneurysm (Fig. 16-21).

Primary retroperitoneal tumors tend to be large when first suspected clinically. When masses are large enough to be detected on physical examination, an ultrasound examination can differentiate a cystic lesion from a solid one. CT is often performed, however, because it can provide additional information about the extent of disease and the relationship to normal structures.

## Pelvis

Ultrasonography remains the primary means of pelvic assessment. The main role of CT in the pelvis, apart from assessment of the bowel and as part of an overall trauma assessment, remains staging the extent of tumor involvement of the bladder (Fig. 16-22), prostate, uterus, and ovaries and documenting any change after treatment. However, MRI, because of its superior soft tissue contrast and multiplanar capability, is assuming a greater role in staging pelvic neoplasms.

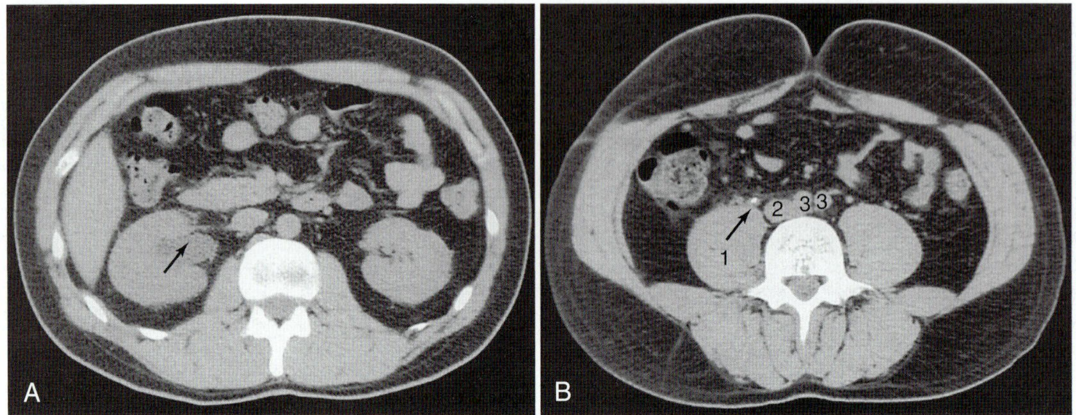


**FIGURE 16-17** **A,** Dilated right renal pelvis (*arrow*). **B,** Calculus (*arrow*) in the right ureter. *1,* Psoas muscle; *2,* inferior vena cava; *3,* iliac arteries.

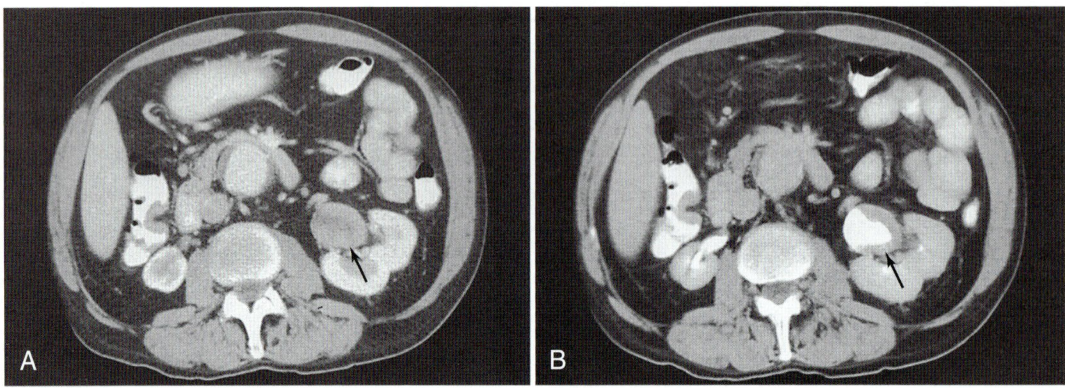


**FIGURE 16-18** Solid mass in the renal pelvis (*arrow*) before **(A)** and after **(B)** contrast opacification of the renal pelvis.

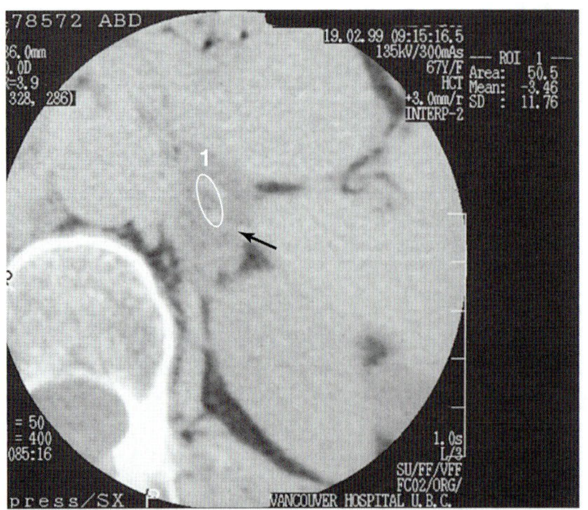


**FIGURE 16-19** Region of interest within an adrenal mass (*arrow*) indicating a negative Hounsfield number, confirming the diagnosis of adenoma. *1,* Left kidney; *2,* aorta.

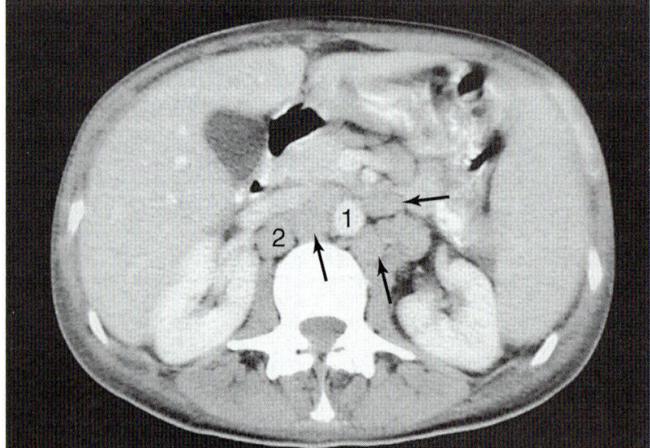


**FIGURE 16-20** Enlarged para-aortic and paracaval lymph nodes (*arrows*). *1,* Aorta; *2,* inferior vena cava.

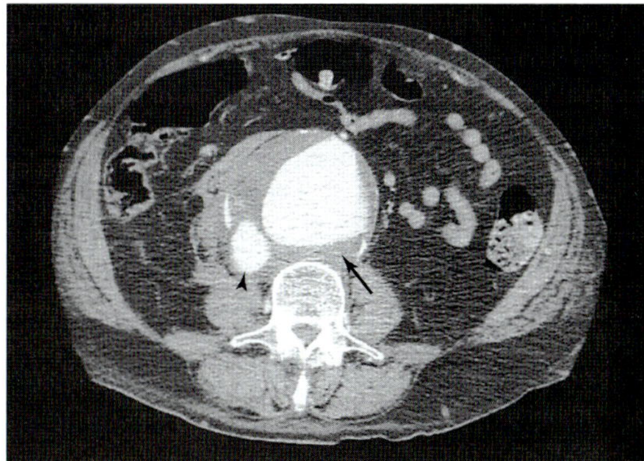

**FIGURE 16-21** Large abdominal aortic aneurysm (*arrow*) that has ruptured into the IVC (*arrowhead*), resulting in abnormally dense contrast within the IVC.

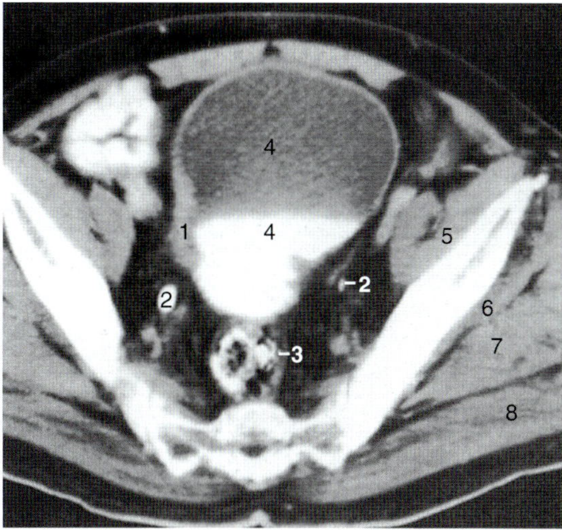


**FIGURE 16-22** Thickening of the bladder wall without evidence of extension into the perivesical fat (proven amyloidosis). *1*, Thickened bladder wall; *2*, ureters; *3*, sigmoid colon; *4*, urine and contrast medium in the bladder; *5*, iliac muscle; *6*, gluteus minimus; *7*, gluteus medius; *8*, gluteus maximus.

## Trauma

Trauma is the leading cause of death of individuals less than age 45 years (Novelline et al., 1999). CNS injuries as the cause of death rank the highest, followed by blunt chest trauma and then blunt abdominal trauma. Because of its high sensitivity, specificity, negative predictive value, speed, and ability to provide comprehensive information about not only abdominal injuries but also extra-abdominal injuries such as pelvic, spinal fractures, skull and facial fractures, pulmonary contusions, and pneumothorax, CT has become an integral component of the assessment of blunt abdominal and chest trauma, especially in specialized trauma centers (Shuman, 1997). A full-body trauma protocol can be completed in minutes, allowing scanning of all but the most hemodynamically unstable patients, who may require immediate surgery. By acquiring very thin helical axial slices (e.g., 0.5 mm), it is possible to subsequently use this same data to acquire MPR images to specifically assess the spine or major vascular structures (e.g., aorta). Grading schemes are available to help determine the extent of injury to various organs, which helps determine whether immediate surgery is required or whether conservative management is appropriate. Findings that are worrisome include evidence of active arterial extravasation, evidence of hypotension such as a collapsed inferior vena cava (IVC) or a small aorta, and the presence of free fluid. Measuring the Hounsfield units (HU) of fluid can be helpful for characterization purposes: extravasated contrast 85 to 350 HU; unclotted blood 25 to 50 HU; clotted blood 40 to 75 HU; and ascites, bile, urine, and bowel contents 5 to 10 HU (Rhea, 2004).

CT has largely replaced other imaging methods and considerably reduced the need for exploratory laparotomies. The so-called *FAST ultrasonography* (focused abdominal sonogram in trauma), which is useful in screening for free intraperitoneal fluid, sometimes is performed first to identify patients more likely to have a positive CT result. However, FAST ultrasonography has a limited ability to define the extent and site of injury and cannot assess the retroperitoneal structures thoroughly (Molina et al., 1998).

## Vascular System

The use of CT for aortic injury, dissection, coronary arteries, pulmonary arteries, renal arteries, and abdominal aortic aneurysms has already been discussed. CTA has largely replaced standard catheter angiography for the diagnosis of peripheral vascular disease. CTA can provide an angiographic caliber study that includes the entire aorta to the digital arteries in the foot (Fig 16-23). Catheter angiography is now largely reserved for **interventional procedures** such as angioplasty or stenting.

## Interventional Applications

### Abscess Drainage

An abscess is a potentially curable condition. Because the morbidity and mortality rates associated with an undrained abscess are high, it is important to use whatever means are available to localize the abscess

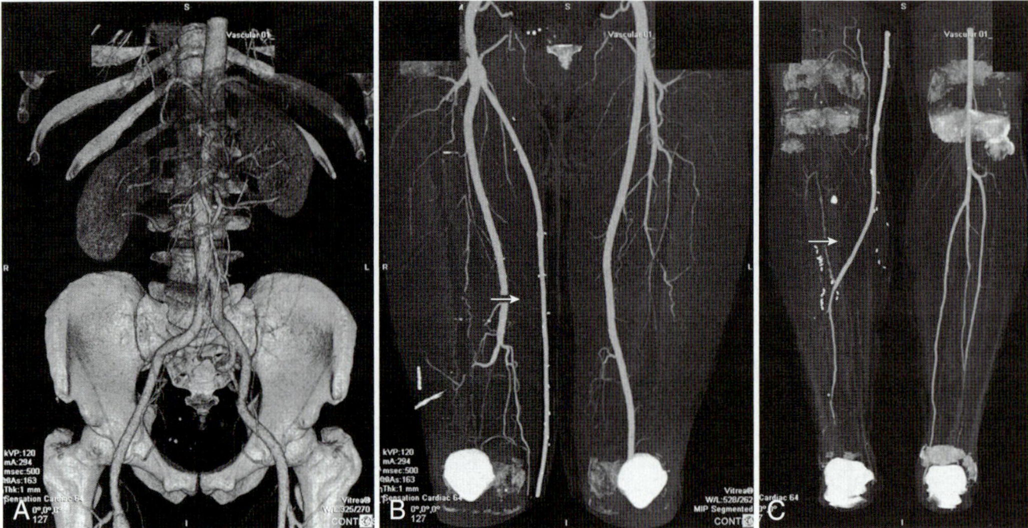

**FIGURE 16-23** CT runoff angiogram demonstrating the entire vascular tree from the aorta to the lower calves. 3D reconstruction of the aorta and iliac arteries **(A)**. Maximum intensity projection image of the thighs **(B)** demonstrating a femoral graft on the right (*arrow*) replacing the occluded superficial femoral artery. Maximum intensity projection image of the calves **(C)** demonstrating that the graft (*arrow*) has been anastomosed to one of the runoff branches. Most of the bony structures have been segmented and removed. (Images courtesy Dr. Mike Martin, Vancouver Hospital.)

accurately, to determine the relationship to adjacent structures, including bowel loops, and to institute prompt treatment through the placement of drainage catheters (Callen, 1979; Gerzof et al., 1981; Halber et al., 1979). The advantage of CT over ultrasonography is that it is not limited by wounds, drains, ostomies, bandages, or bowel gas associated with paralytic ileus, which is common in postoperative patients. Extraluminal gas, although not always present, is the most specific CT sign of an abscess (Fig. 16-24). This may be missed on a sonogram because differentiation from normal bowel gas can be extremely difficult.

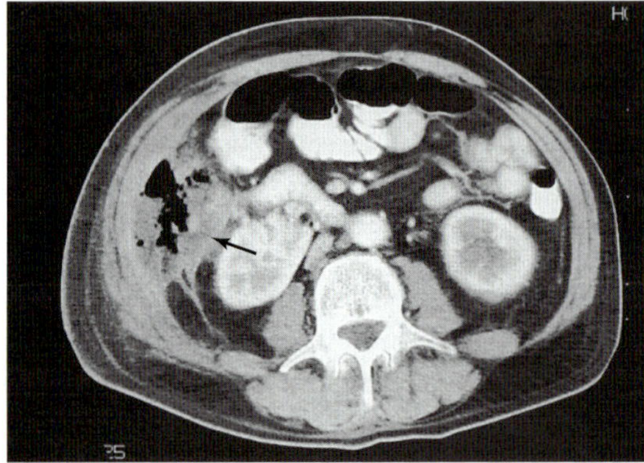

**FIGURE 16-24** Abnormal localized collection of gas and fluid (*arrow*) in a right flank abscess that occurred as a result of a ruptured appendix.

## Biopsy

Cytological aspiration biopsy and core biopsy have proved to be effective, safe, and simple techniques for establishing a cytological or histological diagnosis for masses anywhere in the body (Ferrucci et al., 1980). The exact location of the needle tip relative to the tumor (Fig. 16-19, *B*) can be displayed on CT; therefore even small lesions deep in the abdomen can be approached. This capability was enhanced by the introduction of **CT fluoroscopy,** which allows the radiologist to directly monitor the **position** of the needle tip by continuous scanning. The biopsy thus can be performed under direct vision rather than using the conventional "blind" approach of advancing the needle and then determining its location. Problems arising from erratic patient breathing are diminished, the procedure time is reduced, and the patient's safety and comfort are improved.

## Musculoskeletal System

CT generally is a problem-solving technique. It is often performed after plain films or radionuclide bone scans have already been used. Conventional tomography and arteriography, which formerly were used to determine the extent of disease, are now rarely used. With bony tumors, CT is useful in showing the location of

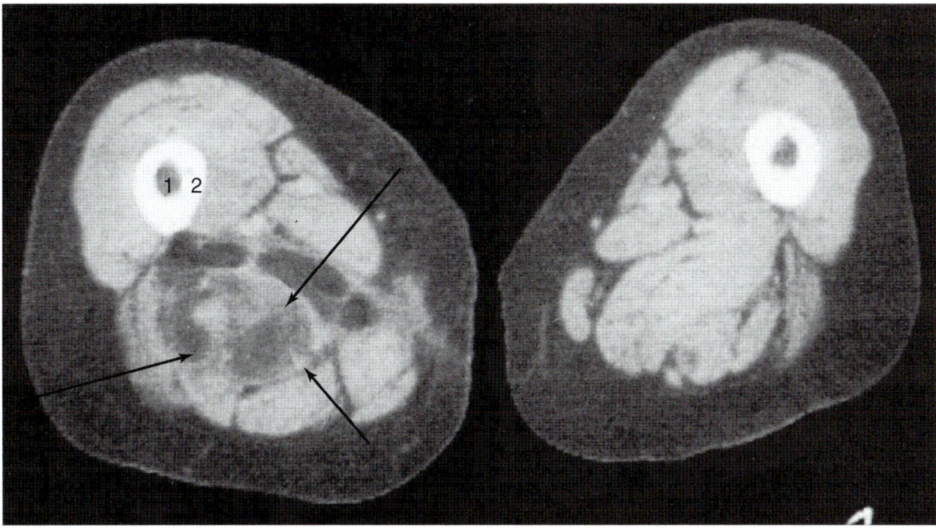


**FIGURE 16-25** Liposarcoma (*arrows*) involving the right adductor magnus muscle. *1*, Medullary canal; *2*, cortex.

the tumor in the bone; evaluating cortical integrity, articular involvement, and intermedullary extent; and defining extraosseous extension (Schreiman et al., 1986). When soft tissues are involved, the relationship of these masses to important neurovascular structures can be determined (Fig. 16-25). However, because of its superior soft tissue contrast resolution (Boyko et al., 1987; Petasnik et al., 1986), MRI has replaced CT for many musculoskeletal applications.

Skeletal trauma generally can be studied by standard radiographs. In complex anatomic regions, however, such as the pelvis, shoulder, foot, and ankle, more precise information about the presence, location, orientation, and relationship of fracture fragments can be obtained with CT (Guyer et al., 1985; Lange & Alter, 1980). In this regard, multiplanar reformations and 3D reconstructions can be extremely useful.

## EXAMINATION PREPARATION

### Planning

After the radiologist has determined that a CT scan is clinically indicated, the radiologist and technologist must plan the patient preparation, including the potential use of oral or IV **contrast media,** and the scanning protocol to be used. This can be done verbally or by written instructions. Patients need to be screened for potential contrast allergies and status of renal function. Patients with compromised renal function generally defined as a calculated glomerular **filtration** rate (GFR) of <60 have a threefold greater risk for development of contrast-induced nephropathy (CIN) compared with healthy individuals (McCullough et al., 1997). Two studies have found that CIN may occur in up to 15% of unselected patients undergoing contrast studies (Iakovou et al., 2003; McCullough et al., 2006). Each site should have in place specific protocols based on the patient's calculated GFR. This may determine whether contrast is administered, which contrast agent is used (i.e., low osmolar or iso-osmolar), whether extra hydration is required, or whether the patient may require *N*-acetylcysteine or sodium bicarbonate infusion.

The use of standard protocol sheets may be helpful. When these instructions are different from those routinely followed, it is important for the technologist to discuss the case individually with the radiologist so that the examination can be tailored specifically to the clinical problem. This is even more crucial with helical multislice scanners, which have a myriad of new and very specialized protocols. After reviewing the initial scans, the radiologist may extend, modify, or terminate the examination.

### Patient Information

The "high-tech" aspect of CT does not diminish the importance of establishing good rapport with the patient. Patient cooperation can mean the difference between a poor-quality examination and a high-quality result. It is essential that the technologist explain procedures clearly before and during the CT study. The explanations should be brief and given in "lay" terms so that patients know what to expect and what is expected of them. A patient information sheet may be helpful, and pictures of scans may be of interest to the person.

Before the examination, the technologist should:

1. Briefly explain the process of CT.
2. Describe the examination to be performed, including the area of the body to be studied, and give an estimate of the duration of the examination.
3. Emphasize the importance of keeping still because of the image degradation that occurs with motion.
4. Give appropriate breathing instructions.
5. Have the patient empty the bladder immediately before the examination so that the patient is more comfortable and less likely to move, especially if the study involves use of an IV contrast medium.
6. If a contrast medium is to be used, explain the reason for its use and question the patient about allergies. A description of any unpleasant sensations the patient may feel from injection of the contrast material also should be given (this is especially important when mechanical power injectors are used).
7. Reassure the patient that the technologist, although not in the room, will be able to see and talk to the patient.

The patient should always be encouraged to ask questions about the examination. If the questions are more medical in nature, the patient should speak directly with the radiologist. It is important to remember that, although the examination is routine to the staff, it is not for the patient. In addition to being anxious and worried about the results of the examination, patients are fearful and concerned about the examination itself. The staff should try to make the "high-tech" study a "high-touch" experience and constantly be sensitive to the patient's feelings.

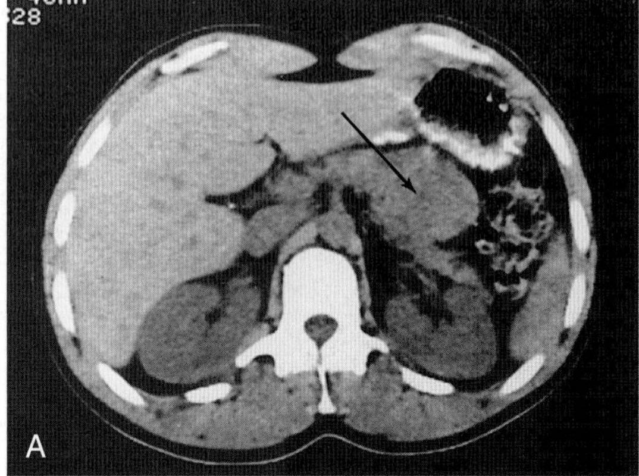


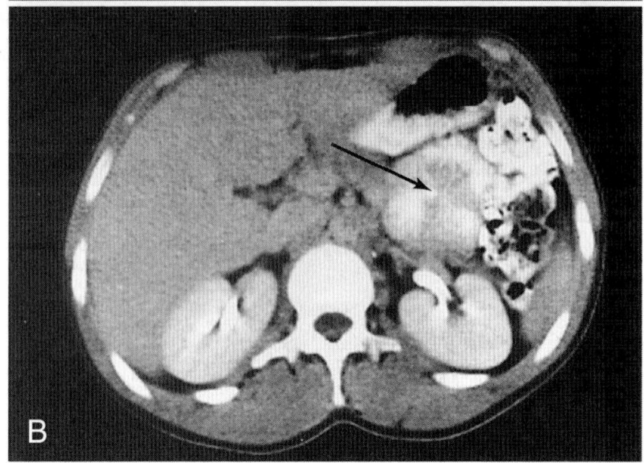


**FIGURE 16-26 A,** An apparent mass of the body of the pancreas (*arrow*). **B,** When an oral contrast medium is used, the mass is revealed to be multiple small bowel loops (*arrow*).

## Oral Contrast Media

The use of dilute oral contrast material to opacify the entire GI tract has been the typical standard of practice so that homogeneous, fluid-filled bowel loops are not mistaken for masses (Fig. 16-26) or gas-filled loops of bowel for abscesses. Proper opacification of the GI tract can be especially valuable in very thin patients who lack the amount of intra-abdominal fat necessary to outline various structures (Fig. 16-13, *B*). To simplify the preparation for outpatients by not requiring them to pick up contrast before the scan and because of the improved resolution and multiplanar capabilities of current CT scanners, some radiologists are now satisfied to only administer water as the sole bowel preparation. A typical regimen is 1 liter (L) of water the night before followed by 1.5 L 1 to 2 hours before the scan and 300 to 400 milliliters (ml) immediately before the scan. If positive contrast agents are required, dilute barium sulfate solution (e.g., Readi-Cat 2.0% weight/weight 225 ml mixed with 275 ml of water and ingested the evening before and again 1 hour before the scan) and water-soluble iodinated contrast solutions (e.g., Telebrix 10 ml diluted in 900 ml of water or juice, 400 ml of this mixture ingested 2 hours before, 400 ml 1 hour before, and the remaining 100 ml immediately before the scan) are commonly used. The latter has the advantage of opacifying the entire small and large bowel more quickly; therefore, it is especially useful for inpatients that may require somewhat more urgent scanning. Barium sulfate suspension should not be used for patients suspected of having a GI perforation. However, when there is concern about a contrast reaction to iodinated compounds, barium sulfate solution should be used instead. Failure to give the patient the first dose, however, is not a reason to cancel or postpone the procedure; a small-volume contrast enema (150 to 250 ml) can be given to opacify the rectum and distal large bowel. The enema also distends the colon, whereas perioral techniques do not.

For assessment of gastric neoplasms, water alone with or without gas may be given instead of a positive contrast medium to distend the stomach. Some

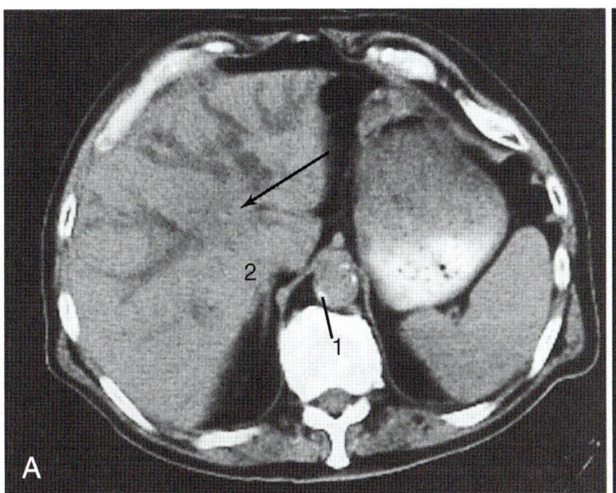


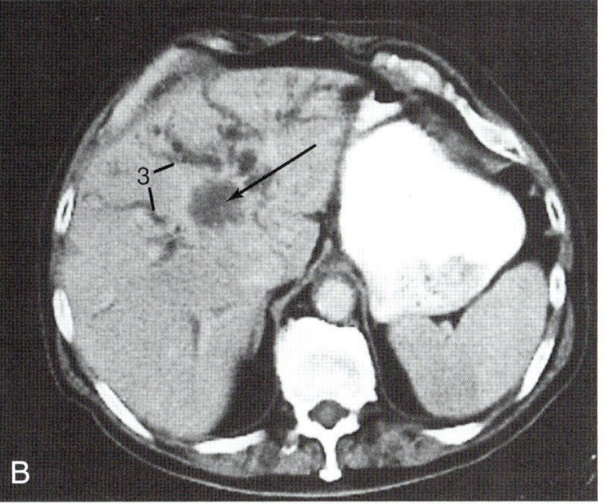


**FIGURE 16-27** Cholangiocarcinoma (*arrow*). **A,** Precontrast scan. **B,** Postcontrast scan. The large mass at the porta hepatis is more evident on the postcontrast scan, which also better differentiates dilated bile ducts from blood vessels. *1,* Aortic calcification; *2,* adrenal gland; *3,* dilated intrahepatic ducts.

investigators distend the stomach with air or gas alone. An effervescent agent similar to that used in double-contrast upper GI examinations can be administered or a carbonated soft drink can be administered. This method allows good visualization of the gastric wall. If a patient cannot drink the oral contrast medium because of nausea and vomiting, air can be introduced through a nasogastric tube. However, the radiopaque markers used in nasogastric tubes to indicate their position on conventional radiographs can produce artifacts on CT; therefore, these should be removed before the examination, if possible, or at least replaced by ones that are not radiopaque.

If the patient has had a recent barium examination of the GI tract, sufficient time should be allowed for elimination of the contrast medium, or the colon can be cleansed of residual barium. Because residual barium can result in considerable image degradation caused by streak artifacts, the technologist should seek the advice of the radiologist if contrast is detected on the scout scan as the examination may need to be postponed.

CT colonography typically requires the use of purgatives, hydration, and dietary restriction to ensure a clean colon, although some recent studies have shown promising results without a full bowel preparation but instead tagging stool with contrast agents.

## Intravenous Contrast Agents

IV contrast material is used for several purposes. The initial vascular opacification may be useful for anatomic localization; distinguishing vessels from a mass; determining the extent of vascular displacement or invasion by a tumor; and assessing specific vascular disease such as aneurysms, stenoses, or loss of vascular integrity resulting in extravasation of the contrast medium. The subsequent extravascular distribution of contrast medium into various tissues helps confirm an intact blood supply of body organs and, to a limited extent, provides some functional assessment such as in opacification of the urinary tract. Often tumors and normal parenchyma do not enhance to the same extent or at the same time. This differential enhancement, which increases the attenuation difference between normal and abnormal tissue (Fig. 16-27), can be used to maximize lesion detectability. However, the timing of the scans and the contrast injection protocols must be chosen carefully because some lesions may be masked by tissue enhancement.

The degree of contrast medium enhancement is the result of a combination of complex factors including the rate, amount, and concentration of contrast material administered; the speed of injection; the timing of the scans; cardiac output; plasma expansion; extravascular redistribution; and renal filtration and excretion of the contrast material. Various approaches to IV administration of contrast material have been used, reflecting the inadequacies of any one method (Nelson, 1991). Drip infusion of contrast medium usually does not result in ideal enhancement because of inconsistent flow rates, which result in too slow a rise in the plasma iodine concentration. This method has largely been replaced by bolus injections, with some notable exceptions such as routine contrast medium–enhanced head scans and postoperative lumbar spine and cervical spine scans.

A mechanical injector is mandatory for use of injection rates as high as 5 or 6 ml/s and to obtain a sustained, reproducible level of contrast medium enhancement. This usually requires insertion of an 18- or 19-gauge short IV needle catheter into a medially directed antecubital vein connected to tubing capable of withstanding the pressures generated in high-flow injections. It is imperative that any air bubbles in the syringe and tubing be cleared before the final connection is made to the needle to prevent the possibility of a potentially fatal cerebral air embolus. The major disadvantage of a power injector is the slight risk of extravasation of contrast material into the soft tissues. It therefore is imperative that the patient be able to alert the technologist immediately if a local "burning" sensation occurs so that the injection can be stopped, preventing tissue damage. Most often the injector is loaded with 100 to 180 ml of 60% contrast medium, with injection rates varying from 1 to 6 ml/s depending on the specific indication.

Different delay times are used to match scanning with the arrival of contrast medium at the appropriate vessels and organs. These delays can be set empirically on the basis of experience and published data, or they can be tailored individually through the use of bolus tracking or automated techniques such as "SmartPrep" (General Electric) or "SureStart" (Toshiba). With use of helical or spiral volumetric acquisition, a large region (typically 30 centimeters [cm] or more) such as the entire liver can be easily examined in several seconds. The latest generation of scanners, with subsecond and multislice technology, enhances this capability (Berland & Smith, 1998) further by allowing even greater ranges or thinner collimation or both.

With a single bolus injection of contrast medium, the pattern of vascular enhancement during the first circulation and the pattern of vascular and tissue enhancement during recirculation can be studied. This method is useful for studying aortic dissection, in which flow in the false lumen is often delayed, and for evaluation of a possible hemangioma (Fig. 16-8). In these a specific area may be examined dynamically and repeatedly over a period of time without table movement.

Other, more specialized techniques include selective catheterization and injection of specific vessels followed by CT scanning such as the proper hepatic artery for CT hepatic arteriography and the superior mesenteric artery or splenic artery for CT arterial portography (Nelson, 1991). These studies are reported to be more sensitive for detecting small liver lesions (<2 cm) than either MRI or biphasic CT (Hori et al., 1998).

## SCANNING PROTOCOLS

Developing routine protocols is helpful. These protocols serve as general guidelines and can be modified as required, tailoring the examination to a particular patient's clinical problem. In addition to the details specific to a region, scanning protocols should optimize the radiographic technique to maximize lesion detection. This requires careful consideration in choosing the appropriate kilovoltage (kV), milliamperage (mA), collimation, reconstruction interval, **pitch,** range, **field of view (FOV),** reconstruction **matrix,** field size, reconstruction **algorithm,** postprocessing filters, and window widths and levels.

Scanning protocols can vary significantly from site to site, primarily on the basis of the type of scanner used and to some extent on the preference of the radiologists. The following protocols deal exclusively with helical (spiral) multislice scanners. Even among multislice scanners significant variations exist between 4-, 8-, 16-, 32-, and 64-slice scanners. Many centers with multislice scanners, especially 16 slice or greater, will use the narrowest detector collimation possible (typically 0.5 to 0.75 mm) to obtain a volume dataset. These initial scans are used to obtain near **isotropic** voxels that enable excellent quality MPRs and 3D images. According to study requirements and department preferences, scans of varying thickness and in the axial, sagittal, or coronal planes may be reconstructed for diagnosis and documentation. Typically these will consist of contiguous or overlapping 2- to 5-mm-thick images that are reconstructed from the initial volume dataset.

### Thorax

In most thoracic examinations, scanning begins superiorly from the level of the clavicles and extends to the posterior costophrenic angle. When a neoplasm is suspected, the scans should include the liver and adrenal glands. Because detection of liver metastases is maximized when scans are obtained immediately after administration of a contrast medium, it may be more appropriate to scan in a caudocranial direction through the liver and adrenal glands first and then superiorly through the remainder of the chest, where a high plasma iodine concentration is not as critical (Foley, 1989). This is not necessary with current multislice scanners.

Scans are typically obtained in full inspiration during a single breath-hold; therefore, misregistration artifacts are no longer a problem (Costello et al., 1991). When the posterior lung base is the region of primary concern, prone scans may be helpful to increase aeration to this area. Lateral decubitus scans also are helpful in rare instances in distinguishing between complex pleural and pulmonary pathological conditions, such as differentiating an empyema from a large lung abscess.

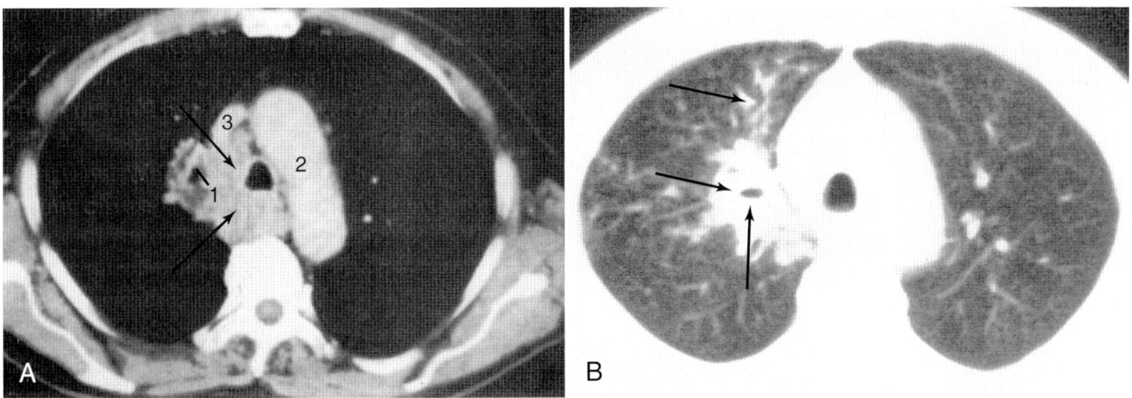


**FIGURE 16-28** Bronchogenic carcinoma (*arrows*) involving the right hilum with mediastinal invasion and distal obstructive pneumonitis in the right upper lobe. **A,** Mediastinal window. **B,** Lung window. *1,* Right superior segmental bronchus of the right upper lobe; *2,* aortic arch; *3,* superior vena cava.

Thoracic CT scans should be viewed with at least two different window width settings (Fig. 16-28). One of these should be optimized for the mediastinum and chest wall and the other for the lungs. If necessary, an additional setting for the bones should be used. The use of higher frequency filters for the lung parenchyma is helpful.

Scans of the chest are generally obtained with the patient supine and the arms elevated. The arms should not be so high as to obstruct the flow of IV contrast material; therefore, some radiologists prefer to leave the arm with the IV line by the patient's side, especially for high flow rate examinations, even though there will be some artifacts.

Some radiologists believe that an IV contrast medium need not be used routinely because the anatomy of the mediastinal structures is not complicated and they are generally well delineated by the mediastinal fat. Contrast medium is useful, however, for better defining the mediastinum, for determining the relationship of the mass to the mediastinal vessels, or for checking for vascular abnormalities.

CT examination of the thorax usually begins with a digital localizing radiograph (e.g., scout view, topogram, or scanogram), typically in the anteroposterior **projection.** Scan levels can be prescribed from this image, and the scans obtained can be displayed on it. This can be helpful in correlating the CT images with a plain film abnormality and may be of some value in planning radiation therapy and guiding biopsy. Thicker slices (2.5 to 7 mm) obtained at 1.25- to 5-mm slice intervals are routinely used. Thinner sections of 1 to 2 mm may be used to improve **spatial resolution,** particularly in assessing the hila, fissures, and airways. When HRCT is used for assessing diffuse lung disease, 1- to 2-mm-thick sections are used, often with a smaller FOV with target reconstruction and a high spatial frequency algorithm to improve spatial resolution (Mayo, 1991; Fig. 16-6).

Before the current generation of multidetector scanners, it was impractical to examine the entire chest by using contiguous thin slices. The examination therefore was tailored to the particular clinical indication. For the assessment of bronchiectasis and diffuse infiltrative lung disease, 1- to 2-mm-thick sections obtained at 10-mm intervals were used most often. In assessing asbestos-related disease, a more limited examination consisting of five to eight scans spaced throughout the middle and lower thorax usually was sufficient. With multidetector scanners it is now feasible to examine the entire chest with contiguous thin slices; the main consideration is to balance benefit with risk with respect to radiation **exposure,** especially with repeated examinations. Because of the high intrinsic contrast, HRCT can be performed by using lower radiation (low mAs) techniques. Occasionally, selected scans obtained in expiration may be useful for determining the presence or extent of air trapping.

## Abdomen and Pelvis

Scans are most commonly obtained with the patient supine. Scanning in the prone position may be useful for biopsy of posterior structures, such as the adrenal glands or retroperitoneal lymph nodes. CT kidneys-ureter-bladder (KUB) studies for renal colic are also typically performed in the prone position because bladder stones that are not impacted at the ureterovesical junction will be located in the dependent portion of the bladder.

All abdominal and pelvic scans are acquired helically using the narrowest detector collimation

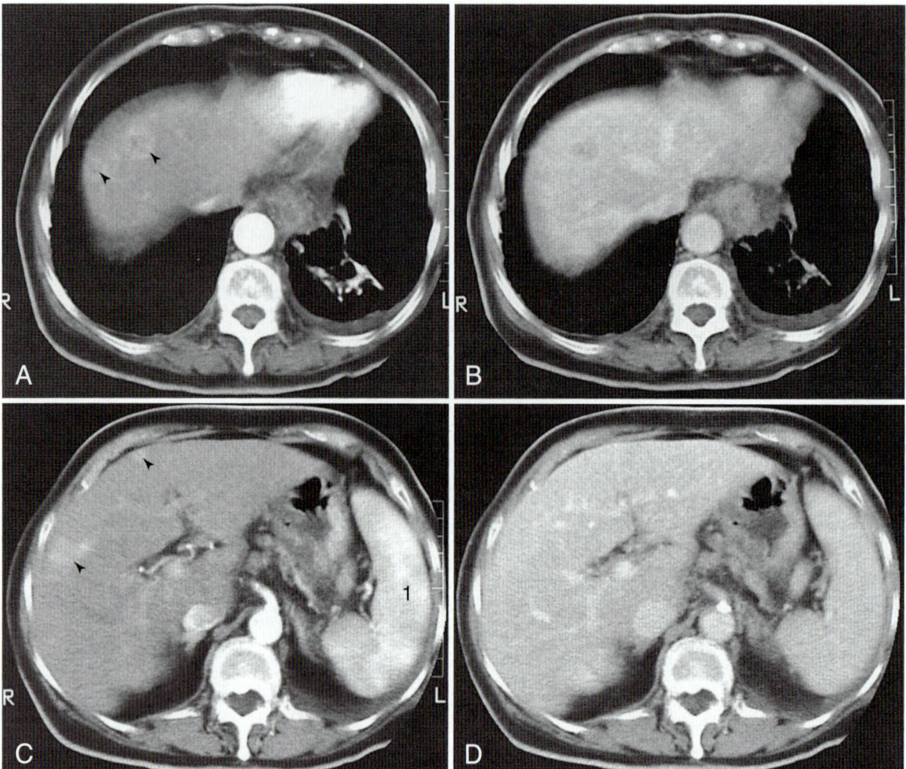


**FIGURE 16-29** **A** and **C,** Scans obtained within 2 minutes of administration of a contrast medium reveal four hypervascular lesions. **B** and **D,** In "early delayed" scans (i.e., scans obtained approximately 5 minutes after injection of the contrast medium), two of the lesions have "disappeared" and two others are much less conspicuous. *1,* Normal inhomogeneous appearance of the spleen during early enhancement by the contrast medium.

available. A general survey type examination generally consists of axial images reconstructed as 5-mm contiguous or overlapping slices. Adrenal and pancreatic studies are reconstructed at 2- to 3-mm thickness and generally with some overlap. Newer multislice scanners permit extended coverage and reduce scan times to 5 to 10 seconds for an average abdominal examination. Helical data acquisition using detector collimation of 0.5 to 0.75 mm allows retrospective reconstruction of varying **slice thickness** at closer intervals, including overlapping slices, if the **raw data** are saved. This provides tremendous flexibility in protocols, largely solves problems of volume averaging, and provides excellent multiplanar reformations.

Images obtained without the use of a contrast medium usually are of limited value with the following exceptions: identification and characterization of calcific masses or renal calculi or to localize a hepatic lesion before rapid, contrast medium–enhanced, dynamic scans are obtained at the same level without table movement.

IV contrast medium generally is essential, particularly for evaluating the liver and pancreas. Several factors are important in the detection and differential diagnosis of liver lesions, including (1) the liver has a dual blood supply, from the hepatic artery and the portal vein; (2) arterial inflow occurs earlier than portal inflow; and (3) most neoplasms receive their blood primarily from the hepatic artery, whereas normal hepatocytes primarily receive their blood from the portal vein.

The early "arterial phase" scans with typical scan delays of 20 to 30 seconds best visualize highly vascular lesions, both benign and malignant, such as focal nodular hyperplasia, hepatic adenoma, hepatocellular carcinoma, and hypervascular metastases such as from the kidney, breast, and islet cell tumors (Fig. 16-29). The later "venous phase" scans with scan delays of 70 to 80 seconds are best suited for studying hypovascular lesions such as colon metastases that, lacking a portal venous supply, enhance much less than normal hepatocytes (Baron, 1994). The trend, therefore, is to perform these so-called *biphasic examinations* for many hepatic studies. In some cases delayed scans (e.g., 10 minutes) may be helpful in studying cholangiocarcinoma, which may show delayed enhancement and hemangioma by demonstrating contrast "filling in."

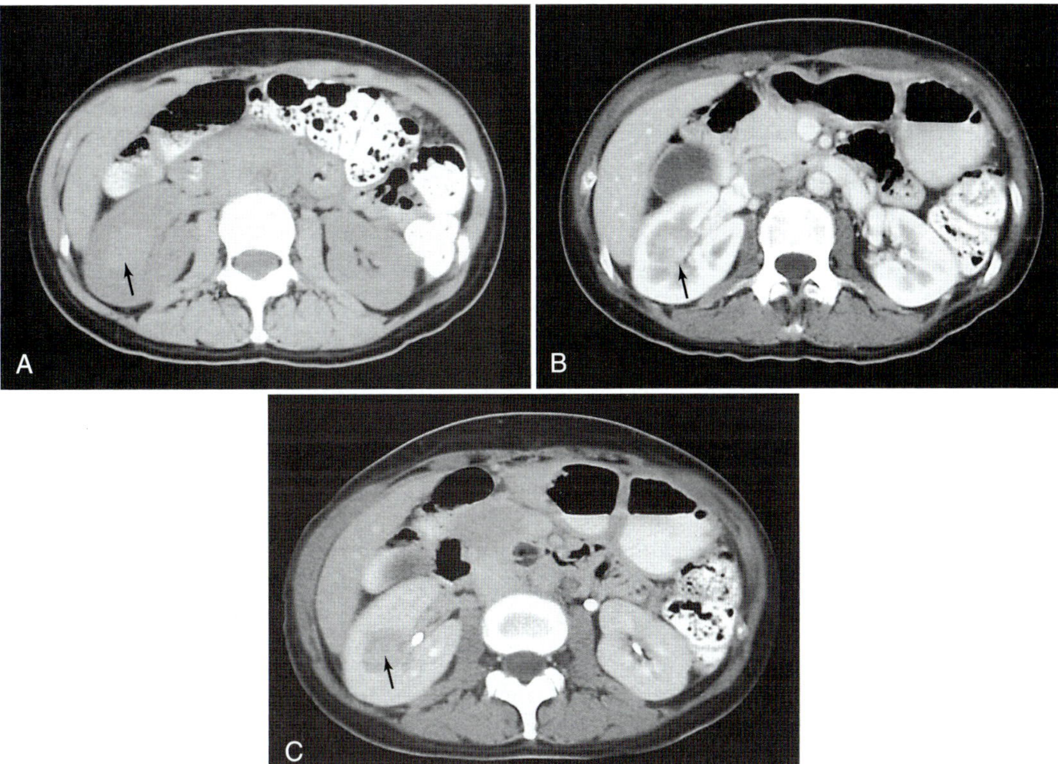


**FIGURE 16-30** Renal carcinoma. **A,** Scan obtained before administration of a contrast medium demonstrates a mass of higher density (*arrow*) than renal parenchyma. This is atypical because most renal carcinomas are isodense or hypodense on studies done without use of a contrast medium; the higher density likely indicates recent hemorrhage. **B,** A corticomedullary phase scan demonstrates that the mass (*arrow*) is enhancing, but less than normal renal cortex. **C,** A nephrographic phase scan demonstrates the mass (*arrow*) with greater conspicuity because of the now homogeneous enhancement of the cortex and medulla. Contrast medium is also seen within the collecting system.

A biphasic protocol for pancreatic scans is also useful. The earlier arterial phase with injection of 100 to 120 ml of contrast medium at a rate of 4 to 5 ml/s, reconstructing thin (2.5 to 3 mm) overlapping images (every 1.5 to 2.5 mm) and a scan delay set to the time of aortic peak plus 5 seconds, optimally enhances the arteries and pancreatic parenchyma, allowing visualization of small hypodense or hyperdense masses (islet cell tumors) and demonstrating any vascular invasion (Hollett et al., 1995). The later venous phase with a scan delay of 70 seconds and 2.5- to 5-mm overlapping reconstructed images through the liver and pancreas delineates the peripancreatic veins, further helping to stage a pancreatic carcinoma. This phase is also best for detecting hepatic metastases from nonislet-cell tumors, which tend to be hypovascular.

Renal CT typically is performed to further characterize a renal mass or to stage a tumor. This is best done with a three-phase study: examination of the kidneys without a contrast medium (0.5-0.75 mm detector collimation, 2.5- to 5-mm slice thickness, 1.25- to 2.5-mm slice intervals) followed by examination after administration of the contrast medium (100 to 120 ml at 3.5 to 4 ml/s) with an early study in the corticomedullary phase (minimum 70-second delay) and by a later scan (3- to 5-minute delay) in the nephrographic or pyelographic phase (Fig. 16-30). The unenhanced scan is useful for detecting stones and fatty tumors (e.g., angiomyolipomas) and for establishing a baseline for determining whether a mass is enhancing. Performing two studies after administration of the contrast medium improves the detection of masses and provides better characterization and more accurate staging (Kopka et al., 1997).

The protocol for the so-called CT KUB is designed specifically to identify renal and ureteral calculi, typically in the acute phase. Neither oral nor IV contrast material is administered. The range scanned extends from the top of the kidneys to the symphysis pubis. Our preferred protocol is to use 0.6-mm detector collimation with 5-mm-thick slices reconstructed every 2.5 mm. The images are transferred to a workstation to be reviewed in cine or movie mode to facilitate interpretation. Only every third image is filmed. The radiation dosage can be significantly diminished by lowering the mA to 80 because more noisy images are adequate for the purposes of this examination.

For "routine" abdominal scans with less specific indications, an adequate protocol generally is 2.5- to 5-mm-thick scans, administration of 100 to 120 ml of contrast medium at a rate of 2.5 ml/s, and a scan delay of 70 seconds.

The use of oral contrast medium has already been emphasized. When the pelvis is examined, use of a tampon is an easy means of anatomic localization of the vagina.

### Musculoskeletal System

Because the anatomy of the musculoskeletal system varies from one region to another, the technique used for each patient should be tailored to the clinical problem. A computed radiograph is helpful for visualizing any bony abnormalities to determine the number, location, and range of images needed and to correlate with plain films.

Precise positioning is important. Whenever possible, the normal extremity should also be examined. The two sides should be symmetrically positioned and displayed to facilitate side-to-side comparison. Slice thickness and interval are determined by the clinical problem. For assessing most tumors and masses, 2.5- to 5-mm slices are adequate. Smaller lesions require 1- to 3-mm slices, and examination of smaller structures such as the ankle and wrist often requires 0.5- to 1-mm slices.

Once the images have been obtained, they should always be displayed and viewed at two window settings, soft tissue and bone settings. In some cases reconstruction of the images with higher resolution algorithms and higher spatial frequency filters may be necessary to improve bony detail. Multiplanar and 3D reconstructions can be helpful with complicated anatomy, particularly in the evaluation of fractures.

When tumors and their relationship to neurovascular structures are assessed, bolus injection of IV contrast material is required. Intra-articular injection of a contrast medium or air can be useful when joints are being evaluated, but these arthrographic examinations are now more often performed as MRI studies.

## REVIEW QUESTIONS

Answer the following questions to check your understanding of the materials studied.

1. Which of the following abnormalities is not seen on CT images?
   A. pulmonary embolism
   B. pleurisy
   C. granulomas
   D. lymphangitic carcinomas
2. High resolution CT has replaced ______ in detecting bronchiectasis.
   A. conventional tomography
   B. angiography
   C. chest radiography
   D. nuclear medicine
3. Which of the following is the most common clinical indication for CT imaging of the spleen?
   A. trauma
   B. lymphoma
   C. metastasis
   D. localized pain in the abdomen
4. The modality of choice to demonstrate intrahepatic and extrahepatic bile ducts in jaundiced patients is:
   A. digital radiography.
   B. nuclear medicine.
   C. CT.
   D. diagnostic medical sonography.
5. The accuracy of needle placement in an examination is best determined with:
   A. quantitative CT imaging.
   B. CT angiography.
   C. CT fluoroscopy.
   D. CT screening.
6. Notable tasks performed by the CT technologist before the CT examination commences include all of the following *except:*
   A. communicate all aspects of the CT examination to be performed.
   B. explain the use of any oral contrast media or any contrast agent.
   C. explain appropriate respiration instructions during the scanning sequence.
   D. ensure that the CT manager and/or radiologist is always present in the room during scanning.
7. A useful tool that is used to tailor the CT examination to the clinical problem of the patient is the:
   A. scanogram.
   B. scanning protocol.
   C. radiation dose computed and displayed on the scanner console.
   D. reconstruction matrix that will be used.

8. Which of the following patient positions is commonplace during a CT examination of the abdomen?
   A. supine position
   B. prone position
   C. decubitis position
   D. any lateral position is acceptable
9. In general, the slice thickness that should be used for an effective examination of the wrist in CT is:
   A. 5 mm.
   B. 3 mm.
   C. 2.5 mm.
   D. 0.5 mm.
10. In an effort to enhance bony detail of the wrist or ankle during a CT examination, the following is (are) useful:
    A. high spatial frequency digital filter
    B. higher resolution algorithm compared to a standard algorithm
    C. coronal multiplanar reconstructions and/or 3D volume rendered images
    D. all are correct

## REFERENCES


Abrams, H. I., Siegelman, S. S., Adams, D. F., Sanders, R., Finberg, H. J., Hessel, S. J., et al. (1982). Computed tomography versus ultrasound of the adrenal gland: a prospective study. *Radiology, 143*, 121–128.

Alpern, M. B., Lawson, T. L., Foley, W. D., Perlman, S. J., Reif, L. J., Arevalos, E., et al. (1986). Focal hepatic masses and fatty infiltration detected by enhanced dynamic CT. *Radiology, 158*, 45–49.

Ambrosetti, P., Grossholz, M., Becker, C., Terrier, F., & Morel, P. (1997). Computed tomography in acute left colonic diverticulitis. *British Journal of Surgery, 84*, 532–534.

Balthazar, E. J. (1994). CT of small bowel obstruction. *American Journal of Roentgenology, 162*, 255–261.

Baron, R. L. (1994). Understanding and optimizing use of contrast material for CT of the liver. *American Journal of Roentgenology, 163*, 323–331.

Baron, R. L., Stanley, R. J., Lee, J. K., Koehler, R. E., Melson, G. L., Balfe, D. M., et al. (1982). A prospective comparison of the evaluation of biliary obstruction using computed tomography and ultrasonography. *Radiology, 145*, 91–98.

Berland, L. L., & Smith, J. K. (1998). Multidetector-array CT: once again, technology creates new opportunities. *Radiology, 209*, 327–329.

Berry, J., Jr., & Malt, R. A. (1984). Appendicitis near its centenary. *Annals of Surgery, 200*, 567–575.

Boyko, O. B., Cory, D. A., Cohen, M. D., Provisor, A., Mirkin, D., & Derosa, G. P. (1987). MR imaging of osteogenic and Ewing's sarcoma. *American Journal of Roentgenology, 148*, 317–322.

Callen, P. W. (1979). Computed tomographic evaluation of abdominal and pelvic abscesses. *Radiology, 131*, 171–175.

Castellino, R. A., Hoppe, R. T., Blank, N., Young, S. W., Neumann, C., Rosenberg, S. A., et al. (1984). Computed tomography, lymphography and staging laparotomy: correlations in initial staging of Hodgkin's disease. *American Journal of Roentgenology, 143*, 37–41.

Chen, M. Y., & Zagoria, R. J. (1999). Can noncontrast helical computed tomography replace intravenous urography for evaluation of patients with acute urinary tract colic? *Journal of Emergency Medicine, 17*, 299–303.

Costello, P., Anderson, W., & Blume, D. (1991). Pulmonary nodule: evaluation with spiral volumetric CT. *Radiology, 179*, 875–876.

Davies, J., Chalmers, A. G., Sue-Ling, H. M., May, J., Miller, G., Martin, I., et al. (1997). Spiral computed tomography and operative staging of gastric carcinoma: a comparison with histopathological staging. *Gut, 41*(3), 314–319.

Fenlon, H. M., Nunes, D. P., Schroy, P. C., Barish, M. A., Clarke, P. D., & Ferrucci, J. T. (1999). A comparison of virtual and conventional colonoscopy for the detection of colorectal polyps. *New England Journal of Medicine, 341*, 1496–1503.

Ferrucci, J. T., Jr., Wittenberg, J., Mueller, P. R., Simeone, J. F., Harbin, W. P., Kirkpatrick, R. H., et al. (1980). Diagnosis of abdominal malignancy by radiologic fine needle biopsy. *American Journal of Roentgenology, 134*, 323–330.

Fielding, J. R., Silverman, S. G., Samuel, S., Zou, K. H., & Loughlin, K. R. (1998). Unenhanced helical CT of ureteral stones: a replacement for excretory urography in planning treatment. *American Journal of Roentgenology, 171*, 1051–1053.

Foley, W. D. (1989). Dynamic hepatic CT. *Radiology, 170*, 617–622.

Fon, G. T., Bein, M. E., Mancuso, A. A., Keesey, J., Lupetin, A. R., & Wong, W. S. (1982). Computed tomography of the anterior mediastinum in myasthenia gravis. *Radiology, 142*, 135–141.

Forster, B. B., & Isserow, S. (2005). Coronary artery calcification and subclinical atherosclerosis: what's the score? *British Columbia Medical Association Journal, 47*, 181–187.

Freeny, P. C., & Marks, W. M. (1986). Hepatic hemangioma: dynamic bolus CT. *American Journal of Roentgenology, 147*, 711–719.

Gamsu, G. (1992). The mediastinum. In A. A. Moss, et al. (Ed.), *Computed tomography of the upper body with magnetic resonance imaging* (2nd ed.). Philadelphia, PA: WB Saunders.

Geisinger, M. A., Zelch, M. G., Bravo, E. L., Risius, B. F., O'Donovan, P. B., & Borkowski, G. P. (1983). Primary hyperaldosteronism: comparison of CT, adrenal venography, and venous sampling. *American Journal of Roentgenology, 141*, 299–302.

Gerzof, S. G., Spira, R., & Robbins, A. H. (1981). Percutaneous abscess drainage. *Seminars in Roentgenology, 16*, 62–71.

Goldman, I. S., Winkler, M. L., Raper, S. E., Barker, M. E., Keung, E., Goldberg, H. I., et al. (1985). Increased hepatic density and phospholipidosis due to amiodarone. *American Journal of Roentgenology, 144*, 541–546.

Gore, R. M., Balthazar, E. J., Ghahremani, G. G., & Miller, F. H. (1996). CT features of ulcerative colitis and Crohn's disease. *American Journal of Roentgenology, 167*, 3–15.

Guyer, B. H., Levinsohn, E. M., Fredrickson, B. E., Bailey, G. L., & Formikell, M. (1985). Computed tomography of calcaneal fractures: anatomy, pathology, dosimetry, and clinical relevance. *American Journal of Roentgenology, 145*, 911–919.

Halber, M. D., Daffner, R. H., Morgan, C. L., Trought, W. S., Thompson, W. M., Rice, R. P., et al. (1979). Intra-abdominal abscess: current concepts in radiologic evaluation. *American Journal of Roentgenology, 133*, 9–13.

Hara, A. K., Johnson, C. D., Reed, J. E., Ahlquist, D. A., Nelson, H., MacCarty, R. L., et al. (1997). Detection of colorectal polyps with CT colography: initial assessment of sensitivity and specificity. *Radiology, 205*, 59–65.

Hessel, S. J., Siegelman, S. S., McNeil, B. J., Sanders, R., Adams, D. F., Alderson, P. O., et al. (1982). A prospective evaluation of computed tomography and ultrasound of the pancreas. *Radiology, 143*, 129–133.

Hollett, M., Jorgensen, M. J., & Jeffrey, R. B., Jr. (1995). Quantitative evaluation of pancreatic enhancement during dual-phase helical CT. *Radiology, 195*, 359–361.

Hori, M., Murakami, T., Oi, H., Kim, T., Takahashi, S., Matsushita, M., et al. (1998). Sensitivity in detection of hypervascular hepatocellular carcinoma by helical CT with intra-arterial injection of contrast medium and by helical CT and MR imaging with intravenous injection of contrast medium. *Acta Radiology, 39*, 144–151.

Iakovou, I., Dangas, G., Mehran, R., Lansky, A. J., Ashby, D. T., Fahy, M., et al. (2003). Impact of gender on the incidence and outcome of contrast-induced nephropathy after percutaneous coronary intervention. *Journal of Invasive Cardiology, 15*, 18–22.

Johnson, C. D., Dunnick, N. R., Cohan, R. H., & Illescas, F. F. (1987). Renal adenocarcinoma: CT staging of 100 tumors. *American Journal of Roentgenology, 148*, 59–63.

Kopka, L., Fischer, U., Zoeller, G., Schmidt, C., Ringert, R. H., & Grabbe, E. (1997). Dual-phase helical CT of the kidney: value of the corticomedullary and nephrographic phase for evaluation of renal lesions and preoperative staging of renal cell carcinoma. *American Journal of Roentgenology, 169*, 1573–1578.

Lane, M. J., Katz, D. S., Ross, B. A., Clautice-Engle, T. L., Mindelzun, R. E., & Jeffrey, R. B., Jr. (1997). Unenhanced helical CT for suspected acute appendicitis. *American Journal of Roentgenology, 168*, 405–409.

Lange, T. A., & Alter, A. J. (1980). Evaluation of complex acetabular fractures by computed tomography. *Journal of Computer Assisted Tomography, 6*, 849–852.

Leschka, S., Alkadhi, H., Plass, A., Desbiolles, L., Grunefelder, J., & Marincek, B. (2005). Accuracy of MSCT coronary angiography with 64-slice technology: first experience. *European Heart Journal, 10*, 1093–1100.

Levine, E., & Grantham, J. J. (1985). High-density renal cysts in autosomal dominant polycystic kidney disease demonstrated by CT. *Radiology, 154*, 477–482.

Manfredi, R., Pirronti, T., Bonomo, L., & Marano, P. (1996). Accuracy of computed tomography and magnetic resonance imaging in staging bronchogenic carcinoma. *MAGMA, 4*, 257–262.

Mayo, J. R. (1991). The high-resolution computed tomography technique. *Seminars in Roentgenology, 26*, 104–109.

Mayo, J. R., Remy-Jardin, M., Muller, N. L., Remy, J., Worsley, D. F., Hossein-Foucher, C., et al. (1997). Pulmonary embolism: prospective comparison of spiral CT with ventilation-perfusion scintigraphy. *Radiology, 205*, 447–452.

Mayo-Smith, W. W., Boland, G. W., Noto, R. B., & Lee, M. J. (2001). State-of-the-art adrenal imaging. *Radiographics, 21*, 995–1012.

McCullough, P. A., Wolyn, R., Rocher, L. L., Levin, R. N., & O'Neill, W. W. (1997). Acute renal failure after coronary intervention: incidence, risk factors, and relationship to mortality. *American Journal of Medicine, 103*, 368–375.

McCullough, P. A., Adam, A., Becker, C. R., Davidson, C., Lameire, N., Stacul, F., et al. (2006). Risk prediction of contrast-induced nephropathy. *American Journal of Cardiology, 98*, 5K–13K.

Molina, P. L., et al. (1998). Computed tomography of thoracoabdominal trauma. In J. K. T. Lee, et al. (Ed.), *Computed body tomography with MRI correlation* (3rd ed.). New York: Raven Press.

Mucha, P., Jr. (1987). Small intestinal obstruction. *Surgical Clinics of North America, 67*, 597–620.

Muhm, J. R., Brown, L. R., Crowe, J. K., Sheedy, P. F., 2nd, Hattery, R. R., & Stephens, D. H. (1978). Comparison of whole lung tomography and computed tomography for detecting pulmonary nodules. *American Journal of Roentgenology, 131*, 981–984.

Muller, N. L. (1991). Differential diagnosis of chronic diffuse infiltrative lung disease on high-resolution computed tomography. *Seminars in Roentgenology, 26*, 132–142.

Munk, P. L., Muller, N. L., Miller, R. R., & Ostrow, D. N. (1988). Pulmonary lymphangitic carcinomatosis: CT and pathologic findings. *Radiology, 166*, 705–709.

Nelson, R. C. (1991). Techniques for computed tomography of the liver. *Radiologic Clinics of North America, 29*, 1199–1212.

Novelline, R. A., Rhea, J. T., & Bell, T. (1999). Helical CT of abdominal trauma. *Radiologic Clinics of North America, 37*, 591–612.

Pang, J. A., Hamilton-Wood, C., & Metreweli, C. (1989). Value of computed tomography in the diagnosis and management of bronchiectasis. *Clinical Radiology, 40*, 40–44.

Petasnick, J. P., Turner, D. A., Charters, J. R., Gitelis, S., & Zacharias, C. E. (1986). Soft tissue masses of the locomotor system: comparison of MR imaging with CT. *Radiology, 160,* 125–133.

Pickhardt, P. J., Choi, J. R., Hwang, I., Butler, J. A., Puckett, M. L., Hildebrandt, M. D., et al. (2003). Computed tomographic virtual colonoscopy to screen for colorectal neoplasia in asymptomatic adults. *New England Journal of Medicine, 349,* 2191–2200.

Pollack, H. M., Arger, P. H., Banner, M. P., Mulhern, C. B., & Coleman, B. G. (1981). Computed tomography of renal pelvic filling defects. *Radiology, 138,* 645–651.

Posniak, H. V., Demos, T. C., & Marsan, R. E. (1989). Computed tomography of the normal aorta and thoracic aneurysms. *Seminars in Roentgenology, 24,* 7–21.

Prince, M. R., Narasimham, D. L., Stanley, J. C., Chenevert, T. L., Williams, D. M., Marx, M. V., et al. (1995). Breath-hold gadolinium-enhanced MR angiography of the abdominal aorta and its major branches. *Radiology, 197,* 785–792.

Raff, G. L., Gallagher, M. J., O'Neill, W. W., & Goldstein, J. A. (2005). Diagnostic accuracy of noninvasive coronary angiography using 64-slice spiral computed tomography. *Journal of the American College of Cardiology, 46,* 552–557.

Rhea, J. T. (2004). CT of abdominal trauma: part 1. In *RSNA categorical course in diagnostic radiology: emergency radiology* (pp. 91–99). Oak Brook, IL: Radiological Society of North America.

Rossi, P., Baert, A., Passariello, R., Simonetti, G., Pavone, P., & Tempesta, P. (1985). CT of functioning tumours of the pancreas. *American Journal of Roentgenology, 144,* 57–60.

Schaner, E. G., Chang, A. E., Doppman, J. L., Conkle, D. M., Flye, M. W., & Rosenberg, S. A. (1978). Comparison of computed and conventional whole lung tomography in detecting pulmonary nodules: prospective radiologic-pathologic study. *American Journal of Roentgenology, 131,* 51–54.

Schreiman, J. S., Crass, J. R., Wick, M. R., Malle, C. W., & Thompson, R. C., Jr. (1986). Osteosarcoma: role of CT in limb sparing treatment. *Radiology, 161,* 485–488.

Shanmuganathan, K. (2004). CT of abdominal trauma: part II. In *RSNA categorical course in diagnostic radiology: emergency radiology* (pp. 102–112). Oak Brook, IL: Radiological Society of North America.

Shuman, W. P. (1997). CT of blunt abdominal trauma in adults. *Radiology, 205,* 297–306 1997.

Siegel, C. L., & Cohan, R. H. (1994). CT of abdominal aortic aneurysms. *American Journal of Roentgenology, 163,* 17–29.

Siegelman, S. S., Copeland, B. E., Saba, G. P., Cameron, J. L., Sanders, R. C., & Zerhouni, E. A. (1980). CT of fluid collections associated with pancreatitis. *American Journal of Roentgenology, 134,* 1121–1132.

Smith, R. C., Rosenfield, A. T., Choe, K. A., Essenmacher, K. R., Verga, M., Glickman, M. G., et al. (1995). Acute flank pain: comparison of noncontrast-enhanced CT and intravenous urography. *Radiology, 194,* 789–794.

Smith, R. C., Verga, M., Dalrymple, N., McCarthy, S., & Rosenfield, A. T. (1996). Acute ureteral obstruction: value of secondary signs on helical unenhanced CT. *American Journal of Roentgenology, 167,* 1109–1113.

Sommer, T., Fehske, W., Holzknecht, N., Smekal, A. V., Keller, E., Lutterbey, G., et al. (1996). Aortic dissection: a comparative study of diagnosis with spiral CT, multiplanar transesophageal echocardiography, and MR imaging. *Radiology, 199,* 347–352.

Stein, P. D., Henry, J. W., & Relyea, B. (1995). Untreated patients with pulmonary embolism. *Chest, 107,* 931–935.

Sundaram, M., Wolverson, M. K., Heiberg, E., Pilla, T., Vas, W. G., & Shields, J. B. (1982). Utility of CT-guided abdominal aspiration procedures. *American Journal of Roentgenology, 139,* 1111–1115.

Swensen, S. J., Brown, L. R., Colby, T. V., Weavher, A. L., & Midthun, D. E. (1996). Lung nodule enhancement at CT: prospective findings. *Radiology, 201,* 447–455.

Swensen, S. J., Jett, J. R., Sloan, J. A., Midthun, D. E., Hartman, T. E., Sykes, A., et al. (2002). Screening for lung cancer with low-dose spiral computed tomography. *American Journal of Respiratory and Critical Care Medicine, 165,* 508–513.

Tateishi, U., Gladish, G. W., Kusumoto, M., Hasegawa, T., Yokoyama, R., Tsuchiya, R., et al. (2003). Chest wall tumors: radiologic findings and pathologic correlation, 2: malignant tumors. *Radiographics, 23,* 1491–1508.

Totty, W. G., McClennan, B. L., Melson, G. L., & Patel, R. (1981). Relative value of computed tomography and ultrasonography in the assessment of renal angiomyolipoma. *Journal of Computer Assisted Tomography, 5,* 173–178.

Weg, N., Scheer, M. R., & Gabor, M. P. (1998). Liver lesions: improved detection with dual-detector-array CT and routine 2.5-mm thin collimation. *Radiology, 209,* 417–426.

Zerhouni, E. A., Stitik, F. P., Siegelman, S. S., Naidich, D. P., Sagel, S. S., Proto, A. V., et al. (1986). CT of the pulmonary nodule: a cooperative study. *Radiology, 160,* 319–327.


## Further Reading

For further exploration of CT of the body, the following should be of interest to readers as an update beyond some of the references listed above.


*An Atlas of CT anatomy of the thorax, abdomen, pelvis and appendicular skeleton (shoulder and arm, elbow and forearm, wrist, hand, and fingers, hip and thigh, knee and leg, and ankle and foot).* (2015). <http://w-radiology.com/chest_ct.php> Accessed January 2015.

Carberry, G. A., Pooler, B. D., Binkley, N., et al. (2013). Unreported vertebral body compression fractures at abdominal multidetector CT. *Radiology, 68*(1), 120–126.

Chen, M. Y., Shanbhag, S. M. M., & Arai, A. E. (2013). Submillisievert median radiation dose for coronary angiography with a second-generation 320-detector row CT scanner in 107 consecutive patients. *Radiology, 267*(1), 76–85.

Dewey, M. (2011). Coronary CT versus MR angiography: pro CT—the role of CT angiography. *Radiology, 258*(2), 329–339.

Fuentes-Orrego, J. M., Pinho, D., Kulkami, N. M., et al. (2014). New and evolving concepts in CT for abdominal vascular imaging. *Radiographics, 34*, 1363–1384.

Gayer, G., Petrovitch, I., & Jeffrey, R. B. (2011). Foreign objects encountered in the abdominal cavity at CT. *Radiographics, 31*, 409–428.

Goshima, S., Kanematus, M., Nishibori, H., et al. (2011). CT of the pancreas: comparison of anatomic structure depiction, image quality, and radiation exposure between 320-detector volumetric images and 64 detector helical images. *Radiology, 260*(1), 139–147.

Holly, B. P., & Steeburg, S. D. (2011). Multidetector CT of blunt traumatic venous injuries in the chest, abdomen, and pelvis. *Radiographics, 31*, 1415–1424.

Jude, C. M., Nayak, N. B., Patel, M. K., Deshmukh, M., & Batra, P. (2014). Pulmonary coccidioidomycosis: pictorial review of chest radiographic and CT findings. *Radiographics, 34*, 912–925.

Lamba, R., Tanner, D. T., Sekhon, S., et al. (2014). Multidetector CT of vascular compression syndromes in the abdomen and pelvis. *Radiographics, 34*, 93–115.

Meyer, C. A., Vagal, A. S., & Seaman, D. (2011). Put your back into it: pathologic conditions of the spine at chest CT. *Radiographics, 31*, 1425–1441.

# 17

# Pediatric Computed Tomography

*Son Nguyen, Scott Lipson*

## OUTLINE



## LEARNING OBJECTIVES

On completion of this chapter, you should be able to:

1. state two basic tenets and other considerations necessary for an effective pediatric CT examination.
2. state the advantages of multidetector CT (MDCT) compared to single-slice spiral CT (SSCT).
3. identify new applications in pediatric CT imaging made possible with MDCT scanners.
4. describe the major tasks of the CT technologist in performing a CT examination on a pediatric patient with respect to:
   - patient management
   - neonatal patients
   - sedation
   - immobilization
   - use of intravenous contrast media
   - radiation protection
   - scan planning and preparation
   - scan parameters.
5. state the advantages of pediatric CT imaging of the brain, face, neck and spine compared with magnetic resonance imaging (MRI).
6. explain critical elements of positioning the pediatic patient for a CT examination.
7. outline the necessary technical aspects of a pediatric CT examination.
8. describe the importance of using protocols in pediatric CT.
9. outline each of the following elements of pediatric CT imaging of the chest and abdomen; musculoskeletal examinations; and CT angiography:
   - indications
   - patient positioning
   - technical considerations
   - scanning protocols.

## KEY TERMS TO WATCH FOR AND REMEMBER

The following key terms/concepts are important to your understanding of this chapter

**immobilization**
**multidetector CT (MDCT)**
**neonatal patient**
**osseous tumors**
**pediatric patient**
**radiation protection**
**scan parameters**
**sedation**

The objective of the pediatric **computed tomography (CT)** examination is to acquire optimum diagnostic images with minimum discomfort and radiation **exposure** to the patient. To this end, two basic tenets apply: (1) the technologist should be knowledgeable and well prepared and (2) the technologist should be honest and upfront with the patient and family. A well-prepared technologist plays an important role in avoiding delays and helps reduce the time the patient must be on the table of the CT scanner.

The CT technologist taking care of children should be honest in terms of the exact details of the CT examination. This helps ensure the cooperation of young patients and their parents during the procedure. The results can be successful, especially when the patient and parents are well informed. In most institutions, parents are encouraged to remain in the CT room during the examination.

In addition, a relaxed, nonthreatening environment helps gain the confidence and cooperation of the **pediatric patient.** Toys, books, and puzzles are a welcome diversion for the child who is waiting for a CT examination. In the CT room, interesting posters (Fig. 17-1) or pictures hung on the walls or ceiling help provide a friendly atmosphere. Young children are encouraged to bring a favorite blanket or cuddly toy with them for reassurance.

Fortunately, the current **generation** of **multidetector CT (MDCT)** scanners has made the CT examination much shorter and better tolerated by children. A trained CT technologist enlisting the cooperation of the parents is now able to scan the majority of children quickly, painlessly, and without sedating them.

## MULTIDETECTOR CT

### Differences Versus Single-Detector CT

MDCT is fundamentally different from single-slice spiral CT (SSCT). With SSCT a single row of detectors is present. The **x-ray** tube rotates around the patient, and a single image is produced for every rotation. The **slice thickness** of the image is determined by beam **collimation** in the "z" direction. An MDCT scanner,

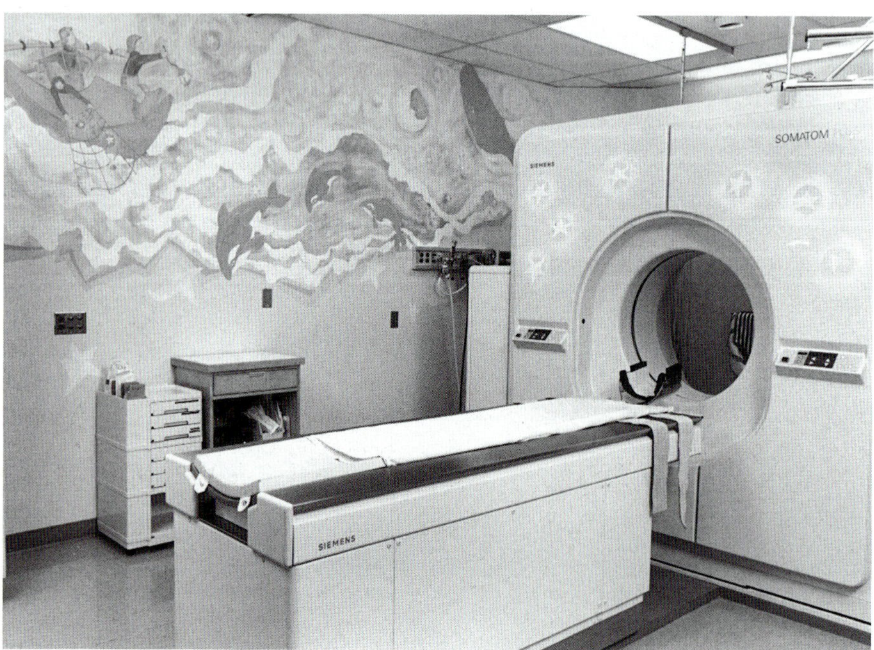


**FIGURE 17-1** An interesting wall mural helps provide a friendly environment.

however, contains multiple rows of detector elements and can therefore generate multiple images from each rotation of the x-ray tube. Current CT scanners can yield up to 320 images per rotation. Image slice thickness is determined not by beam collimation alone but also by the number and size of the detector elements included in the "z" direction and the number of channels into which the system divides the signals collected during the scan acquisition.

The size, number, and arrangement of detector elements are different for each scanner. Some scanners have detector elements that are uniform size throughout the entire detector, whereas other scanners may contain central elements that are smaller and more peripheral elements that are larger. Detector elements may be combined to produce thicker slices and more coverage or used individually for higher resolution images. The number of data channels present in the scanner determines the maximum number of images that can be produced per rotation. Each channel can use information from a single row or multiple detector rows. The scanner is named by the number of data channels present (e.g., a 16-slice scanner has 16 data channels capable of producing up to 16 images per **gantry** rotation). This scanner may have more than 16 rows of detector elements, however, because more than one row may be combined into a single channel.

### Advantages of Multidetector CT in Pediatric Imaging

Advantages of MDCT are substantial for pediatric imaging. Faster scanners allow for substantially more rapid acquisition of data, producing better patient tolerance, reduced motion artifacts, and more efficient use of **contrast media.** This is particularly important in pediatric imaging, where motion is a constant issue and scan time is of the essence. In addition, there is substantial improvement in **spatial resolution.** These qualities make MDCT especially useful in multiplanar and volume reconstructions and have opened up a plethora of new applications. Volumetric data acquisitions with very thin slices produce datasets that can be reconstructed in any plane with virtually no loss in image quality. This makes patient positioning for examinations easier and eliminates the need to obtain direct coronal images for examinations such as sinuses, temporal bone, and extremities. This helps to keep the radiation dose lower in children.

One inherent disadvantage with MDCT **scanning** is that the radiation dose may be increased when submillimeter slices are acquired. These thin slices will increase the effects of dose buildup of the radiation penumbra (the radiation penumbra is that portion of the radiation from a point source that falls outside the detector opening and therefore contributes to patient radiation dose but does not contribute to image formation). The thinner the slices, the more the penumbra effect can increase dose. This effect is dependent on the number of slices acquired per rotation and can be significant with 4-slice scanners but is small with 16-slice scanners and negligible in 32-64-slice and higher configuration scanners.

### New Pediatric Applications Possible with Multidetector CT

Many new applications and techniques for pediatric imaging are now possible with MDCT because of the ability to acquire thinner images in a shorter duration. These include 3D volume- and surface-rendering techniques, allowing the radiologist to look at 3D relationships of anatomical structures, airway reconstructions, virtual bronchoscopy, and colonoscopy. **CT angiography** (CTA) by use of MDCT has blossomed, with detail never before possible. CTA has virtually replaced conventional angiography in many areas, including evaluation of the aorta and pulmonary arteries. CTA is useful in pediatric imaging, especially to delineate aortic arch anomalies, cardiac anomalies (before and after surgery), and aberrant vasculature, such as in cases of pulmonary sequestration or vascular malformations. Cerebrovascular evaluation for aneurysms and vascular malformations is also helpful. Because of the speed of MDCT, it is frequently possible to obtain images with reduced intravenous contrast volumes compared with older scanners. CTA offers many advantages compared with catheter angiography. It is noninvasive and safer, and the radiation dose is lower. CTA also allows evaluation of structures adjacent to and outside of the vasculature.

Another major growth area is orthopedic imaging. Characterization of fractures and congenital abnormalities of the skeletal system is greatly improved with advanced visualization techniques. MDCT allows for a single volumetric dataset to be produced and reconstructed in any plane or **projection.** It is no longer necessary to scan patients in more than one plane. Current-generation scanners generate much less **artifact** in patients with metal **hardware** in place and are useful for evaluating patients who have undergone surgery with internal fixation devices.

## ROLE OF THE CT TECHNOLOGIST

### Patient Management

Pediatric patients need constant attention and monitoring. The technologist should work to ensure that the scanner is ready when the patient arrives and needed information such as clinical history and scan protocol has been determined. This will minimize delays and distractions that can interfere with the technologist's duty to care for the patient (Box 17-1).

The parents are usually an important ally of the technologist and should be included in the process whenever possible. One parent can be given a lead apron and remain in the room with the child during the entire procedure. This frequently helps reduce anxiety of both the child and the parent. If no parent is available, other ancillary staff such as nurses or assistants may be able to fill this role and comfort the child. The principal duty of the technologist, however, is to ensure that the scan is done safely, quickly, and accurately.

## Neonatal Patients

To minimize the risk of infection to the **neonatal patient,** CT personnel who handle the infant should remove rings and watches, wash hands thoroughly with antibacterial soap, and always wear a cover gown. During the scanning procedure, it is important to maintain the infant's body temperature. This can be achieved by increasing the temperature in the CT scanning room before the arrival of the patient, wrapping the infant in a warm blanket, and covering the infant's head with a cap or small towel to prevent rapid heat loss. Equally important is placing a heating blanket under the infant positioned on the scanning table or focusing a heat lamp on the patient with special attention to the correct **distance** of the lamp from the patient. Finally, a nurse who accompanies the patient to the radiology department should monitor the patient's vital signs and body temperature throughout the CT examination.

### BOX 17-1 Procedure Preparation

1. Have the patient's radiographic file available for consultation.
2. Review the order to make sure it is appropriate and that adequate clinical information is available. If there are any questions, contact the radiologist or ordering physician.
3. Obtain a protocol for the examination from the radiologist.
4. Register pertinent patient data into the CT system and select the appropriate parameters under which the CT examination is to be conducted.
5. Prepare the scanning room and have all necessary accessory equipment (e.g., immobilization devices, monitoring equipment) available for the procedure.
6. Prepare the necessary intravenous contrast media, if required.

## Sedation

The use of **sedation** is inevitable in pediatric CT scanning. Image degradation from patient motion remains a problem. The introduction of MDCT has been a tremendous advance in pediatric imaging. Most scans can be completed in less than 30 seconds, and with current 16- to 64-slice and higher scanners, scan times as short as 5 to 10 seconds can be routinely achieved while the highest image quality is maintained. This substantially decreases the need for sedation.

With MDCT sedation is rarely required for routine head and sinus studies, where some motion is tolerable. Sedation may still be required for studies requiring advanced multiplanar and volume reconstructions because motion artifact can significantly reduce the quality of these types of studies. Common examples would include studies of the temporal bone and CTA.

Sedation protocols and standards should be cooperatively established by the departments of radiology and anesthesiology to ensure high-quality care for the sedated patient. Any syndrome or condition with a respiratory risk that contraindicates sedation is recorded and brought to the attention of the radiologist. The decision to sedate a child should be a cooperative effort of the radiologist, the nurse, and a parent. Factors affecting the decision to sedate are summarized in Box 17-2.

**Preparation** for sedation typically requires patients to ingest nothing by mouth 4 to 6 hours for solid foods, 2 to 4 hours for formula or breast milk, and 2 hours for clear liquids before the examination. CT department personnel should inform parents of

### BOX 17-2 Sedation Assessment

1. Consider the complexity of the CT study planned. (Is intravenous contrast required? Will 3D or multiplanar imaging be needed?)
2. Explain the examination to the parents and child.
3. Consider the parents' opinion of the child's ability to cooperate.
4. Evaluate whether babies seem ready to sleep on their own. With older children, a visit to the scan room to observe another child being scanned may be helpful.
5. Observe the child in the scan room. A dry run is often useful to gauge whether the child will be able to cooperate.

the correct preparation and sedation instructions at the time the examination is scheduled to help minimize any misunderstanding on the day of the examination. Any child who potentially may need sedation should be given preparation instructions for this at the time of scheduling. When the patient arrives in the radiology department, the CT technologist or the radiology nurse performs a careful assessment of the child's ability to undergo the CT examination without sedation.

Children less than 6 months of age rarely require sedation. Wrapping them in a warm blanket and providing them with a pacifier and use of a table restraint system to immobilize them can be all that is needed for a successful scan. Sleep deprivation is another technique that can be used with infants. With faster scanners, good patient communication, and the proper use of restraints, the need for sedation can be minimized.

For older infants and toddlers requiring sedation, oral or rectal chloral hydrate is the most commonly used drug. The typical starting dose is 50 to 75 milligrams (mg) per kilogram (kg) to a maximum dose of 100 mg/kg. This is generally effective and can be routinely administered by a radiology nurse under the direction of a radiologist.

Children older than toddler age can usually be talked through a CT study with the help of a parent. When this does not work, oral or intravenous (IV) midazolam (Versed) with or without morphine may be used for conscious sedation. Some children and toddlers may not adequately respond to these drugs and will require deep sedation with drugs such as IV pentobarbital sodium (Nembutal). This group may also include children with delayed development, sleep apnea, or chronic respiratory problems. Pentobarbital is generally administered by specially trained personnel such as a dedicated pediatric sedation team or anesthesiologists.

All sedation patients require continuous monitoring by nursing staff including pulse oximetry, blood pressure, and respiratory rate. Paradoxical hyperactivity and agitation is a side effect of chloral hydrate and also has been reported with pentobarbital sodium. When this does occur, it is necessary to keep the child safely under observation until the effect passes.

Resuscitative supplies are kept in the CT scan room at all times. When the study is completed, the sedated child is moved to the recovery room for monitoring. Patients are discharged when they are easily aroused, have enough muscle tone to hold up their heads, and can drink clear fluids. The parents are given an information sheet about care of the sedated child, which includes a telephone number to call if they have any concerns after their return home.

## Immobilization

**Immobilization** of the child is essential to ensure patient safety and to provide images free of motion artifacts. For patients less than 5 years old, the immobilizer (Fig. 17-2) is a comfortable device that secures the patient's arms beside the head during body examinations. This device is secured to the patient scanning table with adhesive straps after the patient has been positioned.

Larger children are generally immobilized by other methods, such as adhesive straps placed under the mattress and over the patient. After the patient has been immobilized, the CT technologist should still carefully monitor the child by closed-circuit television or direct visualization.

Using some type or method of immobilization is important in nearly every case. Sedated children should be gently immobilized with soft straps or paper tape. Cooperative older children should also have immobilization to help remind them not to move.

## Use of Intravenous Contrast Media

The routine use of nonionic contrast media almost eliminates minor reactions such as pain, nausea, vomiting, and urticaria. This is especially important in pediatric CT, and the use of nonionic contrast media is therefore recommended in those examinations requiring contrast media. The removal of these potential reactions and discomforts helps ensure the cooperation of the patient and provides a safer examination for the sedated child. Fortunately, severe allergic reactions to contrast media are rare in children. Informed consent should be obtained before IV contrast injection.

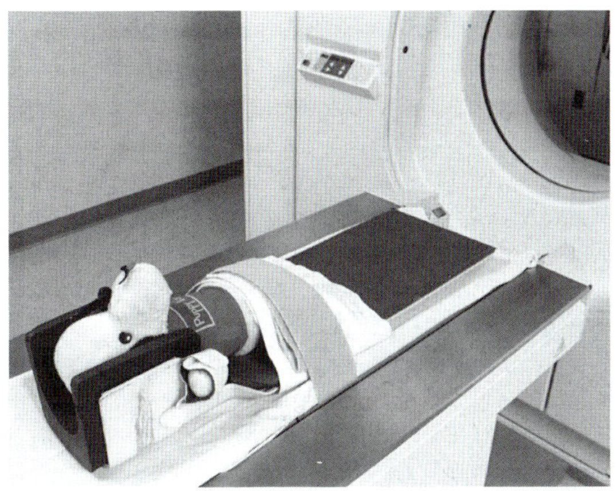

**FIGURE 17-2** A patient immobilizer is a comfortable device to secure the pediatric patient.

The dose of contrast material (which can vary with each manufacturer) for children is 2 to 3 milliliters (ml)/kg to a maximum of 150 ml. Power injectors are now commonly used because they provide a constant rate of injection that allows more accurate timing of the bolus and better organ enhancement. The deciding factor for use of a power injector depends on the IV site and size. Only peripheral IV sites can be obtained on most children. The injection rate is determined by the size of the IV catheter; injection rates of 2 to 3 ml/s can be used with 22-gauge catheters, whereas a 24-gauge catheter can be injected at 1 to 2 ml/s. Butterfly-type needles and percutaneous indwelling central venous catheter lines are almost always hand injected rather than by use of power injectors.

Scan timing is very important for contrast-enhanced imaging, particularly of the neck, chest, and body. Unlike in adult patients where routine scan delays are effective in most people, scan delay in children must be individualized depending on the size of the child, the site of the IV, the injection rate, and the duration of the scan. If a power injector is used, standard delays can be used in most patients. For neck and chest examinations, delays of 35 to 45 seconds are effective. For studies of the abdomen and pelvis, longer delays of 50 to 70 seconds are used. Infants generally require shorter delays because the volume of contrast injected is so small. When hand injection is used, the scan should start when the injection is almost complete. Timing for contrast-enhanced studies of the brain is less critical. These scans are usually begun after all of the contrast has been given.

Another option to determine scan delay to produce optimal vascular enhancement is available on most MDCT scanners (e.g., Toshiba's SureStart, General Electric's SmartPrep, Phillips's Dose-Right). This **software** uses bolus tracking to trigger the start of the scan. The operator places a **region of interest (ROI)** on a vessel or organ at the start of the study. Contrast injection is begun and serial low-dose scans are performed in the same location. The enhancement curve is tracked in real time. The scan can be triggered automatically when the Hounsfield units (HU) reach a predetermined threshold or manually by the technologist on the basis of the visual appearance of the vessel. In children manual triggering is usually preferred because the small size of the vessels may make automatic triggering unreliable if the child moves at all. Bolus tracking is the preferred method to initiate the scan for CT angiography, but it can also be useful for scans of the neck, chest, and abdomen. One disadvantage of this technique is increased radiation dose to the region where the monitoring scan is performed.

Regardless of the injection type, it is important to monitor the IV site during injection. If manual injection is used, filling the contrast medium into smaller syringes facilitates safer injection compared with the use of a large syringe.

## Radiation Protection

Growing cells are the most sensitive to radiation. For any particular milliamperage (mA), pediatric organ doses are higher compared with those of an adult. Because of these factors, and the cumulative effect over a lifetime of exposure, radiation exposure has a potentially higher risk for the pediatric patient than for the adult patient. It has been shown that even small radiation doses carry the same relative risk of cancer mortality as low-dose exposure for atomic bomb survivors. These radiation doses are in the range typically seen with CT scans with adult **scan parameters** not adjusted for children. Therefore, **radiation protection** is an integral part of the pediatric CT examination. The ALARA principle should be followed, in that radiation dose should be kept *as low as can be reasonably achievable.*

This issue has generated substantial interest in both the popular press and the radiology literature. It is the responsibility of every person involved with imaging pediatric patients to make sure that diagnostic scans are obtained with the minimum radiation dose. This goal requires a comprehensive approach that addresses all aspects of the CT examination from ordering procedures to examination planning to specific examination parameters chosen by the technologist at the CT console.

### Scan Planning and Preparation

Controlling radiation exposure begins with a careful review of all orders to ensure that the study is indicated and appropriate. Some requests may need to be redirected to ultrasonography or **magnetic resonance imaging (MRI),** depending on the indication. Additional clinical information from the ordering physician may be needed to ensure that the proper study is performed the first time.

Once it is determined the examination is necessary, the proper protocol must be chosen. Coverage should be limited to the area of interest. Multiphase scans should be minimized in children. Scans both with and without contrast should not be performed routinely. Pediatric-specific examination protocols should be created and used. Lead **shielding** should be routinely used to cover body parts that are outside the ROI. Particular attention should be made to avoid scanning sensitive areas such as the breasts, genitalia, and lenses whenever possible.

### Scan Parameters

Particular attention must be paid to many different scan parameters to minimize dose. Factors such as tube current (mA) and peak kilovoltage (kVp) have an obvious effect on radiation dose, but many other variables used in spiral/MDCT such as **pitch,** slice thickness, and rotation time can also significantly affect dose.

Increasing pitch is an effective way to decrease dose. A pitch of 1.5 can lower the dose by about 25% compared with a pitch of 1, whereas a pitch of 2 can reduce the exposure by approximately 50%. Shorter rotation times will also decrease dose. A rotation time of 0.5 seconds gives half the dose of a 1-second rotation time if all other parameters are constant. With MDCT scanners, very thin slice thickness (less than 1 millimeter [mm]) can result in increased dose secondary to overlapping of the radiation penumbra. This effect can be significant with 4-slice scanners but is minor in scanners with 16 or more slices. Care should be used when acquiring submillimeter scans on a 4-slice machine.

Slice thickness may be a consideration in pediatric patients. One inherent disadvantage with MDCT scanning is that the radiation dose may be increased when submillimeter slices are acquired. These thin slices will increase the effects of dose buildup of the radiation penumbra. The thinner the slices, the more the penumbra effect can increase dose. This effect is dependent on the number of slices acquired per rotation and can be significant with 4-slice scanners but is small with 16-slice scanners and negligible in 32- and 64-slice and higher configuration scanners. In fact, 64-slice scanners can produce images of superior quality compared with scanners with fewer detectors with the same radiation dose (same scan parameters). Facilities using 4-slice scanners should use submillimeter slices with caution in children.

Modification of dose parameters is the most straightforward and important method to reduce dose. There are two primary methods to optimize CT dose parameters. The first way is for the CT technologist to individually tailor the dose parameters for each patient on the basis of the patient's weight and the body part being imaged (Table 17-1). Alternatively, multiple different protocols can be created in the scanner for each type of examination on the basis of the patient's size/weight with appropriate kVp/mA parameters built into each protocol. Although this approach can be effective if the protocols are built and followed correctly, it is somewhat cumbersome and is easily subject to error if the technologist chooses the wrong protocol.

Recognizing the limitations of the previous methods, CT manufacturers have focused much attention on methods to control, monitor, and reduce the radiation dose from CT examinations. As a result, most MDCT scanners now have some form of automatic exposure control available. There are different techniques used by the CT manufacturers, but the basic principles are similar. The most common approach relies on **attenuation** measurements derived from the actual patient obtained during scout image acquisition to create a radiation dose profile for the examination that is individually tailored to that patient. The dose will actually vary during the examination depending on the attenuation of the body. For example, in a chest study the radiation dose will be much higher through the shoulders and much lower through the lungs. The most sophisticated systems now allow the operator to select appropriate image quality on the basis of preset **noise** levels (determined by the radiologist), and the scanner would then apply the appropriate tube current regardless of patient size. This relieves the operator of the need to vary conditions on the basis of patient size or weight.

**TABLE 17-1 Recommended Dose Parameters for Pediatric Multidetector Computed Tomography**

| | DOSE PARAMETERS | | | |
|---|---|---|---|---|
| Weight (kg) | kV | mAs Chest | mAs Abdomen | mAs Head (120 kV) |
| <15 | 80 | 20 | 30 | 100 |
| 15-24 | 80-100 | 30 | 40 | 120 |
| 25-34 | 80-100 | 40 | 60 | 140 |
| 35-44 | 100 | 50 | 80 | 160 |
| 45-54 | 100-120 | 60 | 100 | 180 |
| >55 | 120 | 60+ | 100+ | 200+ |

kV, kilovolts.

**BOX 17-3 Steps to Minimize Radiation Exposure**

1. Review all orders for appropriateness and clinical need.
2. Obtain a pediatric-specific protocol from the radiologist.
   a. Multiphase scanning should be minimized.
   b. Judicious use of very thin slices when a 4-row MDCT is used
3. Shield sensitive areas whenever possible.
4. Select appropriate scan parameters on the basis of patient size and weight or use automatic exposure control methods when available.
   a. Refer to pediatric dose charts for mA and kilovolt values.
   b. Adjust pitch and scan time to minimize dose when appropriate.
5. Maintain a QC program to ensure that the scanner is functioning properly and that the protocols that have been set up are being followed correctly.

Finally, it is important to have a quality assurance program to consistently monitor the entire process to ensure that protocols are up to date, scan techniques are optimized, technologists understand and follow the protocols, and the CT scanner is properly maintained and tested with phantoms. Steps used to minimize radiation dose in children are summarized in Box 17-3.

## CT OF THE HEAD, NECK, AND SPINE

Imaging of the head and spine in children depends on a number of factors, including the age of the child, medical condition, ability to cooperate, and above all the indication for the examination. These factors will determine which modality is best suited to the overall assessment of the patient's medical problem. The majority of neuroimaging examinations in children are performed with CT or MRI. The main exception to this is the neonate, in whom ultrasonography is the dominant imaging technique. Plain films have a small role, usually for the spine. Indications for diagnostic pediatric neuroangiography are limited and have been replaced by magnetic resonance angiography (MRA) and CTA. Catheter angiography is primarily a therapeutic tool used to treat children with aneurysms and vascular malformations.

### Indications

With some exceptions, most indications for examination of the central nervous system (CNS) are best studied by MRI. MRI retains several advantages over CT for neuroimaging; it uses no ionizing radiation and has inherently better soft tissue contrast that can be used to characterize normal anatomy and pathology of the CNS. CT has several advantages over MRI, which are primarily speed of acquisition and accessibility. CT is also superior to identify acute hemorrhage and calcifications and to characterize abnormalities of the bone.

#### CT of the Brain

Primary indications for CT over MRI include assessment of trauma in the acute phase (Fig. 17-3), detection of acute hemorrhage, and the detection of calcification such as in cases of prenatal TORCH (toxoplasmosis, other [congenital syphilis and viruses], rubella, cytomegalovirus, and herpes simplex virus) infections or postnatal infection such as cysticercosis. CT is also recommended for skull lesions and fractures (Fig. 17-3).

Either CT or MRI can adequately evaluate many other indications for brain imaging. In these instances CT is often preferred because it is quicker and easier to obtain and often can be done without sedation. Common indications include evaluation of hydrocephalus and shunt malfunction, **screening** evaluation for children with headaches or abnormal head size, and evaluation and follow-up of children with congenital abnormalities such as Chiari malformations or Dandy-Walker syndrome.

MRI is the preferred modality for evaluation of many other indications such as seizures, known or suspected brain tumors, acute and chronic ischemia, most CNS infections and inflammatory diseases, vascular malformations, congenital syndromes such as neurofibromatosis and tuberous sclerosis, diseases of white matter and demyelination such as acute disseminated encephalomyelitis, and evaluation of the pituitary gland. Although MRI may be the study of choice in most instances, CT is frequently performed in these patients either in the acute setting when the child is in the emergency department or for follow-up after the initial evaluation and treatment. CT can also serve as the primary evaluation modality when MRI is not available.

#### CT of the Face and Neck

Primary indications for CT include assessment of facial and orbital trauma, evaluation of osseous abnormalities of the maxilla or mandible, assessment of the temporal bone and middle ear in children with infection or hearing loss, evaluation of the sinuses for sinusitis, and evaluation of the airway. Either CT or MRI may be performed to evaluate the face and neck to characterize masses, enlarged

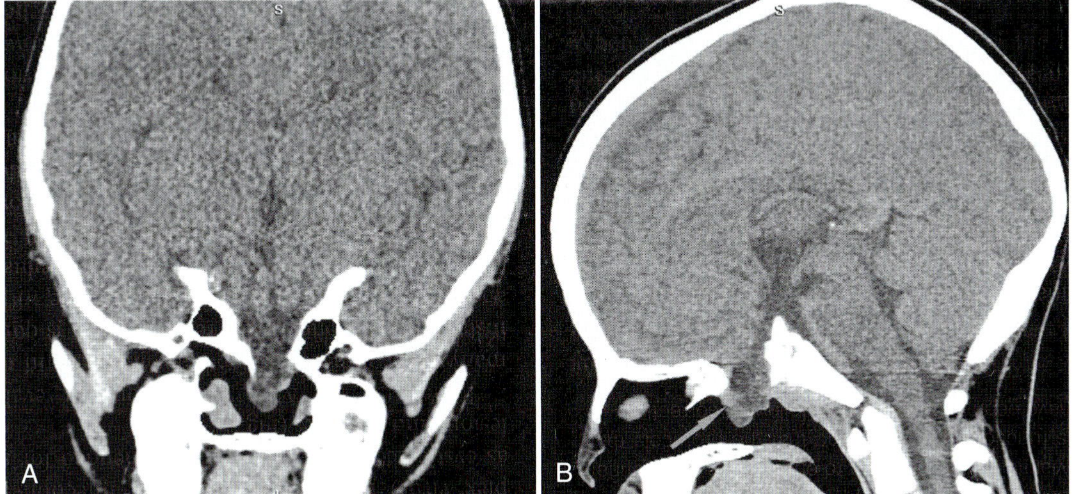


**FIGURE 17-3** Sphenoidal encephalocele. High-resolution 0.5-mm coronal **(A)** and sagittal **(B)** images in soft tissue window. There is a left parasagittal defect in the sphenoid bone with herniation of meninges and cerebrospinal fluid into the sphenoid sinus. The pituitary tissue is shown at the bottom of the encephalocele (*arrow*).

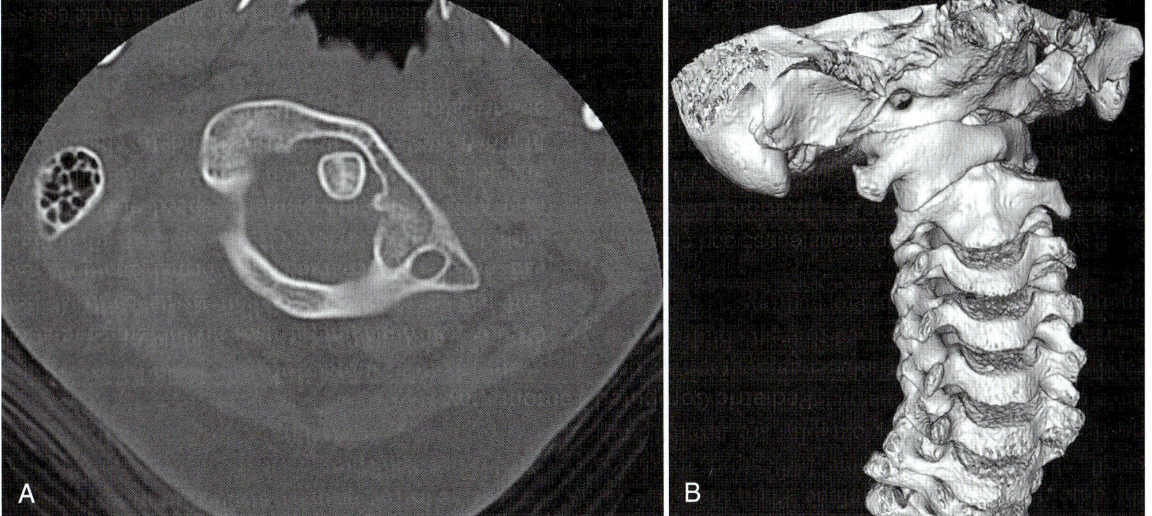


**FIGURE 17-4** Rotary subluxation of C1 vertebral body. Axial image **(A)** demonstrates 30 degrees of clockwise rotation of C1 with respect to C2. The rotation is better demonstrated on the 3D surface-shaded display **(B)**.

lymph nodes, salivary gland evaluation, and infectious processes.

## CT of the Spine

CT is primarily used to evaluate suspected spinal trauma. It is also useful to characterize congenital bony abnormalities such as scoliosis, lesions of the vertebral bodies, and osteomyelitis (Fig. 17-4). MRI is the primary modality for evaluation of the spinal cord and tumors of the cord and canal. Evaluation for disk conditions is uncommon in pediatric patients but is preferable with MRI.

## Patient Positioning

When positioning the patient for CT of the brain and face, it is essential to have the patient's head geometrically centered in the gantry to ensure artifact-free images. In this respect, the patient's head must be centered accurately from right to left in the head holder and from front to back in the gantry. Multiple small positioning sponges can be used to secure the patient's head in the head holder. For the accurate assessment of midline structures, care must be taken to **position** the head so that the right and left sides are symmetrical and not tilted.

Coronal images are important for evaluation of structures such as the orbits, sinuses, and temporal bone. When older-generation scanners are used, it is still important to obtain direct coronal images for these examinations. Newer MDCT scanners, particularly 16- and 64-slice scanners, have obviated the need to obtain direct coronal images, because a single high-resolution dataset can be reconstructed into any plane.

The direct coronal position is usually comfortable for the pediatric patient and is easily achieved with even sedated children. Patients are placed prone with the chin extended forward. The CT gantry is tilted to obtain images in the coronal plane. Occasionally, a patient cannot tolerate the coronal position. An alternate position is a Water's **view,** in which the patient's head is extended to maximum tolerance. With the aid of a scout view, the scans are prescribed as close to 90 degrees to the clivus as possible.

## Technical Considerations

Scans of the brain can be obtained with either conventional sequential axial images or with the helical technique. Some radiologists have traditionally felt that sequential technique produces images that are sharper with better contrast. This technique requires a very cooperative or sedated child and is particularly susceptible to motion artifacts. Helical scanning offers many benefits. The scans are quicker, are less sensitive to motion, and may generate fewer partial volume and streak artifacts, and, above all, high-resolution datasets can be obtained that can be reconstructed into different planes. With current-generation MDCT scanners it is generally possible to obtain image quality from helical scans that is equal or nearly equal to that of sequential scans. For these reasons, we prefer to use helical scanning in the brain for pediatric patients.

Scans of the face, sinuses, temporal bone, neck, and spine should all be obtained helically for obvious reasons. Multiplanar images should routinely be generated and reviewed in these cases.

Most pediatric neurological scans can be performed without contrast. The most common indications such as trauma, headaches, and hydrocephalus do not require contrast. Certain indications such as known or suspected infection or neoplasm do benefit from contrast administration. When the brain is imaged, scans before and after contrast are generally obtained in these patients. However, for evaluation of the face and neck precontrast scans are usually not needed and will needlessly increase the radiation dose to the child.

Timing for contrast studies of the head and face is usually less critical than for body studies and CTA. Contrast can be administered by either hand injection or power injector, and the scan is begun once all the contrast is injected. If a rapid injection is performed, an additional 30- to 60-second delay should be applied before the scan is started.

As in all pediatric CT examinations, the technologist must be careful to ensure that scan parameters chosen for the study are appropriate for the size and age of the child.

## Scanning Protocols

Protocols should be established for each system by a team led by the radiologist, and including techs and equipment applications specialists, to include information such as **data acquisition** and reconstruction and image transfer, etc. These protocols are intended to assist the technologist performing the CT examination and generally help increase the overall **efficiency** of the examination. Comprehensive examination protocols help ensure that the proper study is performed and minimize wasted time for both the technologist and the radiologist.

Acquisition parameters include patient position, prescan localization (scout view), scan range, acquisition slice thickness, pitch, gantry rotation speed, and specific dose parameters. Dose parameters can be determined by the technologist on the basis of the patient's age or weight or automatically chosen by the scanner by use of one of the automated exposure control programs. Reconstruction parameters include reconstruction **algorithm** (e.g., soft tissue or smoothing filter, bone or edge enhancement filter), reconstructed slice thickness, and multiplanar or 3D reconstructions. The protocol should also describe which information is to be archived on the picture archiving and communication system (PACS) or film and whether data should be sent to a 3D workstation for additional postprocessing.

Tables 17-2 through 17-4 are examples of generalized protocols of the head, orbit/sinus, temporal bone/internal auditory canal (IAC), and spine used for 4-, 16-, and 64-slice scanners. These protocols are generalizations and must be modified for each scanner. On 64-slice scanners, the mAs can be decreased slightly compared with 16-slice scanners for a comparable result. All manufacturers have some differences in detector configuration, scan features, and reconstruction options.

# CT OF THE CHEST AND ABDOMEN

Body CT in children (unlike adults) is generally more of an ancillary imaging modality. Ultrasonography remains the primary screening modality for

**TABLE 17-2 Pediatric Neurological Protocols: Techniques for 4-Slice Multidetector Computed Tomography**

| Scan Parameter | Brain | Orbit/Sinus | IAC | Neck | Spine |
|---|---|---|---|---|---|
| Scan mode | Helical | Helical | Helical | Helical | Helical |
| Coverage | Skull base to vertex | Top of orbits through area of interest | Temporal bone | Skull base to lung apex | Spine ROI |
| Gantry rotation speed | 1 second | 0.5 second | 1 second | 0.5 second | 0.5 second |
| Detector slice thickness | 2.5 mm | 2.5 mm | 1.25 mm | 2.5 mm | 2.5 mm |
| Pitch | 1.0 | 1.25 | 1.0 | 1.25 | 1.0 |
| Kilovolts | 120 | 100-120 | 120 | 100-120 | 100-120 |
| mA | 60-100 | 50-100 | 50-100 | 50-100 | 50-100 |
| Reconstruction slice thickness | 3-5 mm | 3 mm | 1-2 mm | 3 mm | 3 mm |
| Reconstruction interval | 3-5 mm | 2 mm | 1 mm | 3 mm | 2 mm |
| Algorithm | Soft tissue | Soft tissue, bone | Bone | Soft tissue | Soft tissue, bone |
| Multiplanar reconstructions | Optional | Coronal | Coronal | Sagittal, coronal | Sagittal, coronal |
| Contrast volume if needed | 2 ml/kg | 2 ml/kg | | 2 ml/kg | 2 ml/kg |

**TABLE 17-3 Pediatric Neurological Protocols: Techniques for 16-Slice Multidetector Computed Tomography**

| Scan Parameter | Brain | Orbit/Sinus | IAC | Neck | Spine |
|---|---|---|---|---|---|
| Scan mode | Helical | Helical | Helical | Helical | Helical |
| Coverage | Skull base to vertex | Top of orbits through area of interest | Temporal bone | Skull base to lung apex | Spine ROI |
| Gantry rotation speed | 0.5 second | 0.5 second | 0.5 second | 0.5 second | 0.5 second |
| Detector slice thickness | 0.5-1.25 mm | 0.5-1.25 mm | 0.5 mm | 0.5-1.25 mm | 0.5-1.25 mm |
| Pitch | 1.0 | 1.25 | 1.0 | 1.25 | 1.0 |
| Kilovolts | 120 | 100-120 | 120 | 100-120 | 100-120 |
| mA | 200+ | 100-200 | 100-200 | 100-200 | 100-200+ |
| Reconstruction slice thickness | 3-5 mm | 2 mm | 1 mm | 3 mm | 2 mm |
| Reconstruction interval | 3-5 mm | 2 mm | 0.5-1 mm | 3 mm | 2 mm |
| Algorithm | Soft tissue | Soft tissue, bone | Bone | Soft tissue | Soft tissue, bone |
| Multiplanar reconstructions | Optional | Sagittal, coronal | Coronal | Sagittal, coronal | Sagittal, coronal |
| Contrast volume if needed | 2 ml/kg | 2 ml/kg | | 2 ml/kg | 2 ml/kg |

the abdomen and pelvis, but CT is a very important modality for many indications.

## Indications

### Trauma

CT is the modality of choice for examination of the abdomen after blunt injury or high-speed trauma to evaluate possible laceration of liver, spleen, pancreas, or kidney (Fig. 17-5). IV and oral contrast (through a nasogastric [NG] tube) should be used in trauma cases. It is usually not possible to give a substantial amount of oral contrast through an NG tube in an unconscious patient because of the risk of aspiration, but a small amount can be given to at least outline the duodenum.

**TABLE 17-4 Pediatric Neurological Protocols: Techniques for 64-Slice Multidetector Computed Tomography**

| Scan Parameter | Brain | Orbit/Sinus | IAC | Neck | Spine |
|---|---|---|---|---|---|
| Scan mode | Helical | Helical | Helical | Helical | Helical |
| Coverage | Skull base to vertex | Top of orbits through area of interest | Temporal bone | Skull base to lung apex | Spine ROI |
| Gantry rotation speed | 0.4-0.5 second | 0.4-0.5 second | 0.4-0.5 second | 0.4-0.5 second | 0.4-0.5 second |
| Detector slice thickness | 0.3-1.25 mm | 0.3-1.25 mm | 0.3-0.5 mm | 0.3-1.25 mm | 0.3-1.25 mm |
| Pitch | 1.0 | 1.25 | 1.0 | 1.25 | 1.0 |
| Kilovolts | 120 | 100-120 | 120 | 100-120 | 100-120 |
| mA | 200+ | 100-200 | 100-200 | 100-200 | 100-200+ |
| Reconstruction slice thickness | 3-5 mm | 2 mm | 1 mm | 3 mm | 2 mm |
| Reconstruction interval | 3-5 mm | 2 mm | 0.5-1 mm | 3 mm | 2 mm |
| Algorithm | Soft tissue | Soft tissue, bone | Bone | Soft tissue | Soft tissue, bone |
| Multiplanar reconstructions | Optional | Sagittal, coronal | Coronal | Sagittal, coronal | Sagittal, coronal |
| Contrast volume if needed | 2 ml/kg | 2 ml/kg | | 2 ml/kg | 2 ml/kg |

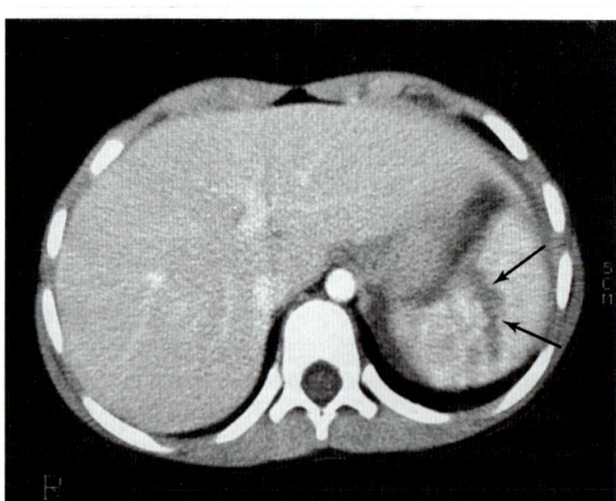

**FIGURE 17-5** Splenic laceration.

## Infections

The most common infections where CT is used in children are pneumonia, pyelonephritis, and appendicitis. IV contrast is needed when there is a pleural effusion or empyema. Oral or rectal contrast, with IV contrast, is needed to evaluate appendicitis and possible abscesses (Fig. 17-6). CT is often used in post-operative patients to look for abscess.

## Tumors

CT is an integral part of the diagnostic workup and post-treatment assessment of pediatric solid tumors, including lymphoma (e.g., Burkitt's or Hodgkin's) and abdominal tumors (e.g., Wilms' tumor of the kidney, neuroblastoma, rhabdomyosarcoma, and hepatoblastoma; Fig. 17-7). The investigation of these oncological diseases generally includes a noncontrast chest CT to look for lung metastases. Chest CT for **mediastinal** disease requires a contrast examination because unenhanced mediastinal vessels may mimic masses or adenopathy on a noncontrast scan.

## CT of the Chest

CT of the chest is used to evaluate central and peripheral airways, pulmonary nodules, vascular anatomy, lung parenchyma, and congenital masses (lung cysts and cystic adenomatoid malformations; Fig. 17-8). CT is an excellent modality to assess foreign body aspirations, when the material is of low density and does not show up well on chest x-ray. MDCT is also used to evaluate the trachea for stenosis, malacia, and atresia with virtual endoscopy (Fig. 17-9). Because these evaluations are limited by the ability of patients to hold their breath for the scan, the use of this technology may be limited in pediatrics. CT for infections, pleural effusions, and malignancy should be with IV contrast.

## High-Resolution CT

High-resolution CT is sometimes performed on pediatric patients for the assessment of parenchymal lung disease such as cystic fibrosis or bronchiectasis

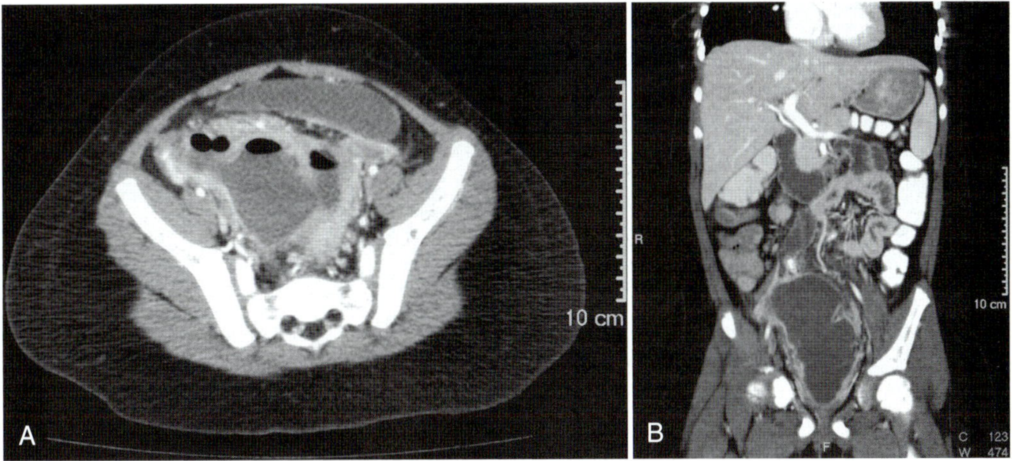


**FIGURE 17-6** **A,** Abscess from perforated appendicitis. **B,** Coronal reformatted image from 3-mm axial images. Complex fluid collections with enhancing walls are present.

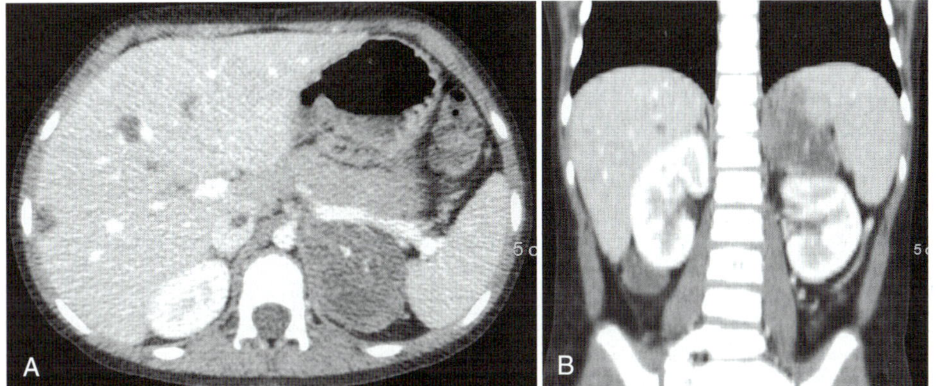


**FIGURE 17-7** **A,** Neuroblastoma of the left adrenal gland. **B,** Coronal reformatted image clearly demonstrates suprarenal location of the calcified mass.

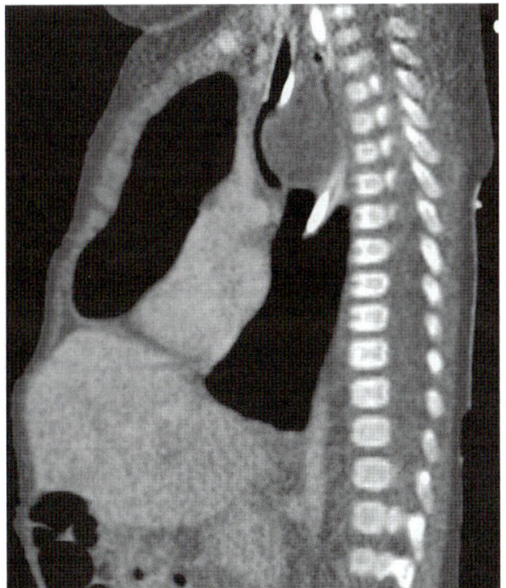

**FIGURE 17-8** Esophageal duplication cyst. Location of cyst posterior to trachea is nicely demonstrated on sagittal image.

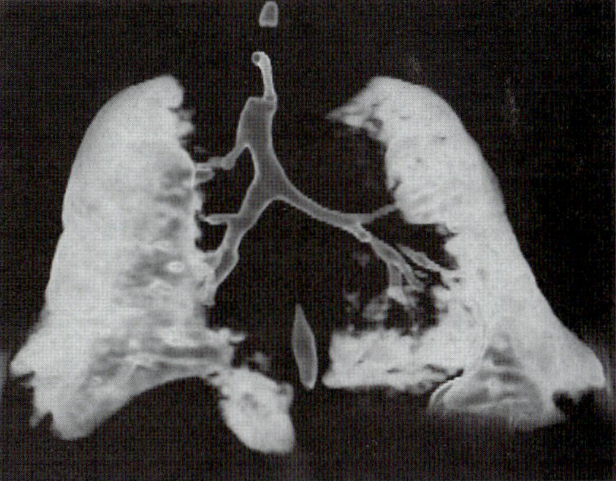

**FIGURE 17-9** Aberrant bronchus (bronchus suis/pig bronchus). Airways reconstruction. Aberrant bronchus to right upper lobe directly from trachea is noted.

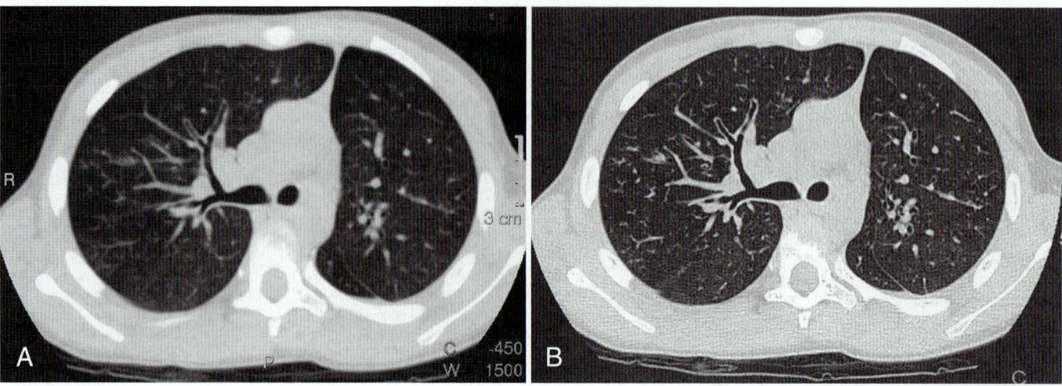


**FIGURE 17-10 A** and **B,** Normal lung, routine CT (3-mm axial slice) versus high-resolution CT (1-mm axial slice). Bronchial walls and diameters can be seen fairly well even with routine imaging.

(Fig. 17-10). However, in most cases bronchiectasis can be well seen by using conventional CT, so high-resolution CT is not necessary. This consideration is important because an increased radiation dose is required to acquire the thinner images in high-resolution CT.

## Patient Positioning

The patient can be placed head or feet first into the scanner. Placing the patient feet first may be less intimidating for young children. This position also allows the parent or technologist a clear view of the child for monitoring and comforting. The patient must be centered correctly in the gantry, which may involve the use of immobilization sponges or blankets and tape.

## Technical Considerations

For chest CT, shallow breathing in the young child will be adequate. Instructions for breath-hold may not work, and misregistration or motion artifacts are risked if the child takes a deep breath. Older children can be instructed to hold their breaths, especially in high-resolution CT. Children on ventilators may be briefly taken off ventilation during image acquisition, provided they are monitored by appropriate medical staff and can tolerate this action.

Scanning of the chest can be initiated by bolus tracking or can be started just before the end of contrast injection. Scans about 30 to 50 seconds after beginning injection will demonstrate adequate vascular enhancement in older children. In infants, this time frame will be shorter, with maximal enhancement probably around 10 to 20 seconds after the beginning of injection. In infants, abdominal scans should begin sooner than the usual 70- to 90-second delay of adult scans, probably right at the end of the contrast bolus.

For abdominal and pelvic CT scans, oral contrast should always be used if the patient can tolerate it. This is especially important in the evaluation of intra-abdominal abscess or bowel obstruction. A long (at least 2-hour) preparation should be performed for studies where there may be conditions of the colon. For trauma patients, a small amount of oral contrast can be injected through the NG tube to delineate the duodenum. Rectal contrast may be used in cases of appendicitis. About 250 ml of contrast is usually adequate to opacify the colon in this patient population (5 to 15 years old), or contrast can be instilled by gravity drip until the patient feels full.

Noncontrast CT scans can be used to evaluate renal stones. Delayed scans (5 to 10 minutes) are needed to evaluate hemangiomas/hemangioendotheliomas. Renal excretion of contrast peaks at around 3 to 5 minutes after injection. Delayed scans to evaluate urinary tract obstruction should therefore be longer than this period (around 10 minutes after injection), with the patient placed prone because the kidneys drain anteriorly.

## Scanning Protocols

Protocols for pediatric CT of the chest, abdomen, and pelvis are summarized in Tables 17-5 through 17-7.

# MUSCULOSKELETAL CT

MDCT has had a significant impact on pediatric orthopedic imaging. **Isotropic** data acquisition with 3D reconstruction techniques has proved valuable for many different indications.

## Indications

### Complex Fractures

MDCT is the study of choice to evaluate complex fractures, particularly of the acetabulum/pelvis and the upper and lower extremities. Surface-rendered and multiplanar reconstructions can give the orthopedic

**TABLE 17-5 Pediatric Chest and Abdomen Protocols: Technique for 4-Slice Multidetector Computed Tomography**

| Scan Parameter | Chest | Abdomen/Pelvis |
|---|---|---|
| Scan mode | Helical | Helical |
| Coverage | Lower neck through lung base | Diaphragm to pubic symphysis |
| Gantry rotation speed | 0.5 second | 0.5 second |
| Detector slice thickness | 2.5 mm | 2.5 mm |
| Pitch | Variable | Variable |
| Kilovolts | 80 (100-120 for >45 kg) | 80 (100-120 for >45 kg) |
| mA | | |
| <15 kg | 40 | 50-70 |
| 15-24 kg | 60 | 80 |
| 25-34 kg | 80 | 100 |
| 35-44 kg | 100 | 120-140 |
| >45 kg | 120-140 | 160-200 |
| Reconstruction slice thickness | 3 mm | 3-5 mm |
| Reconstruction interval | 3 mm | 3-5 mm |
| Algorithm | Soft tissue and lung | Soft tissue and lung |
| Multiplanar reconstructions | Coronal | Coronal |
| Contrast volume (if needed) | 2 ml/kg | 2 ml/kg |

**TABLE 17-6 Pediatric Chest and Abdomen Protocols: Techniques for 16-Slice Multidetector Computed Tomography**

| Scan Parameter | Chest | Abdomen |
|---|---|---|
| Scan mode | Helical | Helical |
| Coverage | Lower neck through lung base | Diaphragm to pubic symphysis |
| Gantry rotation speed | 0.5 second | 0.5 second |
| Detector slice thickness | 0.5-1.25 mm | 0.5-1.25 mm |
| Pitch | Variable | Variable |
| Kilovolts | 80 (100-120 for >45 kg) | 80 (100-120 for >45 kg) |
| mA | | |
| <15 kg | 40 | 50-70 |
| 15-24 kg | 60 | 80 |
| 25-34 kg | 80 | 100 |
| 35-44 kg | 100 | 120-140 |
| >45 kg | 120-140 | 160-200 |
| Reconstruction slice thickness | 3 mm | 3 mm |
| Reconstruction interval | 3 mm | 3 mm |
| Algorithm | Soft tissue and lung | Soft tissue and lung |
| Multiplanar reconstructions | Coronal | Coronal |
| Contrast volume (if needed) | 2 ml/kg | 2 ml/kg |

surgeon a clear 3D picture of the fracture planes and are valuable in planning operative repair (Fig. 17-11). **Segmentation** of the images is very helpful to show the joint surfaces.

### Tumors

**Osseous tumors** (e.g., Ewing's sarcoma and osteogenic sarcoma) are best imaged with MRI, which can delineate soft tissue and marrow involvement much better than CT. CT is used to visualize the cortex itself, or calcifications (Fig. 17-12). It is not good at defining soft tissue involvement.

### Infections

Osseous infections are best evaluated using bone scan or MRI. The infection must be fairly aggressive and advanced to produce bony changes. CT findings may therefore be absent in early stages of an

**TABLE 17-7 Pediatric Chest and Abdomen Protocols: Techniques for 64-Slice Multidetector Computed Tomography**

| Scan Parameter | Chest | Abdomen |
|---|---|---|
| Scan mode | Helical | Helical |
| Coverage | Lower neck through lung base | Diaphragm to pubic symphysis |
| Gantry rotation speed | 0.4-0.5 second | 0.4-0.5 second |
| Detector slice thickness | 0.5-1.25 mm | 0.5-1.25 mm |
| Pitch | Variable | Variable |
| Kilovolts | 80 (100-120 for >45 kg) | 80 (100-120 for >45 kg) |
| mA | | |
| <15 kg | 40 | 50-70 |
| 15-24 kg | 60 | 80 |
| 25-34 kg | 80 | 100 |
| 35-44 kg | 100 | 120-140 |
| >45 kg | 120-140 | 160-200 |
| Reconstruction slice thickness | 3 mm | 3 mm |
| Reconstruction interval | 3 mm | 3 mm |
| Algorithm | Soft tissue and lung | Soft tissue and lung |
| Multiplanar reconstructions | Coronal | Coronal |
| Contrast volume (if needed) | 2 ml/kg | 2 ml/kg |

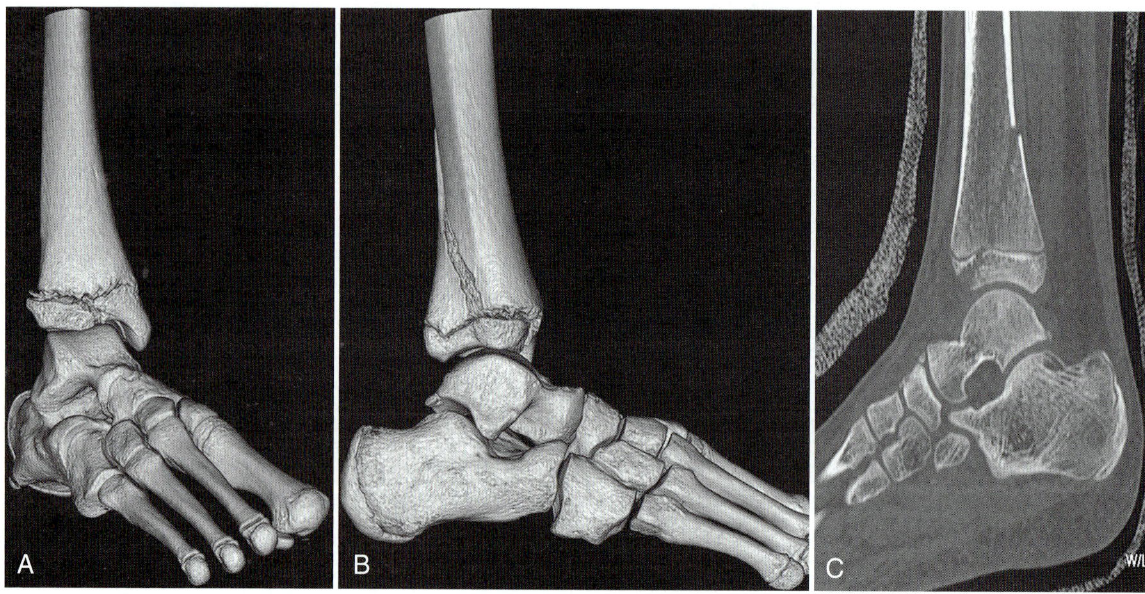


**FIGURE 17-11** Salter 4 fracture of distal tibia. Surface (**A** and **B**) and sagittal reconstructions **(C)** demonstrate fracture line through metaphysis and epiphysis.

infection. Soft tissue infections are also better evaluated by MRI. CT may be used to delineate soft tissue abscesses. IV contrast must be used.

### Deformities

CT can be used to evaluate femoral anteversion or tibial torsion and is also valuable in assessing congenital hip and shoulder dysplasias (Fig. 17-13). CT is also an excellent way to evaluate leg-length discrepancy. Imaging for this purpose can be done by using a low radiation dose method, which imparts lower radiation than the corresponding plain film study.

## Patient Positioning

The area being imaged must be placed as close to the center of the gantry as possible and away from the body (if possible) to minimize scatter artifacts. For studies of deformities or leg-length studies, the ankles should be taped in the neutral (usually with great toes pointing up) position to eliminate movement

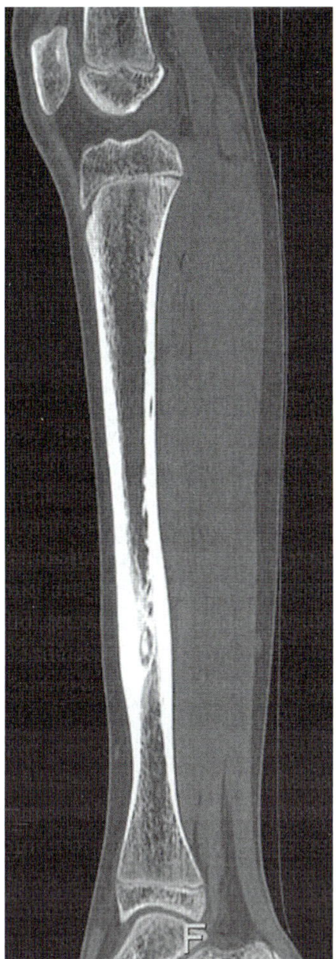

**FIGURE 17-12** Osteoid osteoma. Sagittal reconstruction from 2-mm axial images shows cortical reaction and calcified nidus of lesion.

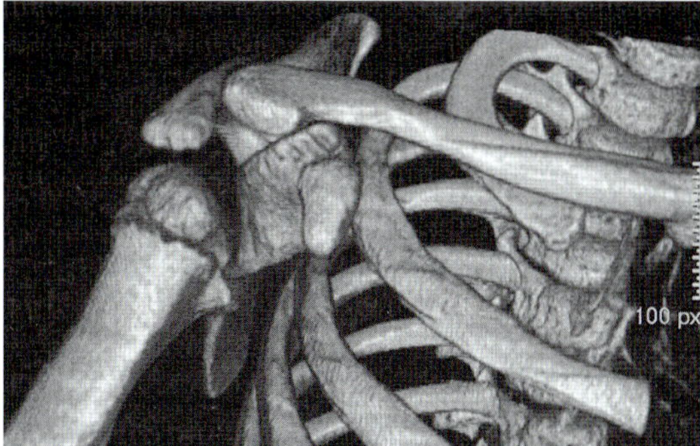


**FIGURE 17-13** Chronic shoulder dislocation. Bone surface reconstruction clearly shows dysplastic glenoid and posterior dislocation of the flattened humeral head.

and artifacts. Both legs should be as parallel to each other as possible. Always scan both extremities at the same time for leg length, tibial torsion, and femoral anteversion studies.

### Technical Considerations

Because most cases of osseous tumors and infections are better evaluated by MRI, it should always be considered whether MRI is the more appropriate examination for the patient. IV contrast should be used whenever there is a question of soft tissue mass or infection. Contrast generally does not help for evaluation of the bone.

MDCT has eliminated the need to scan patients in multiple planes. A single isotropic acquisition can be performed and reconstructed to the desired planes on the scanner or workstation. It is therefore very important to use thin slice images whenever possible. Scans should be reconstructed with both a soft tissue and a bone filter. Bone algorithm produces higher quality multiplanar reconstructions, but the soft tissue algorithm produces smoother, better looking 3D images, with less image noise

Scans for alignment (e.g., tibial torsion) and leg-length studies can be done with a minimal radiation dose because high bone detail is not needed in these types of studies. All patients should have aggressive shielding of the body adjacent to the area being scanned.

### Scanning Protocols

Generalized protocols for musculoskeletal CT are presented in Tables 17-8 through 17-10.

## CT ANGIOGRAPHY

CTA and MRA have replaced diagnostic catheter angiography in children for almost all indications. Advantages of MRA include no ionizing radiation and no need for iodinated contrast. CTA, however, is much faster (better patient tolerance and less motion artifact) and has higher spatial resolution, which is important for evaluating small vessels in infants and children.

### Indications

CTA is useful throughout the head and body primarily to evaluate vascular anomalies such as aberrant vessels, aneurysms and vascular malformations, and manifestations of congenital or acquired diseases such as sickle cell anemia, vasculitis, and thrombotic states (Figs. 17-14 and 17-15). CTA is also the test of choice for traumatic vascular injury.

### Patient Positioning and Preparation

High-quality CTA requires motion-free images for 3D reconstructions. To this end, proper immobilization

**TABLE 17-8 Pediatric Bone Protocol: Technique for 4-Channel Multidetector Computed Tomography**

| Scan Parameter | Infant (<15 kg) | Toddler (15-25 kg) | Child (25-40 kg) | Teenager |
|---|---|---|---|---|
| Scan mode | Helical | Helical | Helical | Helical |
| Coverage | ROI | Same | Same | Same |
| Gantry rotation speed | 0.5 second | 0.5 second | 0.5 second | 0.5 second |
| Detector slice thickness | 0.5-2.5 mm | 0.5-2.5 mm | 0.5-2.5 mm | 0.5-2.5 mm |
| Pitch | Variable | Variable | Variable | Variable |
| Kilovolts | 80 | 80-100 | 100 | 120 |
| mA | 40 | 50-70 | 70-90 | 120+ |
| Reconstruction slice thickness | 2 mm | 2 mm | 2 mm | 2 mm |
| Reconstruction interval | 2 mm | 2 mm | 2 mm | 2 mm |
| Algorithm | Soft tissue, bone | Soft tissue, bone | Soft tissue, bone | Soft tissue, bone |
| Multiplanar reconstructions (as needed) | Coronal, sagittal, 3D | Coronal, sagittal, 3D | Coronal, sagittal, 3D | Coronal, sagittal, 3D |
| Contrast volume (if needed) | 2 ml/kg | 2 ml/kg | 2 ml/kg | 2 ml/kg |

**TABLE 17-9 Pediatric Bone Protocol: Technique for 16- and 64-Channel Multidetector Computed Tomography**

| Scan Parameter | Infant (<15 kg) | Toddler (15-25 kg) | Child (25-40 kg) | Teenager |
|---|---|---|---|---|
| Scan mode | Helical | Helical | Helical | Helical |
| Coverage | ROI | Same | Same | Same |
| Gantry rotation speed | 0.4-0.5 second | 0.4-0.5 second | 0.4-0.5 second | 0.4-0.5 second |
| Detector slice thickness | 0.5-2.5 mm | 0.5-2.5 mm | 0.5-2.5 mm | 0.5-2.5 mm |
| Pitch | Variable | Variable | Variable | Variable |
| Kilovolts | 80 | 80-100 | 100 | 120 |
| mA | 40 | 50-70 | 70-90 | 120+ |
| Reconstruction slice thickness | 2 mm | 2 mm | 2 mm | 2 mm |
| Reconstruction interval | 2 mm | 2 mm | 2 mm | 2 mm |
| Algorithm | Soft tissue, bone | Soft tissue, bone | Soft tissue, bone | Soft tissue, bone |
| Multiplanar reconstructions (as needed) | Coronal, sagittal, 3D | Coronal, sagittal, 3D | Coronal, sagittal, 3D | Coronal, sagittal, 3D |
| Contrast volume (if needed) | 2 ml/kg | 2 ml/kg | 2 ml/kg | 2 ml/kg |

**TABLE 17-10 Special Cases for Musculoskeletal Computed Tomography**

| | Scan Region (Scan Both Extremities at the Same Time) | kV/mA | Detector/Slice Reconstruction Interval |
|---|---|---|---|
| Leg-length discrepancy | Entire leg (above hip through ankle joint) | 80-120 kV<br>40 mA | 2.5-mm detector at 10-mm intervals |
| Femoral anteversion | (1) Femoral head and neck (skip diaphysis)<br>(2) Femoral condyles | Same | Same |
| Tibial torsion | (1) Tibial plateau (skip diaphysis)<br>(2) Tibiotalar joint (include fibula in field of view) | Same | Same |

kV, kilovolts.

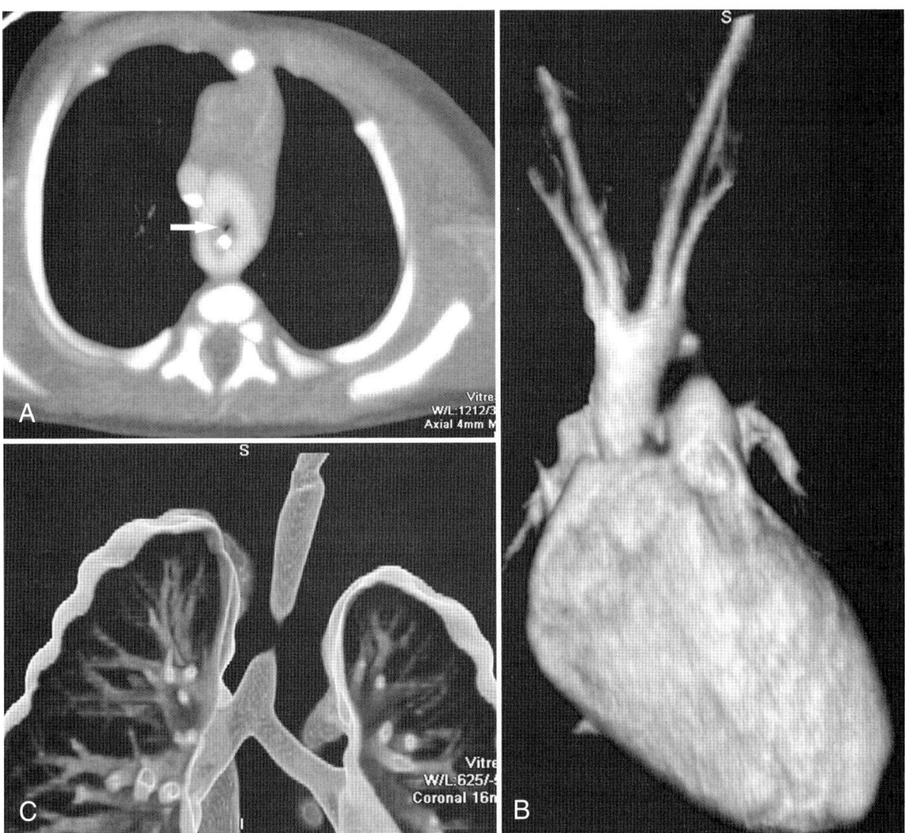


**FIGURE 17-14** Complete vascular ring with tracheal compression. **A,** A 10-mm-thick axial maximum intensity projection image demonstrates a complete vascular ring. The trachea (*white arrow*) is seen as a tiny dot of air. The esophagus has a high-density NG tube within it. The volume-rendered image **(B)** demonstrates a double aortic arch. The two arches are nearly symmetrical and both give rise to a subclavian and a carotid artery. Thin slab (11-mm) volume-rendered image with high transparency **(C)** shows a very high grade tracheal compression resulting from the vascular ring.

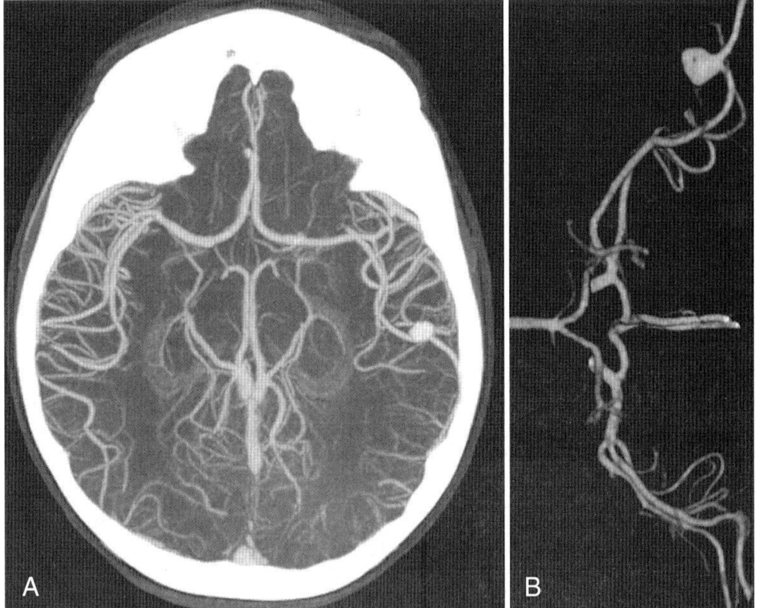


**FIGURE 17-15** Mycotic middle cerebral artery aneurysm. Axial maximum intensity projection image **(A)** shows an aneurysm arising from a left peripheral middle cerebral artery branch artery. The relationship of the aneurysm to the vessel is better demonstrated on the volume-rendered image **(B)**.

TABLE 17-11 **Pediatric Computed Tomography Angiography Protocols: Techniques for 4-Slice Multidetector Computed Tomography**

| Parameters | Cerebral | Cardiothoracic | Abdominal |
|---|---|---|---|
| Detector slice thickness | 1-2.5 mm | 1-2.5 mm | 1-2.5 mm |
| Pitch | 1.2 | 1.2-1.5 | 1.2-1.5 |
| Reconstructed slice thickness | 1-2.5 mm | 1-2.5 mm | 1-2.5 mm |
| Reconstructed slice interval | 1-1.5 mm | 1-1.5 mm | 1-1.5 mm |
| Gantry rotation time | 0.5 second | 0.5 second | 0.5 second |
| Voltage | 120 kV | 120 kV | 120 kV |
| Tube current | 50-120 mA | 50-120 mA | 50-120 mA |
| Injection rate | 2-3 ml/second | 2-3 ml/second | 2-3 ml/second |
| Scan timing | Bolus tracking | Bolus tracking | Bolus tracking |
| Reconstruction algorithm | Soft tissue | Soft tissue | Soft tissue |
| Contrast volume | 2-3 ml/kg | 2-3 ml/kg | 2-3 ml/kg |

kV, kilovolts.

of the patient is essential. Infants can usually be immobilized without the need for sedation. Toddlers and young children may require sedation to obtain a good-quality study. CTA in older children can often be performed without sedation if proper coaching and parental support are provided. Older children should also be coached in breath-holding, which is particularly important in chest studies.

For studies of the abdomen, it is important that patients do not receive any oral contrast because this will interfere with 3D reconstructions.

## Technical Considerations

Successful CTA requires optimization of scan technique and contrast administration. Speed is important for image acquisition to minimize motion artifacts and maximize coverage and contrast density. The shortest rotation time available on the scanner should be used. Pitch values of 1.25 to 1.5 will also reduce scan time. Slice thickness is a trade-off between resolution and scan time (coverage). This can require a difficult decision with a 4-slice scanner but is usually not a factor with 16-slice scanners and higher configuration. In general, the thinnest slice thickness that will allow adequate coverage within an appropriate scan time should be used. Consulting with a radiologist is always appropriate to ensure the best possible image quality with reduced radiation dose.

Proper delivery of contrast media is essential for CTA. Power injection with a rate of at least 2 ml/s (3 ml/s is preferred) is strongly recommended. This can be easily achieved with a 22-gauge peripheral IV and occasionally achieved with a 24-gauge IV if the catheter is in an adequate vein. Hand injection and butterfly needles are not recommended for CTA. High-density contrast such as 350 to 380 mg of iodine per ml is also recommended because this will improve vascular enhancement.

The timing of the scan should be initiated with bolus-tracking software whenever possible, because this will minimize the chance of error caused by mistiming the bolus. Scans can be triggered either manually on the basis of the visual appearance of the vessel or automatically when a certain threshold for HU is achieved. Empirical delays can also be used but will need to be varied depending on the size of the patient, the body part scanned, the IV site, the injection rate, and the presence of certain medical conditions such as heart disease.

After the scan, the thinnest slice thickness available should be reconstructed on the scanner and sent to PACS or the 3D workstation to allow for postprocessing of the images. Overlapping reconstructions are also helpful for improving reconstruction quality if the slice thickness of the data acquisition is greater than 1 mm.

## Scanning Protocols

Generalized CTA protocols for 4-, 16-, and 64-slice scanners are presented in Tables 17-11 and 17-12.

**TABLE 17-12 Pediatric Computed Tomography Angiography Protocols: Techniques for 16- and 64-Slice Multidetector Computed Tomography**

| Parameters | Cerebral | Cardiothoracic | Abdominal |
|---|---|---|---|
| Detector slice thickness | 0.5-0.75 mm | 0.5-1.25 mm | 0.5-1.25 mm |
| Pitch | 1.2 | 1.2-1.5 | 1.2-1.5 |
| Reconstructed slice thickness | 0.5-0.75 mm | 0.5-1.25 mm | 0.5-1.25 mm |
| Reconstructed slice interval | 0.5 mm | 0.5-1 mm | 0.5-1 mm |
| Gantry rotation time | 0.5 second | 0.5 second | 0.5 second |
| Voltage | 120 kV | 120 kV | 120 kV |
| Tube current | 50-120 mA | 50-120 mA | 50-120 mA |
| Injection rate | 2-3 ml/second | 2-3 ml/second | 2-3 ml/second |
| Scan timing | Bolus tracking | Bolus tracking | Bolus tracking |
| Reconstruction Algorithm | Soft tissue | Soft tissue | Soft tissue |
| Contrast volume | 2-3 ml/kg | 2-3 ml/kg | 2-3 ml/kg |

kV, kilovolts.

## REVIEW QUESTIONS

Answer the following questions to check your understanding of the materials studied.

1. Which of the following applies to the two basic tenets and other considerations when imaging the pediatric patient with the CT scanner?
   1. knowledgeable
   2. always prepared and honest with the family of the patient
   3. use of a friendly and an appropriately decorated environment

   A. 1 and 2
   B. 2 and 3
   C. 3 only
   D. 1, 2, and 3
2. The advantages of using MDCT scanners (compared to SSCT scanners) to image the pediatric patient include all of the following *except:*
   A. faster data acquisition.
   B. increased volume coverage.
   C. better patient tolerance and better use of contrast media.
   D. potential increase in radiation dose especially when using imaging thin slices.
3. The introduction of MDCT scanners to image pediatric patients provides the following applications:
   A. volume-rendered 3D images
   B. surface-rendered 3D images
   C. CT angiography and CT colonoscopy
   D. all are correct
4. Sedated pediatric CT patients are monitored for all of the following *except:*
   A. temperature.
   B. respiratory rate.
   C. pulse oximetry.
   D. blood pressure.
5. Which of the following reaction is reduced by using nonionic contrast agents?
   A. vomiting
   B. nausea
   C. urticaria
   D. all of the above
6. Compared to a pitch of 1, a pitch of 1.5 will reduce the dose to the patient by 25%, and a pitch of 2 will reduce the dose by:
   A. 20%.
   B. 30%.
   C. 50%.
   D. Pitch does not affect the dose to the patient.
7. When positioning the pediatric patient for CT of the brain and face in order to reduce artifacts, the head must be:
   A. placed 2-cm from the center of the gantry.
   B. accurately placed in the isocenter of the gantry.
   C. raised 1-cm from center of the gantry.
   D. placed in the Water's position.
8. The following are indications for CT imaging of the musculoskeletal system in children:
   A. complex fractures and deformities
   B. tumors
   C. infections
   D. all are correct
9. Pediatric CTA can demonstrate:
   A. aneurysms and vascular malformations.
   B. vasculitis and thrombosis.
   C. aberrant vessels.
   D. all of the above.

10. Radiation dose to the pediatric CT patient can be reduced by using all of the following *except:*
    A. low pitch ratios.
    B. lead shielding.
    C. low mAs exposure factors.
    D. high kVp exposure techniques.

## BIBLIOGRAPHY

Aitken, G. F., Flodmark, O., Newman, D. E., Kilcoyne, R. F., Shuman, W. P., & Mack, L. A. (1985). Leg length determination by CT digital radiography. *American Journal of Roentgenology, 144*, 613–615.

Brenner, D. J., Elliston, C., Hall, E., & Berdon, W. (2001). Estimated risks of radiation-induced fatal cancer from pediatric CT. *American Journal of Roentgenology, 176*, 289–296.

Chan, F. P., & Rubin, G. D. (2005). MDCT angiography of pediatric vascular diseases of the abdomen, pelvis, and extremities. *Pediatric Radiology, 35*, 40–53.

Daneman, A. (1987). *Pediatric body CT*. New York: Springer-Verlag.

Donelly, L. F., Emery, K. H., Brody, A. S., Laor, T., Gylys-Morn, V. M., et al. (2001). Minimizing radiation dose for pediatric body applications of single-detector helical CT. *American Journal of Roentgenology, 176*, 303–306.

Flodmark, O., Roland, E. H., Hill, A., & Whitfield, M. F. (1978). Periventricular leukomalacia radiologic diagnosis. *Radiology, 162*, 117–124.

Frush, D., & Donnelly, L. F. (1998). Helical CT in children: technical considerations and body applications. *Radiology, 209*, 37–48.

Frush, D., Siegel, M. J., & Bisset, G. S., 3rd (1997). Challenges of pediatric spiral CT. *Radiographics, 17*, 939–959.

Huda, W., Atherton, J. V., Ware, D. E., & Cumming, W. A. (1997). An approach for the estimation of effective radiation dose at CT in pediatric patients. *Radiology, 203*, 417–422.

Jacob, R. P., Haertel, M., & Stussi, E. (1980). Tibial torsion calculated by computerized tomography. *Journal of Bone and Joint Surgery, 62B*, 238–242.

Jacquenier, M., Jouve, J. L., Bollini, G., Panuel, M., & Migliani, R. (1992). Acetabular anteversion in children. *Journal of Pediatric Orthopedics, 12*, 373–375.

Keeter, S., Benator, R. M., Weinberg, S. M., & Hartenberg, M. A. (1990). Sedation in pediatric CT: national survey of current practice. *Radiology, 175*, 745–752.

Ozonoff, M. B. (1992). *Pediatric orthopedic radiology* (2nd ed.). Philadelphia, PA: WB Saunders.

Patterson, A., Frush, D. P., & Donnelly, L. F. (2001). Helical CT scan of the body: are settings adjusted for pediatric patients? *American Journal of Roentgenology, 176*, 297–301.

Siegel, M. J. (2003). Multiplanar and three-dimensional multidetector row CT of thoracic vessels and airways in the pediatric population. *Radiology, 229*, 641–650.

### Further Reading

Riccabona, M. (Ed.). (2013). CT in children: why and what to consider for CT in children. *European Journal of Radiology, 82*(7), 1041–1134.

# 18

# Quality Control for Computed Tomography Scanners

## OUTLINE



## LEARNING OBJECTIVES

On completion of this chapter, you should be able to:

1. explain what is meant by quality control (QC) for CT scanners.
2. state the benefits of a QC program for CT scanners.
3. identify and describe the three essential steps in a QC program.
4. identify the range of QC tests to be done by the technologist as prescribed by the ACR and the IAEA.
5. identify three categories of equipment and phantoms for CT QC tests.
6. describe briefly the features of the ACR phantom.
7. outline the three basic tenets of a QC program for CT.
8. describe briefly each of the following with respect to CT QC:
    - exposure technique selection
    - testing frequency
    - limits of a passing test.
9. outline the visual inspection requirements for CT QC.
10. state the acceptance criteria for the following ACR CT accreditation QC tests using the ACR phantom:
    - light accuracy alignment
    - high-contrast resolution (spatial resolution)
    - low-contrast resolution
    - image uniformity
    - noise
    - CT number accuracy
    - slice thickness.
11. identify other CT QC tests not listed in 10 above.

## KEY TERMS TO WATCH FOR AND REMEMBER

The following key terms/concepts are important to your understanding of this chapter

**acceptance testing**
**acceptance limits**
**dosimetry phantoms and instrumentation**
**error correction**
**generic limits**
**geometric phantoms**
**image performance phantoms**
**quality control (QC)**
**quantitative phantoms**
**routine performance**
**tolerance limits**
**visual inspection**

## WHAT IS QUALITY CONTROL?

What is **quality control (QC),** and how does it relate to **computed tomography (CT)** scanners? For CT scanners, QC may be defined as a program that periodically tests the performance of a CT scanner and compares its performance with some standard. If the scanner is performing suboptimally, then steps must be initiated to correct the problem. The goal of a QC program is to ensure that every image created by the CT scanner is a quality image, with minimum radiation dose to patients and personnel. High-quality images provide the radiologist maximum information, improve the chances for correct diagnosis, and ultimately contribute to quality patient care.

QC deals with the CT imaging equipment and is an essential component of a **radiation protection** program. It includes several principles and concepts that ultimately lead to **dose optimization** as a strategy for radiation protection of patients. Furthermore all CT departments should have a QC program (Nute et al., 2013).

This chapter describes a generic QC program that can be adapted to almost any CT scanner system. As part of the purchase package, CT manufacturers often prescribe a daily QC program for use on their CT systems. Sometimes their QC program includes a specially furnished phantom or test object to be imaged with selected techniques. Descriptions of the testing instruments, an outline of necessary measurements, and hints on interpretation of the results are presented. In some cases, internal **software** is used to interpret the measurements and to notify the operator of unsatisfactory results.

### Essential Steps in a QC Program

Bushong (2013) and others (IAEA, 2012; Papp, 2015) have noted that QC involves three fundamental steps:

1. Acceptance testing
2. Routine performance evaluation
3. Error correction

**Acceptance testing** basically verifies compliance, that is, whether the CT equipment meets manufacturers' specifications (usually as outlined in the hospital's request for proposal to purchase a CT scanner) and ensuring that it operates efficiently in terms of various **outputs,** such as image-quality requirements and dose output. In general, acceptance testing is usually done by qualified medical physicists or others with a firm knowledge of how CT scanners work. Acceptance testing generally includes that the features ordered are delivered and there is mechanical and electrical integrity, **stability,** safety of various components (interlocks and power drives, for example), and CT dose and imaging performance. Acceptance tests, for example, may include verification of **slice thickness,** CT number **linearity,** uniformity, spatial and contrast resolution, **noise,** and dose output.

**Routine performance** *evaluation* refers to monitoring the components of the CT scanner that affect dose and image quality. Monitoring includes QC tests that are performed on a *daily, weekly, monthly,* and *yearly* basis. This is part of an ongoing QC process. In general, technologists are quite active in routine performance testing of the CT scanner. Some tests, however, require the expertise of the medical physicist. Some authorities such as the American College of Radiology (ACR), the International Atomic Energy Agency (IAEA), and Health Canada often prescribe specific tests that should be done by the technologist and those that should be done by the medical physicist. For example, the ACR (2012) suggested that the following tests be done by the CT technologist:

1. CT number for water and standard deviation (noise)
2. **Artifact** evaluation
3. Display monitor QC
4. Visual inspection of certain components of the scanner

In addition, the IAEA noted that the following tests be conducted by the technologist:

1. CT alignment lights
2. Scanned projection radiography (SPR) accuracy, also referred to as "scout view," "topogram," "scanogram," or "pilot" (CT vendor terminology)
3. CT number, image noise, image uniformity, and image artifacts
4. Image display and printing
5. External CT positioning lasers
6. Couch top alignment and positional accuracy
7. CT number of multiple materials

The IAEA (2012) also suggested that the medical physicist should conduct specific QC tests and provide advice to CT departments on the following:

1. CT image quality and radiation protection considerations not only for the patient, but for personnel and members of the public
2. Acquisition and installations of CT scanners, including shielding considerations
3. Performance of specific QC tests (recommended for the medical physicist) on various components of the CT scanner, including acceptance testing and routine performance QC tests
4. Dose optimization
5. The specific responsibilities of the technologist in conducting the tests as required by the QC program

The CT QC tests that should be specifically conducted by the medical physicist (#3 above) as outlined by the IAEA and coincide with those of other radiology authorities such as the ACR and Radiation Protection Bureau-Health Canada (RPB-HC) are as follows:

1. Visual inspection and review of the QC program
2. CT alignment lights
3. SPR accuracy
4. kV and half-value layer
5. Radiation dose
6. CT number accuracy, image noise, image uniformity, and image artifacts
7. Image display and printing
8. Imaged slice width
9. X-ray beam width
10. Spatial resolution (modulation transfer function or modulation)
11. External CT positioning lasers
12. Couch top alignment and index accuracy
13. **Gantry** tilt
14. CT number accuracy

Finally **error correction** deals with the evaluation of the results of the QC tests. If the CT scanner fails to meet the **tolerance limits** or **acceptance limits** (to be described later in the chapter) established for the particular QC test, then the scanner must be serviced to ensure that tolerance limits are met. This is the basic tenet of error correction.

## Equipment and Phantoms for QC Testing

CT QC testing requires a set of test tools that includes special equipment and phantoms, which are used to conduct the QC tests. These phantoms and equipment have been placed in essentially three categories: **image performance phantoms, geometric phantoms,** and quantitative/**dosimetry phantoms and instrumentation** (IAEA, 2012). These phantoms are designed specifically to measure various variables for QC monitoring.

Image performance phantoms are used to verify the performance of the CT scanner on image-quality characteristics such as high- and low-contrast **spatial resolution** and noise. Geometric accuracy phantoms include tools to measure SPR accuracy and CT laser accuracy. On the other hand, dosimetry phantoms are used to assess the CT dose output such as the computed tomography dose index (CTDI). Finally, quantitative CT phantoms are used to measure the accuracy of **CT numbers.**

While some phantoms are included with the CT scanner when delivered to the facility, others are available commercially. Two examples of phantoms include the *ACR CT accreditation phantom*, the Gammex 464 available from Gammex, Middleton, Wisconsin, and the *Catphan 700*, a commercially available phantom from The Phantom Laboratory in New York.

### ACR CT Accreditation Phantom

The ACR accreditation phantom is described in detail by the ACR (2015) for use in their voluntary CT accreditation program, which is intended to demonstrate to patients and personnel operating the CT facility the safety and effectiveness of their CT imaging services.

The phantom is based on Solid Water construction to ensure stability and reproducibility of QC tests conducted over time. An important feature of this phantom is that it consists of the four modules illustrated in Figure 18-1, which are designed to measure positioning accuracy, CT number accuracy, slice thickness, light accuracy alignment, **low-contrast resolution,** CT number uniformity, and high-contrast resolution. Furthermore, the phantom is marked with the words "HEAD," "FOOT," and "TOP" (Fig. 18-1, *A*) to assist with proper alignment during use. An interesting and comprehensive article on the ACR CT accreditation phantom is one by McCollough et al. (2004). This article outlines practical tips, artifact examples, and pitfalls to avoid. Furthermore the essential criteria (tolerance or acceptance limits) are still the same. Last but certainly not least, the essential specifications and characteristics of the ACR CT accreditation phantom are listed in Table 18-1.

### The Catphan 700

There are several CT QC phantoms available for CT QC testing, including those provided by CT manufacturers and included in the purchase of the scanner. It is not within the scope of this chapter to describe details of all of these phantoms; however, essential features of one such commercially available phantom, the Catphan 700, will be highlighted.

The Catphan 700 Phantom (Fig. 18-2, *A*) was designed for The Phantom Laboratory (2015) with the assistance of Dr. David Goodenough for QC of CT volume scanners. As noted by The Phantom Laboratory, ". . . the phantom retains many of the tests and features offered in the other Catphan® models. . . ." This CT QC phantom includes three solid-cast test modules (Fig. 18-2, *B*) positioned inside the housing of the phantom such as sensitometry slice geometry module (Fig. 18-3, *A*), a 30 line pair per centimeter (lp/cm) module (Fig. 18-3, *B*), and a low-contrast sphere array (Fig. 18-3, *C*). In addition, the phantom also contains the new wave insert for measuring slice geometry and resolution across the scan area (Fig. 18-3, *D*). For more complete details of the Catphan 700 Phantom, the interested reader should contact The Phantom Laboratory (2015).

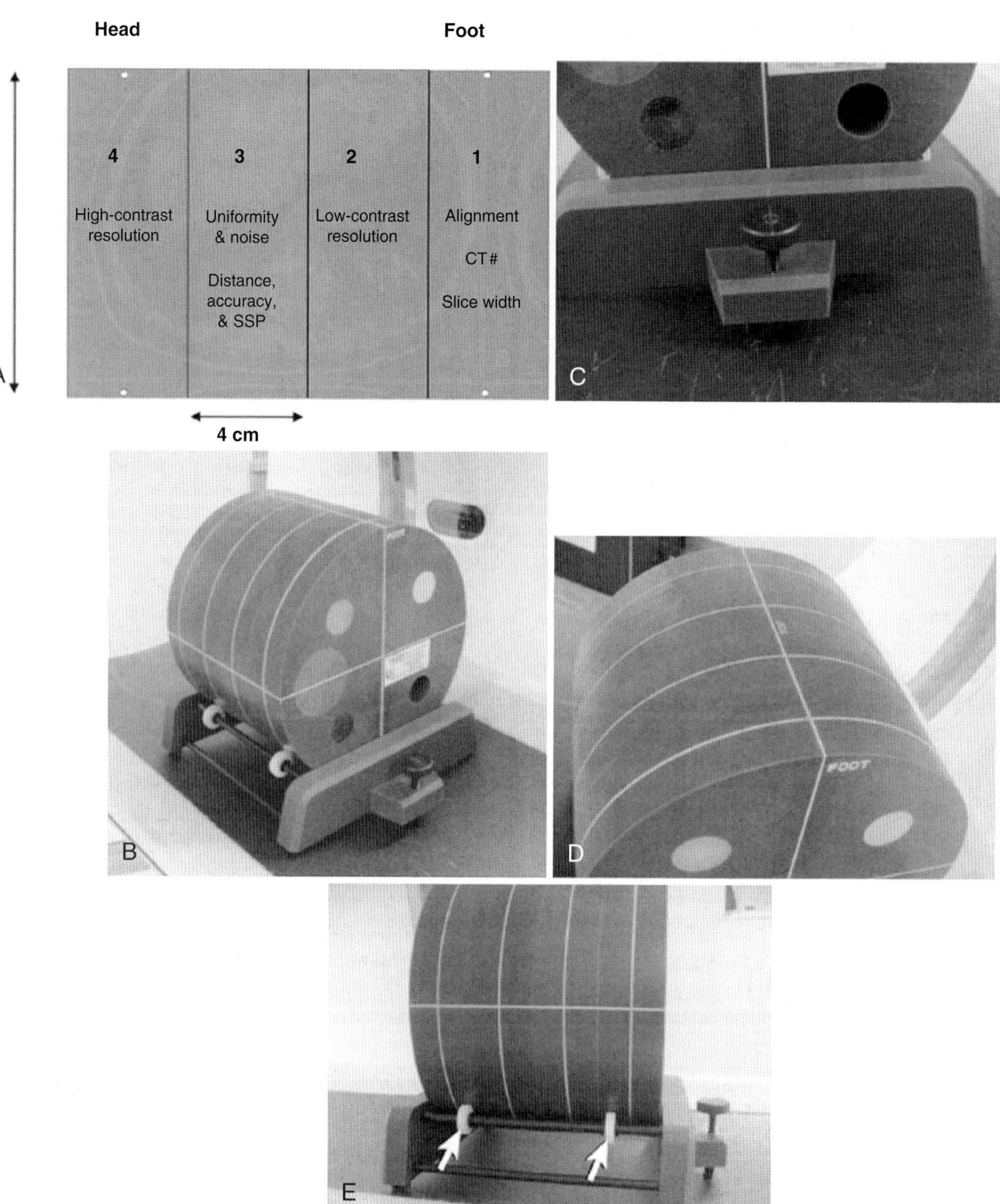


**FIGURE 18-1 A,** Diagram of the four modules of the ACR CT accreditation phantom. **B,** Photograph of a properly aligned phantom. **C,** Centering left to right on both the phantom and the phantom base (optional) substantially simplifies the alignment process. **D,** Top view of a properly aligned phantom. **E,** Side view of a properly aligned phantom. The white Teflon rings on the optional phantom base may cause streak artifacts and should be moved away from the central portions of each module, which are indicated by the four white lines circumscribing the phantom. (From McCollough, C. H., Bruesewitz, M. R., McNitt-Gray, M. F., et al. (2004). *Medical Physics, 31* (9), 2423-2443. Reproduced by permission of the American Association of Physicists in Medicine [AAPM] and the author.)

**TABLE 18-1 Specifications of the ACR CT Accreditation Phantom**

| | |
|---|---|
| **Phantom Construction** | |
| Matrix material | Solid Water, 0 ± 5 HU |
| Length | 16 cm (6.30 inches) |
| Diameter | 20 cm (7.88 inches) |
| Weight | 5.3 kg (11.75 pounds) |
| **Imbedded Test Objects** | |
| Water equivalent linearity rod | Solid Water, 0 HU |
| Bone equivalent linearity rod | 955 HU bone tissue-equivalent material |
| Acrylic linearity rod | Cast acrylic |
| Polyethylene linearity rod | Low-density polyethylene |
| Low-contrast module matrix | Ciba Geigy CB4 epoxy or equivalent |
| Low-contrast rods | Ciba Geigy CB4 epoxy (density adjusted to yield 6 ± 0.5 HU difference) or equivalent |
| Tungsten carbide beads | 0.011 in diameter grade 25 tungsten carbide beads |
| Line pair material | 6061 aluminum and polystyrene |
| Steel beads | 1.00 mm grade 25 chrome steel balls |
| Intramodule homogeneity | The mean ROI values within any module, test objects excluded, can differ by no more than 2 HU |
| Intraphantom homogeneity, modules 1, 3, and 4 | The average CT number of a module must meet the requirements of 0 ± 5 HU |

Optional phantom stand available. Optional hard and soft cases available.
(Courtesy Gammex Inc., Middleton, Wis.)

## WHY QUALITY CONTROL?

The answer to the question, "Is a QC program needed for the CT scanner?" is usually "yes." Modern hospitals and clinics that operate CT scanners and other complex instruments have long recognized the value of QC programs to maintain high performance standards for their patients. In addition, regulatory agencies increasingly demand that some standard of quality be maintained on x-ray units and other equipment that can potentially harm patients if the units are not performing optimally. These agencies frequently require that institutions using CT scanners verify the scanner's performance periodically (e.g., daily, weekly, monthly, annually) and often prescribe alternative measures if the performance standards are not met. To meet these regulatory requirements, a QC program must be operational.

In the case of CT scanners, the engineering is exceedingly complex. With so many mechanical and electronic parts involved in the creation of the images, there are many opportunities for the quality of the images to subtly and unnoticeably degrade. The mechanical parts of these complex, heavy instruments can wear slowly. Electronic parts can change characteristics and drift out of optimal adjustment. When this occurs, the CT scanner may no longer yield the same quality images it did when it was in proper adjustment. Often, this wear and drift can be repaired or compensated, but the suboptimal imaging problems must first be recognized. Comparing modern QC data with past data can demonstrate that the scanner is not performing as well as in the past.

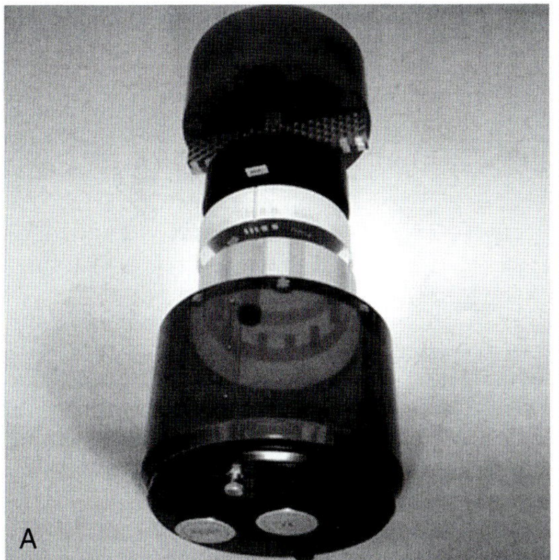


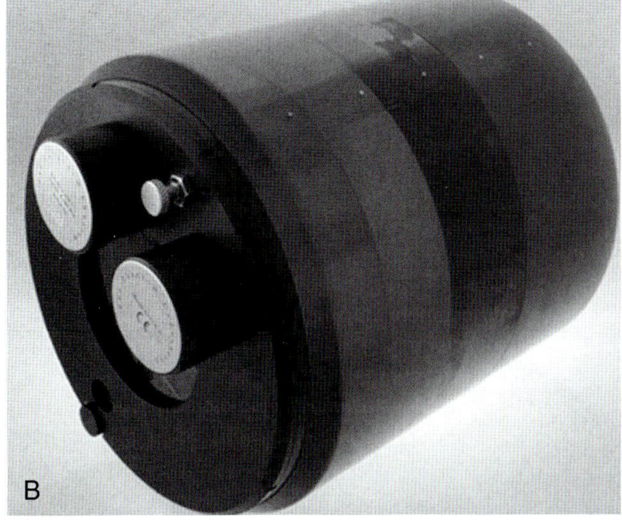


**FIGURE 18-2** The Catphan 700 housing **(A)** and three solid-cast test modules are mounted inside the phantom's housing **(B)**. (Courtesy The Phantom Laboratory, Salem, New York.)

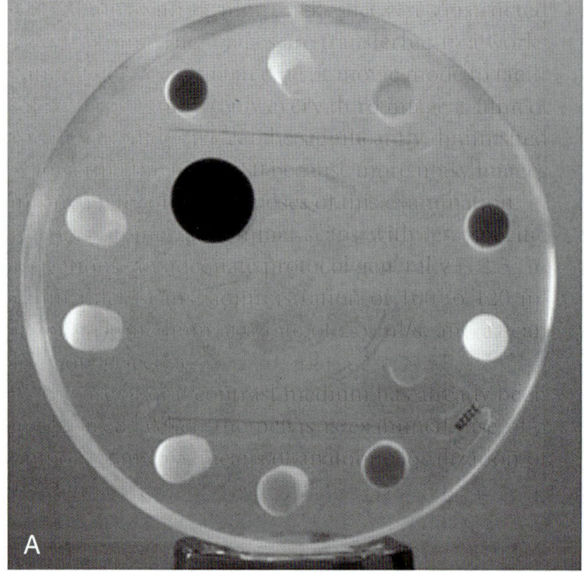

Geometry Sensitometry Module

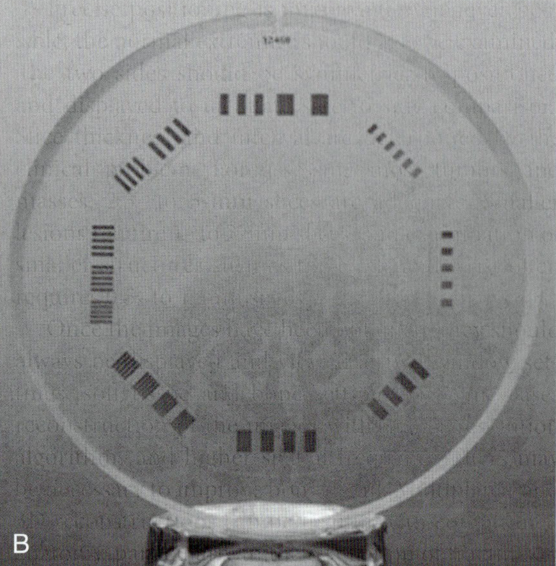

30 Line Pair High-Resolution Module

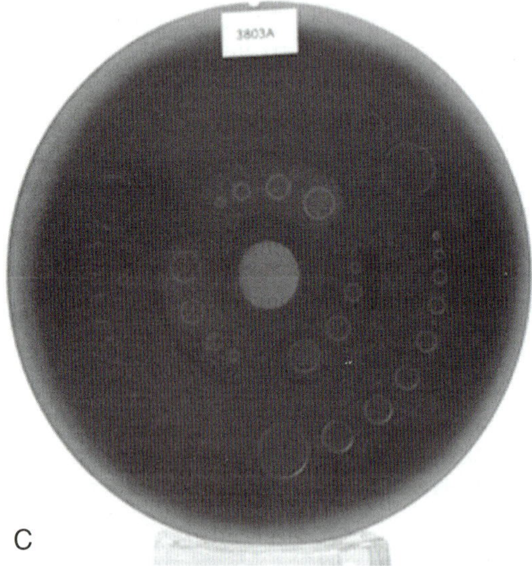

Low-Contrast Module

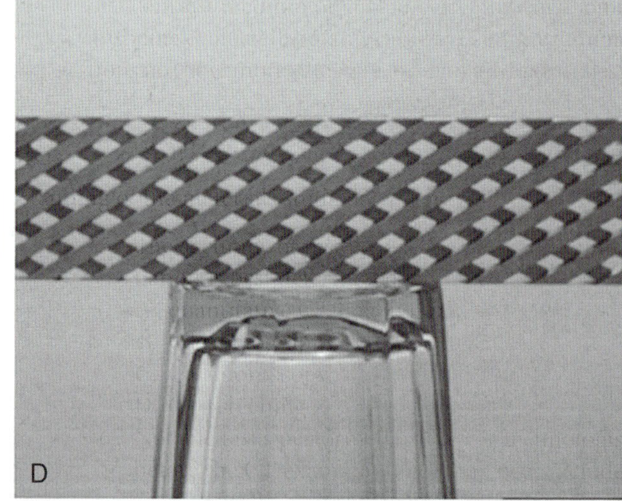

Wave Insert and Bead Blocks

**FIGURE 18-3** The Catphan 700 contains three solid-cast test modules positioned inside the housing of the phantom such as sensitometry slice geometry module **(A)**, a 30 lp/cm module **(B)**, and a low-contrast sphere array **(C)**. In addition, the phantom also contains the new wave insert for measuring slice geometry and resolution across the scan area **(D)**. (Courtesy of the Phantom Laboratory, Salem, New York).

A QC program can be an important ally in many aspects of CT scanner service. For example, if the QC data are used to define the problem and its extent, the service person will be better able to correct a subtle image quality problem. If a measurable change can be quantitatively demonstrated to the service person, the necessity of repair will be more apparent, and the degree to which it should be repaired can be specified (i.e., "we want it to perform like new" or "as good as last August").

Often a QC program can result in reduced downtime. A good QC program may recognize weakened or marginally performing parts before complete failure, and unscheduled service may be avoided.

## THREE TENETS OF QUALITY CONTROL

Three basic tenets of quality control are as follows:

1. *QC must be performed on a regular periodic basis.* Ideally, these tests might be performed between

each patient examination. At this testing frequency, there would be maximal assurance that the CT scanner was always operating correctly. However, in reality, this very frequent QC attention is too costly in terms of the time taken from patient examinations. Some compromises must be made for the sake of time and effort.

It does seem prudent to perform certain quick tests on a daily basis. Less important or more time-consuming tests might be performed less frequently (e.g., monthly), and the most complex tests might be performed semiannually or yearly. The institution's philosophy and its willingness to devote time to periodic QC tests often dictate which tests are performed and how often. To an administrator watching the revenues generated by a CT scanner, QC has a double affliction of requiring labor, which must be paid, and reducing the availability of the CT scanner for patients, which reduces revenue. A compromise must be reached that balances the effort and expense of a QC program with the expected benefits, such as better images, consistent images, reduced downtime, and legal and regulatory dose requirements.

2. *Prompt interpretation of the measurements.* Data usually show that the CT scanner is operating within specified guidelines. But on those occasions when it is not, this fact must be recognized and some remedial action must be taken. This action may be as simple as notifying the physicist, service person, or radiologist, or it may be as aggressive as taking the unit out of service until it is repaired. To institute this facet of the QC program, the person making the test must be able to recognize that the results are outside acceptable limits. Some mechanism should be in place that alerts the QC technologist to errant behavior of the scanner. For example, on the data form for a particular test, acceptable limits of the data may be stated. From an inspection of the measured results, the QC technologist can recognize immediately that the results are out of tolerance. Another method is to enter data into a computer, then instruct the computer to issue an appropriate alert when limits are exceeded. In the latter case, the temptation to sit on data for a few days or weeks before they are entered into the computer must be avoided. If a computer is to be relied on to make the necessary comparisons and if the program is to be effective, the data must be entered promptly.
3. *Faithful bookkeeping.* If time and effort are to be expended to perform the tests, then the results should be recorded. These results should be maintained in a logbook, data form, or computer for a reasonable period, usually as long as the CT scanner is active (i.e., for its lifetime). Keeping good records is not just a tedious exercise. These results will prove invaluable if the unit appears to be malfunctioning in the future. A comparison of past measurements with current results can easily demonstrate a change in performance (usually degradation). These data can also prove important to defend a lawsuit that might arise because of a reading of a CT image. For example, if litigation arises that is dependent on an interpretation (or misinterpretation) of a CT image and data can be produced from the QC logbook to demonstrate that the CT scanner was functioning satisfactorily at the time of interpretation, then the CT scanner is removed as a source of blame for the interpretation.

## QUALITY CONTROL TESTS FOR CT SCANNERS

Historically, current QC tests have evolved from those published in the literature (Burkhart et al., 1987; Cacak, 1985; Cacak & Hendee, 1979; McCollough et al., 2004) and described in Report 99 of the National Council on Radiation Protection and Measurement (1988). More complex physics tests are outlined in Report 39 of the American Association of Physics in Medicine (AAPM, 1993). Additionally, Health Canada (2008) outlined CT QC tests for CT facilities in Canada, for the purposes of ensuring that CT scanners meet national guidelines to protect patients, personnel, and members of the public from radiation dose from CT scanners. Additionally, AAPM Report No. 111: Comprehensive Methodology for the Evaluation of Radiation Dose in X-Ray Computed Tomography (2010) outlined "a new measurement paradigm based on a unified theory for axial, helical, fan-beam, and **cone-beam scanning** with or without longitudinal translation of the patient table." This report, as noted by the AAPM, is to "make available an accurate approach for specifying CT radiation doses based on a theoretically coherent measurement methodology that can be readily implemented by medical physicists and that can be supported by manufacturers, standards developers, and regulators."

More recently, Nute et al. (2013) in a study that examined the "evaluation of over 100 scanner-years of computed tomography daily quality control data." the authors concluded that the

> standard deviation of water is the most important quantitative value to collect as part of a daily QC program. Uniformity and linearity tests have

relatively low failure rates and, therefore, may not require daily verification. While its failure rates were moderate, daily artefact analysis is suggested due to its potentially high impact on clinical image quality. Weekly or monthly large phantom artifact analysis is encouraged for those sites possessing an appropriate phantom. Although the tests are similar to those described in these references, the types and frequency of the QC tests may vary somewhat to reflect advances in CT scanner technology.

The methods described in the remainder of this chapter provide some details of the testing procedure, the equipment required, interpretation of the results, some suggestions for acceptable limits, and how often the tests should be performed. The tests are listed in approximate order of importance, with some weighting of the tests according to the ability to perform the test quickly and easily.

## Choosing a Technique for Quality Control Measurements

The selection of technique for the QC tests depends on the type of CT scanner and the test being performed. Many variables can be selected for each test, including peak kilovoltage (kVp), milliamperage (mA), scan time, **slice width,** type of **algorithm,** x-ray filter type, and focal spot size. The number of possible combinations of techniques is usually overwhelming, and the best that can be done is to select one or two representative techniques. In general, the technique should remain the same for a specific test from day to day. However, the technique for one test does not have to be the same as the technique for other tests. A good rule of thumb is to use a technique that matches a frequently used clinical technique. One way to select a QC technique is to choose the most frequently used head or body technique and use it for the tests. As many tests as possible should be performed with this technique, with the understanding that deviations may be required for some tests.

## Test Priority and Test Frequency

It is usually necessary to limit the more complex tests to annual surveys, those occasions when the CT scanner is initially tested for acceptance, and subsequent occasions when the deterioration of image quality is suspected. It is good practice to repeat appropriate tests after replacement of a major component such as an **x-ray tube** or after the performance of extensive service or adjustments. If data from CT scanner images are used quantitatively or if the precision of an image is used for accurately localizing tissue (e.g., to perform biopsies or plan radiation therapy treatment), the frequency of appropriate tests should be increased.

The IAEA, for example, classifies QC tests into two types that define their priority: those that are essential and those that are desirable. While *essential* tests must be conducted by CT departments, *desirable* tests are those that should be done, if practical (IAEA, 2012).

## Limits of a "Passing" Test

What are *acceptable limits*? How big should the window of acceptable values be for each test described here before the CT scanner is considered "out of tolerance"? These complex questions depend on the technology of the unit tested, the type of test instrument used, and the imaging technique.

Perhaps more important than the actual value of the measured variable is a change in the variable between measurements. A CT scanner that is operating the same today as it did yesterday should produce nearly the same results when the test is repeated. After acceptable limits are established, a quick inspection of the measurements can identify deviant values. Past history can provide good insight into what the values have been. A range that includes most values when the unit was operating optimally can be easily determined from an inspection of past values. Of course, it is never absolutely certain that the CT scanner was operating optimally in the past when these supposedly "good" readings were taken. But if the readings were taken when the unit was new or believed to be functioning well, then they can be presumed to be "good" readings and used as a standard.

The IAEA (2012) provided two "performance standards" for QC test results. These include acceptable and achievable. While *acceptable* "indicates that performance must be within certain tolerances, and if it is not, the equipment should not be used," *achievable* "indicates the level of performance that should be attained under favorable circumstances, which is the level at which a facility should work if feasible."

It is important to realize that various authorities such as the ACR, the IAEA, and RPB-HC provide acceptance or tolerance limits that may not exactly be the same as the generic ones mentioned earlier. For example, the acceptable limits for three QC tests (CT number accuracy, CT number uniformity, and radiation dose) from these three organizations are given in Table 18-2.

## Quality Control Tests

QC tests described in this section include **visual inspection** of the various components of the CT scanner and those that address the *routine performance* of the scanner. For routine performance, the acceptance

**TABLE 18-2 Acceptance Criteria or Tolerance Limits for Three CT QC Tests from one International Organization (IAEA) and Two National Organizations (ACR and RPB-HC)**

| | ACCEPTANCE CRITERIA OR TOLERANCE LIMITS | | |
|---|---|---|---|
| **QC Tests** | **ACR** | **IAEA** | **RPB-HC** |
| CT number accuracy | 0 ± 7 HU (±5 HU preferred) | 0 ± 5 HU | 0 ± 4 HU |
| CT number uniformity | The center CT number must be between ±7 HU (±5 HU preferred) Adult abdomen protocol must be used | ±10 HU | CT number for water must not be greater than ±5 HU from the center of the phantom to the periphery |
| Radiation dose | The $CTDI_W$ should not exceed 35 mGy for the adult abdomen protocol and CTDI | ±20% of manufacturer's specification | $CTDI_W$, which must be within ±20% of the established baseline values and the manufacturer's specifications; it is highly recommended to strive for an agreement with manufacturers' specification of ±10% |

criteria for the ACR CT Accreditation tests will be outlined, followed by a set of proposed routine performance QC tests. For the routine performance QC tests, suggestions are given regarding the following: phantom or equipment, expected results, acceptance limits, possible causes of failure, and frequency of tests.

Some **generic limits** are suggested for these QC tests, and CT departments must decide upon the specific tolerance limits for their QC program, based on the requirements of the related national authorities. For example, if a CT facility participates in the ACR CT Accreditation program, then it is clear that the ACR phantom and the associated tolerance limits must be used. A Canadian CT facility must use the acceptance or tolerance limits provided in Safety Code 35: Radiation Protection in Radiology—Large Facilities (Health Canada, 2008).

## ACR CT Accreditation QC Tests

These tests are described in detail by the ACR (2012) and by McCollough et al. (2004). As noted earlier in the chapter, the ACR CT Accreditation program requires the use of the ACR phantom and the following QC tests using the four modules that make up the phantom. These tests include CT number accuracy, slice thickness, light accuracy alignment, low-contrast resolution, CT number uniformity, and high-contrast resolution. The essential acceptance criteria for these tests are provided in Table 18-3.

Furthermore, CT number linearity and radiation dose must also be included in these tests. As described in Chapter 9, *linearity* refers to the relationship of CT numbers to the **linear attenuation coefficients** of the

**TABLE 18-3 Acceptance Criteria for the ACR CT Accreditation QC Tests Using the ACR Phantom**

| ACR QC Tests | Essential Acceptance Criteria |
|---|---|
| Light accuracy alignment | The light field and x-ray field should coincide to within 2 mm |
| High-contrast resolution (spatial resolution) | 1. For the adult abdomen: 5 lp/cm must be clearly seen<br>2. For the adult chest: 6 lp/cm must be clearly seen |
| Low-contrast resolution | All four 6 mm cylinders must be clearly seen when using the adult abdomen and head CT protocols |
| Image uniformity | 1. ±7 HU (±5 HU preferred) for adult protocol<br>2. Edge to center mean CT number difference must be less than 5 HU for the four edge locations |
| Noise | Results should be compared with the specifications of the Manufacturer |
| CT number accuracy | • Bone = +850 and +970 HU<br>• Acrylic = +110 and +130 HU<br>• Water = ±7 HU (±5 HU preferred)<br>• Polyethylene = −107 and −87 HU<br>• Air = −1005 and −970 HU |
| Slice thickness | Must be within 1.5 mm of the prescribed slice width |

Data from ACR. (2012). *2012 computed tomography manual: radiologic technologists' section.* <http://www.acr.org/Quality-Safety/accreditation/CT> Accessed February 2015.

object to be imaged. The average CT numbers can also be plotted as a function of the attenuation coefficients of the phantom materials. The relationship should be a straight line (see Fig. 9-26) if the scanner is in good working order (Bushong, 2013). For radiation dose the $CTDI_{vol}$ should be measured and should be below the pass/fail criterion of 80 milligray (mGy) for the adult head protocol, 30 mGy for the adult abdomen protocol, and 25 mGy for the pediatric abdomen protocol (ACR, 2012; Papp, 2015; Wolbarst et al., 2013).

## Visual Inspection

A visual inspection component of a CT QC program ensures that the integrity of radiation protection considerations, including patient safety concerns (ACR 2012; IAEA, 2012), is maintained. In general, a checklist of items should be used since it provides a good tool to record the status of the scanner components. While the ACR assigns this task to the technologist, the IAEA assigns this task to the medical physicist.

The ACR (2012) recommended that visual inspection be performed on a monthly basis and should include items such as the following:

1. Check the functioning of the table height indicator, the table **position** and angulation indicators, laser localization light, x-ray on indicator, **exposure** switch, door interlocks, control panel switches, lights and meters, and the intercom system.
2. Check high voltage and other cables for fraying.
3. Check the window width and window level display.
4. Check for the presence of warning labels and availability of all service records.

The IAEA (2012), on the other hand, suggested that the following items be evaluated:

1. Scan protocol book
2. Items (such as QC tests performed and corrective action taken) in the quality control log book are well documented for currency
3. Cleanliness of the scanner room
4. Door of the scanner room operates properly
5. Radiation protection lead shields are available
6. Emergency equipment is available
7. Window between operator's room and scanner room provides clear view of patient (no clutter on the window)
8. Image headers are correct, including patient identification, date, and time
9. Written radiation safety procedures up to date
10. Staff (including radiologists) understands and follows radiation safety procedures (IAEA, 2012)

## Artifact Evaluation

The ACR also requires the CT technologist to be able to identify and correct image artifacts from a water phantom, on a daily basis. These artifacts include both linear streak and ring artifacts (see Chapter 9).

## Proposed QC Tests

There are 18 QC tests described below ranging from CT number calibration, standard deviation of CT number in water, high-contrast resolution, low-contrast resolution, accuracy of distance-measuring device, uniformity or flatness of CT number, hard copy output, accuracy of localization device, CT bed indexing and CT bed backlash, and light field accuracy to **pitch** and slice width (spiral/helical scanner), CT number versus patient position, CT number versus patient size, CT number versus algorithm, CT number versus slice width, noise characteristics, and radiation scatter and leakage. Each of these is described next. It is important to note that since the use of film has become obsolete, computed radiography (CR) cassettes can be used in the tests that mention the use of film.

- TEST 1: Average CT number of the water (CT number calibration)

  Phantom or equipment: A simple water-filled cylindrical plastic container approximately 20 cm in diameter. Commercial phantoms are available for this test and are often provided by the CT manufacturer, but some institutions have used 1-gallon plastic containers from liquid laundry bleach. The bleach, of course, is replaced with water.

  Measurement: Take an axial scan through the water phantom at the usual technique. Reconstruct the image of the water phantom. Examine the **region of interest (ROI)** feature available on the imaging monitor of most scanners to verify that the scanner can measure the average of the CT numbers of the pixels inside the ROI. Enlarge the ROI area to include an area of about 2 to 3 $cm^2$ (or about 200 to 300 pixels). Position the ROI near the center of the phantom image and measure the average CT number (Fig. 18-4).

  Two media that serve as calibration points for CT numbers are water and air. Occasionally (e.g., once a month), move the ROI outside the phantom into the region of the image that is known to contain air. Check the average CT number of air. It should be −1000 if the CT scanner is calibrated properly.

  Expected results: The average CT number of water should be very close to zero.

  Acceptance limits: If the average CT number of water is more than three CT numbers away from 0 (i.e., outside the range −3 to +3

Hounsfield units [HU]), the CT scanner fails the test. The CT number of air should be −1000 ± 5 HU.

Possible causes of failure: Miscalibration of the algorithm that generates the CT number. If a recalibration does not help, notify the service person. Usually the manufacturer provides a procedure to recalibrate the CT number scale.

Frequency: This should be performed at the time of installation as part of acceptance test and daily thereafter.

- TEST 2: Standard deviation of computed tomography number in water

Phantom or equipment: A simple water-filled cylindrical plastic container about 20 cm in diameter (the same phantom used in Test 1).

Measurement: Use the same image as in Test 1 (Fig. 18-4). Position the ROI near the center of the phantom image and measure the standard deviation of the CT number.

Expected results: Typical values are in the range of two to seven CT numbers. The actual value will depend on the dose at the location of the ROI, which depends on the kVp, mA, scan duration, slice width, and phantom size. The standard deviation of the CT number also depends on the type of reconstruction algorithm (can be higher with sharp algorithm compared with smooth algorithm) and the position of the ROI (slightly smaller at the edge of the phantom compared with the center). Ensure that the technique is the same each day and that the standard deviation is measured at the same place each time (e.g., the center of the phantom).

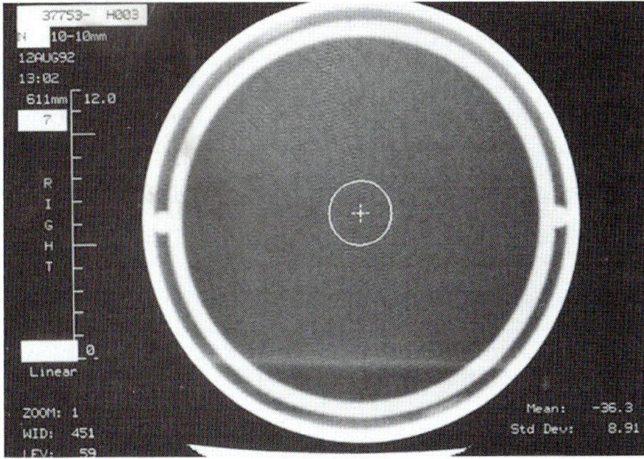


**FIGURE 18-4** CT scanner image of a uniform water phantom. The ROI is placed in the center of the water-filled phantom to measure the average CT number and the standard deviation of the CT numbers inside the ROI. In this case, the average or "mean" CT number measures –36.3, which is not acceptable.

Acceptance limits: Ideally, the standard deviation should be very small. The actual acceptance limits must be determined by examination of past measurements that were presumably performed when the performance of the CT scanner was good. The technique must stay the same for this measurement from day to day. If the standard deviation starts to increase, this indicates a "noisier" image with more variation in pixel-to-pixel CT numbers and poorer low-contrast resolution.

Possible causes of failure: Something is causing a noisier image, such as decreased dose (x-ray tube output) or increased electronic noise of the x-ray detectors, amplifiers, or analog-to-digital (A/D) converters. Notify the service person.

Frequency: This should be performed at the time of installation as part of the acceptance test and daily thereafter.

- TEST 3: High-contrast resolution

Phantom or equipment: High-contrast (contrast difference of 10% or greater) resolution pattern in an imaging phantom. Although a variety of patterns are available to perform high-contrast tests, including patterns for generating modulation transfer function measurements, a quick and easy test pattern is most suitable for QC tests. One such pattern consists of a series of rows of holes drilled in plastic (Fig. 18-5).

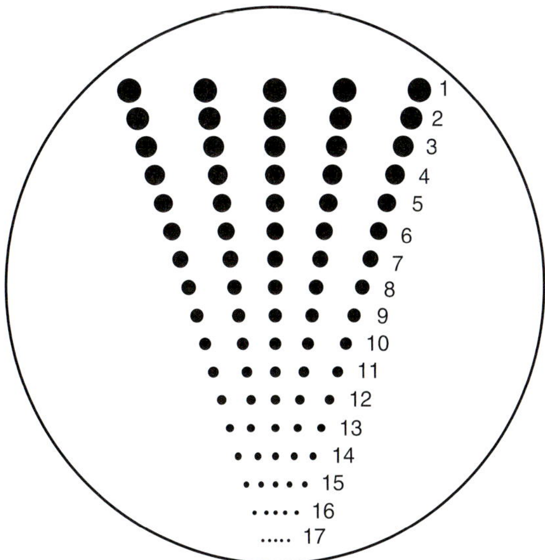


**FIGURE 18-5** Hole pattern for a high-contrast phantom test object. The test pattern consists of rows of holes of various sizes drilled in plastic. Each row contains five holes of the same diameter. In a row of constant sizes, the holes are separated by two diameters from center to center.

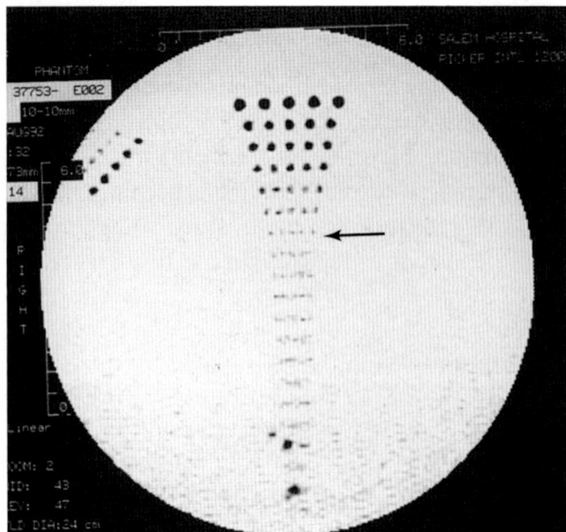

**FIGURE 18-6** CT image of the high-contrast test pattern shown in Figure 18-5. The CT scanner is judged by the smallest row in which all five holes can be seen (*arrow*).

Each row contains a set of holes (usually five) of constant diameter with the centers of the holes two diameters apart. The holes decrease in size from one row to the next. If the holes are drilled in acrylic and filled with water, the contrast is about 20%. If the holes are filled with air, the contrast is about 100%. Either filling is satisfactory. Another pattern consists of eight aluminum bar patterns (4 to 12 lp/cm) embedded in a tissue equivalent material.

Measurement: On the axial CT image (Fig. 18-6), determine the smallest row of holes in which all holes can be clearly seen. The smaller the holes that can be clearly seen, the better the performance of the CT scanner. Be certain that all holes can be seen in the image. Sometimes it appears that one fewer hole is seen in the row than is actually in the phantom. This is usually a phase-reversal phenomenon and should not be counted as a complete set of holes. On the other hand, the bar pattern where the bars and spaces are distinctly visualized indicates the level of high-contrast resolution.

Expected results: Most modern CT scanners have a high-contrast resolving power slightly smaller than 1 millimeter (mm) by using a typical head image technique. Therefore, they will be able to visualize a complete set of holes in some of the rows in the range of 0.75 to 1.0 mm. With the highest resolution technique available to a particular scanner, some CT scanner manufacturers claim to be able to visualize holes as small as 0.25 mm.

Acceptance limits: This baseline number should be established at the time of the acceptance test when the CT scanner is working well by scanning the phantom and noting the smallest set of holes that can be seen. This initial measurement becomes the baseline for future tests. Subsequent tests can be compared with this baseline. Alternatively, the manufacturer's specifications for this test can be used to verify that the performance of the CT scanner is at least as good as the specifications.

Possible causes of failure: Enlarged focal spot in the x-ray tube, excessive mechanical wear in the motion of the gantry, mechanical misalignments or poor registration of electromechanical components, vibrations, or detector failures. If the resolution has degraded from the baseline, inform the service person.

Frequency: This should be performed at the time of installation as part of the acceptance test and biannually thereafter.

- TEST 4: Low-contrast resolution

Phantom or equipment: Low-contrast resolution pattern in imaging phantom. A quick and easy test pattern of low-contrast test objects consists of a series of holes (2 to 8 mm diameter) drilled in polystyrene. The holes are filled with liquid (often water) to which has been added a small amount of some other material (usually methanol or sucrose) to bring the liquid's CT number close (about 0.5% different) to that of the plastic itself. One such pattern (Fig. 18-7) consists of a series of rows of holes drilled in relatively thick plastic. Each row contains holes of a constant diameter. The holes decrease in size from one row to the next. In a CT image, the holes appear to have a density similar to their surround (i.e., the holes have low contrast).

Another technique is to use **partial volume averaging** by making the plastic very thin (e.g., a plastic membrane). Low contrast in the image is achieved by a different principle than the solid plastic type of low-contrast phantom. The membrane type of phantom consists of a thin membrane containing a pattern of holes (the same pattern shown in Fig. 18-7). The membrane is stretched across a plane of the phantom and is then immersed in water. The CT x-ray beam, as visualized from its edge (Fig. 18-8), strikes mostly water. But a small fraction of the beam is absorbed by the plastic, forming a faint (low-contrast) image of the hole pattern. By varying the thickness of the plastic relative to the width of the x-ray beam, the contrast can be varied.

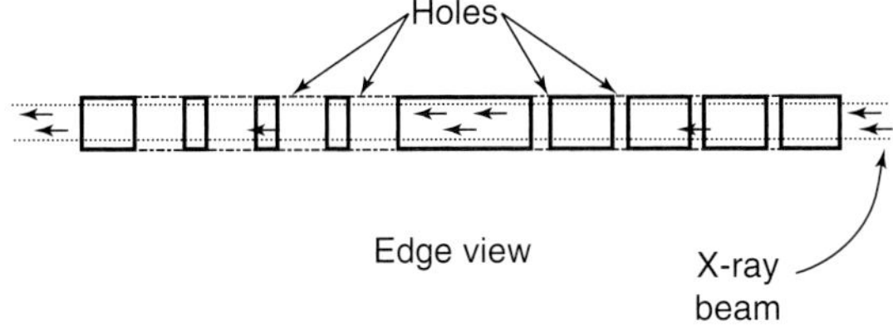


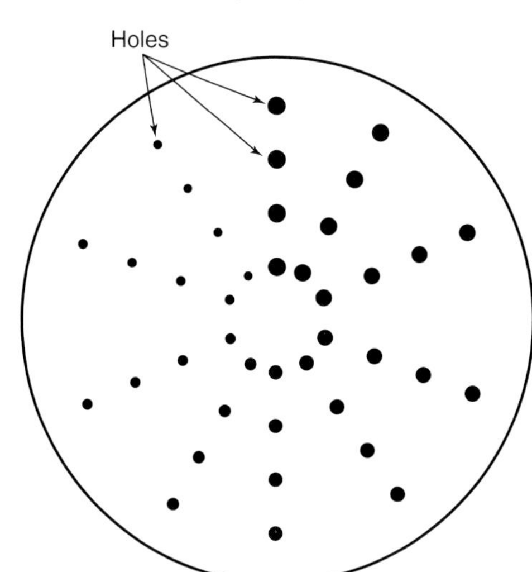


**FIGURE 18-7** "Solid plastic" type of low-contrast phantom test object that consists of a pattern of holes (face view) drilled in a piece of plastic with the holes filled with liquid. The low-contrast aspect of this test object is achieved by adjusting the absorption characteristics of the water solution to nearly match (about 0.5% difference) the absorption of the plastic.

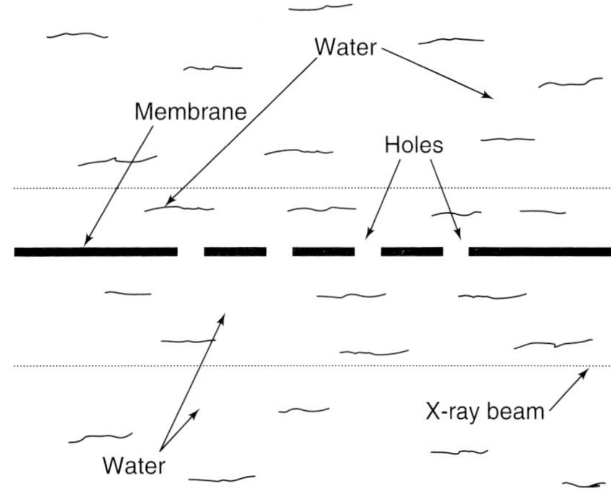


**FIGURE 18-8** Edge view of a membrane of partial-volume type of low-contrast test object. The presence of the thin membrane alters the absorption characteristics very slightly wherever there is membrane. Where the membrane is not present (i.e., in the holes), just water is absorbed. The slight difference in absorption characteristics between the water and the water-plus-membrane combination produce a low-contrast test pattern that appears as the hole pattern in the membrane.

In both techniques, the contrast of the object is difficult to calculate. In QC testing, it is sufficient that the contrast be constant between tests. The contrast should be selected so that the standard test image shows about 50% of the holes. At that level of hole imaging, a decrease in low-contrast imaging performance will result in the visualization of fewer rows of holes.

Measurement: On the CT image, determine the smallest row of holes in which all holes can be clearly seen. The smaller the holes that can be seen at a particular technique, the better the performance of the CT scanner. A sample of a "low-noise" (high-dose) image and a "high-noise" (low-dose) image is shown in Figure 18-9. In the low-noise image, more sets of smaller objects can be seen.

Expected results: The smallest holes that can be imaged by modern CT scanners should be 4 to 5 mm in diameter or smaller for 0.5% contrast objects. Perhaps more important, the minimum size of holes visualized should not increase over the life of the scanner.

Acceptance limits: The number of holes that can be visualized varies widely between techniques. For example, if a partial volume phantom is used, the apparent contrast of the object depends on the thickness of the membrane and the slice width of the image. In addition, an increase in mA value of the scan technique will usually reduce the noise in the image and will permit smaller holes to be visualized. Therefore a baseline scan at a chosen technique (usually a commonly used head technique) performed when the scanner is functioning well can serve as baseline against which future images can be compared. This technique, once chosen, should not be changed from day to day.

A smoothing algorithm filter can also reduce the apparent statistical fluctuations between pixels. These algorithms produce images with smaller standard deviations and usually permit visualization of smaller low-contrast objects by sacrificing some high-contrast resolution. Therefore it is important to always use the same reconstruction algorithm to compare repeated results from this test.

Possible causes of failure: A higher noise level in the image usually causes reduced low-contrast resolution. Some possible sources of increased noise are decreased dose, decreased mA values, or any other factor that will reduce the x-ray tube output, such as a tungsten coating build-up on the inside of older x-ray tubes. Increased electronic noise is also possible and may arise from noise in the x-ray detectors, amplifiers, or A/D converters. The service person should be informed of decreasing low-contrast resolution and asked to perform further diagnosis.

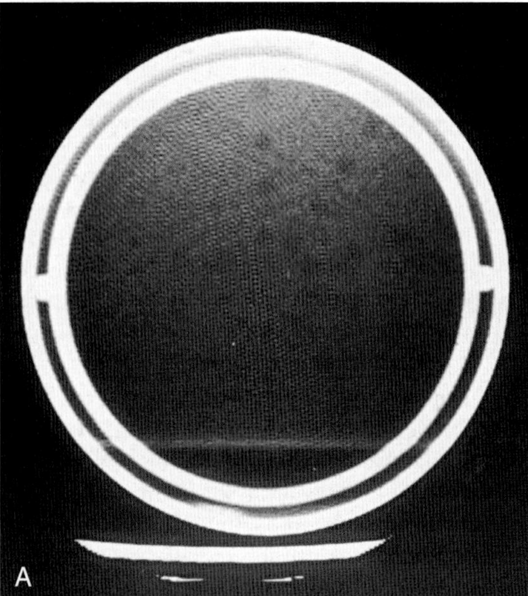


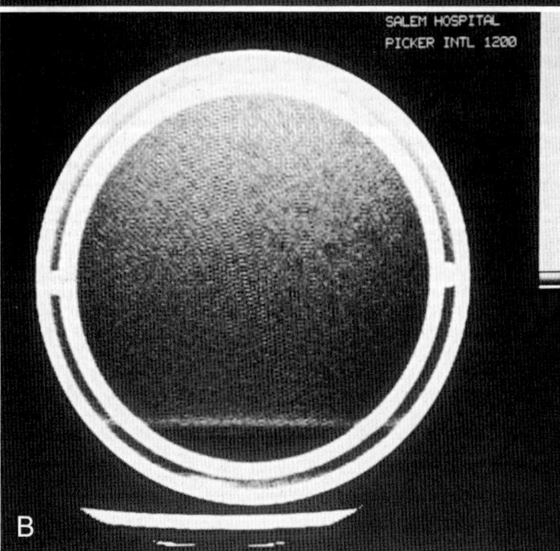


**FIGURE 18-9** Low-noise **(A)** and high-nose **(B)** low-contrast images produced with a membrane-type low-contrast test object obtained from a high-dose (low-noise) CT scan and a low-dose (high-noise) type of scan.

Frequency: This should be performed at the time of installation as part of the acceptance test and biannually thereafter.

- TEST 5: Accuracy of distance-measuring device

Phantom or equipment: An object with two or more small objects (this is a part of ACR phantom) that have a precisely known spatial relationship (i.e., the distance between them is precisely known). One such object is a large "+" pattern of small holes in a plastic phantom (Fig. 18-10). The holes are precisely 1 cm apart, and the size of the "+" is large enough to fill most of the image.

Some institutions have used an image of a regular square grid that covers most of the field of view. One source of square grids is a type of fluorescent light fixture that uses square grid light diffusers made of plastic with a square spacing of about 0.5 inch (12 mm). With a moderate amount of effort, the grids can be cut to fit inside a phantom or scanned in air (no phantom).

Measurement: With use of the distance-measuring feature available on the video monitors of most scanners, measure the **distance** between two well-visualized holes near the periphery of the phantom, one near the top and one near the bottom (Fig. 18-11). Repeat the measurement between two holes, moving right to left. If required, a diagonal measurement between two holes can be made and the true distance can be calculated by the Pythagorean Theorem.

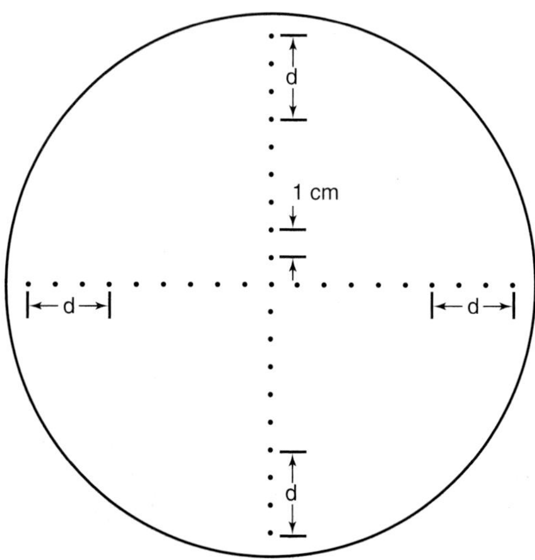


**FIGURE 18-10** A pattern of holes to measure image distortion. The pattern consists of a series of holes arranged in a "++" pattern that spans the diameter of the phantom. The holes are exactly 1 cm apart.

Expected results: The distance indicated by the CT scanner should agree with the true distance as determined by counting the spaces between the two holes.

Acceptance limits: Disagreement of 1 mm or less is good. Disagreement of greater than 2 mm should be corrected.

Possible causes of failure: Reconstruction algorithm may be improperly calibrated. If the manufacturer has not provided the user with a means to recalibrate the algorithm, a service person should be notified.

Frequency: This should be performed at the time of installation and annually thereafter.

- TEST 6: Uniformity or flatness of CT number

Phantom or equipment: A simple cylindrical plastic container about 20 cm in diameter (the same phantom used for Test 1).

Measurement: Using the ROI feature available on most CT scanners, measure the CT number of water near the top, bottom, right, and left of the phantom (Fig. 18-12). Use an ROI large enough to cover an area of 200 to 300 pixels. Compare with the measurement in Test 1.

Expected results: Ideally, the CT number of water will be zero at all points in the phantom.

Acceptance limits: If the CT number anywhere in the phantom differs by more than five CT numbers from the average CT number collected from all measurements, then the CT image does not have a uniform or *flat* image. If the CT number is high in the center and low near the perimeter of the phantom, the image exhibits *capping*. A low value in the center relative to the edges exhibits *cupping*.

Possible causes of failure: Often capping and cupping are the result of the hardening of the x-ray beam as it penetrates the phantom. Near the edges of the phantom, the x-ray beam does not penetrate as much phantom material, and the beam is softer (i.e., it has a lower average energy). To arrive at the center, the x rays must penetrate more phantom material and are harder near the center of the phantom. Because the effective energy of the x rays determines the absorption characteristics of the x rays, the absorption characteristics of water change slightly from center to edge in the phantom. Because the CT number is calculated from the number of x rays absorbed, slight differences in CT number may indicate differences of the average energy of the x-ray beam at various points in the phantom. Some CT scanners have software corrections built into the algorithm that compensate for these x-ray beam-hardening effects, and these corrections sometimes overcompensate or undercompensate for the **beam hardening.** The service person may be able to adjust the algorithm to compensate for an unflat image.

Frequency: This should be performed at the time of installation as part of the acceptance test and monthly/biannually thereafter. Furthermore, this may be done daily or weekly on many scanners,

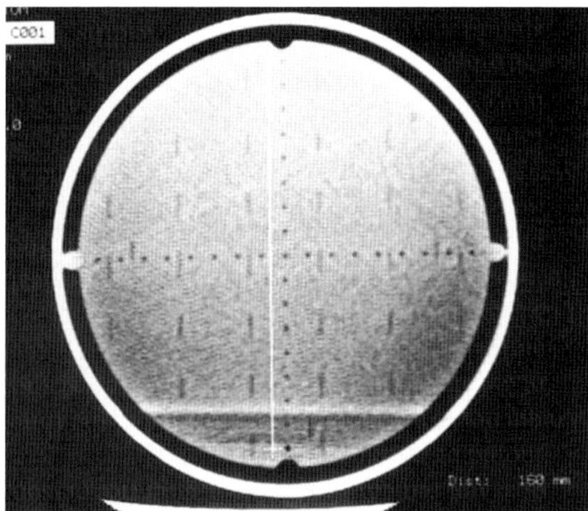


**FIGURE 18-11** Testing the distance-measuring device by measuring the distance between two holes separated by a precisely known distance. In this case the measured distance (*Dist*) between two holes spaced 16 cm apart is 160 mm (perfect).

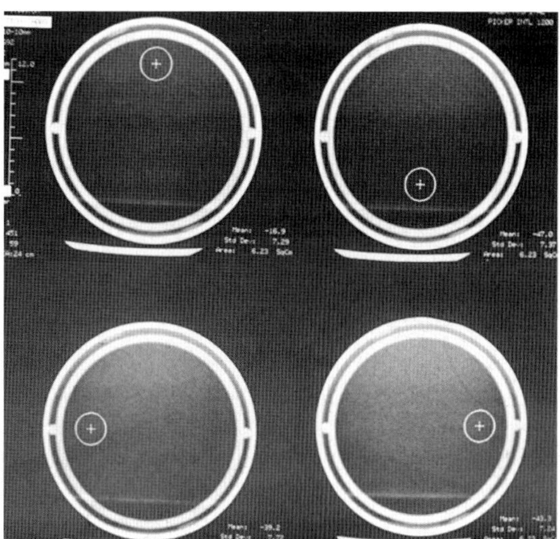

**FIGURE 18-12** Use several ROIs to measure flatness. In a homogeneous water phantom, the CT number should measure zero at any location in the phantom. In these images, the CT number at the top measures −16.9 and the rest of the image has values in the range of −37 to −47. This image is unacceptable because it is not "flat."

as with water HU and SD, since it serves to cover HU, SD, and uniformity at one time.

- TEST 7: Hard copy output

  Phantom or equipment: A stepped grayscale image generated by the computer such as Society of Motion Picture and Television Engineers (SMPTE) pattern and a film densitometer.

  Measurement: Display the SMPTE pattern on the display monitor. Adjust the display contrast so that both 95% and 100% patches are clearly separated. The 5% patch should just be visible inside of the 0% patch. The area of the 0% patch should be almost black. The 95% patch should be visible inside the 100% patch. Print the image and display on a viewbox to ensure the visibility of the 5% and 95% patch (McCollough et al., 2004; Fig. 18-13).

  Expected results: The same image should be reproduced with a the hard copy device each time the image is recorded.

  Acceptance limits: If the hard copy image is unable to display both 5% and 95% patches, examine the display setting and also the printer setting. If the condition still exists, then investigate further with a service person to reset the hard copy printer settings.

  Possible causes of failure: Most frequently, drifts in the optical density of films from the camera can be traced to problems in the film processing. However, if the processor has been eliminated as a source of the problem, then the camera must be assumed to be the errant instrument. Sometimes the video monitor, laser, or other light device used to expose the film has changed its output. In this case a service person should be called for repairs.

  Frequency: This should be performed at the time of installation as part of the acceptance test and annually thereafter.

- TEST 8: Accuracy of localization device

  Phantom or equipment: A test object with a target that can be aimed for in the localization image and a gauge that indicates how far the resulting CT images fall from the target. One example of this phantom is a set of two small holes drilled in plastic that are perpendicular to each other but at 45 degrees to the plane of the image. A cross-sectional drawing of the device is shown in Figure 18-14. The two

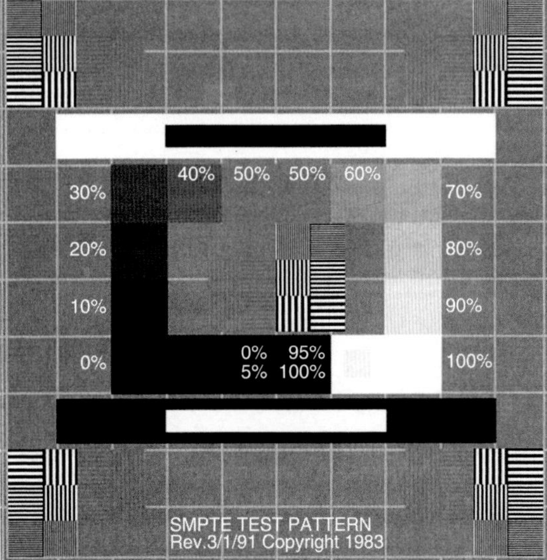


**FIGURE 18-13** SMPTE image for checking hard copy output. A film image of this pattern is processed and visualized to examine the visibility of 5% and 95% squares. (From Carter, C. E., & Veale, B. L. (2008). *Digital radiography and PACS*. St. Louis, MO: Mosby/Elsevier.)

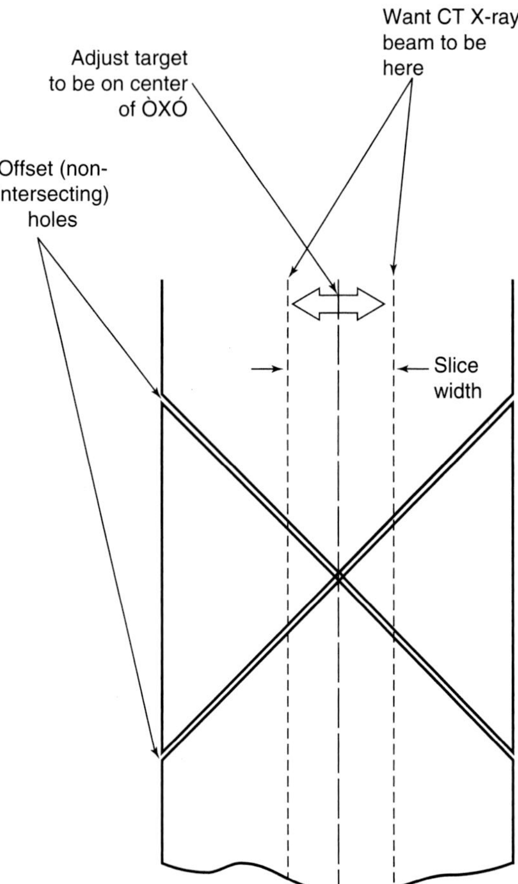


**FIGURE 18-14** Target pattern to test localization device. After this section is imaged with the localization image, the CT image is targeted directly on the spot where the two holes tilted 45 degrees to the scan plane appear to cross. Then a scan is performed and an image at the targeted location is reconstructed. In the image, the relative location of the two slanted holes indicates the position of the scan relative to the target.

holes are offset slightly and do not intersect. The localization target is centered on the point where the two holes appear to intersect in the localization image, and a scan is performed. After the CT image is reconstructed, the holes should appear directly opposite each other with perfect alignment between the holes. If there is offset in the holes, the scan is not being performed where the localization image shows it to be.

Measurement: Image the phantom by using the localization device (sometimes called a *scout* or *targeting* image). With this localization image, set up the scanner to make a single scan at a certain thickness so that the center of the scan is directly on the intersection of the holes. Make a scan and reconstruct the image. At the very least, both holes should appear in the CT image. If they do not, then the localization device is so poorly adjusted that the width of the x-ray beam does not intersect the plastic section in which the holes are drilled. If the localization device is working properly, the image of the two holes should appear exactly side by side (Fig. 18-15). If the holes are not aligned, then the center of the slice is off target. The distance that the center of the CT image is located from its targeted position (the intersection of the holes) can be quantified by measuring the amount of offset of the two holes in the image. By using the distance-measuring device on the video monitor (the measurement can be made with a ruler on the video monitor or on the hard copy image if there is no distortion in these devices and if appropriate compensation for the magnification of the image is made), measure the distance from the tip of one hole to the tip of the other hole (Fig. 18-16). The

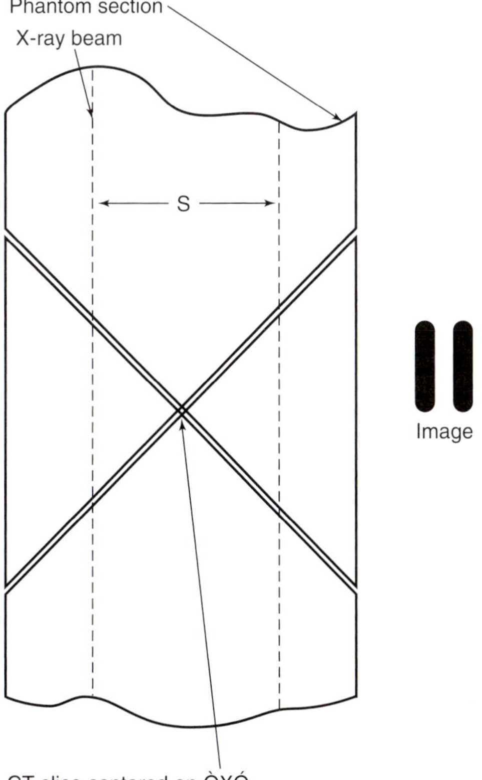


**FIGURE 18-15** Example of CT slice centered on the spot where the holes appear to cross. If the two holes are aligned as shown, the localization feature is on target.

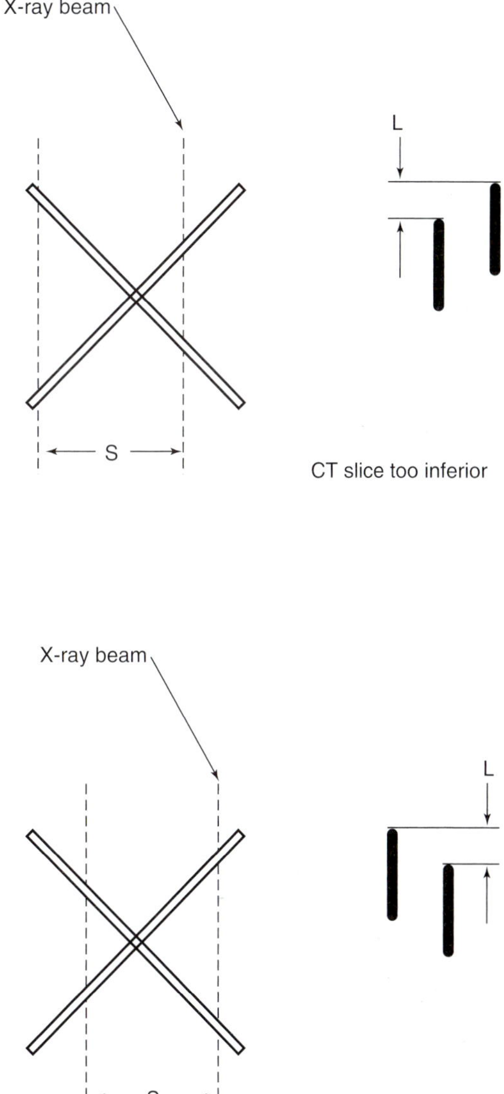


**FIGURE 18-16** Measurement of *L* for slice localization accuracy. If the two holes appear offset in the image, the error in the localization feature can be determined by measuring the offset of the lines *L*.

distance that the center of the CT slice is from the targeted location is equal to the length $L$.

Repeat the test at other slice widths.

Note that the lengths of the holes on the image, measured from end to end, are a direct measurement of the width of the CT slice. See Test 12 for a more thorough description of why this is so.

Expected results: In the ideal case, the holes should be exactly aligned.

Acceptance limits: If the measured value of $L$ is 3 mm or greater, the localization device is out of adjustment and a service person should be called.

Possible causes of failure: Miscalibration of the patient bed-positioning mechanisms is usually the cause, although a software problem is also possible.

Frequency: This should be performed at the time of installation as part of acceptance test and annually thereafter.

- TEST 9: Bed indexing

Phantom or equipment: A single piece of x-ray film or a Computed Radiography (CR) cassetteA 10 × 12-inch "Ready-pak" film (Kodak) works particularly well.

Measurement: The x-ray film is taped to the patient table; the length of the film is parallel to the length of the bed. The scanner is programmed to perform a series of 10 to 12 scans; each scan is 10 mm from the preceding scan with the slice width set to the smallest width available (less than 5 mm). The bed is loaded with at least 100 pounds (50 kilograms [kg]) of material to simulate the weight of a patient. When the scan is initiated, the x-ray beam exposes a series of narrow bands on the film (Fig. 18-17). With a ruler, measure the distance between the bands to determine how much the film (and bed) has moved between each scan.

Expected results: The distance from center to center of the exposed bands on the film is expected to be 10 mm, or whatever the scan spacing was chosen to be.

Acceptance limits: A series of 10 scans (nine interscan spacings) should create a series of exposed bands exactly 90 mm from the first to the last band. If the measured length of this band distance differs by more than 1 mm, the bed movement is not accurate and a service person should be notified.

Possible causes of failure: Excessive slippage in the bed drive mechanism or miscalibration of the bed position indicators. Notify a service person.

Frequency: This should be performed at the time of installation as part of the acceptance test and annually thereafter.

- TEST 10: Bed backlash

Phantom or equipment: Two small lengths of masking tape, a pencil, and a ruler.

Measurement: The patient bed is loaded with at least 100 pounds (50 kg) of material to simulate the weight of a patient. The bed is moved to a convenient location to serve as a zero point. Two strips of masking tape are placed adjacent to each other, one on the edge of the movable part of the bed, the other on a part of the bed that does not move (Fig. 18-18). A pencil mark is placed on each piece of tape so that the two marks are exactly opposite each other. The CT scanner is programmed to move the bed automatically about 150 to 200 mm in 10- or

**FIGURE 18-17** Measurement of bed indexing from an exposed x-ray film. The series of dark lines on the film are produced by several scans through a piece of x-ray film, moving the bed after each scan. The distance between the lines (*B*) is a measure of the distance that the patient bed has moved between scans.

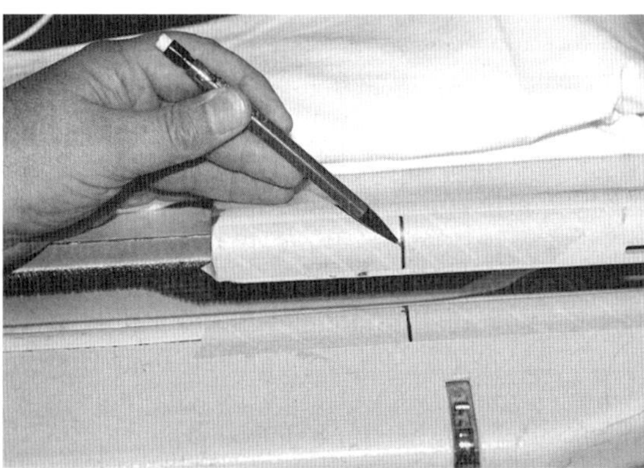

**FIGURE 18-18** Two strips of tape on the bed to determine bed backlash for both the moveable and stationary parts of the bed. The two pencil marks opposite each other define the starting or zero location of the bed.

20-mm increments in one direction (for example, bed into scanner), and then return to its original (zero) starting location. After all the motions, the mark on the moving bed should return to its original position opposite the stationary mark. A measurement of the distance between the two marks indicates if there are mechanical discrepancies ("backlash") in the patient bed.

This measurement should be repeated driving the bed in the opposite direction as the first test.

If there is a position readout on the bed, the readout should be tested by driving the bed in and out about 200 to 300 mm and then returning the bed to its original position, as determined by the readout. Again, the marks on the tape should align if there is no backlash.

Expected results: The marks on the two pieces of tape should always align when the bed is returned to its starting (zero) location.

Acceptance limits: If the bed does not return to its starting position within 1 mm, then a service person should be notified.

Possible causes of failure: Various types of mechanical backlash in the gears, belts, and pulleys driving the table, or slippage of the sensors that indicate the position of the bed. A service person can usually adjust the bed drive mechanism to eliminate this problem.

Frequency: This should be performed at the time of installation as part of the acceptance test and annually thereafter.

- TEST 11: Light field accuracy

Phantom or equipment: A piece of x-ray film or a CR cassette. The same piece of film used for Test 9 can be used for this test.

Measurement: Tape a sheet of Ready-pak film to the patient bed. Raise the patient bed so that the film is approximately centered (vertically) in the gantry opening. Turn on the external or internal light field (some CT scanners use a laser beam) that indicates the location of the first scan. With a needle or other sharp object (e.g., a penknife), poke two very small holes through the paper wrapper of the film and into the film (Fig. 18-19). The two holes should be exactly on top of the light field, with one hole near the left edge of the film and the other on the right edge. These holes, which will be visible after the film is processed, will indicate the location of the light field.

If an external light field was used, move the bed into position for the first scan. Make a medium-technique scan with the slice width set to the minimal width. The radiation should produce a narrow dark band on the film that indicates where the radiation struck the film. Process the film and examine the location of the dark band relative to the two pinholes.

Expected results: If the light field is correctly centered on the radiation field, which is also the position of the image, the dark exposed band caused by the radiation should be centered on both pinholes.

Acceptance limits: The light field should be coincident with (i.e., on top of) the radiation field to within 2 mm.

Possible causes of failure: Often the optical field light system is out of alignment. Less frequently, the x-ray tube may have been installed off center. Notify your service person.

Frequency: This should be performed at the time of installation as part of the acceptance test and annually thereafter.

- TEST 12: Pitch and slice width (spiral/helical scanner)

Note: A single test may be used to determine both the slice width and pitch of spiral/helical CT scanners. For a CT scanner with a single array of detectors, the *pitch* is defined as the ratio of bed movement (mm) that occurs during one complete revolution to the slice width (mm). For CT scanners with a single array of detectors, the slice width is determined by collimator spacing.

In the case of CT scanners with multidetector arrays that enable several slices of data to be

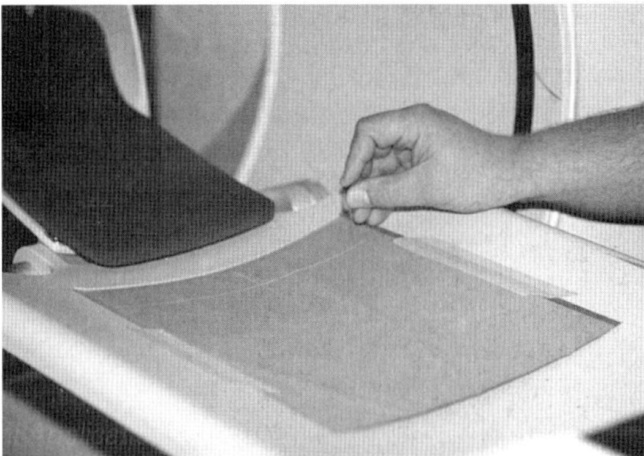

**FIGURE 18-19** Marking the light field position on film with a needle. Two small holes are poked into the film at the center of the light field. The film is then scanned (exposed) with a narrow beam slice to produce a darkened stripe of the film where the radiation field hit the beam. The needle marks indicate the location of the light field. The position of the light field and the radiation field should coincide.

acquired simultaneously, the definition of pitch must be clarified. In these multidetector cases the IEC definition (Pitch (P) = Distance the table travels per rotation (d)/Total **collimation** (W)) would apply.

Phantom or equipment: A phantom with a small diameter wire, several centimeters long, placed in the center of the scan plane at 45 degrees to the scan plane. This test involves several adjacent scans, which may be either single scans separated by bed indexing between scans or, if the scanner is capable of spiral/helical scanning, several revolutions of the x-ray tube while the bed moves several centimeters.

*Do not* rely on the measurement of the width of the radiation bands on the film to determine the slice width.

Measurement: For an axial scanner, set up the scanner to perform a series of five or six single scans with a constant bed indexing between the scans. Analysis of this test is easier if the slice width is selected to be the same as the bed indexing (e.g., set the bed indexing = slice width = 10 mm). For spiral/helical scans from a single array CT scanner, set the bed index the same as the slice width (pitch = 1). For a multidetector CT scanner, set the bed indexing equal to the slice width multiplied by the number of detector arrays used. Perform the scans of the wire and reconstruct the images. For spiral/helical scans, make sure that the data from the same 360-degree arc are used to reconstruct each image. To measure the slice width, use the distance-measuring device on the reconstructed image. Measure the length of the wire visible on the image. When the wire is oriented at 45 degrees to the incoming radiation beam, the **projection** of the wire onto the CT image is the same length as the width of the x-ray beam that strikes the wire (Fig. 18-20, *A*).

From this same set of images, the slice overlap or gap may be determined. To do this, overlay any two adjacent images, electronically if possible. If the images cannot be added electronically (some scanners do not have this feature), then make a film copy of the two images. Cut the adjacent images from the hard copy film and manually overlay them on a viewbox.

Expected results: First, the beam width measured from the image should agree with the set or nominal beam width by use of a technique similar to that described in Test 12. Next, examine the images for correct pitch by looking at the overlaid images. The image of the wires (inclined at 45 degrees) should appear in different positions in the two images. If the bed indexing is exactly the same as the slice width, the images of the wire segments should just touch at the two ends of the wire that are closest to each other. If the ends of the wire seem to overlap as shown in Figure 18-20, *B*, this indicates that the adjacent slices also overlap. If the two images of the wires do not touch at the ends as shown at the bottom of Figure 18-20, *C*, the adjacent slices also have a gap between them. Ideally, the ends of the wires will just touch. Either overlap or a gap indicates that the bed indexing is not the same as the slice width. If the bed-indexing test (Test 9) verifies the bed-indexing accuracy, then the slice width is usually at fault.

Acceptance limits: For slice widths 7 mm and greater, the measured slice width should agree with the nominal slice width to within 2 mm or less. The gap or overlap between adjacent slices should be less than 3 mm. Unfortunately, at narrower slice widths and bed-index settings, the discrepancy between nominal and measured often becomes greater and these values may be relaxed somewhat.

Possible causes of failure: Errors in beam width are usually caused by miscalibration of the mechanism (e.g., shutters or collimators) that collimates the portion of the x-ray beam reaching the detectors. Overlap or gaps in adjacent images or improper pitch settings may be caused by inaccuracies in the bed indexing (see Test 9) or more frequently, inaccuracy in the slice width setting. In either case, notify a service person.

Frequency: This should be performed at the time of installation as part of the acceptance test and annually thereafter.

- TEST 13: CT number versus patient position

Phantom or equipment: A simple cylindrical plastic container about 20 cm in diameter (the same phantom used for Test 1).

Measurement: At least five scans of the same phantom at the same technique are performed. However, the position of the phantom in the gantry should be changed for each scan. Place the phantom near the center of the gantry (use this image as the "standard"), top, bottom, and right and left sides. Set the ROI feature available on the video monitor to about 200 to 300 $mm^2$ (or 200 to 300 pixels) and measure the average

CT number of water at the center of the phantom (not the center of the image) in each image.

Expected results: The average CT number of water should always be zero, independent of the position of the phantom in the CT scanner.

Acceptance limits: If the average CT number varies by more than five CT numbers from the CT number at the center of the CT scanner, there may be a problem with the symmetry of the CT scanner.

Possible causes of failure: Various asymmetries in the CT scanner system. Consult a service person.

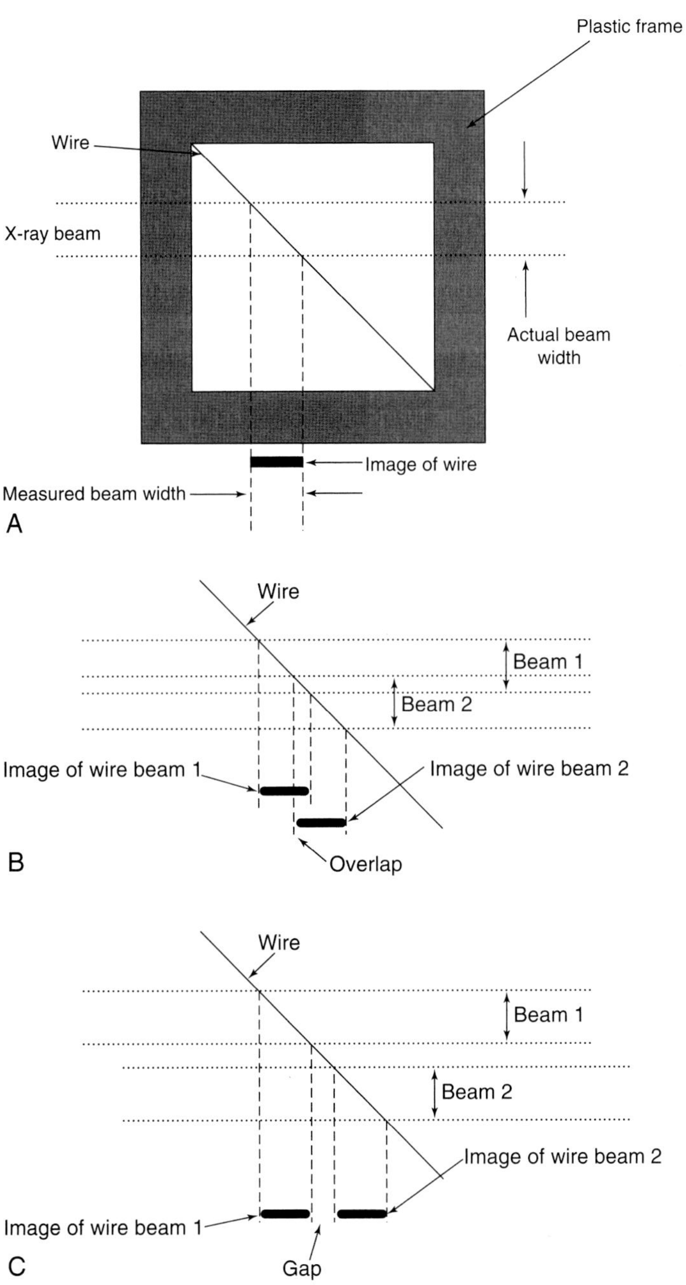


**FIGURE 18-20 A,** A several centimeters long (e.g., 10 cm) piece of wire stretched 45 degrees diagonally across a plastic frame serves as an object that projects the beam width directly to the CT scanner image. **B,** Overlaying the images from adjacent slices allows a comparison of the relative location of the adjacent slices. If adjacent slices overlap, the ends of the wire on the overlaid images will also overlap. **C,** If the adjacent slices are too far apart, a gap will appear in the overlaid images.

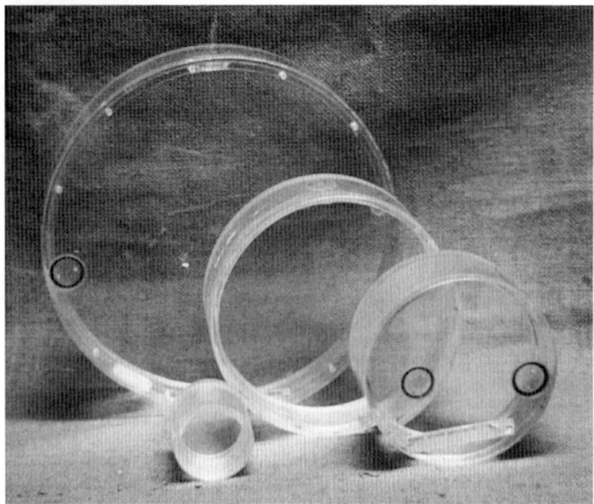

**FIGURE 18-21** Water phantoms of several diameters. A selection of water phantom sizes is used to test whether the CT number of water changes as the phantom (patient) size changes.

Frequency: This should be performed at the time of installation as part of the acceptance test and annually thereafter.

- TEST 14: CT number versus patient size

Phantom or equipment: Three or four water-filled phantoms, each of different diameters (Fig. 18-21). Typical diameters are 30 cm (body), 20 cm (adult head), and 15 cm (pediatric head). Figure 18-21 also shows a very small phantom (8 cm in diameter) that models extremities.

Measurement: A scan of each phantom size at the same technique is performed. The size of the phantoms should cover the sizes of the anatomy used clinically. For each CT scan, set the CT scanner field of view just large enough to view the entire phantom. Set the ROI feature available on the video monitor to about 200 to 300 mm$^2$ (or 200 to 300 pixels) and measure the average CT number of water at the center of each phantom image.

Expected results: The average CT number of water should always be zero, independent of the size of the phantom.

Acceptance limits: The average CT number of water should vary no more than 20 CT numbers from the smallest to the largest phantom.

Possible causes of failure: Some CT scanners have electronic circuitry that compensates for the wide range of x-ray intensities that activates the detectors. The intensity of the x-ray signal depends on the amount of tissue that the x rays penetrate before they strike the detector. Improper compensation for the number of x rays that reach the detector may cause the calibration of CT for water and other materials to shift from the ideal value. A service person is usually required to trace the problem.

Frequency: This should be performed at the time of installation as part of the acceptance test and annually thereafter.

- TEST 15: CT number versus algorithm

Phantom or equipment: A simple cylindrical plastic container about 20 cm in diameter (the same phantom used for Test 1).

Measurement: Perform a single scan of the phantom. If possible, use the same **raw data** to construct the image several times, each time using a different reconstruction algorithm or filter. If it is not possible to use the same data for several reconstructions, rescan the phantom using a different algorithm for each image.

Expected results: The average CT number of water should always be zero, independent of the type of algorithm used to reconstruct the image.

Acceptance limits: The average CT number should vary no more than three CT numbers from one algorithm to the next.

Possible causes of failure: Miscalibration of the algorithm. If a recalibration of the CT scanner does not remedy the problem, a service person should be notified.

Frequency: This should be performed at the time of installation as part of the acceptance test and annually thereafter.

- TEST 16: CT number versus slice width

Phantom or equipment: A simple cylindrical plastic container about 20 cm in diameter (the same phantom used for Test 1).

Measurement: A few scans of the water phantom are performed at the same technique; however, the nominal slice width is changed between each scan. The slice widths used should cover the sizes of slice widths used clinically. Set the ROI feature available on the video monitor to about 200 to 300 mm$^2$ (or 200 to 300 pixels) and measure the average CT number of water at the center of each phantom image.

Expected results: The average CT number of water should always be zero, independent of the slice width.

Acceptance limits: The average CT number should vary no more than three CT numbers from one slice width to the next.

Possible causes of failure: Miscalibration of the electronic detection circuitry or algorithm, especially the part that compensates for changes in x-ray intensity striking the detectors. Notify the service person.

Frequency: This should be performed at the time of installation as part of the acceptance test and annually thereafter.

- TEST 17: Noise characteristics

Phantom or equipment: A simple cylindrical plastic container about 20 cm in diameter (the same phantom used for Test 1).

Measurement: A few scans of the water phantom are performed at different mAs and different slice widths, with all other parameters constant. The settings should start at the smallest mA value available and fast scans (low mAs) and increase to the highest mA value and slow scans (high mAs). Set the ROI feature available on the video monitor to about 200 to 300 $mm^2$ (or 200 to 300 pixels) and measure the standard deviation (not the average) of the CT number of water at the center of each phantom image.

Expected results: The noise in the image is proportional to the standard deviation of the CT number measured in a homogeneous medium (water). Generally, the standard deviation of the CT numbers in the ROI (σ) should decrease as the mA values and slice width are increased, keeping all other parameters constant (Brooks & Di Chiro, 1976). At lower mA values, the dependence is σ ∞ (mA • Slice width) – 1/2.

The low mA region is called the *photon noise region* and is statistical in nature. On a sheet of graph paper, plot the standard deviation versus (*mAs* × *Slice width*) – 1/2 (Fig. 18-22). As the mA value is increased, the standard deviation will decrease; eventually the image noise will not be limited by the number of photons. At that point, the noise will become more or less constant and characteristic of the inherent electronic noise of the CT scanner.

Acceptance limits: The noise curve that was obtained when the CT scanner was new should not change appreciably with age. Be especially sensitive to increased standard deviation as the CT scanner ages in the high mA portion of the curve, in which the noise is dominated by electronic components.

Possible causes of failure: Anything that can cause the noise of the system to change, such as

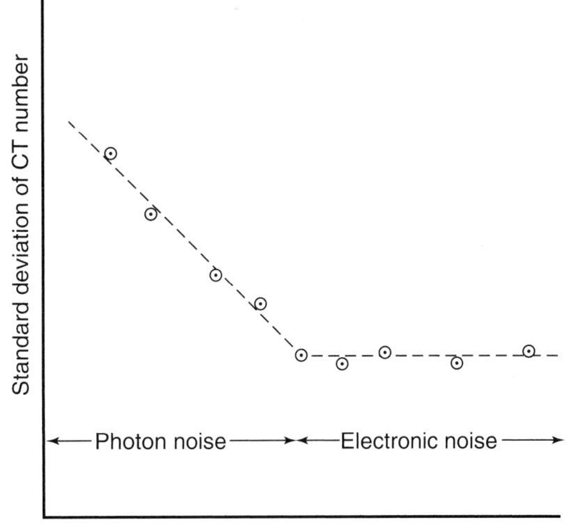


**FIGURE 18-22** Standard deviation of CT number (*Noise versus mA × slice width*) – 1/2. The noise decreases gradually in the photon noise (low-dose) region and assumes an approximately constant value at high-dose levels. In the high-dose region, the noise is mostly inherent electronic noise that cannot be easily reduced.

changed **sensitivity** of the detectors, increased noise in the detector amplification circuits, or reduced photon output per mA. Notify the service person.

Frequency: This should be performed at the time of installation as part of the acceptance test and annually thereafter.

- TEST 18: Radiation scatter and leakage

Phantom or equipment: An integrating or total exposure/dose survey meter (Geiger counter) or large volume ion chamber and a head-size water phantom. An integrating exposure meter is essential for these measurements. A simple dose-rate meter is not very satisfactory because of the wide variation in dose received as the CT gantry rotates.

Measurement: Insert the head phantom into the scan plane to provide radiation scatter for the measurements. Put on a lead apron normally used for fluoroscopic procedures. Position the radiation detector at the location where the radiation measurement will be performed, and initiate a scan. It may be helpful to have a colleague initiate the scan during these measurements. Measure the total radiation emitted at that location per one complete scan. Repeat the measurements for several locations, paying particular attention to locations where attending personnel might stand during a scan. To determine an attendant's total radiation dose, simply multiply the number of attending scans by the dose per scan at the attendant's location during the scans.

Expected results: The results will vary according to location and distance from the scanner. Usually, the highest exposure rate will be next to the patient and close to the scanner (Fig. 18-23).

Acceptance limits: None.

Possible causes of failure: If the exposure rate is exceedingly high (>25 milliroentgens per scan), there may be a problem with the collimation system or the x-ray tube **shielding.** In that case, notify the service person.

Frequency: This should be performed at the time of installation as part of the acceptance test and annually thereafter.

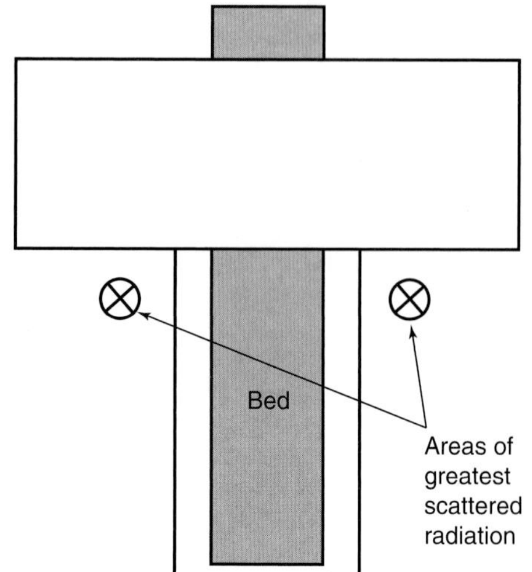


**FIGURE 18-23** Top view of a CT scanner suite showing areas of highest radiation intensity near a CT scanner (*f*).

## REVIEW QUESTIONS

Answer the following questions to check your understanding of the materials studied.

1. Which of the following refers to ensuring that the CT scanner performance and various parameters fall within established acceptable limits?
   A. quality control
   B. quality administration
   C. quality assurance
   D. preventive maintenance
2. A term used to describe the monitoring of the components of the CT scanner that affect dose and image quality is:
   A. acceptance testing.
   B. routine performance.
   C. error correction.
   D. preventive maintenance.
3. Which of the following CT phantoms is used to assess the CTDI?
   A. image performance phantom
   B. geometric phantom
   C. instrumentation phantom
   D. dosimetry phantom
4. The ACR CT accreditation phantom is designed to perform QC measurements of:
   A. positioning accuracy and light accuracy alignment only.
   B. CT number accuracy and slice thickness only.
   C. low-contrast resolution, CT number uniformity, and high-contrast resolution only.
   D. all are correct.
5. The following are all basic tenets of a QC program for computed tomography scanners *except:*
   A. all phantoms must be kept in an air conditioning room.
   B. all test results must be interpreted promptly.
   C. faithful record keeping.
   D. QC tests must be conducted regularly.
6. The QC test for the average CT number for water should be done:
   A. daily.
   B. weekly.
   C. monthly.
   D. yearly.
7. The ACR tolerance limit for the CT number accuracy for water is:
   A. ± 7 HU (± 5 HU preferred).
   B. ± 3 CT numbers.
   C. no tolerance limit has been established.
   D. ± 10 HU (± 2 preferred).
8. The following are possible causes of the failure for the standard deviation of the CT number for water *except*:
   A. electronic noise from the amplifiers.
   B. decreased dose.
   C. reconstruction algorithm miscalibration.
   D. electronic noise from the analog-to-digital converters.

## REVIEW QUESTIONS—cont'd

9. The following QC test should be done on a monthly basis:
   A. CT number calibration.
   B. standard deviation of the CT number in water.
   C. high-contrast resolution.
   D. noise.
10. The ACR tolerance limit for the CT number uniformity is:
    A. ± 10 HU.
    B. CT number for water must not be greater than ± 5 HU from the center of the phantom to the periphery.
    C. 0 ± 4 HU.
    D. the center CT number must be between ±7 HU (±5 HU preferred). Adult abdomen protocol must be used.

## REFERENCES


American Association of Physics in Medicine (AAPM). (1993). *Specifications and acceptance testing of computed tomographic scanners*, Report 39. New York: American Association of Physics in Medicine.

American Association of Physicists in Medicine (AAPM). (2010). *Comprehensive methodology for the evaluation of radiation dose in x-ray computed tomography*, Report No 111. College Park, MD: American Association of Physics in Medicine.

American College of Radiology (ACR). (2012). *2012 computed tomography manual: radiologic technologists' section*. http://www.acr.org/Quality-Safety/accreditation/CT. Accessed February 2015.

American College of Radiology (ACR). (2015). <http://www.acr.org/Quality-Safety/accreditation/CT> Accessed February 2015.

Brooks, R. A., & Di Chiro, G. (1976). Statistical limitations in x-ray reconstructive tomography. *Medical Physics*, *3*, 237–240.

Burkhart, R. L., McCrohan, J. L., & Shuman, F. G. (1987). CT quality assurance in the mid-1980s. Part 1. *Applied Radiology*, *25*, 28–30.

Bushong, S. (2013). *Radiologic science for technologists* (10th ed.). St. Louis, MI: Elsevier.

Cacak, R. K. (1985). *Design of a quality assurance program. The selection and performance of radiographic equipment*. Baltimore, MD: Williams & Wilkins.

Cacak, R. K., & Hendee, W. R. (1979). Performance evaluation of a fourth-generation computed tomography (CT) scanner. *Proceedings of the Society of Photo-optic Instruments and Engineering*, *173*, 194–207, 1979.

Carter, C. E., & Veale, B. L. (2008). *Digital radiography and PACS*. St. Louis, MO: Mosby/Elsevier.

Health Canada. (2008). *Radiation protection in radiology—large facilities: Safety code 35* Government of Canada. http://www.hc-sc.gc.ca/ewh-semt/pubs/radiation/safety-code_35-securite/index-eng.php.

International Atomic Energy Agency (IAEA). (2012). *Quality assurance programme for computed tomography: diagnostic and therapy applications*. Vienna, Austria: IAEA Human Health Series No 19.

McCollough, C. H., Bruesewitz, M. R., McNitt-Gray, M. F., Bush, K., Ruckdeschel, T., Payne, J. T., et al. (2004). The phantom portion of the American College of Radiology (ACR) computed tomography (CT) accreditation program: practical tips, artifact examples, and pitfalls to avoid. *Medical Physics*, *31*, 2423–2441.

National Council on Radiation Protection and Measurements. (1988). *Quality assurance for diagnostic imaging, Report 99*. Bethesda, MD: National Council on Radiation Protection and Measurements. 120–124.

Nute, J. L., Rong, J., & Stevens, D. M. (2013). Evaluation of over 100 scanner-years of computed tomography daily quality control data. *Medical Physics*, *40*(5) 051908-1 to 051908-11.

Papp, J. (2015). *Quality management in the imaging sciences* (5th ed.). St. Louis, MI: Elsevier.

The Phantom Laboratory. (2015). *The Catphan® 700 Phantom*. www.phantomlab.com. Accessed February 2105.

Wolbarst, A. B., Capasso, P., & Wyant, A. R. (2013). *Medical imaging: essentials for physicians*. Hoboken, NJ: Wiley-Blackwell.

A APPENDIX

# Spiral Versus Helical

## *Spiral or helical CT: right or wrong?*

*Willi A. Kalender*

The term spiral computed tomography (CT) was first made public at the 1989 RSNA scientific assembly (Kalender et al., 1989). Peter Vock, MD, from Switzerland and myself, not native speakers of the English language, had had some trouble in deciding on the name for the technique. Both spiral and helical appeared to be acceptable to us—helical was possibly more precise (which is very important to the Swiss), and spiral was more readily understandable. Authoritative dictionaries of the English language told us that both terms were correct. Having walked up and down spiral staircases with spiral binders under our arms without any problems, we believed that the term spiral might be more readily understood and accepted intuitively. Indeed, the term was accepted. However, in several of our communications, we stressed that spiral and helical can be considered as synonyms (Kalender, 1994).

Apparently, a controversy arose in the past 1-2 years, as documented by letters to editors of scientific journals (Mintz, 1994; Towers, 1993). The authors made very intelligent and acceptable statements voting for either one of the terms. I think that the discussion is unnecessary. There is no right or wrong term; both terms should be kept as synonyms.

Last, but not least, for yet another reason I recommend that the scientific community and their journals stay away from deciding that one term is right and the other one is wrong. There are some commercial implications and interests connected to the terms, and any decision might be misinterpreted. For what I hope are understandable reasons, I will continue to use the original term spiral CT in my communications; however, it shall not imply a decision about which term is right and which term is wrong.

## REFERENCES

Kalender, W. A. (1994). Technical foundations of spiral CT. *Seminars in Ultrasound, CT, and MR*, *15*, 81–89.

Kalender, W. A., Seissler, W., & Vock, P. (1989). Single-breathhold spiral volumetric CT by continuous patient translation and scanner rotation (abstr). *Radiology*, *173*, 414.

Mintz, R. D. (1994). Spiral vs helical: a matter of precision (letter). *American Journal of Roentgenology*, *162*, 1507.

Towers, M. J. (1993). Spiral or helical CT? (letter). *American Journal of Roentgenology*, *161*, 901.

*Editor's note*. We concur; hereafter, *Radiology* will accept either term.
Stanley S. Siegelman, MD
Editor, *Radiology*
Letter to editor, *Radiology*, *193*, 583, 1994.

APPENDIX B

# Cardiac Computed Tomography: Essential Technical Considerations

Cardiac computed tomography (CT) imaging is described briefly in Chapter 9, along with factors that affect temporal resolution and techniques used to reduce the effect of the beating heart on image quality, including the use of electrocardiographic (ECG) signal during the data acquisition process through synchronization with the image reconstruction (see Fig. 9-21).

The essentials of cardiac CT have been described by Wolbarst et al. (2013), Bushberg et al. (2012), and Mahesh (2009) in three seminal papers on the physical principles of CT imaging of the heart, including one by Mahesh and Cody (2007), one by Flohr and Ohnesorge (2008), and another by Bardo and Brown (2008). The paper by Mahesh and Cody is titled "Physics of Cardiac Imaging with Multiple-Row Detector CT," and the papers by Flohr and Ohnesorge and Bardo and Brown are called "Imaging the Heart with Computed Tomography" and "Cardiac Multidetector Computed Tomography: Basic Physics of Image Acquisition and Clinical Applications," respectively. These articles describe the important general technical elements required for cardiac CT imaging, including a description of temporal resolution, spatial resolution, pitch, radiation risk, geometric efficiency, and artifacts. Furthermore, while the paper by Flohr and Ohnesorge (2008) outlined the role of CT of the heart with area detectors and the dual-source CT (DSCT) scanner, the paper by Bardo and Brown (2008) outlined the clinical applications of cardiac CT imaging.

## BRIEF HISTORY

The history of CT imaging of the heart can be traced back to 1979, when Robb and Ritman (1979) worked on the development of the Dynamic Spatial Reconstruction System (DSR). They described the system as follows:

> ...fully electronic high-speed whole-body computed tomography system is being developed to provide accurate dynamic visualization and measurement of the vital functions of the heart based on rapid changes in its shape, dimensions, and perfusion. This Dynamic Spatial Reconstruction System (DSR) will provide stop-action (1/100 sec.), rapidly sequential (60/sec.) synchronous volume (240 simultaneous, 1mm-thick cross sections) reconstructions and display of the full anatomic extent of the internal and external structures of the heart throughout successive cardiac cycles, and will permit visualization of the three-dimensional vascular anatomy and circulation throughout the myocardium.

This was followed by the invention of the electron-beam CT scanner introduced in 1984. This scanner was briefly described in Chapter 4. Subsequently, third-generation single-slice CT scanners were used to image the heart. However, since these third-generation CT scanners failed to provide the essential requirements for an accurate and efficient way to image the beating heart without artifacts from motion, for example, various efforts were made using multislice CT (MSCT) scanners ranging from 4-slice to 64-slice CT scanners, with improved results compared with the earlier systems. For a more detailed account of the history and the improvement potential of CT imaging of the heart, the reader should refer to the paper by Flohr and Ohnesorge (2008).

## ESSENTIAL TECHNICAL CONSIDERATIONS FOR CARDIAC COMPUTER TOMOGRAPHY IMAGING

To image the beating heart using a CT scanner, there are several challenges that must be addressed related to image quality considerations, including high temporal resolution, high spatial resolution, adequate contrast-to-noise ratio, and keeping the radiation dose within the as low as reasonably achievable (ALARA) philosophy of the International Commission on Radiological Protection. This means that the dose must be kept as low as possible and not compromise the diagnostic quality of the images.

## Temporal Resolution

*Temporal resolution* was described in Chapter 9 as it relates to cardiac CT imaging. The word "temporal" refers to time and the temporal resolution refers to the operation of the CT scanner in a way that can freeze the motion of the beating heart. As noted by Mahesh and Cody (2007):

> with rapid heart rates, the diastolic phase narrows to such an extent that the temporal resolution needed to image such subjects is less than 100 msec. The desired temporal resolution for motion-free cardiac imaging is 250 msec for heart rates up to 70 beats per minute and up to 150 msec for heart rates greater than 100 beats per minute. Ideally, motion-free imaging for all phases requires temporal resolution to be around 50 msec…Therefore the demand for high temporal resolution implies decreased scan time required to obtain data needed for image reconstruction and is usually expressed in milliseconds.

There are several factors affecting temporal resolution including the gantry rotation time, the data acquisition mode, and reconstruction method. The *gantry rotation time* refers to the time it takes the x-ray tube and detectors to rotate 360° around the patient. The faster the gantry rotation time the greater is the temporal resolution. However, faster rotation times can create stress force problems on the gantry; therefore, methods such as different types of scan acquisitions or image reconstruction may be used to address these problems (Bardo and Brown, 2008; Mahesh and Cody, 2007).

## Data Acquisition Mode

The *data acquisition mode* for cardiac CT imaging must be as fast as possible to freeze the beating heart in an effort to obtain good image quality. In this regard, two methods of ECG gating (see Fig. 9-21) are used in cardiac CT imaging: prospective ECG gating and retrospective ECG gating (Chapter 9). It is not within the scope of this appendix to describe the details of ECG gating; however, the following is noteworthy: while prospective gating refers to "a technique used with cardiac computed tomography (CT) that uses forward-looking prediction of R wave timing, step-and-shoot nonspiral acquisition with no table motion during imaging, and unique cone beam reconstruction" (Shuman et al., 2008), retrospective gating "uses backward-looking measurement of R wave timing, spiral scanning during table motion, and more traditional cone beam reconstruction." Additionally, "with prospective gating, the x-ray beam is turned on for only a short portion of diastole, and it is turned off during the rest of the R-R cycle, whereas with retrospective gating, the x-ray beam is turned on throughout the R-R interval" (Shuman et al., 2008).

An interesting study is done by Shuman et al. (2008) who compared prospective ECG gating with retrospective ECG gating on image quality and patient dose using a 64-slice MSCT scanner. The researchers concluded that "use of 64-detector CT coronary angiography performed with prospective ECG gating has similar subjective image quality scores but 77% lower patient radiation dose when compared with use of retrospective ECG gating."

In an effort to freeze the beating heart completely, the acquisition data can be reconstructed by using either partial scan (or half-scan) reconstruction algorithm or the multisegment reconstruction algorithm (Chapter 9). While the former algorithm uses data collected through 180° plus the fan angle (about 220°) and result in a 40% improvement in temporal resolution, the latter algorithm uses 220° datasets obtained over multiple cardiac cycles. In this manner, this multisegment algorithm provides additional improvements in temporal resolution compared with the half-scan algorithm, and as such optimize performance.

## Spatial Resolution

The spatial resolution of a CT scanner was described in detail in Chapter 9. Essentially, spatial resolution is the ability of the CT scanner to discriminate closely spaced objects that are significantly different from their background. A major concern in CT imaging of the beating heart is that to demonstrate small vessels, such as the coronary arteries, it is vital that the spatial resolution be high enough to demonstrate these very small vessels.

Discussed in detail in Chapter 9 are several factors affecting the spatial resolution in CT: the collimation, slice width (thickness), reconstruction interval (increment), and patient motion (Mahesh and Cody, 2007). Typical acquisition parameters including collimation, slice width/spatial resolution, rotation time/temporal resolution, and scan time to cover the heart volume and typical contrast protocol are provided in Table B-1 for 4-slice, 16-slice, and 64-slice CT scanners. "The gold standard for spatial resolution has been set by conventional angiography which has a spatial resolution capable of less than 0.2 mm" (Bardo and Brown, 2008). Furthermore, Mahesh and Cody (2007) noted that while the spatial resolution in the *x-y* plane is about 10 to 20 line pairs per centimeter (lp/cm), it is about 7 to 15 lp/cm in the *z*-axis.

**TABLE B-1 Typical Acquisition Parameters for Cardiac Computed Tomography Imaging with Three Different Multislice Computed Tomography Scanners**

| | Four Slices | Sixteen Slices | Sixty-Four Slices |
|---|---|---|---|
| Collimation | 4 × 1/4 × 1.25 mm | 16 × 0.5/16 × 0.625/16 × 0.75 mm | 64 × 0.5/64 × 0.625/2 × 32 × 0.6 mm (double z-sampling) |
| Slicewidth/Spatial resolution | 1.3/1 mm | 0.8-1/0.6 mm | 0.6-0.8/0.4-0.6 mm |
| Rotation time/Temporal resolution | 0.5 s/250 ms | 0.375-0.42 s/188-210 ms | 0.33-0.4 s/165-200 ms |
| Scan time to cover the heart volume | 40 s | 15-20 s | 6-12 s |
| Contrast protocol (typical) | ~150 ml @ 3.5 ml/s | ~110 ml @ 4 ml/s | ~80 ml @ 5 ml/s |

From Flohr, T. G., & Ohnesorge, B. (2008). Imaging the heart with computed tomography. *Basic Research in Cardiology, 103* (2), 161-173. Reproduced by permission.

The American College of Radiology (ACR) also noted that for cardiac CT, the scanner must meet or exceed an "in-plane spatial resolution ≤ 0.5 × 0.5 mm axial, z-axis spatial resolution ≤ 1 mm longitudinal, and a temporal resolution ≤ 0.25 sec" when performing contrast-enhanced cardiac CT and CT coronary arteriography (ACR, 2014).

## Pitch

Another important technical factor used in cardiac CT imaging is the pitch, since it affects image quality (both temporal resolution and spatial resolution) and patient dose. Pitch was described in detail in Chapter 11. In summary, the pitch (P) for MSCT scanners is a ratio of the distance the table travels per rotation (d) to the total collimation (W). In cardiac CT imaging pitch values from 0.2 to 0.4 are typical (Mahesh and Cody, 2007). To optimize image quality and dose to the patient, the pitch factor must be carefully selected, since the dose is inversely related to the pitch.

## Radiation Dose Considerations

The dose in CT has been described in detail in Chapter 10, which includes not only the dose quantities, such as effective dose (a quantity that relates exposure to risk), but also CT dose metrics (CT dose index and dose length product), the factors affecting the dose to the patient and the ways in which dose optimization can be achieved. Dose optimization allows users to operate within the ALARA principle by carefully planning the examination so the lowest possible dose is used without compromising the image quality needed for accurate diagnosis.

In cardiac CT, the dose essentially is related to the scan protocol (Chinnaiyan et al., 2014; Eisentopf et al., 2014). For example, for calcium scoring the effective dose is about 1 to 3 milliSieverts (mSv; Mahesh, 2009). Sun (2012) examined doses in CT coronary angiography through an examination of several systematic and meta-analyses reports and summarized this issue as follows:

> ...the mean effective radiation dose for prospective ECG-triggered coronary CT angiography in patients with a low and regular heart rate ranges from 2.7 to 4.5 mSv which is significantly lower than that for retrospective ECG-gated coronary CT angiography. Further reduction of radiation dose can be achieved in prospective ECG-triggered coronary CT angiography with use of lower kVp values and high-pitch mode. A reduction of effective dose by up to 55% has been reported in prospective ECG-triggering with application of 80 and 100 kVp without compromising image quality. Therefore, a combination of prospective ECG-triggering with a low kVp protocol should be recommended in patients with body mass index (BMI) less than 25 kg/m$^2$, since changing tube voltage needs to be correlated with the patient's BMI. The prospective ECG-triggered high-pitch mode further and significantly lowers the radiation dose to less than 1 mSv while maintaining the image quality and high diagnostic performance, as reported in some studies). This technique can only be achieved with the second generation of DSCT as it requires high temporal resolution to allow single cardiac cycle reconstruction without motion artefacts. For the high-pitch mode, only patients with a low and stable heart rate (<65 bpm) and BMI <30 kg/m$^2$ are eligible to accommodate the long image acquisition window and allow accurate triggering of the image acquisition process. Both high and irregular heart rates preclude the use of high-pitch coronary CT angiography because inconstant heart rates would compromise image quality by causing data acquisition in an unfavourable segment of the cardiac cycle. In addition, the broader detector width of 128-slice scanner reduces the misalignment artefacts that are observed in 64-slice CT scanners.

In an effort to scan the heart more efficiently and effectively, two new CT scanners with alternative designs were introduced. These include the 320-slice dynamic volume high-speed scanner (see Figure 11-56) that features a rotation time of 350 milliseconds, which is needed to provide a temporal resolution for imaging the entire heart in one heartbeat with excellent spatial and contrast resolution at lower doses, and the DSCT scanner (see Figure 11-57) primarily "well-suited" for cardiac imaging (Cody and Mahesh, 2007), including coronary angiography. The essential features of these scanners are described in Chapter 11. Dose studies have been performed with these two scanners and the results demonstrate that the doses are indeed low.

The *DSCT experts community* (2015; DSCT.com) features a number of studies on dose in cardiac CT imaging and the interested reader should refer to this site for further explorations of dose-image quality studies. One such study, for example, reported that in prospectively triggered cardiac CT, a dose below 1 mSv for a coronary CT angiography (CTA) is possible, while "a sub-mSv coronary CTA protocol using prospectively ECG-triggered high-pitch spiral acquisition provides good image quality at a consistent dose below 1.0 mSv. The use of iterative reconstruction algorithms can further reduce the radiation dose for cardiac imaging, including coronary CT angiography without impairing image quality" (DSCT.com). In another example, Engel et al. (2012) performed a study using a second-generation DSCT scanner comparing the image quality obtained with an iterative reconstruction (IR) algorithm with that of the filtered back-projection (FBP) algorithm in cardiac CTA. The researchers found that "in all evaluated coronary artery locations, the CNR was significantly improved with iterative reconstruction when compared to conventional FBP (improvement: 39.5 ± 2.8%, $p<0.05$). Iterative reconstruction demonstrated less image noise across all cardiac phases (reduction: 22.1 ± 4.0%, $p<0.05$)." Furthermore, another study was done by Glöcklera et al. (2014) using a low-dose, high-pitch DSCT scanner to examine aortic arch malformations in children with congenital heart disease. The results showed that the use of the DSCT scanner "was successful in all patients, image quality was rated 1.34 on the 4-point scale and the impact of the 3D reconstructions for surgical planning was 2.05 on the 5-point scale. Mean dose-length product was 6.8 ± 2.6 mGy cm, and the effective dose was 0.45 ± 0.13 mSv (0.21-0.74)."

Eisentopf et al. (2014) performed another study using the DSCT scanner to evaluate not only image quality, but also diagnostic accuracy at a very low dose, in imaging coronary stents. The investigators found that "the median dose-length product was 23.0 (22.0; 23.0) mGy cm (median estimated effective dose of 0.32 [0.31; 0.32] mSv)" and that "prospectively electrocardiography-triggered image acquisition with 80-kV tube voltage and low current in combination with IR permits the evaluation of patients with implanted coronary artery stents with reasonable diagnostic accuracy at very low radiation exposure."

An example of the dose from the 320-slice dynamic volume CT scanner is one reported by the National Institutes of Health (NIH). The report showed that

> the median effective radiation dose for the new scanner was 0.93 millisieverts (mSv), compared to 2.67 mSv for the first-generation scanner, and almost every patient (103 of 107) received less than 4 mSv of radiation. (millisieverts reflect how much radiation a body absorbs, so it can help determine potential health risks. The average person receives about 2.4 mSv of background radiation each year.) Nationwide, coronary CT angiography typically involves effective radiation doses between 5 and 20 mSv, depending on the patient's body type and the quality of the machine (NIH, 2015).

Yet another example of a study conducted with a second-generation 320-detector row CT scanner was done by Chen et al. (2013) who examined dose optimization in coronary CTA by comparing the dose and image quality with that of a first-generation 320 CT scanner. The results demonstrated that while the median dose was 0.93 mSv for the second-generation 320 CT scanner, it was 2.67 mSv for the first-generation 320 CT scanner, with excellent image quality and low doses.

## REFERENCES

*American College of Radiology: ACR manual—NASCI–SPR practice parameter for the performance and interpretation of cardiac computed (CT) tomography (CT).* (2015). < http://www.acr.org/~/media/f4720a18f03b4a26a0c9c3cc18637d87.pdf> Accessed June 11, 2105.

Bardo, D. M. E., & Brown, P. (2008). Cardiac multidetector computed tomography: basic physics of image acquisition and clinical applications. *Current Cardiology Review*, *4*(3), 231–243.

Bushberg, J. T., et al. (2012). *The essential physics of medical imaging.* Philadelphia, PA: Wolters Kluwer/Lippincott Williams & Wilkins.

Chen, M., et al. (2013). Submillisievert median radiation dose for coronary angiography with a second-generation 320–detector row CT scanner in 107 consecutive patients. *Radiology, 267*(1), 76–85.

Chinnaiyan, K. M., et al. (2014). CT dose reduction using prospectively triggered or fast-pitch spiral technique employed in cardiothoracic imaging (the CT dose study). *Journal of Cardiovascular Computed Tomography, 8*(3), 205–214.

*DSCT Experts Community: Low dose CT*. (2015). <DSCT.com> Accessed June 2015.

Edyvean, S. (2013). *Cardiac CT physics—the basics*. <https://vimeo.com/78021186> Accessed October 2013.

Engel, L.-C., et al. (2012). Effects of iterative reconstruction technique on image quality in cardiac CT angiography: initial experience. *Journal of Biomedical Graphics and Computing, 2*(1), 80–88.

Eisentopf, J., et al. (2013). Low-dose dual-source CT angiography with iterative reconstruction for coronary artery stent evaluation. *JACC: Cardiovascular Imaging*, 6(4), 458–465.

Flohr, T. G., & Ohnesorge, B. (2008). Imaging the heart with computed tomography. *Basic Research in Cardiology, 103*(2), 161–173.

Glöcklera, M., et al. (2014). Preoperative assessment of the aortic arch in children younger than 1 year with congenital heart disease: utility of low-dose high-pitch dual-source computed tomography. A single-centre, retrospective analysis of 62 cases. *European Journal of Cardiothoracic Surgery, 45*, 1060–1065.

Halliburton, S. S., Abbara, S., Chen, M. Y., Gentry, R., Mahesh, M., Raff, G. L., et al. (2011). SCCT guidelines on radiation dose and dose-optimization strategies in cardiovascular CT. *Journal of Cardiovascular Computed Tomography, 5*(4), 198–224.

Hammer, M. (2014). *CT physics: cardiac CT*. <http://xrayphysics.com/cardiac_ct.html> Accessed June 2014.

Mahesh, M. (2009). *MDCT physics: the basics-technology, image quality and radiation dose*. Philadelphia, PA: Wolters Kluwer/Lippincott Williams & Wilkins.

Mahesh, M., & Cody, D. D. (2007). Physics of cardiac imaging with multiple-row detector CT1. *Radiographics, 27*, 1495–1509.

NIH. (2015). *Next-generation CT scanner provides better images with minimal radiation*. <http://www.nih.gov/news/health/jan2013/nhlbi-31.htm> Accessed June 2015.

Rob, R. A., & Ritman, E. L. (1979). High speed synchronous volume computed tomography of the heart. *Radiology, 133*(3 Pt 1), 655–656.

Shuman, W. P., et al. (2008). Prospective versus retrospective ECG gating for 64-detector CT of the coronary arteries: comparison of image quality and patient radiation dose. *Radiology, 248*, 431–437.

Silva, A. C., Lawder, H. J., Hara, A., Kujak, J., & Pavlicek, W. (2010). Innovations in CT dose reduction strategy: application of the adaptive statistical iterative reconstruction algorithm. *American Journal of Roentgenology, 194*(1), 191–199.

Sun, Z. (2012). Coronary CT angiography with prospective ECG-triggering: an effective alternative to invasive coronary angiography. *Cardiovascular Diagnosis and Therapy, 2*(1), 28–37.

Wolbarst, A. B., et al. (2013). *Medical imaging: essentials for physicians*. Hoboken, NJ: Wiley-Blackwell.

# Answers to Review Questions

## CHAPTER 1

The answers to the review questions are:

1. C
2. B
3. B
4. D
5. C
6. A
7. C
8. A
9. C
10. D

## CHAPTER 2

The answers to the review questions are:

1. A
2. C
3. D
4. A
5. C
6. B
7. D
8. B
9. D
10. C

## CHAPTER 3

The answers to the review questions are:

1. C
2. D
3. C
4. A
5. D
6. A
7. D
8. A
9. B
10. D

## CHAPTER 4

The answers to the review questions are:

1. B
2. C
3. A
4. C
5. D
6. D
7. D
8. B
9. A
10. D

## CHAPTER 5

The answers to the review questions are:

1. A
2. C
3. D
4. C
5. D
6. D
7. B
8. B
9. B
10. D

## CHAPTER 6

The answers to the review questions are:

1. C
2. A
3. A
4. D
5. D
6. B
7. D
8. C
9. C
10. A

## CHAPTER 7

The answers to the review questions are:

1. D
2. A
3. A
4. D
5. B
6. C
7. D
8. D
9. B
10. D

## CHAPTER 8

The answers to the review questions are:

1. C
2. C
3. C
4. A
5. B
6. D
7. A
8. B
9. D
10. C

## CHAPTER 9

The answers to the review questions are:

1. D
2. A
3. B
4. D
5. A
6. D
7. A
8. C
9. D
10. C

## CHAPTER 10

The answers to the review questions are:

1. C
2. A
3. C
4. B
5. A
6. D
7. D
8. D
9. D
10. C

## CHAPTER 11

The answers to the review questions are:

1. D
2. D
3. A
4. B
5. B
6. A
7. B
8. A
9. B
10. C

## CHAPTER 12

The answers to the review questions are:

1. C
2. D
3. A
4. A
5. C
6. A
7. C
8. C
9. D
10. B

## CHAPTER 13

The answers to the review questions are:

1. A
2. B
3. C
4. D
5. D
6. C
7. C
8. A
9. B
10. A

## CHAPTER 14

The answers to the review questions are:

1. B
2. D
3. A
4. D
5. C
6. A
7. C
8. B
9. A
10. D

## CHAPTER 15

The answers to the review questions are:

1. D
2. C
3. A
4. B
5. D
6. D
7. B
8. B
9. A
10. D

## CHAPTER 16

The answers to the review questions are:

1. B
2. C
3. A
4. D
5. C
6. D
7. B
8. A
9. D
10. D

## CHAPTER 17

The answers to the review questions are:

1. D
2. D
3. D
4. A
5. D
6. C
7. B
8. D
9. D
10. A

## CHAPTER 18

The answers to the review questions are:

1. A
2. B
3. D
4. D
5. A
6. A
7. A
8. C
9. C
10. D

# GLOSSARY

## A

**absorbed dose** the amount of energy absorbed per unit mass of material; expressed as the gray in SI unit or rad; the energy imparted by ionizing radiation per unit mass of irradiated material at the place of interest

**absorption efficiency** the number of photons absorbed by the detector; dependent on the atomic number, physical density, size, and thickness of the detector face

**acceptance limits** performance standard range of values for a QC test indicating what performance readings are within certain tolerances, and if outside this range, the equipment should not be used; issued by various authorities such as the ACR, the IAEA, and RPB-HC

**acceptance testing** process performed by a qualified medical physicist that verifies compliance of the CT equipment with manufacturers' specifications and ensures that it operates efficiently in terms of various outputs, such as, for example, image quality requirements and dose output; generally includes checking that the features ordered are delivered, mechanical and electrical integrity, stability, safety of various components (interlocks and power drives, for example), and CT dose and imaging performance like CT number linearity, uniformity, spatial and contrast resolution, noise, and dose output, to mention only a few

**accessories** devices that support and provide excellent immobilization of the patient to enhance the overall efficiency of the CT examination; include pediatric cradles, arm and leg supports, elevated and flat head holders, table mattresses, side rails, table extenders, knee supports, head pillows with hand rests, axial and coronal head holders, and radiation therapy table tops, to mention only a few

**adaptive array detector** arrangement of multirow detectors that are anisotropic in design

**adaptive section collimation** technique used to solve the problems encountered with overscanning and overbeaming in MSCT scanners by allowing parts of the x-ray beam exposing tissue outside of the volume to be imaged to be blocked in the z-direction by dynamically adjusted collimators at the beginning and at the end of the CT scan

**advanced quantitative measurement tools** tools used to facilitate measurements such as distances, angles, areas, mean, standard deviation, minimum and maximum voxel values, density value in HU, density histogram for a particular ROI, and volume of 3D objects

**advanced visualization tools** techniques that require powerful computer workstations with advanced image processing capabilities and increased memory to handle the vast amount of data used to create 4D angio, vessel tracking, multimodality image fusion, etc.

**afterglow** the persistence of the image even after the radiation has been turned off

**algorithm** a set of rules or directions for getting a specific output from a specific input and terminates after a finite number of steps rules that must describe operations that are so simple and well defined, they can be executed by a machine

**americium** a synthetic radioactive element of the actinide group whose atomic number is 95 and atomic mass is 243

**analog processing** type of image processing where both the input image and converted output image are in analog form

**analog signal** a continuous electric signal representing a specific condition, such as temperature, electrocardiogram waveforms, telephones, or computer modems

**analog-to-digital converter (ADC)** component of the digital acquisition system that converts analog signals to digital information for processing by a digital computer

**analytic reconstruction algorithms** developed to overcome the limitations of back-projection and iterative algorithms and are used in modern CT scanners; two examples of analytic reconstruction algorithms are the Fourier reconstruction algorithm and filtered back-projection

**applications software** programs developed by computer systems users to solve specific problems

**array processor** a dedicated electronic circuit capable of the high-speed calculations that feature key elements such as speed, power, flexibility, and expandability making it an important component of computer processing architectures for CT and magnetic resonance imaging

**artifact** a distortion or error in an image that is unrelated to the subject being studied; any discrepancy between the reconstructed CT numbers in the image and the true attenuation coefficients of the object

**as low as is reasonably achievable (ALARA)** philosophy advocated by the International Commission on Radiological Protection (ICRP) to be considered for dose reduction to patients

**attenuation** the reduction of the intensity of a beam of radiation as it passes through an object—some photons are absorbed, but others are scattered

**attenuation correction** calculation process used in PET and SPECT imaging of applying corrections to each line of response (LOR) prior to image reconstruction in order to achieve uniform quantitative accuracy despite photon attenuation or object thickness; effective approach to attenuation correction for PET or SPECT is to use the data from a registered CT scan; that is, it is the same size and in the same orientation and sliced along the same planes as the PET or SPECT scan and CT inherently provides images of the attenuation properties of the object being imaged

**automatic exposure control (AEC)** concept used to provide a level of image quality in which there is consistent optical density for any examination regardless of the thickness (small, medium, and large) of the patient; image quality is controlled by varying the duration of the exposure on the basis of the size of the patient being imaged

**automatic tube current modulation (ATCM)** manufacturer developed scheme whereby milliamperage (mA) is optimized to the patient characteristics (diameter and absorption) to reduce radiation dose in CT

**average intensity projection (AIP)** an algorithm that is intended to create a thick multiplanar reformation (MPR) image by using the average of the attenuation through the tissues of interest to calculate the pixel viewed on the computer

## B

**back-projection** third step in the IR loop of iterative reconstruction algorithm that is applied to the updated image to result in the final volumetric CT image

**basic visualization tools** basic computer programs integrated into the CT system with the capabilities of image magnification, distance evaluation, highlighting, ROI statistics and transfer, split imaging, etc.

**beam geometry** the size, shape and motion of the x-ray beam emanating from the x-ray tube and passing through the patient to strike a set of detectors that collects radiation attenuation data

**beam hardening** an increase in the mean energy of the x-ray beam as it passes through the patient

**bit** abbreviation for binary digit, the smallest unit of information in a computer. the building blocks for all information processing in digital electronics and computers Eight bits equals one byte

## C

**capture efficiency** the effectiveness with which detectors can obtain photons transmitted from the patient

**cine visualization tools** advanced computer software that allows the user to view a large set of images very quickly

**coincidence detection** a phenomenon that occurs if a positron-electron pair annihilates and converts its mass into two photons back to back in opposite directions and then interacts with detectors on opposite sides of the PET scanner with a short window of time

**collimation** restriction of the x-ray beam to the anatomy of interest only and to define the beam width for the examination; in CT collimation is crucial not only in affecting patient dose but along image quality because CT has three types of collimators; prepatient, postpatient, and predetector

**communications** the electronic transmission of text data and images from the CT scanner to other devices such as laser printers; diagnostic workstations; display monitors in the radiology department, intensive care unit, and operating and trauma rooms in the hospital; and computers outside the hospital electronic networking or connectivity by using a local-area or wide-area network

**computed tomography (CT)** the Radiological Society of North America's established term for the radiographic technique discovered by Hounsfield that produces an image of a detailed cross section of tissue

**computer architecture** the general structure of a computer and includes both the elements of hardware and software specifically referring to computer systems, computer chips, circuitry, and systems software

**computer system** a problem solving machine that consists of at least hardware, software, and computer users; a high-speed electronic computational machine that accepts information in the form of data and instructions through an input device and processes this information with arithmetic and logic operations from a program stored in its memory

**cone-beam** beam geometry seen with scanners capable of imaging 16 or greater slices per 360-degree rotation; beam geometry term for the shape of the x-ray beam when it diverges along the z-axis in multiple detector CT scanners

**connectivity** a measure of the effectiveness and efficiency of computers and computer-based devices to communicate and share information and messages without human intervention networking

**constant milliamperage-seconds (mAs)** refers to the selection of milliamperage and time (in seconds) separately or mAs on some scanners before the scan begins, keeping all other technical factors constant

**continuous rotation** capability made possible through the use of slip-ring technology that allowed the x-ray tube, detectors, and other gantry components to no longer stop during scanning to unwind long high-tension cables thus eliminating interscan delay

**contrast factor** scaling factor used in the formula to calculate CT numbers from the linear attenuation coefficients, and numbers obtained with this factor are referred to as the Hounsfield scale; represented by the constant value K

**contrast media** a substance that is injected into the body, introduced via catheter, or swallowed to facilitate radiographic imaging of internal structures that otherwise are difficult to visualize on x-ray films. Contrast media may be either radiopaque or radiolucent; also called contrast agent

**convolution** a general-purpose processing algorithm technique of filtering in the space domain

**convolution kernel** group of pixels used in determining the weighting factors that average the value of each pixel from input to output mathematical filter

**convolution method** process of applying a mathematical filter or kernel to raw data

**CT angiography** CT imaging of blood vessels opacified by contrast media

**CT dose index (CTDI)** CT dose descriptor developed by the U.S. FDA that represents the mean absorbed dose in the scanned object volume; dose descriptor used in CT dose studies and reports providing a measurement of the exposure per slice of tissue

**CT fluoroscopy** Continuous imaging that allows for the reconstruction and display of images in real-time with variable frame rates; discovered to be a useful clinical tool in interventional procedures

**CT numbers** the numeric information contained in each pixel of a CT image related to the composition and nature of the tissue imaged and is used to represent the density of tissue; another term for Hounsfield unit

**CT screening** controversial concept of using CT for imaging healthy people as a means of detecting disease early

## D

**D(z)** symbol used to represent dose distribution in the CTDI equation

**data acquisition** the systematic collection of information from the patient to produce the CT image; the method by which the patient is scanned to obtain enough data for image reconstruction

**data acquisition geometry** the way that the x-ray tube and detectors are arranged to collect transmission measurements

**data acquisition system (DAS)** the detector electronics positioned between the detector array and the computer that performs three major functions: (1) it measures the transmitted radiation beam, (2) it encodes these measurements into binary data, and (3) it transmits the binary data to the computer; a radiation detection system that measures the amount of radiation passing through a patient. In computed tomography, the system also converts analog signals to digital data that can be analyzed by a computer

**data processing** the techniques and practices involved in the manipulation of information by a computer

**data sample** each transmission measurement obtained as part of a signal profile by each detector

**deterministic effects** those effects for which the severity of the effect (rather than the probability of the effect) increases with increasing dose and for which there is a threshold dose; referred to as early effects nonstochastic effects

**digital imaging system** a scheme in its generic form that uses computers to process images by data acquisition, image processing, image display/storage/archiving, and image communication

**digital processing** method through specific operations of a digital computer processing and manipulating an input of a digital image to produce an output image that is different from and more useful than the input image; subjecting numerical representations of objects to a series of operations in order to obtain a desired result

**digital signal** the characterization or measurement of a signal in terms of a series of numbers rather than some continuously varying value. Use of the binary system in computer technology, or computerized communications

**digital-to-analog converter (DAC)** component of the data acquisition system that converts digital information to analog signals

**digitization** process of converting an analog imaging into numerical data for processing by a computer; consists of three distinct steps: scanning, sampling, and quantization

**distance** a major dose reduction action that is inversely related to dose

**dose descriptors** metrics and calculation terms used to describe CT doses as approved in the Federal Performance Standard; include the single-scan dose profile, multiple-scan dose profile, CT dose index, multiple-scan average dose, and isodose curves

**dose optimization** a radiation protection principle that is intended to ensure that doses delivered to patients are kept as low as is reasonably achievable (ALARA) while maintaining the required image quality needed for making a diagnosis

**dose-length product (DLP)** a CT dose descriptor that provides a measurement of the total amount of exposure for a series of scans; calculated by using the following relationship:

$$DLP = CTDI_{volume} \times \text{Scan length}$$

**dosimeters** devices utilized to measure dose in CT; examples include film dosimeters, thermoluminescent dosimeters (TLDs), and specially designed ionization chambers

**dosimetry phantoms and instrumentation** a mass of material ranging from water to complex chemical mixtures that faithfully mimic the human body as it would interact with radiation thus allowing assessment of the CT dose like CTDI for example

**dynamic range** the ratio of the largest signal to be measured to the precision of the smallest signal to be discriminated by a CT detector

## E

**effective dose** used to quantify the risk from partial-body exposure to that from an equivalent whole-body dose; the old unit is the rem, the SI unit is the Sievert (Sv), where 1 Sv = 100 rems relates radiation exposure to risk, and it takes into account that different tissues have different radiosensitivities

**effective milliamperage-seconds (mAs)** term used for multislice CT scanners that denotes the mAs per slice, thus meaning that mAs is in a direct relationship with pitch

**efficiency** the ability to capture, absorb, and convert x-ray photons to electrical signals

**electrometer** a very sensitive instrument used to measure the charge in an ionization chamber

**electron beam CT scanner (EBCT scanner)** high-speed computed tomography scanner in which the patient is surrounded by a large circular anode that emits x rays as the electron beam is guided around it; used to image the cardiovascular system without artifacts caused by motion

**emission CT** collective reference of PET/CT and SPECT/CT imaging where fusion imaging provides an image with clear anatomical landmarks and functioning metabolic rate

**energy dependence** the relationship of the linear attenuation coefficient with the energy of the x-ray beam that ultimately affects the CT numbers of imaged tissue

**error correction** the process used to ensure that QC test results are evaluated and confirm that service is performed if a CT scanner fails to meet the tolerance limits or acceptance limits established for a particular QC test

**exposure** the concentration of radiation at a particular point on the patient; unit of measure is the Roentgen (R), the conventional unit, or the coulomb per kilogram (C/kg), the SI unit

## F

**field of view (FOV)** a circular region from which the transmission measurements are recorded during scanning; scan FOV vs display FOV

**filtered back projection (FBP)** a mathematical technique used in magnetic resonance imaging and computed tomography to create images from a set of multiple projection profiles

**filtration** the addition of sheets of metal to a beam of x rays for the purpose of altering the energy spectrum and thus the imaging characteristics and penetrating ability of the radiation

**fixed array detector** multirow CT detector system that contains channels that are equal in all dimensions or isotropic in design; more commonly referred to as matrix array detectors

**flat-detector CT** CT imaging using C-arm systems built for radiography and fluoroscopy which are equipped with a flat panel digital detector and prepared to take projection data over an angular range of 180° or more

**flat-panel digital detector** used in digital projection radiography and fluoroscopy that overcome the limitations of image intensifier-based C-arm units in showing low-contrast resolution of soft tissues; used in interventional and intraoperative imaging, radiation therapy, maxillofacial scanning, micro-CT imaging, and breast CT imaging

**flight path** the pathway created by navigational markers along the anatomy of interest to display hollow anatomical structures in a manner that appears as a "fly through"; beneficial in CT virtual endoscopy

**fluorine-18 ($^{18}F$;FDG)** the most commonly used radiopharmaceutical for PET imaging a radioactive analog of glucose that distributes in tissues that are actively metabolizing glucose making it a useful radiopharmaceutical for a number of very different clinical applications including neurology, cardiology and, most importantly, oncology

**forward projection** first step in the IR loop that is the basis of the iterative reconstruction; the application to the initial CT image to create artificial raw data in the IR loop

**Fourier coefficients** constants used in the Fourier series making reconstruction of a CT image possible and easy

**Fourier transform** a function that describes the amplitude and phases of each sinusoid, which corresponds to a specific frequency; a mathematical function that converts a signal in the spatial domain to a signal in the frequency domain

**frequency domain** space that digital imaging processing can transform image data with the use of the Fourier transform preferred domain by physicists and engineers to view images because it is displayed as a the number of times a signal changes per unit length, thus allowing image processing to enhance or suppress certain features of the image

**full-width at half-maximum (FWHM)** a measure of resolution equal to the width of an image line source at points where the intensity is reduced to half the maximum; represents the distance between two points on the slice sensitivity profile curve whose intensity is 50% of the peak

**full-width at tenth-maximum (FWTM)** a measure of resolution equal to the width of an image line source at points where the intensity is ten percent of the peak; represents the distance between two points on the slice sensitivity profile whose intensity is 10% of the peak

## G

**gallium-68 ($^{68}Ga$)** a radionuclide used for oncologic PET imaging

**gamma camera** a device used in nuclear medicine, PET, and SPECT imaging that can localize each detection of a gamma ray incident upon it; SPECT instrumentation consisting of two rectangular, large field of view camera heads composed of a thallium-drifted sodium iodide scintillating crystal mounted opposite each other on a rotating gantry

**gamma ray** also called gamma radiation; a very-high-frequency form of electromagnetic radiation consisting of photons emitted by radioactive elements in the course of nuclear transition; the wavelength of gamma radiation is characteristic of the radioactive elements involved and ranges from about 4 · 10–10 to 5 · 10–13 m. Gamma radiation can penetrate thousands of meters of air and several centimeters of soft tissue and bone. It is more penetrating than alpha radiation and beta radiation but has less ionizing power and is not deflected in electric or magnetic fields. Like x radiation, gamma radiation can injure and destroy body cells and tissue, especially cell nuclei. However, controlled application of gamma radiation is important in the diagnosis and treatment of various conditions, including skin cancer and malignancies deep within the body

**gantry** a mounted framework surrounding the patient that contains a rotating scan frame onto which the x-ray generator, x-ray tube, detectors, and other components of the data acquisition system

**gas-ionization detectors** consists of a series of individual gas chambers, usually separated by tungsten plates carefully positioned to act as electron collection plates when x rays fall on the individual chambers, ionization of the gas results and produces positive and negative ions. The positive ions migrate to the negatively charged plate, whereas the negative ions are attracted to the positively charged plate. This migration of ions causes a small signal current that varies directly with the number of photons absorbed

**generation** term used to refer to the method of scanning in computed tomography

**generic limits** suggested performance ranges for QC tests based on the requirements of the related national authorities that CT departments use a resource or reference when deciding upon specific tolerance limits for their QC program

**geometric operation** algorithm that modifies the spatial position or orientation of the pixels in an image

**geometric phantoms** a mass of material ranging from water to complex chemical mixtures that act as tools to evaluate specific quality controls in CT; specifically geometric phantoms measure SPR accuracy and CT laser accuracy

**global operation** algorithm based process in which the entire input image is used to compute the value of the pixel in the output image; example is Fourier domain processing

**graphics pipeline** main feature of graphics processing units that can perform mathematically intensive operations by decomposing graphics computation into a sequence of stages that exposes both task parallelism and data parallelism

**graphics processing unit (GPU)** computer processor capable of fast mathematical processing that is necessary in rendering the vast datasets generated by CT imaging

**gray-level mapping** the most commonly used point processing technique that uses a look-up table that plots the output and input gray levels against each other; referred to as contrast enhancement, contrast stretching, histogram modification, histogram stretching, or windowing

## H

**hardware** the physical components of the computer machine

**heterogeneous beam** the photons in the x-ray beam have different energies; a polychromatic beam

**high-frequency generator** a small, compact, efficient device located inside the CT gantry whose circuit converts the main power's low-frequency current supply to a high-voltage, high-frequency current used by the x-ray tube and other CT components

**high-speed CT** scanner introduced as an evolved multislice CT scanner that uses higher pitch ratios and larger area detectors to scan larger volumes at high speeds as a means to improve volume coverage speed performance to image the entire heart in one complete rotation and subsequently display all images in 3D

**high-voltage slip-ring system** arrangement of the AC delivers power to the high-voltage generator, which subsequently supplies high voltage to the slip ring then being transferred to the x-ray tube; AC power travels by the chain of high-voltage generator → slip ring → x-ray tube

**histogram** a graph of the pixels in all or part of the image, plotted as a function of the gray level

**homogeneous beam** all the photons in the x-ray beam have the same energy; a monochromatic or monoenergetic beam

**host computer** a primary component in the data acquisition system that is capable of reading and writing the data in the image, storing and providing for archival storage on tape and disk storage systems, and transmitting images to another location

## I

**image fusion** registering two datasets from two different modalities and display as a single image to aid in adequate diagnosis

**image performance phantoms** tools used to verify the performance of the CT scanner on image quality characteristics such as high- and low-contrast spatial resolution and noise

**image postprocessing** the use of various techniques (image processing software or algorithms) that modify the reconstructed images displayed for viewing and interpretation by an observer

**image processing** performance of a digital computer that takes an input digital image and processes it to produce an output digital image by using the binary number system

**image processing hardware** several interconnected physical components of an imaging system whose major components include the ADC, image storage, image display, image processor, host computer, and DAC

**image reconstruction** mathematical construct applied to projections to produce sharp, clear images of cross-sectional anatomy; the process of producing an image of a two-dimensional distribution (usually some physical property) from estimates of its line integrals along a finite number of lines of known locations; process used by CT scanner to produce a variety of images ranging from cross-sectional two-dimensional images and three-dimensional (3D) images to virtual reality images of the anatomy or organ system under study; special mathematical techniques to reconstruct the CT image in a finite number of steps

**imaging system** a system that uses a computer to process images and is able to perform data acquisition, image processing, image display/storage/archiving, and image communication

**immobilization** methods or devices that ensure patient comfort and safety while also providing a manner of providing images free of motion artifact; types of devices vary based on age and size of the patient

**input** devices that acquire data

**input hardware** devices such as a keyboard that can send information to the processor

**integrated control console** multimedia concept that allows the operator full control of the entire physical system (e.g. gantry control) and enables the operation of various functions; consists of the following components: floating keyboard, touch panel, window controls, image display, optical disk drive and CD writer, and various automated control functions

**interactive visualization tools** computer programs that provide the observer-diagnostician with the following features in any 3D rendering mode: window/level adjustment, volume of interest adjustment, scan information display, movie creation and playback, split screen presentation, zoom, and measurements

**interpolation** a mathematical technique to estimate the value of a function from known values on either side of the function

**interscan delay time (ISD)** a sum of time where data collection is halted in single-slice CT scanning so that the cables within the gantry can unwind from the previous 360-degree rotation of the x-ray tube and detector and the patient table can move to the next contiguous slice to be scanned; imposes longer CT examination times and increased slice-to-slice misregistration

**interventional procedures** exams such as abscess drainages and biopsies that have benefited from CT fluoroscopy's real-time display of images therefore limiting movement associated with certain body regions and improving localization of the lesions of interest

**intravenous (IV) contrast agents** contrast media that is delivered directly into the blood stream via a vein during scanning to improve visualization of normal and abnormal structures

**isotropic** term used to describe a voxel of equal length, width, and height; a voxel that is a perfect cube

**iterations** a calculation process using a series of operations that are repeated several times

**iterative reconstruction (IR)** algorithms developed with the primary goal of reducing image noise when using lower exposure technique factors and at the same time preserving image quality (namely spatial resolution and low-contrast detectability) as well as reducing artifacts due to the presence of metal implants, beam hardening effects, and photon starvation; different IR algorithms are available based on CT scanner manufacturers, but all can be placed in three categories based on different physical methods and concepts; iterative methods without modeling, statistical methods with modeling, model-based methods

**iterative reconstruction (IR) loop** a three-step process that begins, first, with the initial CT image having a forward projection applied to create artificial raw data, second, an updated image is created from raw data and measured projection raw data being compared, third, back-projection occurs to the updated image; this process is continued until a predefined quality criterion is met or a fixed number of iterations is reached; forms the basis of the iterative reconstruction

**iterative reconstruction (IR) process** fundamental process of three typical steps; input, IR loop, and output; in iterative reconstruction algorithms

## L

**Lambert-Beer Law** an exponential relationship that describes what happens to photons as they travel through the tissues based on their attenuation of $I = I_0e^{-\mu x}$; I is the transmitted intensity, $I_0$ is the original intensity, x is the thickness of the object, e is Euler's constant (2.718), and μ is the linear attenuation coefficient

**linear attenuation coefficient** indicator of the amount of attenuation that has occurred for a block of tissue and is directly related to CT numbers (Hounsfield units) through the following calculation:

$$\text{CT number} = \frac{\mu_t - \mu_w}{\mu_w} \bullet K$$

represented by the symbol μ; known linear attenuation coefficients used for reference are water at 0.19 $cm^{-1}$ and bone at 0.38 $cm^{-1}$

**linearity** parameter in CT image quality that refers to the relationship of CT numbers to the linear attenuation coefficients of the object to be imaged

**local operation** an image processing operation in which the output image pixel value is determined from a small area of pixels around the corresponding input pixel

**longitudinal tube current modulation (z-axis TCM)** technique based on differences in the attenuation among body parts and designed to change the mA automatically as the patient is scanned along the z-axis while maintaining a uniform noise level for different thicknesses

**look-up table (LUT)** used in gray-level mapping to plot the output and input gray levels against each other for gray-level transformation

**low-contrast resolution** the smallest object that can be visualized at a given contrast level and dose low-contrast detectability (LCD)

**low-voltage slip-ring system** arrangement of the AC power and x-ray control signals being transmitted to slip rings by means of low-voltage brushes, and then the slip ring providing power to the high-voltage transformer, which ultimately transmits high voltage to the x-ray tube; AC power travels by the chain of slip ring → high-voltage transformer → x-ray tube

**lymphadenopathy** any disorder characterized by a localized or generalized enlargement of the lymph nodes or lymph vessels

**lymphoscintigraphy** a diagnostic technique using scintillation scanning of technetium-99m antimony trisulfide colloid in a noninvasive test for primary and secondary lymphedema. The radiopharmaceutical is injected subcutaneously in the interdigital space of the hands and feet

## M

**magnetic resonance imaging (MRI)** medical imaging based on the resonance of atomic nuclei in a strong magnetic field; the magnetic field causes those nuclei with an odd number of protons to align and rotate around the axis of the field. Application of a radiofrequency pulse causes the protons to resonate. When the pulse is terminated, the protons "relax" back toward equilibrium. As they do so, they release energy that is detected as a radio signal. Analysis of the amplitude and frequency of the signal yields information about the number and position of nuclei in the tissue, from which the image is produced

**mammography** the radiographic examination of the soft tissues of the breast and is used to identify various benign and malignant neoplastic processes and may show conclusively that a lesion is malignant

**matrix** two-dimensional array of numbers consisting of columns (M) and rows (N) that define small square regions called picture elements, or pixels, that ultimately make up a digital image

**maximum intensity projection (MIP)** a volume-rendering 3D technique in which the algorithm ensures only the tissues with the greatest attenuation will be displayed for viewing by an observer

**measured projection data** raw data produced by the CT scanner that is subject to calibrations, corrections, and the standard filtered back-projection algorithm to generate the initial CT image

**mediastinal** pertaining to a median septum or space between two parts of the body, such as the interval between the pleural sacs

**minimum intensity projection (MinIP)** an algorithm ensures that only the tissues with the minimum or lowest attenuation will be displayed for viewing by an observer; provides valuable information for defining lesions for surgical planning or detecting subtle small airway diseases

**modeling** generation of a 3D object using computer software using mathematics to describe physical properties of an object; a computer simulation of a physical object in which length, width, and depth are real attributes

**modular design concept** model used and intended to simplify the upgrading of scanners

**modulation transfer function (MTF)** a quantitative measure of the ability of an imaging system to reproduce patterns that vary in spatial frequency useful in predicting image degradation in a series of radiographic components

**multidetector CT (MDCT)** CT system that has a detector array consisting of four or more detectors coupled to the x-ray tube resulting in multiple slices produced in one 360-degree rotation of the system; another term for multislice CT (MSCT)

**multimodality image fusion tools** allow the user to combine images from a wide variety of imaging modalities such as CT, MR imaging, positron emission tomography, and single-photon emission computed tomography to facilitate diagnosis of tumor localization and quantification, surgical planning, and oncology planning

**multiplanar reconstruction (MPR)** a technique used in two-dimensional tomographic imaging (computed tomography and magnetic resonance) to generate sagittal, coronal, and oblique views from axial sections

**multirow detector designs** unique feature and enabling component in multislice computed tomography that influences the speed of acquisition, resolution, and thickness of the acquired slices

**multislice CT (MSCT)** generation of CT scanner that uses multidetector technology to scan four or more slices per revolution of the x-ray tube and detectors; another term for multidetector CT (MDCT)

**myocardial perfusion SPECT** the most commonly performed nuclear medicine study accounting for close to 50% of radiopharmaceutical imaging procedures; imaging method that uses $^{99m}$Tc sestaMIBI to directly assess the blood flow or perfusion to the myocardium and determine if the patient's myocardium is normal, ischemic, or infarcted

## N

**neonatal patient** subcategory of the pediatric community involving infants that requires additional care and precautions when delivering preventative or primary health care treatment

**noise** random variation of CT numbers; image-quality metric that is dependent on both the quality (beam energy) and quantity (number of x-ray photons) of the radiation beam; random signals or disturbances that interfere with the normal flow of data through pathways of computers and other electronic devices

**noise statistics (noise model)** one modeling approach in iterative reconstruction that takes into consideration the x-ray photon statistics (x-ray flux at the source and detector)

## O

**object and physics models** one modeling approach in iterative reconstruction that deals with radiation attenuation through the patient object representation

**object delineation** portrayal of an object by drawing it

**operating mode** various methods by which the CT scanner has the capability of acquiring data for various clinical examinations; these methods include routine scan mode, rapid or dynamic scan mode, and various spiral/helical scan modes (e.g. overlap scan, skip scan, tilt scan, etc.)

**osseous tumors** clinical indication in pediatric musculoskeletal imaging that is best imaged with MRI; however, CT is used to visualize the cortex of the bone or calcifications; includes pathologies such as Ewing's sarcoma and osteogenic sarcoma

**output** devices that display, view, or record completed processes of data; final step of the IR loop that results in the final volumetric image

## P

**parallel processing** method of processing that can run only on a type of computer containing two or more processors running simultaneously

**partial volume averaging** occurs when multiple tissues with varying linear attenuation coefficient values are contained within the same voxel resulting in an inaccurate calculation of the voxel's CT number

**pediatric patient** a person of age 17 or younger that is seen for preventative or primary health care and treatment

**picture archiving and communication systems (PACS)** a computer system that is used to capture, store, distribute, and then display medical images

**pipeline processing** method of fetching and decoding instructions in which, at any given time, several program instructions are in various stages of being fetched or decoded; a method in which instructions are passed from one processing unit to another, as on an assembly line, and each unit is specialized for performing a particular type of operation

**pitch** a ratio of the distance the table travels per revolution (in millimeters) to the total nominal beam collimation (in millimeters)

**pixel** picture element

**pixel size** determined by the calculation of FOV / Matrix size has a direct relationship with spatial resolution; smaller the pixel size, the larger the matrix size, the better the spatial resolution

**point operation** image processing technique that scans the input image matrix pixel by pixel and maps it to the corresponding output image pixel until the entire image is transformed; the least complicated and most frequently used image processing technique; most commonly used point operation technique is gray-level mapping

**portable MSCT scanners** system that is compact and mounted on wheels to facilitate transportation of the unit to remote locations in the hospital such as the operating room, intensive care unit, and emergency trauma unit by technologists

**positron** a positively charged beta particle that has the same mass as an electron but with a positive charge

**positron emission tomography (PET)** a computerized radiographic technique that uses radioactive substances to examine the metabolic activity of various body structures. The patient either inhales or is injected with a metabolically important substance such as glucose, carrying a radioactive element that emits positively charged particles, or positrons; when the positrons combine with electrons normally found in the cells of the body, gamma rays are emitted, then detected and constructed into color-coded images that indicate the intensity of metabolic activity throughout the organ involved

**positron emission tomography (PET) scanner** a machine that provides functional information such as the metabolic rate of tumors versus normal tissue; however, its images lack in anatomical detail; this machine is currently only marketed as a hybrid PET/CT scanner due to the beneficial nature of registering two datasets and displaying a single fused image

**preparation** process prior to imaging that educates the patient about different aspects of the exam (i.e. allergies, renal function, etc.) and provides the technologist with key information about which protocol needs to be used to best diagnosis the patient's primary complaints (i.e. use of contrast media)

**preprocessor** optimizes images before processing

**processing hardware** the CPU and internal memory of a computer

**processing operations** methods used to modify the CT images in order to make them more useful to the observer for diagnostic interpretation; common image processing operations include windowing, magnification, surface and volume rendering, image smoothing, edge enhancement, gray-scale manipulation, 3D image processing, etc.; create images from other images or non-image data; used when a desired image is either physically impossible or impractical to acquire or does not exist in a physical form at all; image reconstruction techniques that are the basis for the production of CT and MRI images and 3D visualization techniques

**projection** a set of ray sums

**projection profile** datasets produced from x ray passing through an object to reconstruct an image of that object, these datasets are then filtered and back-projected to create an image free of blurring that represents the originally scanned object

## Q

**qualitative information** data used to compare how observers perform on a specific task to demonstrate the diagnostic value of 3D imaging

**quality control (QC)** a program that periodically tests the performance of a CT scanner and compares its performance with some standard

**quantitative CT (QCT)** a type of computed tomography that calculates and displays bone density in three dimensions. QCT is used mainly for lumbar spine studies but can also be applied in hip and peripheral bone mineral evaluations

**quantitative information** data are used to assess three elements of the technique: precision (reliability), accuracy (true detection), and efficiency (feasibility) of the 3D imaging procedure

**quantitative phantoms** tool used to conduct the QC test of measuring the accuracy of CT numbers

**quantization** final step in image digitization method of a brightness value of each sampled pixel being assigned an integer (0, or a positive or negative number) called a gray level

## R

**radiation protection** the principles, considerations, and actions that encourage the use of devices, equipment, distance, and barriers to reduce the risk of exposure to ionizing radiation in a health care facility, research center, or industrial site where radiation-emitting devices are operated

**radioactive radionuclide** an isotope that undergoes radioactive decay; any element with an excess of either neutrons or protons in the nucleus is unstable and tends toward radioactive decay, with the emission of energy that may be measurable with a detector; the processes of radioactive decay include beta particle emission, electron capture, isomeric transition, and positron emission; important component in positron emission tomography and in medical research

**radiopharmaceutical** a drug that contains radioactive atoms

**random coincidences** process that occurs in PET scanning when two independent events occur simultaneously and that two annihilation photons are randomly detected in coincidence; the line of response (LOR) cannot accurately localize either annihilation event resulting in increase of background activity and image contrast reduction

**raw data** the result of preprocessed scan data that are subjected to the image reconstruction algorithm used by the scanner

**ray** the part of the radiation beam that falls on one detector

**ray sum** a measure of the total absorption along a straight line (radiation beam)

**ray tracing** a popular method of image projection in which a mathematical ray is sent from the observer's eye through the 2D computer screen to pass through the 3D volume that contains opaque and transparent objects; the pixel intensity on the screen for that single ray is the average of the intensities of all the voxels through which the ray travels

**reference point** location(s) on the CT number scale that represent key values; for example, water and air

**region of interest (ROI)** an area on a digital image that circumscribes a desired anatomical location; image processing systems permit drawing of ROIs on images and computing the average parametric value for all pixels within the ROI and returning that value to the operator

**relative transmission**

$$\text{Relative Transmission} = \text{Log}\frac{\text{Intensity of x-rays at the source } (I_0)}{\text{Intensity of x-rays at the detector } (I)}$$

attenuation measurements collected by the detectors as the radiation transmitted through the patient from various locations and stored as raw data by the computer

**rendering** the final step in 3D image production that adds lighting, texture, and color to the final 3D image; a computer program used to transform 3D space into simulated 3D images to be displayed on a two-dimensional computer screen

**response time** the speed with which the detector can detect an x-ray event and recover to detect another event

**routine performance** refers to monitoring the components of the CT scanner that affect dose and image quality; includes QC tests that are performed on a daily, weekly, monthly, and yearly basis as part of an ongoing QC process

**rubidium-82 ($^{82}$Rb)** radionuclide used for cardiac PET imaging

## S

**sampling** second step in image digitization measuring of the brightness of each pixel in an entire image

**scan parameters** factors that are within the CT technologist's control that affect image quality and patient dose; examples include constant and effective mAs, kVp, collimation, pitch, number of detectors, overranging, patient centering, ATCM

**scanning** process of the x-ray tube and the detector(s) translating and/or rotating around the patient to collect views; the division of the picture into small regions

**scattered coincidence** process that occurs in PET scanning when one of the annihilation photons undergoes Compton scattering prior to exiting the patient resulting in an inaccurate localization of the annihilation event

**scintillation detectors** solid-state detectors that consist of a scintillation crystal coupled to a photodiode tube; when x-rays fall onto this type of detector flashes of light are produced, measured by a photomultiplier, the electrons are released as a result of the strength of light

**screening** a preliminary procedure, such as a test or examination, to detect the most characteristic sign or signs of a disorder that may require further investigation; the examination of a large sample of a population to detect a specific disease or disorder, such as hypertension

**sedation** an induced state of quiet, calmness, or sleep, as by means of a sedative or hypnotic medication

**segmentation** a 3D processing technique used to identify the structure of interest in a given scene; it determines which voxels are a part of the object and should be displayed and which are not and should be discarded; editing

**sensitivity** ability to observe low-contrast objects whose density is slightly different from the background

**shaded surface display (SSD)** 3D processing method in which the computer creates an internal representation of surfaces that will be visible in the displayed image then highlighting them according to a standard protocol, and displays an image according to its calculation of how the light rays would be reflected to the viewer's eye surface rendering

**shielding** a radiation protection action that can be utilized by both patient and personnel that alleviates fears about risk of exposure to radiosensitive areas like the gonads, breast, eyes, and thyroid

**simulated projection data** artificial raw data result of a forward projection being applied to the initial CT image in the IR loop process

**single-photon emission tomography (SPECT)** a variation of computed tomography in which the ray sum is defined by the collimator holes on the gamma-ray detector rotating around the patient; SPECT units usually consist of large crystal gamma cameras mounted on a gantry that permits rotation of the camera around the patient

**single-slice CT (SSCT)** CT scanners that acquire a volume dataset by scanning a volume of the patient's anatomy using a one-dimensional (1D) detector array

**slice sensitivity profile (SSP)** a curve showing the effect of broadening of the computed tomography slice thickness along the patient axis in helical CT

**slice thickness** an imaging parameter selected by the operator used in CT defined by the collimators to determine a dimension of depth adapted to the area of interest; thinner slices improve spatial resolution with cost of decreases signal-to-noise ratio, thicker slices decrease radiation dose; average slice thickness in CT imaging today is 2.5 to 5 mm

**slice width** determined by collimator spacing in single array of detectors determined by the number and size of detector elements grouped into each data channel and defined at the center of gantry rotation in multidetector arrays; one of the required quality control tests that verifies bed indexing is the same as beam width in order to eliminate overlaps or gaps when not warranted

**slice-by-slice data acquisition** method of information collection in which data are collected through different beam geometries to scan a patient; method of information collection where essentially the x-ray tube rotates around the patient and collects data from the first slice, next the tube stops and the patient moves into position to scan the next slice; this process continues until all slices have been individually scanned

**slice-to-slice misregistration** the omission of anatomy caused by the patient respiration phase not always being consistent between scans in single-slice CT data acquisition

**software** the computer instructions that make the hardware work to solve problems

**spatial domain** place in which spatial frequency filtering is performed in which pixel values, gray levels, are used to alter images by image sharpening, image smoothing, image blurring, noise reduction, and feature extraction

**spatial frequency filtering** an example of a local operation that concerns brightness information in an image

**spatial resolution** the ability to resolve closely placed objects that are significantly different from their background

**specificity** the likelihood that a test will be negative in an individual who has no disease (i.e. the ability to detect normalcy)

**spectral CT imaging** addresses how best to utilize the broad energy spectrum (from the x-ray tube) reaching the detector to optimize the demonstration and visualization of structures in the object being imaged; exploits the transmitted x-ray photons through the patient by energy weighting and material decomposition; used synonymously to refer to dual-energy CT

**spiral-helical scanning** a technique in which a volume of tissue is scanned by moving the patient continuously through the gantry of the scanner while the x-ray tube and detectors rotate continuously for several rotations

**stability** the steadiness of the detector response

**stochastic effects** effects for which the probability (rather than the severity) of the effect occurring depends on the dose; probability increases with increasing dose, and there is no threshold dose for these effect to as late effects

**system optics (optics model)** type of modeling used in iterative reconstruction that addresses the x-ray source, image voxel, and detectors

**systems software** programs that start up the computer and coordinate the activities of all hardware components and applications software

## T

**technetium-99m ($^{99m}Tc$) sestaMIBI** radionuclide used in the imaging of parathyroid adenomas; the radionuclide most commonly used to image the body in nuclear medicine scans. It is preferred because of its short half-life and because the emitted photon has an appropriate energy for normal imaging techniques

**temporal resolution** an indication of a CT system's ability to freeze motions of the scanned object; performance parameter that deals in time or speed of data acquisition; important parameter when wanting to minimize motion

**thresholding** a 3D processing method of classifying the types of tissues, such as bone, soft tissue, or fat, represented by each of the voxels

**time-of-flight PET** a specified approach in PET imaging that requires a fast enough temporal resolution so that one might be able to time the detection of the annihilation photons and discern not only the LOR of a particular annihilation event, but where along the LOR the event occurred leading to a more accurate reconstruction of the PET data

**tolerance limits** used synonymously with acceptance limits to describe a required performance range for a CT QC test as provided by an accreditation program

**transmission CT** type of CT system in which the radiation source is outside the patient e.g. x-ray imaging

**transverse axial tomography** a tomographic technique in which the imaged sections are cross sections

**true coincidence** action in PET scanning that occurs when both annihilation photons exit the patient without incident and are detected in coincidence

## U

**updated image** resultant image when simulated raw data and measured projection raw data are compared in the IR loop of the iterative reconstruction process; image in the iterative reconstruction process that is subjected to back-projection to create the current CT image modification

## V

**view** a collection of rays for one translation across an object

**virtual reality (VR) imaging** a branch of computer science that immerses the users in a computer-generated environment and allows them to interact with 3D scenes processing method that creates the perception of 3D anatomy from a set of two-dimensional images

**virtual reality visualization tools** tools that create 3D and 4D images of tubular structures such as the colon and bronchi and allow the user to "fly through" the images of hollow organs in a technique referred to as CT virtual endoscopy

**visual inspection** task performed by the CT technologist to be done on a monthly basis as a part of the CT AC program ensuring the integrity of radiation protection considerations such as patient safety concerns is maintained; typically a checklist that includes items such as checking high-voltage cables for fraying, checking window width and window level displays, checking availability of all service records, and checking proper functioning of all CT gantry and table operations

**visualization tools** computer programs that provide the observer-diagnostician with additional information to facilitate diagnosis

**volume CT** term used synonymously with spiral-helical beam geometry because as the tube rotates, the patient is transported through the gantry aperture for a single breath hold resulting in a volume of the patient being scanned

**volume data acquisition** method of data collection using a special beam geometry referred to as spiral or helical geometry; is used to scan a volume of tissue rather than one slice at a time; method of data collection where the x-ray tube rotates around the patient and traces a spiral/helical path to scan an entire volume of tissue while the patient holds a single breath generating a single slice per one revolution of the x-ray tube

**volume rendering** postprocessing technique that uses all the data in 3D space to provide additional information by allowing the observer to view more details inside the object

**volume scanning** scheme that allows a volume of tissue to be acquired from rotating the x-ray tube and detectors continuously as the patient moves through the scanner simultaneously

**volume visualization** computer program tools used to provide an observer-diagnostician with additional information from the image to better facilitate diagnosis; examples of this include image contrast and brightness (windowing tools)

## W

**window level (WL)** the center or midpoint of the CT number range that composes a CT image's gray scale; controls the CT image brightness

**window width (WW)** range of CT numbers that compose a CT image's gray scale; controls the CT image contrast

**windowing** a method by which the CT image gray scale can be manipulated with the CT numbers of the image

## X

**x-ray tube** a large vacuum tube containing a tungsten filament cathode and an anode that often is a tungsten disk. When heated to incandescence, the cathode emits a cloud of electrons that produce x rays when they strike the surface of the anode at high speed. The anode is designed to deflect the x rays toward an object to be radiographed. X-ray tubes are produced in a variety of designs for different purposes. Low-kilovoltage x-ray tubes may contain anodes made of molybdenum rather than tungsten. Some anodes are stationary and others rotate at high speed. Because of the intense heat generated by x-ray production, the specific design usually includes devices to help dissipate the heat

## Z

**z-axis** longitudinal direction

**z-flying focal spot technique** innovation that provides doubling sampling where two overlapping slices for each detector row are obtained at the same time per 360-degree rotation, thus creating a sharper CT image with improved image quality; referred to as the z-Sharp technology

# INDEX



Page numbers followed by f indicate figures; t, tables, b, boxes.

J



K



L

**S**